THE PSYCHOLOGY OF DESIRE

The Psychology of Desire

Edited by
Wilhelm Hofmann
Loran F. Nordgren

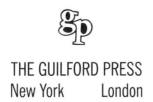

THE GUILFORD PRESS
New York   London

© 2015 The Guilford Press
A Division of Guilford Publications, Inc.
370 Seventh Avenue, Suite 1200, New York, NY 10001
www.guilford.com

Paperback edition 2016

Printed in the United States of America

This book is printed on acid-free paper.

Last digit is print number: 9   8   7   6   5   4   3   2

Library of Congress Cataloging-in-Publication Data

The psychology of desire / edited by Wilhelm Hofmann, Loran F. Nordgren.
    pages cm
  Includes bibliographical references and index.
  ISBN 978-1-4625-2160-9 (hardback)
  ISBN 978-1-4625-2768-7 (paperback)
  1. Desire. I. Hofmann, Wilhelm, 1976- II. Nordgren, Loran F.
  BF575.D4P79 2015
  153.8--dc23
                                                    2015023076

About the Editors

Wilhelm Hofmann, PhD, is Professor of Social and Economic Cognition at the University of Cologne, Germany. He also has taught and conducted research at the University of Würzburg (Germany), the University of Amsterdam (The Netherlands), and the University of Chicago Booth School of Business. Dr. Hofmann has written more than 60 professional publications, including two books. His research is concerned with desire, self-control, and moral behavior, particularly the emergence of impulses and desires, the role of executive functioning in self-control and health behavior, and the connection among self-control, morality, and happiness. In his methodological approach, he strives to combine the rigor of experimental research with the ecological validity and richness of behavioral data from everyday life.

Loran F. Nordgren, PhD, is Professor of Management and Organizations at Northwestern University's Kellogg School of Management and Codirector of the Human Ecology Lab at Northwestern, which aims to develop, extend, and test psychological theory through immersive field research. His research broadly considers the basic psychological processes that guide how we think and act. Much of Dr. Nordgren's research examines how people maintain self-control in the face of desire, how people think about desire, and how people's beliefs about desire inform their self-control strategies. He is a recipient of the Theoretical Innovation Award in Social Psychology from the Society for Personality and Social Psychology.

Contributors

Jackie Andrade, PhD, School of Psychology, Plymouth University, Plymouth, United Kingdom

Lawrence W. Barsalou, PhD, Department of Psychology, Emory University, Atlanta, Georgia

Roy F. Baumeister, PhD, Department of Psychology, Florida State University, Tallahassee, Florida

Kent C. Berridge, PhD, Department of Psychology, University of Michigan, Ann Arbor, Michigan

T. Bradford Bitterly, BA, Operations and Information Management Department, The Wharton School, University of Pennsylvania, Philadelphia, Pennsylvania

Hengchen Dai, PhD, Operations and Information Management Department, The Wharton School, University of Pennsylvania, Philadelphia, Pennsylvania

Thomas F. Denson, PhD, School of Psychology, University of New South Wales, Sydney, Australia

Denise T. D. de Ridder, PhD, Department of Clinical and Health Psychology, Utrecht University, Utrecht, The Netherlands

Jessie C. de Witt Huberts, PhD, London School of Hygiene and Tropical Medicine, London, United Kingdom

Utpal M. Dholakia, PhD, Marketing Area, Jones Graduate School of Business, Rice University, Houston, Texas

Catharine Evers, PhD, Department of Clinical and Health Psychology, Utrecht University, Utrecht, The Netherlands

Emma C. Fabiansson, PhD, School of Psychology, University of New South Wales, Sydney, Australia

Ingmar H. A. Franken, PhD, Institute of Psychology, Erasmus University Rotterdam, Rotterdam, The Netherlands

Philip A. Gable, PhD, Department of Psychology, The University of Alabama, Tuscaloosa, Alabama

Adriana Galván, PhD, Department of Psychology, University of California, Los Angeles, Los Angeles, California

Cindy Harmon-Jones, PhD, School of Psychology, University of New South Wales, Sydney, Australia

Eddie Harmon-Jones, PhD, School of Psychology, University of New South Wales, Sydney, Australia

Todd F. Heatherton, PhD, Department of Psychological and Brain Sciences, Dartmouth College, Hanover, New Hampshire

Wilhelm Hofmann, PhD, Department of Psychology, University of Cologne, Cologne, Germany

Katrijn Houben, PhD, Department of Clinical Psychological Science, Maastricht University, Maastricht, The Netherlands

David J. Kavanagh, PhD, Institute of Health and Biomedical Innovation and School of Psychology and Counselling, Queensland University of Technology, Kelvin Grove, Australia

Asuka Komiya, MA, Department of Psychology, University of Virginia, Charlottesville, Virginia

Hiroki P. Kotabe, MA, Booth School of Business, University of Chicago, Chicago, Illinois

Morten L. Kringelbach, PhD, Department of Psychiatry, University of Oxford, Oxford, United Kingdom

Richard B. Lopez, PhD, Department of Psychological and Brain Sciences, Dartmouth College, Hanover, New Hampshire

Jon May, PhD, School of Psychology, Plymouth University, Plymouth, United Kingdom

Katherine L. Milkman, PhD, Operations and Information Management Department, The Wharton School, University of Pennsylvania, Philadelphia, Pennsylvania

Robert Mislavsky, MBA, Operations and Information Management Department, The Wharton School, University of Pennsylvania, Philadelphia, Pennsylvania

Hannah U. Nohlen, MSc, Deparament of Psychology, University of Amsterdam, Amsterdam, The Netherlands

Loran F. Nordgren, PhD, Management and Organizations Department, Kellogg School of Management, Northwestern University, Evanston, Illinois

Shigehiro Oishi, PhD, Department of Psychology, University of Virginia, Charlottesville, Virginia

Esther K. Papies, PhD, Department of Social and Organizational Psychology, Utrecht University, Utrecht, The Netherlands

Joseph P. Redden, PhD, Marketing Department, Carlson School of Management, University of Minnesota, Minneapolis, Minnesota

Pamela C. Regan, PhD, Psychology Department, California State University, Los Angeles, California

Anne Roefs, PhD, Department of Clinical Psychological Science, Maastricht University, Maastricht, The Netherlands

Rachel L. Ruttan, PhD, Management and Organizations Department, Kellogg School of Management, Northwestern University, Evanston, Illinois

Michael A. Sayette, PhD, Department of Psychology,
University of Pittsburgh, Pittsburgh, Pennsylvania

Iris K. Schneider, PhD, Department of Clinical Psychology,
VU University, Amsterdam, The Netherlands

Timothy P. Schofield, PhD, School of Psychology,
University of New South Wales, Sydney, Australia

Diana I. Tamir, PhD, Department of Psychology, Princeton University,
Princeton, New Jersey

Michael T. Treadway, PhD, Department of Psychology,
Emory University, Atlanta, Georgia

Jane Tucker, MA, Department of Psychology, University of Virginia,
Charlottesville, Virginia

Lotte van Dillen, PhD, Department of Social and Organizational
Psychology and Leiden Institute for Brain and Cognition,
Leiden University, Leiden, The Netherlands

Frenk van Harreveld, PhD, Department of Psychology,
University of Amsterdam, Amsterdam, The Netherlands

Kathleen D. Vohs, PhD, Carlson School of Management,
University of Minnesota, Minneapolis, Minnesota

Dylan D. Wagner, PhD, Department of Psychological and Brain
Sciences, Dartmouth College, Hanover, New Hampshire

Adrian F. Ward, PhD, McCombs School of Business, University of Texas
at Austin, Austin, Texas

Jessica Werthmann, PhD, Department of Clinical Psychological
Science, Maastricht University, Maastricht, The Netherlands

Erin Westgate, MA, Department of Psychology, University of Virginia,
Charlottesville, Virginia

Stephen J. Wilson, PhD, Department of Psychology,
The Pennsylvania State University, University Park, Pennsylvania

Contents

PART II

Neuroscience of Desire and Desire Regulation

PART III

Desire, Judgment, and Decision Making

Introduction

Wilhelm Hofmann
Loran F. Nordgren

Desire is our innumerable king.
—FERNAND GREGH

Just think back about the things you did during the last couple of hours. Chances are that you had a desire of some sort, be it for delicious food, a freshly brewed cup of coffee, a quick "surf" on Facebook, or for someone else you simply find "irresistible." As humans, we spend enormous amounts of time experiencing and dealing with desire. Desire floods our senses, occupies our thoughts. Desire propels us to action. And, in doing so, desire touches us emotionally: at first, by promising pleasure (or relief), making us feel that we lack something important; and then, during or after the desired act, by providing us with the actual pleasures of desire satisfaction—and sometimes also a good dose of guilt. Accordingly, our language is filled with expressions of how we experience and deal with desire: We burn with desire, are tormented by it; we "resist, and struggle with, or succumb, surrender to, and indulge our desires" (Belk, Ger, & Askegaard, 2000, p. 99).

Desires are among the most universal human experiences. Across cultures and continents we may crave different foods and go weak at the knees through different routes of seduction, but the basic desire is largely unchanged. The shared nature of desire extends beyond human experience and connects us to much of the animal kingdom. Understanding the basic needs and wants of your cat or dog at home doesn't require much perspective taking on your part because they aren't so very different from your own.

Desires are key motivators in our lives, often rooted in evolutionary old systems that secure our own and our species' survival. And yet, our relationship with desire is complicated, as the unfettered enactment of desire can be self-harming or interfere with the freedom and well-being of our fellow citizens. Just imagine a world in which every physical desire was enacted right away and right on the spot. The capacity to regulate our desire is a prerequisite for participating in society, and those who chronically fail to regulate their desires often find themselves removed from free society. Not surprisingly, our legal, religious, and educational systems are all heavily involved in the regulation of (problematic) desire. To illustrate, just take the well-known joke about Moses trudging down Mount Sinai, tablets in hand, announcing to the assembled crowd: "I've got good news and bad news to share. The good news is that I got Him down to 10. The bad news: Adultery is still in."

Legal, religious, and educational systems promote the "proper" way to deal with certain urges and desires and punish those who cross the boundaries of what is considered appropriate. Even beyond those institutionalized influences, there are often additional moral (e.g., "Should I suppress my desire for meat in light of all that animal suffering and become a vegetarian?"), health-related (e.g., "Should I cut down on my soft drink consumption?"), financial (e.g., "Do I really need a seventh pair of boots?"), or other "common sense" considerations that motivate us to keep our desires in check—sometimes to no avail.

Accordingly, the aggregated effects of poor desire regulation can be enormous. Public health figures suggest that 40% of deaths in the United States each year are associated with behaviors that are at least partially attributable to the way people deal with desires such as those for unhealthy foods, tobacco, alcohol, unprotected sex, aggressive urges, and illicit drugs (Schroeder, 2007). Viewed from that perspective, gaining a better understanding of desire and its regulation is clearly warranted.

The Need for an Integrated Book on Desire

The study of desire has an incredibly long and rich intellectual history that would deserve a book of its own. It dates back all the way to milestone insights by Sigmund Freud, and even far beyond to the writings of Western philosophers such as Plato, Hume, and Schopenhauer, as well as Buddhist philosophy. In the history of psychology, desire is a central part of motivational theories built around the concepts of drives, needs, and incentives. In modern psychology, the role of desires and cravings has been studied in isolated domains such as sexual desire (e.g., Baumeister, Catanese, & Vohs, 2001; Buss, 2003) or addiction (e.g., Field, Munafo, & Franken, 2009; Franken, 2003; Robinson & Berridge, 1993). Desire is also implicit as a "driving force" in many areas of psychology, such as self-regulation (Vohs & Baumeister, 2011), health psychology (Kemps, Tiggemann, & Grigg, 2008; Lowe & Butryn, 2007), and consumer research

(Belk, Ger, & Askegaard, 2003; Hoch & Loewenstein, 1991). However, the origin, phenomenological nature, and motivational power of desire has rarely been studied as a topic worthy of its own volume.

We believe the time is ripe for it. There has been a recent surge in desire-related themes in many subdisciplines of psychology, including behavioral neuroscience (e.g., Heatherton & Wagner, 2011; Kringelbach & Berridge, 2010), self-control research (e.g., Hofmann, Baumeister, Förster, & Vohs, 2012; Hofmann & Van Dillen, 2012; Nordgren & Chou, 2011), consumer psychology (e.g., Belk et al., 2003; Redden & Haws, 2013), addiction (e.g., Kavanagh, Andrade, & May, 2004, 2005), and health research (e.g., Hofmann, Friese, & Wiers, 2008; Hollmann et al., 2012; Lawton, Conner, & McEachan, 2009). The insights gained in these areas have never been pulled together, though, into an integrated and comprehensive volume.

Central Themes in Desire Research

The primary goal of this book is to provide a broad, stimulating, and cross-cutting perspective on human desire. To this end, we invited an interdisciplinary team of experts to address a number of core questions about desire, and from a variety of angles. The authors in this book draw on a wide variety of experimental and field methods from neuroscience, social and cognitive psychology, motivation research, behavioral economics, consumer psychology, personality psychology, and clinical psychology. Together, they cover a large number of interrelated questions and general themes found throughout human desire research:

- *How does desire emerge, wax, and wane?* What renders some things so attractive that they grab our attention, occupy our thoughts, and fuel our desire? Which mechanisms magnify desire, and according to which principles does desire satiate? Theories of desire need to address the often complex interplay of stimulus features in the environment and the predispositions within ourselves (i.e., need states, learning history) that provide the "fertile ground" against which these external stimuli can have their powerful effects.
- *How is desire experienced?* What are the affective, cognitive, and motivational components that define the experience of desire? How are conscious desires mentally represented? What is the role of mental simulation and cognitive elaboration in the generation of desire experiences? Which aspects create the difference between unproblematic desire and problematic desire (i.e., temptation)?
- *How does desire influence judgments and behavior?* What are the mechanisms through which desires can color and bias behavioral

decision making? What does current desire research have to say about Hume's famous dictum that "reason is the slave of passion"? Through which processes of motivated reasoning does desire accomplish that feat? More broadly, how can psychological models account for the wide range of behaviors driven by desire, sometimes in more rash, impulsive ways, and sometimes supported by (motivated) reasoning and cognitive elaboration?

• *How can unwanted desires be effectively controlled?* Given that desire is sometimes problematic, leading to the interesting phenomenon of "unwanted" wants, how can desire be effectively down-regulated or otherwise controlled through inhibitory processes?

• *What underlying brain mechanisms cause desire and are involved in its control?* The science of desire would lack an important ingredient without support from neuroscience. The neuroscientific perspective greatly enriches our understanding of desire by showing how desire is grounded in reward-processing areas in the brain, how these and other areas evolved and develop to contribute to desire experiences and their control.

• *How do these aspects differ across domains, people, and situations?* Not all desires are created equal, some people are more passionate or impulsive than others, and not all situational contexts are equally conducive to experiences of desire and its enactment. How can these various differences be accounted for? Why, for instance, are some people more sensitive to immediate rewards in their environment, and why are some better at resisting desire? How do such differences develop?

• *What is the connection between desire and well-being?* Satisfying one's desire is typically a pleasurable momentary experience, but does more pleasure necessarily lead to more happiness? In other words, are desires a blessing or a curse when taking a broader perspective on human well-being? To quote the Bard: "Can one desire too much of a good thing?" And what would an optimal approach to dealing with desire look like?

• *What are pathological forms of desire?* How and why does too much desire lead to problematic, sometimes pathological outcomes such as extreme overweight, antisocial personality, and progressively burdensome addictions? And what about the opposite problem: too little desire (anhedonia), a common symptom in many psychological disorders including major depression and schizophrenia?

Conceptual Issues

The Scope of Desire

As with many constructs in psychology, there is considerable (and unavoidable) leeway in definition and scope. The construct of "desire" is no exception. The term can be understood quite narrowly (in the sense of passionate sexual desire) as well as very broadly, including all sorts of ideals and wishes. In the present volume, most authors adopt a middle-ground definition of desire as those wants and urges that are intricately linked to motivation, pleasure, and reward. Such a middle-ground definition encompasses what is often referred to as *appetitive* desires—those motivations that propel us to approach certain stimuli in our environment and engage in activities with them that provide us with a relative gain in immediate pleasure (including relief from discomfort). Some of these desires are linked to primary physiological need states, such as the desires for food, drink, sex, and rest, while many others are acquired through processes of reinforcement learning. The purpose of this book is not to chart the entire landscape of human desire—an impossible task— but rather to provide an in-depth analysis of the common mechanisms and processes that underlie these everyday varieties of desire.

"Desires" and "Goals"

Another important conceptual issue with psychological constructs such as "desire" concerns their overlap with other constructs. One question that presents itself in light of much current theorizing in psychology is how desires are different or similar to goals. The contributors to this volume did not have the task of addressing this thorny issue explicitly, so we would therefore like to use this opportunity to offer some brief thoughts that have emerged during the reviewing process and through conference and workshop interactions with the authors.

The goal construct is an incredibly useful concept for understanding behavior (e.g., Moskowitz & Grant, 2009a). In the increasingly broad sense in which this construct has been used in recent years, it can refer to all those responses that are intentionally performed to bring about a desired state and response, and those intentionally performed to control or prevent an undesired state (aka willpower). The "new look" at motivation, driven by the cognitive revolution in psychology, has greatly advanced our understanding of how motivation is colored by cognition (or how motivation may be understood as some form of cognition). For instance, the conceptualization of goals as knowledge structures has advanced our understanding of how the desired end states, means, and obstacles involved in goal pursuit are mentally represented and interconnected in memory (Kruglanski et al., 2002). Other groundbreaking developments in the field have integrated both conscious and unconscious goal strivings, extrinsic and intrinsic goals, and many more distinctions to cover an ever more expansive territory in human motivation (see Moskowitz & Grant, 2009b). The goal construct thus offers a huge conceptual toolbox with which to analyze people's behavior, from short-term task performance to long-term goals, ideals, and strivings.

However, such breadth and near-universal applicability may also come at a cost, especially when one seeks to identify and understand how certain subtypes of human motivation may differ systematically from others. Hence, despite the search for the unifying principles of goal pursuit, it is also important to keep asking how a motivational phenomenon such as the stated long-term goal to lose weight over the next year may differ from a motivational phenomenon such as the short-term inclination to consume this incredibly delicious dessert in front of you in a devil-may-care manner. We believe that the desire concept may fulfill a useful and complementary function here (when used in its more narrow sense to refer to appetitive desire).

As Figure I.1 shows, we believe that such a desire construct is narrower in scope and partially overlaps with the goal construct. (Think of the center of the "goal" circle as representing the features of the "prototypical" goal in the empirical distribution of all goals in a multidimensional space representing features such as intentionality, controllability, intrinsicness, and time frame; think of the center of the "desire" circle as representing the features of the "prototypical" desire in the empirical distribution of all desires in the same multivariate space.) The substantial overlap in the distribution of goals and desires implies that most desires can be reframed within a goal language. For instance, we can reframe intense chocolate craving as the *goal* to consume sweet foods, the urge to fall asleep during a lecture with the *goal* to get some rest, a one-night stand as the *goal* to have sex with a stranger after having drunk too much, problems with quitting smoking as too much commitment to the *goal* to smoke one last cigarette, and so forth. The question is whether such a terminology is always the most useful or fruitful—and whether, in some cases, it may even obscure a more precise analysis and understanding of the motivational phenomenon at hand.

Why would that be? First, the terms *goal* and *desire* may refer to different prototypes in the landscape of human motivation (and thus tend to evoke different conceptual ideas in researchers and laypeople alike).

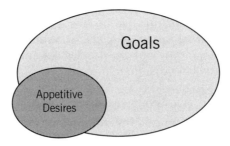

FIGURE I.1. Proposed overlap and nonoverlap of the psychological constructs of goals and desires.

For instance, the prototypical goal—we are thinking all kinds of work goals, important life projects, self-regulatory goals here—may be experienced as being higher in intentionality, personal control, temporal scope, and meaning (Moskowitz & Grant, 2009a) when compared to the prototypical desire. The prototypical desire, in contrast, may be higher on aspects such as intrinsic reward and affective "hotness" when compared to the prototypical goal. Recognizing such differences—through the use of a more narrow terminology—may advance our understanding of the variety in human motivation and direct research in novel ways. To name just a few:

1. Consider the many fruitful links between neuroimaging research on reward processing in the brain and the psychology of desire (e.g., Chapters 6, 7, 9, 15, 19); such a collaboration does not automatically flow from a knowledge-structure perspective on goals, but it is almost inherent in the conceptual link between desire and pleasure.
2. Or consider the emerging cross-fertilization between the emotion-regulation literature and the literature on self-control that flows from the idea of likening desire, an inherently "hot" construct, to emotion (e.g., Chapters 3 and 19). Again, such a connection is not as apparent when recasting desires as short-term goals.
3. Innovative interventions on how to improve long-term goal pursuit (e.g., Chapter 1) may stem from a comparison of (prototypical) desires and goals: Why is it that, often, the goals we believe will lead to important changes in our life do *not* feel like a prototypical desire, and how can we make them more like one?

Second, we believe that the desire concept may be useful in preventing an overextension of the goal concept to those more extreme cases of impulsive behavior that are hard to reconcile with the idea of goals as intentional and meaning-providing responses (Moskowitz & Grant, 2009a) (indicated in Figure I.1 as those desire cases that fall outside the goal circle). Equating desires with goals implies that even unintended, spontaneous, utterly nonendorsed urges at one extreme end of the desire distribution should be included in the goal category. For instance, it would seem to require a very expansive definition of the goal concept to account for the nicotine addict trying to quit, wishing she'd not feel such a strong desire to smoke yet another cigarette. Sometimes, a desire is the very thing we do not even want to experience, let alone have it affect our behavior, and we use all our self-regulatory powers to control it. Should the goal concept include such *unintended* forms of motivation? (Try substituting the word *desire* for *goal* in the preceding sentence.) Whereas such cases could still be framed as a conflict between goals, of course, one could argue that the structural asymmetry in the two opponents of the

conflict may be sufficiently large to not put them on an equal conceptual footing. Despite the high usefulness of the goal concept, we thus
hope that the present volume, through its emphasis on desire, will offer a
refreshing new look at the phenomenon of appetitive motivation.

Organization of the Book

The Psychology of Desire is organized into five parts. Part I, "Basic Processes
and Mechanisms," sets the conceptual foundation that will help the
reader get an up-to-date understanding of desire. Andrade, May, van Dillen, and Kavanagh (Chapter 1) provide an updated of the elaborated intrusion theory of desire, at its 10th anniversary (Kavanagh et al., 2005). The
theory highlights the role of cognitive elaboration and imagery in desire.
It also provides a useful basis on which to develop innovative behavior
change strategies. Papies and Barsalou (Chapter 2) introduce a sophisticated grounded-cognition theory of desire, centered on the idea of mental
simulation. According to this framework, desire arises from the multimodal simulation (i.e., reenactment) of past consumptive experiences,
stored in memory as a "situated conceptualization" that can be triggered
in line with principles of pattern completion. The theory offers a broad,
learning-based account of how desire emerges and motivates behavior
from the interplay of stimulus environments and past experience. Hofmann, Kotabe, Vohs, and Baumeister (Chapter 3) ask about the various
reasons that desire may be problematic. They liken desire regulation to
emotion regulation to derive a taxonomy of desire control that helps distinguish among those strategies that constrain the emergence of desire,
those that support its down-regulation, and those that serve to inhibit or
override desire-related behavior. Redden (Chapter 4) delves deeply into
the dynamic nature of desire resulting from satiation and recovery by
surveying a large range of accelerants and retardants of satiation. To fully
account for the range of satiation effects found in the literature, Redden
proposes a novel taxonomy that integrates homeostatic, perceptual, and
reflective components that each contribute to satiation. Part I concludes
with an up-to-date review of desire and craving assessment by Sayette and
Wilson (Chapter 5). They highlight conceptual issues and provide practical recommendations desire researchers should consider when choosing
among the large range of self-report and nonverbal measures available.

Part II, "Neuroscience of Desire and Desire Regulation," assembles
recent insights into the biobehavioral foundations of desire and its control. Kringelbach and Berridge (Chapter 6) provide an introduction to
"evolution's boldest trick" (Kringelbach, 2005)—the motivating power of
pleasure-generating reward circuits in the brain. In their phasic model of
pleasure, they carefully distinguish wanting, the motivation for reward,
from liking, the actual pleasure of a reward, and from the ensuing satiety

or learning phase during which reward predictions are updated. Lopez, Wagner, and Heatherton (Chapter 7) start out by reviewing how meso-limbic dopamine pathways promotes reward-seeking behavior and then discuss how prefrontal cortex regions can be recruited to curb desires and reduce the likelihood of acting upon desire. They also touch on situational triggers of poor desire regulation and on whether desire control may be improved through cognitive training. Harmon-Jones, Gable, and Harmon-Jones (Chapter 8) focus on individual differences in desire from the broader perspective of approach motivation, as measured via the behavioral activation system (BAS) sensitivity scale (Carver & White, 1994). Of particular interest is how individual differences in BAS sensitivity relate to electrophysiological indices (such as EEG, startle eyeblink, and fMRI activity) and influence cognitive and emotive responses. Galván (Chapter 9) concludes this part by reviewing cognitive neuroscience research on the development of brain regions implicated in desire, with an emphasis on how significant changes in the reward network during adolescence, in combination with the lagging development of cognitive control regions, can bring about a greater sensitivity to rewards observed during this critical developmental phase.

Part III, "Desire, Judgment, and Decision Making," illuminates the various ways by which desire can bias judgment and decision making. De Ridder, de Witt Huberts, and Evers (Chapter 10) set the stage by spelling out means by which short-term desires may direct reflective thinking processes toward justifying indulgence. One key insight gained through their analysis of such motivated reasoning processes is that the failure to regulate problematic desire is not solely the consequence of a "breakdown" of control capacities, but that reflective processes can contribute as well by providing people with a "license to sin." Ruttan and Nordgren (Chapter 11) show that despite the central role of desire in daily life, people have tremendous difficulties imagining how they or others will behave in a state of desire that is different from what they are currently experiencing. This hot–cold empathy gap can lead to a number of distortions in the way people think, evaluate, and decide about desire—most typically an underestimation of how much desire will influence their attitudes, preferences, and behavior. Bitterly, Mislavsky, Dai, and Milkman (Chapter 12) provide a utility-based synthesis of *want–should* conflicts—struggles between choosing what we desire in the heat of the moment and more "prudent" options that would be best for us in the long run. Drawing on decision-making research and the behavioral economics literature, they review a large range of factors that can tip the balance between *want* and *should* options and discuss a series of interventions and "nudges" (Thaler & Sunstein, 2008) that policy makers, organizations, and individuals can use to promote more future-oriented (*should*) choices.

The goal of Part IV, "Desire, Affect, and Well-Being," is to more closely link desire with affective states as well as to address the complex relationship between desire (satisfaction) and well-being. Van Harreveld, Nohlen, and Schneider (Chapter 13) place a fine-grained focus on the nature of ambivalence toward desires—the psychological state in which a person holds mixed feelings toward the object of temptation. They show that the experience of ambivalence is inherently unpleasant, discuss its relation to regret, and illuminate how ambivalence affects information processing and triggers emotion-focused and problem-focused strategies as people attempt to reduce the psychological discomfort of ambivalence. Oishi, Westgate, Tucker, and Komiya (Chapter 14) examine the link between desire and happiness by asking "Are desires a blessing or a curse?" and "Does the satisfaction of desires lead to happiness?" Integrating positive psychology insights and ethical thinking from the Aristotelian conception of happiness with Puritan and Buddhist approaches to dealing with temptation, they provide a thought-provoking analysis of the—perhaps never fully solvable—dilemma of human desire. Part IV concludes with a contribution by Treadway (Chapter 15) on anhedonia, the lack of motivation and pleasure, which is a frequent aspect of psychopathologies such as major depressive disorder and schizophrenia. Treadway makes a convincing case for distinguishing more clearly among subcomponents of abnormal reward seeking (i.e., "wanting" vs. "liking") and shows how disturbances in distinct underlying neural circuits may be responsible for the observed differences among normal and abnormal reward motivation.

Part V, "Applied Content Domains," highlights a number of specific desire domains from areas that have witnessed a lot of progress in recent years and that serve as great examples of how a desire perspective can enrich our understanding of (often problematic) human behavior in those domains. Roefs, Houben, and Werthmann (Chapter 16) survey food desires against the background of the rising obesity crisis. They integrate separate lines of research on reward processing, attentional bias, and associative learning with a focus on how restrained and unrestrained eaters may differ in those areas and discuss the moderating role of top-down factors such as current processing goals. Next, Regan (Chapter 17) explores the complex phenomenon of sexual desire. She provides a broad framework for understanding the interplay among physical and social environmental factors (e.g., seductive settings, norms and regulations), personal factors (e.g., hormonal activity, sex appeal), and relational factors (e.g., proximity, mutual attraction) in determining sexual desire. Denson, Schofield, and Fabiansson (Chapter 18) review research suggesting how aggressive desires emerge and are maintained over time by angry rumination. They discuss the latest research suggesting that aggressive desires are accompanied by neural changes associated with reward processing, conflict detection, and approach motivation, as well as reduced inhibitory control. They conclude with psychological strategies that may prevent aggressive desires from emerging and help people control those aggressive desires that have already entered consciousness. Franken (Chapter 19) reviews the central role of appetitive desire in substance (ab)use and relapse in addiction: What are the genetic and neuroanatomical substrates of drug craving? How is drug craving shaped by learning experiences and outcome expectations? And how can behavioral therapy, pharmacological approaches, neuromodulation, and neurofeedback all be used to treat addiction by curbing drug cravings? Dholakia (Chapter 20) provides a lucid analysis and review of three senses in which desire has been studied in consumer research: as the motivational impetus for engaging in decision making and effortful goal pursuit, as the countervailing force that opposes self-control, and as a sudden, spontaneous buying impulse. He demonstrates the many important insights that each of these perspectives has contributed to consumer psychology and marketing research and addresses exciting questions and suggestions for future research. Tamir and Ward (Chapter 21) conclude the book with a new look at the modern desire for social media use. The authors cover novel ground by exploring how our evolutionarily old social minds contribute to the new desire to find and create social connection through television and social media. They also critically ask whether our old adaptive systems acting in new technological environments may result in "easy solutions" that lead to maladaptive outcomes in the long run.

The breadth and organization of this volume are designed to provide the reader with a deep understanding of the literature to date as well as the emerging themes in the vibrant science of human desire.

Acknowledgments

We conclude by acknowledging the effort and dedication of all our contributors, without whom this long-desired project would never have become a reality. We would also like to extend our gratitude to Seymour Weingarten and Carolyn Graham at The Guilford Press. From beginning to end, this handbook is better because of their outstanding support at all stages of the project. In particular, we would like to thank Seymour Weingarten for pointing out that our initially proposed title for this book, *The Handbook of Desire*, would likely have ended up on the wrong bookshelf and attracted readers we didn't intend.

REFERENCES

Baumeister, R. F., Catanese, K. R., & Vohs, K. D. (2001). Is there a gender difference in strength of sex drive? Theoretical views, conceptual distinctions, and a review of relevent evidence. *Personality and Social Psychology Review, 5*(3), 242.

Belk, R. W., Ger, G., & Askegaard, S. (2000). The missing streetcar named desire.

In S. Ratneshwar, D. G. Mick, & C. Huffman (Eds.), *The why of consumption* (pp. 98–119). London: Routledge.

Belk, R. W., Ger, G., & Askegaard, S. (2003). The fire of desire: A multisited inquiry into consumer passion. *Journal of Consumer Research, 30*(3), 326–351.

Buss, D. M. (2003). *The evolution of desire.* New York: Basic Books.

Carver, C. S., & White, T. L. (1994). Behavioral inhibition, behavioral activation, and affective responses to impending reward and punishment: The BIS/BAS scales. *Journal of Personality and Social Psychology, 67,* 319–333.

Field, M., Munafo, M. R., & Franken, I. H. A. (2009). A meta-analytic investigation of the relationship between attentional bias and subjective craving in substance abuse. *Psychological Bulletin, 135*(4), 589–607.

Franken, I. H. (2003). Drug craving and addiction: Integrating psychological and neuropsychopharmacological approaches. *Progress in Neuropsychopharmacological Biological Psychiatry, 27*(4), 563–579.

Heatherton, T. F., & Wagner, D. D. (2011). Cognitive neuroscience of self-regulation failure. *Trends in Cognitive Sciences, 15*(3), 132–139.

Hoch, S. J., & Loewenstein, G. F. (1991). Time-inconsistent preferences and consumer self-control. *Journal of Consumer Research, 17*(4), 492.

Hofmann, W., Baumeister, R. F., Förster, G., & Vohs, K. D. (2012). Everyday temptations: An experience sampling study of desire, conflict, and self-control. *Journal of Personality and Social Psychology, 102*(6), 1318–1335.

Hofmann, W., Friese, M., & Wiers, R. W. (2008). Impulsive versus reflective influences on health behavior: A theoretical framework and empirical review. *Health Psychology Review, 2,* 111–137.

Hofmann, W., & Van Dillen, L. F. (2012). Desire: The new hotspot in self-control research. *Current Directions in Psychological Science, 21,* 317–322.

Hollmann, M., Hellrung, L., Pleger, B., Schlogl, H., Kabisch, S., Stumvoll, M., et al. (2012). Neural correlates of the volitional regulation of the desire for food. *International Journal of Obesity, 36*(5), 648–655.

Kavanagh, D. J., Andrade, J., & May, J. (2004). Beating the urge: Implications of research into substance-related desires. *Addictive Behaviors, 29*(7), 1359–1372.

Kavanagh, D. J., Andrade, J., & May, J. (2005). Imaginary relish and exquisite torture: The elaborated intrusion theory of desire. *Psychological Review, 112,* 446–467.

Kemps, E., Tiggemann, M., & Grigg, M. (2008). Food cravings consume limited cognitive resources. *Journal of Experimental Psychology: Applied, 14*(3), 247–254.

Kringelbach, M. L. (2005). The orbitofrontal cortex: Linking reward to hedonic experience. *Nature Reviews Neuroscience, 6,* 691–702.

Kringelbach, M. L., & Berridge, K. C. (Eds.). (2010). *Pleasures of the brain.* Oxford, UK: Oxford University Press.

Kruglanski, A. W., Shah, J. Y., Fishbach, A., Friedman, R., Chun, W. Y., & Sleeth-Keppler, D. (2002). A theory of goal systems. In M. P. Zanna (Ed.), *Advances in experimental social psychology* (Vol. 34, pp. 331–378). San Diego, CA: Academic Press.

Lawton, R., Conner, M., & McEachan, R. (2009). Desire or reason: Predicting health behaviors from affective and cognitive attitudes. *Health Psychology, 28*(1), 56–65.

Lowe, M. R., & Butryn, M. L. (2007). Hedonic hunger: A new dimension of appetite? *Physiology and Behavior, 91*(4), 432–439.

Moskowitz, G. B., & Grant, H. (2009a). Introduction. In G. B. Moskowitz & H. Grant (Eds.), *The psychology of goals* (pp. 1–26). New York: Guilford Press.

Moskowitz, G. B., & Grant, H. (Eds.). (2009b). *The psychology of goals.* New York: Guilford Press.

Nordgren, L. F., & Chou, E. Y. (2011). The push and pull of temptation: The bidirectional influence of temptation on self-control. *Psychological Science, 22*(11), 1386–1390.

Redden, J. P., & Haws, K. L. (2013). Healthy satiation: The role of desire in effective self-control. *Journal of Consumer Research, 39,* 1100–1114.

Robinson, T. E., & Berridge, K. C. (1993). The neural basis of drug craving: An incentive-sensitization theory of addiction. *Brain Research Review, 18,* 247–291.

Schroeder, S. A. (2007). We can do better: Improving the health of the American people. *New England Journal of Medicine, 357,* 1221–1228.

Thaler, R., & Sunstein, C. (2008). *Nudge: Improving decisions about health, wealth, and happiness.* New Haven, CT: Yale University Press.

Vohs, K. D., & Baumeister, R. F. (Eds.). (2011). *Handbook of self-regulation: Research, theory, and applications* (2nd ed.). New York: Guilford Press.

PART I

Basic Processes and Mechanisms

CHAPTER 1

Elaborated Intrusion Theory

*Explaining the Cognitive
and Motivational Basis of Desire*

**Jackie Andrade
Jon May
Lotte van Dillen
David J. Kavanagh**

In 2005, we published a new theory of desire (Kavanagh, Andrade, & May, 2005). Although there was plenty of prior research on desire, that research typically focused on specific drug or food cravings, or on sexual desire. With elaborated intrusion (EI) theory, we aimed to provide a coherent theory of desire that integrated the diverse literature on drug cravings and was applicable to the entire range of desires experienced in everyday life. We wanted to explain desire itself, rather than its precursors, correlates, or behavioral consequences. This chapter provides an overview of EI theory and of research testing its key predictions, ending with a discussion of the implications of the theory for measurement of desire, and for interventions to tackle unwanted desires and strengthen desired desires.

Understanding desire is important because many behaviors are driven by moment-to-moment decision making that involves choices between competing goals. Those choices are influenced by desire, thus strong desires—cravings—to smoke are associated with relapse after a quit attempt (Shiffman, Engberg, Paty, Perz, Gnys, et al., 1997), and cravings for food are associated with binge eating (Ng & Davis, 2013) and failed weight-loss attempts (Sitton, 1991). Desire may influence choices between a longer-term healthy goal and an immediate temptation (e.g., a goal to lose weight vs. the hedonic pleasure derived from eating; Stroebe, van Koningsbruggen, Papies, & Aarts, 2013), and may also influence choices when there is conflict between goals with similar timescales. Being fitter and spending more time with the family may seem compatible, but the actions required to reach these goals can prove incompatible—exercise can be hard to fit into days full of work and child care commitments— and a person may opt for the one that he or she desires more strongly at the moment of deciding which path to take. Desires and goal conflicts are common events, forming a major feature of people's conscious mental lives. Hofmann, Baumeister, Förster, and Vohs (2012; see also Hofmann, Kotabe, Vohs, & Baumeister, Chapter 3, this volume) showed that people experience desires to do or consume something during half their waking hours, and half of these desires conflict, to varying degrees, with other goals: respondents actively tried to resist a desire for 40% of the time. A theory of desire can thus potentially account for a substantial part of people's everyday experience.

EI theory views desire as a conscious wanting, an affectively charged cognitive event that can vary in intensity, duration, and frequency and "in which an object or activity that is associated with pleasure or relief of discomfort is in focal attention" (Kavanagh et al., 2005, p. 447). Desires are not exclusively physiological events. Desires to eat chocolate or drink coffee are not the same thing as hunger or thirst, and cravings for heroin are not the same thing as opiate withdrawal, though they may be triggered by these deficits. EI theory explains the cognitive processes that lead from a trigger to the desire itself. As the name suggests, the key tenet of the theory is that desire is the experience of cognitively elaborating a verbal thought or image, of a target associated with pleasure or reward, which intrudes into conscious awareness. This cognitive elaboration involves affectively charged sensory imagery of the target of desire, which motivates further desire thoughts and imagery, and behavior, through contrasting of that imagery with one's current state. Figure 1.1 illustrates the main components of EI theory.

A Cognitive Approach to Desire

Any view that desires are purely biologically determined underestimates the important and often overriding role of cognitive factors in basic, appetitive behaviors. Asking people to recall what they ate for lunch reduces the amount that they eat on a subsequent "taste test" (Higgs, 2005), and amnesic patients will eat again even if they have only just finished a meal (Rozin, Dow, Moscovitch, & Rajaram, 1998). Cravings for addictive substances are often attributed to withdrawal or opponent processes, but these physiological effects often follow a different time course to that of drug craving. Dar, Rosen-Korakin, Shapira, Gottlieb, and Frenk (2010) found that flight crews' cravings to smoke are determined by the proximity of landing rather than duration since takeoff, showing that cognitive

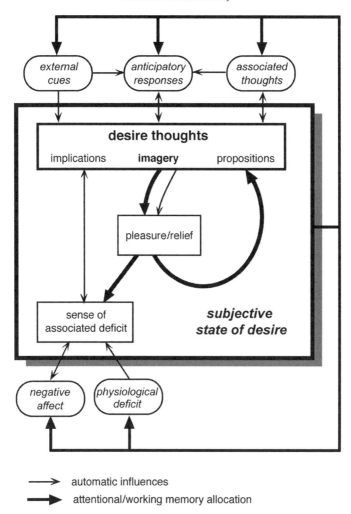

automatic influences
attentional/working memory allocation

FIGURE 1.1. The elaborated intrusion theory of motivation, showing the contribution of triggers (rounded external boxes), intrusive thoughts ("desire thoughts"), and sensory imagery to desire (central square box). Thick arrows show the controlled processing cycle of conscious imagery and associated affect; thin arrows represent automatic influences on desire. From Kavanagh, Andrade, and May (2005). Reprinted by permission. Copyright 2005 by the American Psychological Association.

factors such as expectations can be more important determinants of craving than nicotine deprivation or physiological withdrawal.

If desires were merely automatic or visceral processes that must be opposed by effortful willpower, impairing willpower should leave us at the mercy of our desires. In fact, cognitive loads that interfere with other conscious and controlled tasks do not increase the risk of indulging a desire: they weaken the desire (e.g., Van Dillen & Koole, 2007; Van der Wal & Van Dillen, 2013). In one recent study (Van Dillen, Papies, & Hofmann, 2013), participants exposed to tempting food cues were less likely to select a more attractive snack over a less tasty one when they performed a high working memory load task during the exposure than if the load was low.

Research outside the laboratory also highlights the beneficial potential of cognitive load for self-regulation: Van Dillen and Andrade (under review) asked commuters on a train to choose a three-course meal from a menu. Those who said they were easily tempted by foods subsequently desired food more strongly and chose a high-calorie reward more often than those who said they were less easily tempted. However, this difference vanished when they completed word puzzles after making selections from the menu: when cognitive resources were unavailable, participants were not tempted to choose chocolate over a pen. Notably, when people are instructed to quickly categorize appetitive and neutral images (Van Dillen et al., 2013), working memory load reduces selective attention to more attractive food pictures and (for male participants) to pictures of more attractive female faces.

These findings are consistent with the idea that desire involves cognitive processing. EI theory explains the nature of that processing, from the automatic triggering of desire via associative processes to the cognitive elaboration of desire thoughts using controlled working memory processes.

Triggers of Desire

In EI theory, desires are activated by a range of triggers, often outside awareness, including associated thoughts, physiological cues (e.g., hunger pangs or drug withdrawal symptoms), or awareness of conditioned responses such as salivation. Negative mood can be a cue, as it broadly triggers desires to act to improve one's current state (Petty & Cacioppo, 1984).

Triggers do not always lead to an episode of desire, and when they do, the nature of the desire is not always predictable. Physiological deficits can be misattributed to a particular source. For example, cocaine users who are shown erotic pictures experience increased craving for cocaine (Bauer & Kranzler, 1994). Environmental cues have been given a particularly prominent role in the literature on drug craving, for example in provoking conditioned withdrawal (Ludwig & Wikler, 1974). However, a given environmental cue can trigger multiple goals, whereas desires are specific to a particular target. While chocolate-related cues often trigger desires to eat chocolate (Kemps, Tiggemann, & Grigg, 2008), Fishbach, Friedman, and Kruglanski (2003) showed that they can also trigger weight-loss goals in those wanting to diet, and can do so as effectively as explicit diet and fitness cues. In EI theory, whether a particular trigger leads to a desire depends on a sequence of cognitive processes that begins with priming of mental representations.

Desire-Related Thoughts

Triggers of desire activate or prime desire-related representations in memory. We assume that these representations are embodied, in the sense that they incorporate sensory, affective, and motor output information (e.g., Barsalou, 2008; see also Papies & Barsalou, Chapter 2, this volume), and are activated by automatic associative processes operating outside conscious awareness. This activation or priming of representations increases the likelihood of an apparently spontaneous desire thought intruding into awareness (*I need a cigarette* or *I want lunch*). Supporting this assumption is research that shows associations between the extent of priming of food-related words on a lexical decision task and the frequency of intrusive thoughts about eating experienced by participants while completing the task (Berry, Andrade, & May, 2007).

The apparent spontaneity of intrusions is a key feature of the phenomenology of desire for food, cigarettes, alcohol, and physical exercise (May, Andrade, Kavanagh, Feeney, Gullo, et al., 2014), with most respondents feeling that their desire began with a thought popping into mind, and not being able to report why their desire arose. As with other intrusive thoughts, attempted suppression of desire-related thoughts can be counterproductive, leading to stronger desire (Salkovskis & Reynolds, 1994) and increased behavior (e.g., increased chocolate consumption after suppression of thoughts about chocolate; Erskine, 2008; Erskine & Georgiou, 2010). Interventions that instead encourage participants to accept intrusive thoughts and focus on unrelated imagery (Hamilton, Fawson, May, Andrade, & Kavanagh, 2013; May, Andrade, Willoughby, & Brown, 2012) lead to weaker desire and lower consumption.

Elaboration of Intrusions

Desire-related intrusions are common, but they do not inevitably lead to an episode of desire. Whether they are elaborated is critical in their influence upon an individual's experience and behavior. Thoughts alone do not always elicit the anticipated pleasure or relief that is required for them to constitute a desire. Even in people starting to address alcohol-related problems, when we might expect thoughts about drinking to capture attention, 87% reported that the thoughts sometimes popped into mind but then vanished without effort (Kavanagh et al., 2009). Self-report data on desires confirm that the occurrence of thoughts about a target and elaborated imagery of that target form separate factors, although the hypothesized causal chain between them means the factors are correlated (May et al., 2014; Statham et al., 2011). Elaborated images can also lead to further intrusions, strengthening activation of the current goal or activating a new goal. Intrusions about hunger might lead to an initial image of a meal, but then to elaborated imagery of appetizing foods, and lead to a goal to eat the specific imagined food.

Elaboration has to compete with ongoing cognitive activity for limited-capacity resources. When people are engaged in information-rich, conceptually coherent tasks, there is less opportunity for the mind to wander in any way, including elaboration of task-unrelated thoughts (Smallwood & Schooler, 2006), among which are desire-related cognitions. As discussed above, food cravings are less intense when high competing cognitive loads reduce the opportunity to elaborate thoughts about eating (Van Dillen & Andrade, 2014; Van Dillen et al., 2013). In a study using a primed lexical decision task (Van Dillen et al., 2013), participants were faster to recognize hedonic food-related words (e.g., *delicious*) than irrelevant words (*cozy*) when these were primed by tasty food pictures, suggesting that participants spontaneously formed hedonic associations in response to the pictures. However, this advantage disappeared when participants were placed under high concurrent working memory load, and participants reported fewer food cravings. These findings are consistent with the idea that cognitive loads prevent the elaboration of desire-related representations, which weakens priming, even when those representations are associated with pleasure or reward.

Cognitive load inductions can also then reduce approach behavior. In one study on alcohol consumption (Sharbanee, Stritzke, Jamalludin, & Wiers, 2014), an approach–avoidance test (AAT) was used to assess people's approach tendencies, while cognitive load was varied. During low cognitive load, there was a positive relationship between an alcohol-related approach bias on the AAT and subsequent drinking on a taste test. During high cognitive load, this relationship disappeared. While Sharnabee et al. (2014) attributed the result to inhibition of an alcohol-related action tendency, the result is also consistent with inhibition of elaborative processing of alcohol as an attractive target, which then also impedes the amount of alcohol that is consumed.

Complementary evidence that desires involve cognitive elaboration comes from studies of the effects of desire on cognitive performance:

while cognitive load can interfere with desire, desire can also interfere with concurrent tasks. People perform more poorly on tasks assessing reaction speed, arithmetic, language, and memory performance when craving cigarettes (Madden & Zwaan, 2001; Sweet et al., 2010; Zwaan, Stanfield, & Madden, 2000; Zwaan & Truit, 1998) or food (Green, Rogers, & Elliman, 2000; Kemps et al., 2008; Meule, Skirde, Freund, Vögele, & Kübler, 2012). The findings for food craving are often limited to those with high trait craving or restricted diets: since food is readily available in well-resourced societies, deprivation is usually low, so that effects of elaboration of food-related desires may be restricted to subgroups. Overall, this body of research shows mutual interactions between desire and cognitive performance, consistent with the assumption that desire involves cognitive elaboration that taps limited-capacity working memory processes.

Elaboration Involves Affectively Rich Embodied Sensory Imagery

Elaboration may involve generating expectancies ("A drink would make me feel better") or evaluating self-efficacy ("I can resist" or "I can stop at a bar on my way home"), but EI theory uniquely proposes that the core component is affectively charged sensory imagery that emulates the experience of achieving one's desire. This mental imagery of the target and its acquisition serve to ready the individual for target-directed behavior.

Advertisements for food often use slogans such as "finger-lickin' good" or "snap, crackle, and pop" that encourage rich, multisensory imagery—and, through repetition, link it to a specific product. In EI theory, such imagery is at the heart of desire. It is embodied and thus affectively charged (e.g., Moulton & Kosslyn, 2009; Schendan & Ganis, 2012); imagining consuming a delicious treat is itself a pleasurable experience, not just a neutral anticipation of future pleasure. The more vivid and realistic the image, the greater the pleasure: a smoker said to us that the cigarettes he imagined were always perfect—better than the actual cigarette he later had. In line with this, Elder and Krishna (2010) demonstrated that multisensory advertisements for food products resulted in higher taste perceptions than ones focusing on taste alone, and that restricting cognitive resources (imposing cognitive load) attenuated the enhancing effect of the multiple-sense advertisement.

Strong desires are characterized by sensory imagery (Kavanagh et al., 2009; Tiggemann & Kemps, 2005; May et al., 2004, 2008, 2014; Statham et al., 2011). In a questionnaire study of triggers and experiences of craving, respondents endorsed items relating to sensory imagery more than items relating to habit, stress, or attempted abstinence (May et al., 2004), and an EI theory factor combining sensory imagery and intrusiveness questions is the strongest unique predictor of craving strength (May et al., 2008). People with alcohol problems who were trying to control their drinking frequently imagined a drink, tasting and swallowing it, with an average of 2.3 sensory modalities represented (Kavanagh et al., 2009). More frequent sensory imagery was associated with stronger and longer-lasting episodes of alcohol craving. Jauregui-Lobera, Bolanos-Rios, Valero, and Prieto (2012) similarly found that vivid sensory imagery was associated with strength of desire for food.

Imagery is also important in desires for nonconsummatory behaviors. Research in sport and exercise shows close associations between imagery and motivation to exercise (Hall, Rodgers, Wilson, & Norman, 2010). The extent to which players imagine themselves playing hockey explains a substantial portion of the difference between their weakest and strongest desires to play over the week (May et al., 2008). Consistent with the focus of EI theory on embodied, affectively charged imagery, it is especially imagery of the positive benefits of exercising, such as enjoyment and feeling energized, that is important for motivation (Stanley & Cumming, 2010).

Studies on the interference of concurrent tasks with desires also provide evidence on the specific sense domains that are implicated in desire imagery. Given the evidence that substance cravings involve more visual than auditory imagery (Jauregui-Lobera et al., 2012; May et al., 2008, 2004, 2014; Tiggemann & Kemps, 2005), and evidence that imagery requires modality-specific working memory resources (Baddeley & Andrade, 2000), EI theory predicts that a concurrent visuospatial task will have a greater impact on appetitive desires than would an auditory task. Findings are consistent with this prediction, for example showing that imagined neutral visual scenes reduce desires for smoking (May et al., 2010; Versland & Rosenberg, 2007) and eating (Kemps & Tiggemann, 2007), more than do imagined neutral sounds. Other visuospatial tasks that require working memory capacity (e.g., molding clay out of sight) reduce desire more than verbal tasks (Andrade, Pears, May, & Kavanagh, 2012; May, Andrade, Panabokke, & Kavanagh, 2010). Showing that these findings generalize to naturally occurring cravings, Knäuper, Pillay, Lacaille, McCollam, and Kelso (2011b) found that imagining a positive activity whenever food cravings struck helped to reduce the intensity of food cravings over a 4-day period, compared with reciting the alphabet or forming intentions to reduce cravings.

Olfactory imagery is also reported as part of the phenomenology of substance cravings (e.g., Kavanagh et al., 2009; May et al., 2004, 2008, 2014; Tiggemann & Kemps, 2005). Again there is evidence that experimentally interfering with olfactory imagery leads to weakened desire: Versland and Rosenberg (2007) found that neutral olfactory imagery reduced craving for cigarettes, while Kemps and Tiggemann reported similar findings for food (2007) and coffee (2009) cravings. Smelling a nonfood scent also reduced strength of desire for food and coffee (Kemps & Tiggemann, 2013).

Because EI theory assumes that desires are embodied and that desire imagery emulates the sensory qualities of the desired behavior, auditory or verbal tasks are predicted to reduce the strength of desires to engage in activities where sound is an integral part of the pleasure and reward of the activity. Examples may include racetrack betting, gambling on jackpot machines, video gaming, and noisy sports such as hockey where players report auditory imagery as a feature of their desire to play (May et al., 2008).

Initially, desire imagery is pleasurable, which is why people persist in it even if they are trying to avoid indulging. However, if a strong desire cannot immediately be fulfilled (as in a desire to smoke during a lecture), awareness of the gap between our current and imagined states becomes unpleasant unless it can be reinterpreted as evidence that we are reaching another highly valued goal (e.g., abstinence). Blackburn, Thompson, and May (2012) found that restricted eaters elaborated cues about being hungry in ways that emphasized their personal success in not eating, rather than as cues to eat. Normally, though, negative emotions arising from unfulfilled desires motivate us to inspect our current situation (Schwarz & Clore, 1983), enhancing the salience of the desired target.

Imagery Motivates Behavior

The research reviewed in the previous section supports EI theory by showing how sensory imagery is closely linked with desire. We contend that desire is not epiphenomenal, but rather drives behavior toward the desired goal, by keeping the goal active until it is attained. Studies of substance craving support our claim that imagery is associated with goal-directed behavior: there are positive associations between the intensity and frequency of desire imagery and drug use (Kavanagh et al., 2009; May et al., 2014; Connor et al., 2014).

As shown in Figure 1.1, EI theory assumes that desire imagery increases awareness of current deficit. Oettingen and colleagues have argued that mentally contrasting an image with one's current state is an important part of the motivational power of imagery, thus Achtziger, Fehr, Oettingen, Gollwitzer, and Rochstroh (2009) reported MEG (magnetoencephalography) data consistent with mental contrasting involving imagery, and Oettingen, Mayer, and Thorpe (2009) showed that mentally contrasting instructions increased success at quitting smoking.

However, correlations between desire strength and behavior are not always strong (Maude-Griffin & Tiffany, 1996), because successful goal acquisition is also strongly influenced by factors such as opportunity, acquisition and control skills, and related self-efficacy (Bandura, 1986). Furthermore, predictions from a particular desire are often moderated by the presence of competing desires. Thoughts about a drug, for example, might trigger both approach and avoidance responses, because they activate goals to use it, but also goals to avoid drugs in order to become healthy, save money, or retain a valued relationship or job (Krieglmeyer, Deutsch, De Houwer, & De Raedt, 2010).

Implications of EI Theory

Measuring Desire

In a recent review of tools for measuring drug craving, we concluded that measures often confound desire with behavioral intentions, expectancies, and self-efficacy (Kavanagh et al., 2013; see also Sayette & Wilson, Chapter 5, this volume). For example, the Questionnaire on Smoking Urges includes expectancy items (e.g., "I would enjoy a cigarette right now") and behavior items (e.g., "I will smoke as soon as I get the chance"), potentially giving a high score to people who intend to smoke soon—perhaps because they know they will not have another opportunity for some time—even though they are not experiencing a strong desire for a cigarette.

We developed the Alcohol Craving Experience (ACE) questionnaire (Kavanagh et al., 2009; Statham et al., 2011) to help disentangle desire from these confounds, using EI theory to help formulate items assessing the intensity, vividness, and intrusiveness of desire for alcohol. In a recent study of young adults, scores on the imagery component of the ACE predicted 12–16% of the variance in alcohol consumption (Connor et al., 2014), supporting the inclusion of imagery in measures of desire. The Craving Experience Questionnaire (CEQ) is a generalized version of the ACE designed to measure strength and frequency of desires for various substances over variable timescales ranging from the past week or month to the past few minutes of an experimental lab session. The CEQ has a consistent three-factor structure, comprising desire intensity, imagery, and intrusiveness, and has undergone preliminary validation against measures of nicotine dependence and obsessional drinking (May et al., 2014).

Changing Behavior

Laboratory studies on cognitive interference with desires for food or drugs suggest that simple tasks can weaken desires if they load the working memory processes that support desire imagery. Recent research extends these findings to real-world settings. Knäuper et al.'s (2011b) study, cited above, showed selective reductions in food cravings over four days when people imagined a favorite activity whenever cravings struck. Skorka-Brown, Andrade, Whalley, and May (in press) used SMS messages to prompt participants seven times a day for a week to report cravings and, in the experimental group, to play Tetris for 3 minutes before reporting craving strength again. Playing Tetris weakened cravings by approximately 13 percentage points, similar to the reduction seen in laboratory research with a range of desires for food, physical activity, and addictive substances (Skorka-Brown, Andrade, & May, 2014). Also building on lab studies, Kemps and Tiggemann (2013) found that undergraduates experienced less intense food cravings over 4 weeks and consumed fewer calories when they used a handheld device to display dynamic visual noise in response to food cravings. Hsu et al. (2013) tested a smartphone app (iCrave) that provided written cues to imagine neutral visual scenes whenever users craved snacks and asked users to record both snacking and successful behavioral control. Over a week, community volunteers using iCrave ate fewer unhealthy snacks (but similar amounts of healthy snacks) than those who simply tracked their snacking.

Rodríguez-Martín, Gómez-Quintana, Díaz-Martínez, and Molerio-Perez (2013) reported that a self-help manual based on EI theory helped overweight and obese people to manage their cravings. "Imagery diversion" techniques such as imagining a pleasant activity (Knäuper et al., 2011b) or neutral scene (May et al., 2010), and olfactory or visual imagery interference techniques were particularly helpful. Over 3 months, BMI decreased by 6% for participants randomly allocated to the manual condition, compared to no change in the control group who were asked to use their willpower to control their cravings.

Changing behavior in the long term is not just a matter of maintaining abstinence by managing cravings. Rather, there is a need to shift the balance of desire from immediate rewards to the long-term goal. EI theory predicts that people's behavior can be shifted toward functional goals by encouraging vivid, emotive imagery of those goals. Although imagery of the negative consequences of continuing a behavior might also be effective (Giuliani, Calcott, & Berkman, 2013; Kober, Kross, Mischel, Hart, & Ochsner, 2010; Szasz, Szentagotai, & Hofmann, 2012), there is a risk that thinking about negative future consequences will lead people to avoid thinking about the future because it is unpleasant, or because they assume that something so bad would never happen to them (Ruiter, Abraham, & Kok, 2001). EI theory predicts that behavior change interventions will be most effective when they encourage people to imagine positive benefits of change, which is a more rewarding mental exercise, rather than negative consequences of not changing. This strategy shifts attention from present to future rewards in a way that strengthens desire for the future goal while also absorbing the imagery capacity that would otherwise support desire for immediate rewards.

Consistent with this prediction, Daniel, Stanton, and Epstein (2013) showed that positive future imagery aided motivation as well as decision making. Overweight and obese women who were cued to imagine personally relevant positive future events before making decisions showed less delay discounting and consumed fewer calories on a taste test compared with women who imagined events described by a travel writer. In this study, imagining personal future events helped focus attention on future rather than immediate rewards, and this increased decisions in favor of the future rewards.

Goals in the distant future can be motivating if vivid imagery about them can be generated, but often it cannot—future events are not typically construed in sufficient detail to support vivid imagery (Trope & Liberman, 2003). We suggest that motivation will be maximized if distal goals are linked to proximal steps that also provide valued outcomes. Highly realistic imagery for proximal outcomes is easier to elicit, and this imagery serves as an effective contrast against one's current state. Greater likelihood of achieving the goal may also be inferred when an expected outcome is proximal. Both elements augment the affective charge of the functional stepwise goals.

A related point is that more vivid imagery for the functional behavior and for the context in which it is required is also likely to assist in ensuring that it occurs. Implementation intentions (Gollwitzer & Sheeran, 2006) can be seen as a way of lowering the construal level of goals. Implementation intentions are detailed behavioral plans for achieving a goal, which specify how, when, and where goal-directed behaviors take place. They are argued to work in part by strengthening and automatizing links between cues and goal-related actions, so that cues for desired behaviors become more salient among the multitude of cues for other behaviors, and ambiguous cues become more likely to trigger the desired rather than alternative behavior.

EI theory predicts that implementation intentions will be more effective when they encourage the generation of detailed vivid imagery. If people imagine possible scenarios while constructing their plan ("Which day shall I go to the gym?" "How will I get there?"), this imagery would be expected to contribute to the memorability and motivational power of the plan. This may be especially true of implementation intention interventions in field settings with complex behavioral choices, for example, when planning how to raise the issue of condom use with one's partner (Martin, Sheeran, Slade, Wright, & Dibble, 2009). Explicit instructions to imagine carrying out a plan or overcoming present obstacles increase goal achievement compared with simply making an implementation intention (Adriaanse et al., 2010; Knäuper et al., 2011a), consistent with EI theory's prediction.

A problem with making plans to achieve future rewards is that people's estimates of how they will feel in the future tend to be biased by how they feel right now (see also Ruttan & Nordgren, Chapter 11, this volume). For example, someone who has just eaten Christmas dinner might underestimate the difficulty of sticking to their New Year's resolution to diet. Sayette, Loewenstein, Griffin, and Black (2008) found that smokers who had just smoked a cigarette underestimated the value they would place on smoking in the future, compared with smokers who had abstained from smoking for 12 hours before the study. In EI theory, a reason for this so-called empathy gap is that images are constructed from all the information available, and it is hard to prevent current sensory information being incorporated into an image of a future self or situation. We predict that explicitly instructing participants to generate and rehearse detailed images of the future that incorporate information from past experiences as well as present feelings will help them make more realistic and detailed plans for behavior change and increase their chance of success.

There is also a need to weaken desires for immediate temptations. The laboratory studies discussed above show that any competing sensory imagery can reduce cravings, and future-goal-related imagery will also do this. Strategies that seek to enhance awareness of other bodily sensations from competing behaviors, such as body scanning (Hamilton et al., 2013), mindful attention (Westbrook, Creswell, Tabibnia, Julson, Kober, & Tindle, 2013), or more extended mindfulness training (Witkiewitz & Bowen, 2010) may also help block craving imagery, not only by competition for modality-specific working memory resources, but also by drawing attention to competing sensations. Another advantage of these strategies is that they typically involve instructions to notice but ignore sensations and thoughts, encouraging mental detachment from immediate bodily sensations and tempting thoughts that should help prevent elaboration of goals to indulge immediate temptations (see also Hofmann, Kotabi, Vohs, & Baumeister, Chapter 3, this volume). Papies, Pronk, Keesman, and Barsalou (2014) have shown that brief training in mental detachment from (or "mindful attention" to) responses to food cues can reduce consumption of unhealthy foods, while Bowen and Marlatt (2009) reported reduction in smoking in the 7 days following mindfulness instructions (although they did not find decreases in self-reported craving in response to smoking cues). Mindfulness-related approaches may also therefore find a place in a motivational intervention inspired by EI theory, although extended training and practice may be needed for optimal results from this specific strategy.

Putting It All Together: Functional Imagery Training

In sum, desire to pursue a future goal requires vivid, detailed, and positively affectively charged imagery of goal success and the behavioral path toward that success. Engaging in such imagery also brings the benefit of diverting cognitive resources from imagery of immediate rewards, protecting the good intention from temptation. A corollary for treatment is that this functional imagery needs to be made salient in temptation situations. We suggest that three strategies can help with this task: repeated rehearsal in clinical sessions of the imagery about valued outcomes, past successes, and detailed plans; linking home practice to a frequent routine task; and setting reminders to practice imagery in situations where the functional behavior is most needed.

Based on EI theory and the above findings, we have developed a new motivational intervention to support functional behavior change, which we call functional imagery training (FIT). FIT uses a motivational interviewing style (Miller & Rollnick, 2012) to encourage people to develop vivid imagery about both distal and proximal positive consequences of behavior change, past relevant successes, and detailed hypothetical plans. People who elect to commit to the functional goal are encouraged to rehearse imagery about their plan and its likely benefits whenever they undertake a particular routine task such as washing their hands. Brief phone sessions over the next weeks reinforce the imagery. They also set reminders on their mobile phone to practice imagery in the form of a televised advertisement about their plan and its outcomes, where they feature in the advertisement. They record or write a statement about their goal, why they have adopted it, and the reason they believe they can do it, and are encouraged to share the statement with a person who will give nonintrusive support, and to read or replay the statement, imagining its elements whenever their motivation flags. In some versions of FIT, they can also access audios that guide them in mindful body scanning and attention to environmental stimuli, and help them view temptations as just one part of their total experience. We predict that FIT will promote sustained behavior change by developing habits of vividly imagining future goals rather than immediate pleasures. Trials of FIT for a range of functional behaviors are currently under way.

Conclusion

According to EI theory, desire is what we feel when making a controlled, cognitive response to a seemingly spontaneous thought about a target associated with pleasure or reward. Embodied sensory imagery, which emulates attainment of the target, is central to desire cognition. Such imagery is reported as a potent feature of desire and correlates with desire strength. EI theory has stimulated development of tools for measuring desire in its own right, distinguished from correlates such as behavioral control and intention. It provides a framework for developing strategies to support people quitting addictions, maintaining a healthy weight, or getting more physical exercise. Behavior change interventions need to develop habits of vividly imagining future goals and the paths to their achievement: we argue that future-focused imagery can divert cognitive resources from imagery associated with immediate desires and can help strengthen desire for future goals. Future-focused imagery should be positive and vivid, personally relevant, and detailed. Distant events can be difficult to imagine vividly because they are underspecified—uncertain and abstract—so interventions should help people to identify proximal subgoals that are easier to imagine vividly and more likely to be achieved. Seen through the lens of EI theory, self-regulation might be partly a matter of adopting the mental habit of vividly imagining the benefits of change toward, or maintenance of, healthy goals. Our new intervention, functional imagery training, helps people use imagery to maintain this self-regulation.

REFERENCES

Achtziger, A., Fehr, T., Oettingen, G., Gollwitzer, P. M., & Rockstroh, B. (2009). Strategies of intention formation are reflected in continuous MEG activity. *Social Neuroscience, 4*(1), 11–27.

Adriaanse, M. A., Oettingen, G., Gollwitzer, P. M., Hennes, E. P., de Ridder, D. T., & Wit, J. B. (2010). When planning is not enough: Fighting unhealthy snacking habits by mental contrasting with implementation intentions (MCII). *European Journal of Social Psychology, 40*, 1277–1293.

Ajzen, I. (1991). The theory of planned behavior. *Organizational Behavior and Human Decision Processes, 50*, 179–211.

Anderson, C. A. (1983). Imagination and expectation: The effect of imagining behavioral scripts on personal intentions. *Journal of Personality and Social Psychology, 45*, 293–305.

Andrade, J., Pears, S., May, J., & Kavanagh, D. J. (2012). Use of a clay modeling task to reduce chocolate craving. *Appetite, 58*, 955–963.

Baddeley, A. D., & Andrade, J. (2000). Working memory and the vividness of imagery. *Journal of Experimental Psychology: General, 129*, 126–145.

Bandura, A. (1996). *Self-efficacy: The exercise of control.* New York: Freeman.

Bandura, A., & Simon, K. M. (1977). The role of proximal intentions in self-regulation of refractory behavior. *Cognitive Therapy and Research, 3*, 177–193.

Barsalou, L. W. (2008). Grounded cognition. *Annual Review of Psychology, 59*, 617–645.

Bauer, L., & Kranzler, H. R. (1994). Electroencephalographic activity and mood in cocaine-dependent outpatients: Effects of cocaine cue exposure. *Biological Psychiatry, 36*, 189–197.

Berry, L.-M., Andrade, J., & May, J. (2007). Hunger-related intrusive thoughts reflect increased accessibility of food items. *Cognition and Emotion, 21*, 865–878.

Blackburn, J. F., Thompson, A. R., & May, J. (2012). Feeling good about being hungry: Food-related thoughts in eating disorder. *Journal of Experimental Psychopathology, 3*, 243–257.

Bowen, S., & Marlatt, A. (2009). Surfing the urge: Brief mindfulness-based intervention for college student smokers. *Psychology of Addictive Behaviors, 23*, 666–671.

Connor, J. P., Kavanagh, D. J., Andrade, J., May, J., Feeney, G. F. X., Gullo, M. J., et al. (2014). Alcohol consumption in young adults: The role of multisensory imagery. *Addictive Behaviors, 39,* 721–724.

Daniel, T., Stanton, C., & Epstein, L. (2013). The future is now: Reducing impulsivity and energy intake using episodic future thinking. *Psychological Science, 24,* 2339–2342.

Dar, R., Rosen-Korakin, N., Shapira, O., Gottlieb, Y., & Frenk, H. (2010). The craving to smoke in flight attendants: Relations with smoking deprivation, anticipation of smoking, and actual smoking. *Journal of Abnormal Psychology, 119,* 248–253.

Elder, R. S., & Krishna, A. (2010). The effects of advertising copy on sensory thoughts and perceived taste. *Journal of Consumer Research, 36,* 748–756.

Erskine, J. A. K. (2008). Resistance can be futile: Investigating behavioural rebound. *Appetite, 50,* 415–421.

Erskine, J. A., & Georgiou, G. J. (2010). Effects of thought suppression on eating behaviour in restrained and non-restrained eaters. *Appetite, 54,* 499–503.

Fishbach, A., Friedman, R. S., & Kruglanski, A. W. (2003). Leading us not into temptation: Momentary allurements elicit overriding goal activation. *Journal of Personality and Social Psychology, 84,* 296–309.

Giuliani, N. R., Calcott, R. D., & Berkman, E. T. (2013). Piece of cake: Cognitive reappraisal of food craving. *Appetite, 64,* 56–61.

Gollwitzer, P. M., & Sheeran, P. (2006). Implementation intentions and goal achievement: A meta-analysis of effects and processes. *Advances in Experimental Social Psychology, 38,* 69–119.

Green, M. W., Rogers, P. J., & Elliman, N. A. (2000). Dietary restraint and addictive behaviors—The generalizability of Tiffany's Cue Reactivity Model. *International Journal of Eating Disorders, 27,* 419–427.

Hall, C. R., Rodgers, W. M., Wilson, P. M., & Norman, P. (2010). Imagery use and self-determined motivations in a community sample of exercisers and non-exercisers. *Journal of Applied Social Psychology, 40,* 135–152.

Hamilton, J., Fawson, S., May, J., Andrade, J., & Kavanagh, D. J. (2013). Brief guided imagery and body scanning interventions reduce food cravings. *Appetite, 58,* 955–963.

Higgs, S. (2005). Memory and its role in appetite regulation. *Physiology and Behavior, 85,* 67–72.

Hofmann, W., Baumeister, R. F., Förster, G., & Vohs, K. D. (2012). Everyday temptations: An experience sampling study of desire, conflict, and self-control. *Journal of Personality and Social Psychology, 102,* 1318–1335.

Hsu, A., Yang, J., Yilmaz, Y., Haque, M. S., Can, C., & Blandford, A. (2014). Persuasive technology for overcoming food cravings and improving snack choices. *Proceedings of the SIGCHI Conference on Human Factors in Computing Systems* (pp. 3403–3412). New York: ACM.

Jauregui-Lobera, I., Bolanos-Rios, P., Valero, E., Prieto, I. R. (2012). Induction of food craving experience: The role of mental imagery, dietary restraint, mood and coping strategies. *Nutricion Hospitalaria, 27,* 1928–1935.

Kavanagh, D. J., Andrade, J., & May, J. (2005). Imaginary relish and exquisite torture: The elaborated intrusion theory of desire. *Psychological Review, 112,* 446–467.

Kavanagh, D. J., May, J., & Andrade, J. (2009). Tests of the elaborated intrusion theory of craving and desire: Features of alcohol craving during treatment for an alcohol disorder. *British Journal of Clinical Psychology, 48,* 241–254.

Kavanagh, D. J., Statham, D. J., Feeney, G. F. X., Young, R. McD., May, J., Andrade,

J., et al. (2013). Measurement of alcohol craving, *Addictive Behaviors, 38*, 1572–1584.

Kemps, E., & Tiggemann, M. (2007). Modality-specific imagery reduces cravings for food: An application of the elaborated intrusion theory of desire to food craving. *Journal of Experimental Psychology: Applied, 13*, 95–104.

Kemps, E., & Tiggemann, M. (2009). Attentional bias for craving-related (chocolate) food cues. *Experimental and Clinical Psychopharmacology, 17*, 425.

Kemps, E., & Tiggemann, M. (2013). Olfactory stimulation curbs food cravings. *Addictive Behaviors, 38*, 1550–1554.

Kemps, E., Tiggemann, M., & Grigg, M. (2008). Food cravings consume limited cognitive resources. *Journal of Experimental Psychology: Applied, 14*, 247–254.

Knäuper, B., McCollam, A., Rosen-Brown, A., Lacaille, J., Kelso, E., & Roseman, M. (2011a). Fruitful plans: Adding targeted mental imagery to implementation intentions increases fruit consumption. *Psychology and Health, 26*, 601–617.

Knäuper, B., Pillay, R., Lacaille, J., McCollam, A., & Kelso, E. (2011b). Replacing craving imagery with alternative pleasant imagery reduces craving intensity. *Appetite, 57*, 173–178.

Kober, H., Kross, E. F., Mischel, W., Hart, C. L., & Ochsner, K. N. (2010). Regulation of craving by cognitive strategies in cigarette smokers. *Drug and Alcohol Dependence, 106*, 52–55.

Krieglmeyer, R., Deutsch, R., De Houwer, J., & De Raedt, R. (2010). Being moved: Valence activates approach-avoidance behavior independently of evaluation and approach-avoidance intentions. *Psychological Science, 21*, 607–613.

Ludwig, A. M., & Wikler, A. (1974). "Craving" and relapse to drink. *Quarterly Journal of Studies on Alcohol, 35*, 108–130.

Madden, C. J., & Zwaan, R. A. (2001). The impact of smoking urges on working memory performance. *Experimental and Clinical Psychopharmacology, 9*, 418–424.

Martin, J., Sheeran, P., Slade, P., Wright, A., & Dibble, T. (2009). Implementation intention formation reduces consultations for emergency contraception and pregnancy testing among teenage women. *Health Psychology, 28*, 762–769.

Maude-Griffin, P., & Tiffany, S. T. (1996). Production of smoking urges through imagery: The impact of affect and smoking abstinence. *Experimental and Clinical Psychopharmacology, 4*, 198–208.

May, J., Andrade, J., Kavanagh, D. J., Feeney, G. F. X., Gullo, M., Statham, D. J., et al. (2014). The Craving Experience Questionnaire: A brief, theory-based measure of consummatory desire and craving. *Addiction, 109*, 728–735.

May, J., Andrade, J., Kavanagh, D., & Penfound, L. (2008). Imagery and strength of craving for eating, drinking, and playing sport. *Cognition and Emotion, 22*, 633–650.

May, J., Andrade, J., Panabokke, N., & Kavanagh, D. J. (2004). Images of desire: Cognitive models of craving. *Memory, 12*, 447–461.

May, J., Andrade, J., Panabokke, N., & Kavanagh, D. (2010). Visuospatial tasks suppress craving for cigarettes. *Behaviour Research and Therapy, 48*, 476–485.

May, J., Andrade, J., Willoughby, K., & Brown, C. (2012). An attentional control task reduces intrusive thoughts about smoking, *Nicotine and Tobacco Research, 14*, 472–478.

Meule, A., Skirde, A. K., Freund, R., Vögele, C., & Kübler, A. (2012). High-calorie food-cues impair working memory performance in high and low food cravers. *Appetite, 59*, 264–269.

Miller, W. R., & Rollnick, S. (2012). *Motivational interviewing: Helping people change* (3rd ed.). New York: Guilford Press.

Moulton, S. T., & Kosslyn, S. M. (2009). Imagining predictions: mental imagery as mental emulation. *Philosophical Transactions of the Royal Society B: Biological Sciences, 364*(1521), 1273–1280.

Ng, L., & Davis, C. (2013). Cravings and food consumption in binge eating disorder. *Eating Behaviors, 14*(4), 472–475.

Oettingen, G., Mayer, D., & Thorpe, J. (2010). Self-regulation of commitment to reduce cigarette consumption: Mental contrasting of future with reality. *Psychology and Health, 25*, 961–977.

Papies, E. K., Pronk, T. M., Keesman, M., & Barsalou, L. W. (2014). The benefits of simply observing: Mindful attention modulates the link between motivation and behavior. *Journal of Personality and Social Psychology, 108*, 148–170.

Petty, R. E., & Cacioppo, J. T. (1984). Source factors and the elaboration likelihood model of persuasion. *Advances in Consumer Research, 11*, 668–672.

Rodríguez-Martín, B. C., Gómez-Quintana, A., Díaz-Martínez, G., & Molerio-Perez, O. (2013). Bibliotherapy and food cravings control. *Appetite, 65*, 90–95.

Rozin, P., Dow, S., Moscovitch, M., & Rajaram, S. (1998). What causes humans to begin and end a meal?: A role for memory for what has been eaten, as evidenced by a study of multiple meal eating in amnesic patients, *Psychological Science, 9*, 392–396.

Ruiter, R. A. C., Abraham, C., & Kok, G. (2001). Scary warnings and rational precautions: A review of the psychology of fear appeals. *Psychology and Health, 16*, 613–630.

Salkovskis, P. M., & Reynolds, M. (1994). Thought suppression and smoking cessation. *Behaviour Research and Therapy, 32*, 193–201.

Sayette, M. A., Loewenstein, G., Griffin, K. M., & Black, J. J. (2008). Exploring the cold-to-hot empathy gap in smokers. *Psychological Science, 19*, 926–932.

Schendan, H. E., & Ganis, G. (2012). Electrophysiological potentials reveal cortical mechanisms for mental imagery, mental simulation, and grounded (embodied) cognition. *Frontiers in Psychology, 3*, 329.

Schwarz, N., & Clore, G. L. (1983). Mood, misattribution, and judgments of well-being: Informative and directive functions of affective states. *Journal of Personality and Social Psychology, 45*, 513–523.

Sharbanee, J. M., Stritzke, W. G. K., Jamalludin, M. E., & Wiers, R. W. (2014). Approach-alcohol action tendencies can be inhibited by cognitive load. *Psychopharmacology, 231*, 967–975.

Shiffman, S., Engberg, J., Paty, J., Perz, W. G., Gnys, M., Kassel, J., et al. (1997). A day at a time: Predicting smoking lapse from daily urge. *Journal of Abnormal Psychology, 106*, 104–116.

Sitton, S. C. (1991). Role of craving for carbohydrates upon completion of a protein-sparing fast. *Psychological Reports, 69*, 683–686.

Skorka-Brown, J., Andrade, J., & May, J. (2014). Playing "Tetris" reduces the strength, frequency and vividness of naturally occurring cravings. *Appetite, 76*, 161–165.

Skorka-Brown, J., Whalley, B., Andrade, J., & May, J. (in press). Does playing Tetris decrease cravings in real world situations? The application of laboratory findings to ecologically valid settings. *Addictive Behaviors*.

Smallwood, J., & Schooler, J. W. (2006). The restless mind. *Psychological Bulletin, 132*, 946–958.

Stanley, D. M., & Cumming, J. (2010). Are we having fun yet?: Testing the effects of imagery use on the affective and enjoyment responses to acute moderate exercise. *Psychology of Sport and Exercise, 11*, 582–590.

Statham, D. J., Connor, J. P., Kavanagh, D. J., Feeney, G. F. X., Young, R. M. D., May, J., et al. (2011). Measuring alcohol craving: Development of the Alcohol Craving Experience questionnaire. *Addiction, 106*, 1230–1238.

Stroebe, W., van Koningsbruggen, G. M., Papies, E. K., & Aarts, H. (2013). Why most dieters fail but some succeed: A goal conflict model of eating behavior. *Psychological Review, 120*, 110–138.

Sweet, L. H., Mulligan, R. C., Finnerty, C. E., Jerskey, B. A., David, S. P., Cohen, R. A., et al. (2010). Effects of nicotine withdrawal on verbal working memory and associated brain response. *Psychiatry Research, 183*, 69–74.

Szasz, P. L., Szentagotai, A., & Hofmann, S. G. (2012). Effects of emotion regulation strategies on smoking craving, attentional bias, and task persistence. *Behaviour Research and Therapy, 50*(5), 333–340.

Tiggemann, M., & Kemps, E. (2005). The phenomenology of food cravings: The role of mental imagery. *Appetite, 45*, 305–313.

Trope, Y., & Liberman, N. (2003). Temporal construal. *Psychological Review, 110*, 403–421.

Van der Wal, R., & Van Dillen, L. F. (2013). Leaving a flat taste in your mouth: Task load reduces taste perception. *Psychological Science, 24*, 1277–1284.

Van Dillen, L. F., & Andrade, J. (under review). *Derailing the streetcar named desire: Cognitive distractions disrupt cravings and unhealthy snacking in response to a temptation.* Manuscript submitted for publication.

Van Dillen, L. F., & Koole, S. L. (2007). Clearing the mind: A working memory model of distraction from negative mood. *Emotion, 7*, 715–723.

Van Dillen, L. F., Papies, E. K., & Hofmann, W. (2013). Turning a blind eye to temptation: How cognitive load can facilitate self-regulation. *Journal of Personality and Social Psychology, 104*, 427–443.

Versland, A., & Rosenberg, H. (2007). Effect of brief imagery interventions on craving in college student smokers. *Addiction Research and Theory, 15*, 177–187.

Westbrook, C., Creswell, J. D., Tabibnia, G., Julson, E., Kober, H., & Tindle, H. A. (2013). Mindful attention reduces neural and self-reported cue-induced craving in smokers. *Social Cognitive and Affective Neuroscience, 8*, 73–84.

Witkiewitz, K., & Bowen, S. (2010). Depression, craving, and substance use following a randomized trial of mindfulness-based relapse prevention. *Journal of Consulting and Clinical Psychology, 78*, 362–374.

Zwaan, R. A., Stanfield, R. A., & Madden, C. J. (2000). How persistent is the effect of smoking urges on cognitive performance? *Experimental and Clinical Psychopharmacology, 8*, 518–523.

Zwaan, R. A., & Truitt, T. P. (1998) Smoking urges affect language processing, *Experimental and Clinical Psychopharmacology, 6*, 325–330.

CHAPTER 2

Grounding Desire and Motivated Behavior

A Theoretical Framework and Review of Empirical Evidence

Esther K. Papies
Lawrence W. Barsalou

Experiencing and dealing with desire is a central part of human existence. Whether it is for food, drink, sex, fame, social connectedness, or world peace, our desires shape and energize much of our daily life. A large literature, especially in social and health psychology, has focused on the ways in which desires affect our cognition and behavior. Similarly, many studies have outlined ways of handling such desires responsibly, for example, by planning in advance how to respond to them (e.g., Adriaanse, de Ridder, & de Wit, 2009), by thinking about one's long-term goals when tempted to give in to short-term temptations (Fishbach, Friedman, & Kruglanski, 2003; Papies, Potjes, Keesman, Schwinghammer, & van Koningsbruggen, 2014), or by applying mental strategies such as mindfulness (e.g., Alberts, Thewissen, & Raes, 2012; Jenkins & Tapper, 2014; Papies, Barsalou, & Custers, 2012).

We know less, however, about how desire arises in the first place. What are the actual psychological mechanisms that produce desires and consequently affect our behavior to fulfill them? What neural mechanisms underlie the psychological processes that lead to desire, and that are associated with behaviors such as indulging in tasty food, drinking expensive wine, or driving across the state to see a loved one? To answer these questions, we develop a grounded theory of desire and motivated behavior, and we review empirical work consistent with it. Our theory does not aim to replace earlier accounts. Instead, we further develop the cognitive, affective, and neural mechanisms that underlie desire, together

36

with the motivated behavior that can follow, attempting to integrate and shed new light on earlier findings, especially in the domains of nonconscious goal pursuit, habits, and self-regulation.

We define desire as a psychological state of motivation for a specific stimulus or experience that is anticipated to be rewarding. This state may or may not be consciously experienced. Explaining desire is particularly important given that it often arises and motivates appetitive behavior in the absence of physiological deprivation. Most of us will be familiar with the experience of desire for a certain food, drink, or activity, despite not being hungry, not being thirsty, and actually being quite immersed in another activity. Indeed, there is ample evidence showing that desires can arise purely due to cognitive processes, often in response to environmental cues (see also Kavanagh, Andrade, & May, 2005). Much research has shown, for example, that exposure to attractive food can trigger desire to eat and increase eating behavior (e.g., Hill, Magson, & Blundell, 1984; Tetley, Brunstrom, & Griffiths, 2009), along with physiological responses preparing the body to eat (Nederkoorn, Smulders, & Jansen, 2000). Similarly, cue reactivity research has shown that across a variety of substances, substance-related cues reliably trigger cravings (Carter & Tiffany, 1999; see also Sayette & Wilson, Chapter 5, and Franken, Chapter 19, this volume).

Furthermore, desires arising from cognitive processes and physiological deficits are not always aligned. Conditioning the concept of drinking water, for example, has been shown to increase how much water participants drink, in similar ways but independent of participants' thirst (Veltkamp, Custers, & Aarts, 2011). Smokers attempting to quit often experience cravings in response to smoking cues, even when they wear a nicotine patch that reduces the nicotine deficit and thus eliminates the physiological base for cravings (Tiffany, Cox, & Elash, 2000). What processes produce these powerful desires that do not result from physiological deprivation? In this chapter, we introduce a grounded theory to explain the emergence of desire and its effects on motivated behavior, integrating psychological and neural mechanisms.

Introducing a Grounded Theory of Desire and Motivated Behavior

The theory that we propose makes use of three central constructs that have been suggested to play roles in grounded accounts of conceptual processing more generally, namely, situated conceptualization, pattern completion inference, and simulation (Barsalou, Niedenthal, Barbey, & Ruppert, 2003; Barsalou, 1999, 2003, 2008, 2009, 2011, 2013; Lebois, Wilson-Mendenhall, Simmons, Barrett, & Barsalou, 2015; Wilson-Mendenhall, Barrett, Simmons, & Barsalou, 2011). Specifically, we argue that desire arises when an internal or external cue triggers a *simulation*, or partial reenactment, of an earlier appetitive experience that was rewarding. Simulating the past experience of eating a delicious scone in a coffeehouse, for example, could create a strong desire to consume another scone in a coffee shop now. Because the simulation includes psychologically compelling hedonic and reward qualia (see also Kavanagh et al., 2005), it can motivate consuming a scone even when not hungry.

We assume that such reward simulations are typically situated. When reexperiencing the past consumption of a delicious scone, for example, it is simulated in a background situation, such as a coffeehouse, including a setting, people, object, action, events, emotions, mentalizing, self-attributions, and so forth. In our theory, all of this situational content is captured and integrated at the time of the original experience in a comprehensive representation that we refer to as a *situated conceptualization*. We assume that situated conceptualizations of experience are constantly stored in memory, representing the myriad types of situations that people experience, including pleasurable and rewarding appetitive events.

Once a situated conceptualization of a past experience exists in memory, perceiving one of its elements in the current situation can reactivate other elements of the situated conceptualization via *pattern completion inferences*. In other words, perceiving part of the pattern (e.g., a scone in a coffeehouse display case) can reactivate a larger pattern containing it (e.g., a situated conceptualization established while eating a scone on a previous occasion). Once a pattern is completed in this manner, a multimodal simulation of the previous experience is created. If this situated conceptualization contains experiences of pleasure and reward, these experiences are likely to be reactivated during the pattern completion process. As a result, these pattern completion inferences may lead to appetitive behavior, such as consuming the entity that triggered the inference process. Although pattern completion inferences of reward may be experienced consciously, as in cravings, they may often not reach conscious awareness, leading to motivated behavior that can be experienced as unintentional or impulsive.

In the next section, we elaborate the mechanisms in this grounded theory of desire and motivated behavior. We begin by describing the situated conceptualizations of reward experiences that constitute the basic representations underlying desire. We then describe how the mechanism of pattern completion inference functions to reinstate a situated conceptualization in the brain and body once perceiving one of its elements triggers its activation. Finally, we address how simulations function to reenact reward experiences that engender motivated behavior. We then turn to empirical evidence from the domains of desire for food and alcohol to support the key components of our theory. Finally, we briefly address theoretical and practical implications, together with challenges for further research.

Mechanisms in the Grounded Theory of Desire and Motivated Behavior

Situated Conceptualization

Our theory assumes that people's rewarding experiences become stored in memory as situated conceptualizations. Once stored, a situated conceptualization represents the past situation as a memory. The situated conceptualization can also serve to interpret relevant situations in the future, and to support situated action in them.

Within our theoretical framework, we define a situation broadly, including internal states (e.g., cognitive, affective), bodily states (e.g., interoception, taste), and actions (e.g., executive, motoric); in other words, situations are much more than just environmental settings. Most critically, we assume that a situated conceptualization arises from the situated processing architecture of the brain (Barsalou, 2003, 2009, 2011, 2013; Lebois et al., 2015; Wilson-Mendenhall et al., 2011; Yeh & Barsalou, 2006). In a given situation, as someone perceives and conceptualizes the broadly defined elements of the situation, multiple neural systems simultaneously process these situational elements in parallel. Different neural systems, for example, process objects visible in the environment (the ventral stream), one's own motor behavior (motor and somatosensory cortices, cerebellum, basal ganglia), one's cognitive, affective, and interoceptive states and responses, including goals, reward, and physiological deprivation (lateral prefrontal, anterior cingulate, medial prefrontal, posterior cingulate, orbitofrontal cortices, amygdala, insula), and the external setting (parietal lobe, parahippocampal gyrus, retrosplenial cortex).

We assume that each system provides perceptual analysis and qualia of its respective information, as well as conceptual analyses of it. On seeing a scone in a coffeehouse, for example, the ventral stream performs visual analysis of the physical object and categorizes it as a scone. We similarly assume that perceptual and conceptual analysis occurs on all other aspects of the situation in the respective neural systems. We refer to the conceptualizations that result as "local," given that they process and evaluate one given element of the situation.

We further assume that a coherent global representation of the situation is constructed that integrates these streams of information and interprets them at a higher conceptual level. At the global level of analysis, relations between local situational elements are established (e.g., viewing an object as desirable for oneself; performing actions to possess and consume the object). A wide variety of relational concepts may become active to represent global conceptual structure in the situation, such as verbs and event concepts. In general, such relations may establish the significance of an object for oneself; they may explain the relation between having a goal and acting on it; they may help understand how an action produces an outcome in the situation; and so forth. Together, these global conceptualizations create the experience of a coherent meaningful situation.

We refer to the combined local and global conceptualizations of a situation's elements as a *situated conceptualization*. Most basically, a situated conceptualization supports understanding a situation at both the local and global levels, thereby allowing a person to interpret what is going on in a situation and to produce relevant cognitive, affective, and bodily processes, and importantly, behavior. At a general level, we assume that situated conceptualization underlies all cognitive activity, not just desire (e.g., Barsalou, 2013). Within the domain of desire, a situated conceptualization of a reward experience is the distributed pattern of information that was processed earlier during the rewarding event, now represented and grounded in the brain in terms of various situated elements and their conceptual integration. We suggest that such situated conceptualizations of rewarding experiences play a key role in desire.

As an example, consider the experience of spending an evening with some friends while watching a George Clooney movie. In this situation, all of the neural systems described above produce perceptual experience, along with conceptual interpretation that will help you understand the situation and regulate your behavior. Some of these neural systems may be producing streams of information about the environment you are in, for example, your living room, sitting on the sofa, next to your friends, with a bowl of chips on the table. Another neural system may be controlling your motor actions, such as leaning forward and grabbing chips to eat, along with taste, somatosensory, and visual feedback. At the same time, neural systems processing affective and bodily states may produce various related experiences, such as reward from eating the chips and excitement from suspense in the movie. Another neural system may continually establish the self-relevance of the events, reflecting your identity and goals, such as being a good host and feeling socially connected. All these elements are grounded in perceptual, interoceptive, and motor systems and become stored together as an integrated distributed pattern in memory. This pattern can later be reactivated by relevant cues, for example, when you walk through the grocery store, see a bag of potato chips somewhere, and think about the pleasure and fun of eating chips together with friends (see Papies, 2013).

Pattern Completion Inferences within Situated Conceptualizations

An important function of situated conceptualizations is to provide us with relevant information about the current situation and to facilitate situated action by retrieving information from similar earlier experiences. Once stored as a distributed memory pattern, a situated conceptualization can potentially be cued by any of its elements later on, and can then reinstate itself by reactivating other elements and triggering simulations of these perceptions, bodily states, and actions. This activity may then color our experience, control our behavior, and influence our subjective experience in the current situation. We suggest that pattern completion inferences produce these effects (Barsalou, 2003, 2009, 2013; Barsalou et al., 2003).

When you encounter a situation that shares features with situated conceptualizations stored in memory, a Bayesian retrieval process may be triggered to find the situated conceptualization that best fits the current situation (Barsalou, 2011; cf. Chater, Tenenbaum, & Yuille, 2006; M. Jones & Love, 2011). From the Bayesian perspective, the best-fitting situated conceptualization reflects both the frequency with which it has been relevant in the past and the quality of its fit to the current situation.

Once a situated conceptualization has been retrieved, elements that are not directly activated by the current situation itself may be inferred as pattern completion inferences. In other words, various elements of a situated conceptualization can become active without being triggered directly by anything present in the current situation. Returning to our example, just seeing chips in the grocery store may not only reactivate the mouthfeel of consuming snacks rich in salt and fat, but also its hedonic pleasure, the positive affect of feeling connected with one's friends, and the desire to see another George Clooney movie. Desire, as we will argue in more detail below, may often be the result of this pattern completion process, with external cues inducing motivation for a stimulus that was previously part of a rewarding experience.

A key assumption of our approach is that any element of a situated conceptualization can serve as a cue for retrieving the rest; no one part of the conceptualization is privileged (although some parts may function more effectively under specific conditions, for a wide variety of reasons; see Papies & Barsalou, 2014). Under some conditions, appetitive desires could be triggered when the sight, smell, sound, or feel of an appetitive object activates a situated conceptualization of previously consuming the object (e.g., foods, drinks, drugs). Under other conditions, various other elements from the same situated conceptualizations could also activate them, including the associated settings, people, objects, emotions, self-attributions, bodily states, actions, and so forth (see Papies, 2013). Regardless of the initial trigger of the situated conceptualization, once it's running, the pattern completion inferences it produces have the ability to motivate appetitive behavior in the current situation, independently of any physiological need state. This may also explain why desires are so prevalent in daily life (e.g., Hofmann, Vohs, & Baumeister, 2012), as their numerous triggers in our living environment are hard to control.

Simulation

We assume that when pattern completion inferences are produced, they are realized as simulations of the inferred situational elements, rather than as symbolic descriptions of them. Thus, our grounded theory of desire and motivated behavior is built on the assumption that the various elements comprising situated conceptualizations are grounded in the neural and peripheral bodily systems that produce perception and action, including the production and perception of internal states (Barsalou, 1999). When, for example, a scone activates a situated conceptualization of eating a scone previously, the taste, reward, and actions inferred from the pattern completion process are reenacted in the gustatory, reward, and motor systems. In other words, the brain and body begin operating as if one were eating the scone. Because the same systems are running to produce the inferences that were running during consumption, the inferences that result often appear highly realistic, thereby becoming motivationally compelling.

Simulation can be viewed as the result of two basic processes: capture and reenactment (Barsalou, 1999, 2008). During an actual experience in a situation, representational states in feature areas of relevant neural systems capture these states using associative mechanisms, as described earlier for situated conceptualization. Over time, as the same kind of experience occurs repeatedly, related memories become captured across the same systems, such that an increasingly entrenched network becomes established. After eating many scones, for example, a network becomes established that aggregates the accumulated experience of eating scones into a distributed conceptual structure that represents the category (e.g., Barsalou, 2012; Martin, 2001, 2007). In other words, this increasingly entrenched network captures the aggregated experience of the category across all of the brain areas that process elements of the relevant situations. Although the resultant network reflects extensive experience, we assume that it also reflects strong genetic constraints on the underlying architecture that processes situation elements and links them together in association areas (Barsalou, 1999, 2008; Simmons & Barsalou, 2003). Thus, this account reflects both nativist and empiricist contributions.

Once the network representing a category becomes established, it can then be used to reenact instances of the category in their absence. By reactivating the network, it can reproduce the kind of brain state active when experiencing a category member. Reactivating the network of situated processing areas active when eating scones, for example, partially reproduces the type of brain states active when actually experiencing scones. We refer to these reproduced brain states as "simulations," given that the brain is simulating the kind of state that it would be in if it were experiencing a category instance.

We do not assume that a simulation ever reinstates a previous experience exactly. Instead, we assume that simulations typically reenact previous experiences partially, and that they can be biased and distorted in a variety of ways. We further assume that simulations can take diverse forms, ranging from simulating a specific category instance to simulating an average prototype, or simulating specific features of the category in rule-like manners (Barsalou, 1999). Importantly for our account here, we assume that simulations often operate unconsciously and implicitly, independent of intentional executive processing. When simulations do become conscious, they produce the diverse forms of imagery reported across multiple literatures (e.g., Jeannerod, 1995; Kosslyn, 1980, 1994), which have been suggested to play a role in desire for appetitive stimuli, too (Kavanagh et al., 2005; see also Andrade, May, Van Dillen, & Kavanagh, Chapter 1, this volume). Finally, we assume that simulations support diverse forms of cognitive processing, including high-level perception, categorization, attention, working memory, long-term memory, language, thought, emotion, and social cognition (Barsalou, 2008).

Much empirical evidence supports diverse forms of simulation across the modalities (e.g., Barsalou, 2008; Kiefer & Barsalou, 2013; Pulvermueller, 2013). When people represent visual features during conceptual processing, in the absence of physical objects, they often represent them with simulation in visual areas (e.g., Goldberg, Perfetti, & Schneider, 2006; Hsu, Frankland, & Thompson-Schill, 2012; Kellenbach, Brett, & Patterson, 2001; Martin, 2007). For example, when people are asked to verify that an object has a particular form or color, they represent these form and color properties with visual simulations. Similarly, when people represent the auditory properties of objects conceptually, they often represent them with simulations in auditory areas (e.g., Kiefer, Sim, Herrnberger, Grothe, & Hoenig, 2008). Finally, research indicates that when people conceptually represent the functions of objects and the actions performed on them, they do so with motor simulations (e.g., Pulvermueller, 2013).

Increasing research demonstrates that simulations may also represent more abstract concepts, both literally (e.g., Wilson-Mendenhall, Simmons, Martin, & Barsalou, 2013) and metaphorically (e.g., Lacey, Stilla, & Sathian, 2012). Similarly, when people encounter affective stimuli and experience emotion as pattern completion inferences, these inferences are realized as simulations of previous emotion, both cognitively and bodily (e.g., Barrett, 2006, 2013; Lench, Flores, & Bench, 2011; Wilson-Mendenhall et al., 2011). Finally, and most importantly for our account here, much research demonstrates that when people encounter food stimuli, they simulate the experience of eating them (e.g., Barrós-Loscertales et al., 2012; Simmons, Martin, & Barsalou, 2005; van der Laan, de Ridder, Viergever, & Smeets, 2011). As people encounter a picture of a tasty dessert, for example, they simulate the experience of eating it, and how rewarding it would be to consume, especially if hungry.

The Motivational Potential of Simulated Bodily States in Grounded Desire

Once a simulated experience of consuming something is running, it has the potential to be highly motivating, especially for appetitive stimuli, for which the situated conceptualizations triggered are particularly likely to lead to simulations of behavior that has earlier produced rewarding experiences. As several lines of research show, for example, perceiving a tasty food induces automatic approach impulses (Papies et al., 2012; Seibt, Häfner, & Deutsch, 2007; Veling, Aarts, & Papies, 2011). Similarly, as people become more motivated to consume food or pursue casual sex, for example, they become increasingly likely to choose appetitive stimuli (Papies, Pronk, Keesman, & Barsalou, 2015; Seibt et al., 2007; Simpson & Gangestad, 1992). We suggest that as pattern completion inferences from situated conceptualizations for past experiences become active, the simulations that express these inferences can induce appetitive behavior.

Even though physiological deprivation may often contribute to the emergence of desire (e.g., Veltkamp, Aarts, & Custers, 2009), desire can also develop when situational cues trigger a situated conceptualization of a reward experience in the absence of deprivation. Because situational simulations, together with the bodily reenactments they include, re-create hedonic experiences, they can be so compelling and motivating that they induce appetitive behavior on their own. If, for example, one typically eats chips on relaxed Friday nights with friends while sitting on the sofa, these situated conceptualizations become stored in memory, together with the bodily states associated with desiring chips, tasting their crunchy saltiness, and feeling satisfaction on having consumed them. When experiencing any of these situational elements on a future occasion, one of these situated conceptualizations is likely to become active, thereby reproducing many aspects of these earlier situations, including the associated internal states. Just relaxing on the sofa alone on a Tuesday night might then be enough to make one wander toward the kitchen cabinet in search of a salty snack, independent of one's hunger.

Explaining Individual and Situational Differences in Grounded Desire

This grounded theory of desire naturally explains situational and individual differences in desire that people experience. Specifically, both situational and individual differences in desire can be understood as differences in situated conceptualizations that have become established in memory, as a function of the different motivational states and resulting reward experiences stored at the time of the respective experiences.

Central to this account is our assumption that different levels of reward value become represented in situated conceptualizations, resulting from different levels of internal motivational states, such as hunger, thirst, and sexual motivation, at the time (Papies et al., 2015). Consider the different situated conceptualizations that result when different states are associated with the same appetitive behavior. For example, one might have a highly rewarding pizza experience when very hungry, but only a mildly rewarding pizza experience when slightly hungry. Later, the different internal states encoded in the resulting two situated conceptualizations may serve as cues for retrieving these situated conceptualizations. Thus, when one encounters pizza while very hungry versus mildly hungry, the best-fitting situated conceptualization will be retrieved, namely, the one that best matches one's current hunger. As a result, a pizza may appear highly attractive or only mildly attractive, reflecting the prior reward experience simulated.

Effects of more enduring individual differences, such as reward sensitivity or sexual motivation, may similarly be explained by differences in situated conceptualizations (see also Papies et al., 2015). To the extent that different individuals vary in motivation at the trait level, the respective differences in motivational states and resulting reward experiences will become stored in their situated conceptualizations associated with appetitive behavior. Whereas some individuals might experience intense hedonic pleasure on consuming highly sweet deserts, other individuals might experience queasiness on consuming such desserts. As a result, when these two groups of individuals encounter the same sweet dessert, the pattern completion inferences that result may simulate very different bodily experiences, differentially motivating approach versus avoidance responses toward it.

In this manner, situated conceptualizations reflect variations in reward representations and desire across situations and across individuals, thereby having the potential to explain the statistical subtlety that characterizes individual differences in desire and motivated behavior.

Empirical Evidence

We now turn to evidence that speaks to the situated nature of desire and to the possible roles of situated conceptualizations, pattern completion inferences, and simulation. Focusing on the domains of food and alcohol, this review does not aspire to be exhaustive, but merely to give a brief overview of research that is relevant for our account. The studies we discuss originate from diverse areas and theoretical backgrounds, but we suggest that their findings can be understood and integrated coherently by means of the theoretical framework suggested here.

Desire for Food

Various studies suggest that representations of desirable foods are situated. From the perspective of our account, we expect that food memories are embedded in situated conceptualizations that become established during eating experiences. We further predict that cuing these situated representations will trigger simulations of rewarding eating experiences in neural and bodily systems as pattern completion inferences.

A large set of behavioral findings supports the situated nature of food representations. When categorizing foods, people make use of categories that describe when or how one typically eats a food (e.g., appetizers, snack foods; foods you eat with a spoon; Blake, Bisogni, Sobal, Devine, & Jastran, 2007; Ross & Murphy, 1999). Similarly, when describing eating and food in general, people refer to situated features of consuming it, such as hunger, eating with family and friends, enjoyment, and comfort (Keller & van der Horst, 2013). Specific types of foods are even referred to by their situated function as "comfort foods," implying that these are food items typically eaten in times of distress. While preferences for comfort foods differ between different individuals and groups (e.g., between men and women), such foods tend to be high in fat and/or sugar, and are heavily associated with memories of earlier rewarding eating situations (e.g., Locher, Yoels, Maurer, & van Ells, 2005; Wansink, Cheney, & Chan, 2003). These findings suggest that attractive foods are represented in relevant eating situations, including internal bodily and affective states, as well as features of the eating environment.

A recent study using a feature-listing task confirms these findings and further demonstrates the richness of the situated representations that people have of food, particularly when this food is highly rewarding (Papies, 2013). In this study, participants were presented with words for four tempting foods (e.g., chips, cookies) and four neutral foods (e.g., apple, rice), and listed "features that are typically true of these concepts." In line with the earlier findings described above, participants listed various features describing the situated nature of food, such as when, where, why, and with whom one eats the foods (e.g., TV; on the sofa; to treat yourself; eat sociably together) and the hedonic pleasure that results (e.g., tasty, delicious). Both hedonic and situation features were listed more often for tempting compared to neutral foods, and the situation features were much more varied and detailed for tempting foods. In addition, participants heavily made use of features describing the sensory experience of eating a tempting food, such as its taste, texture, and temperature (e.g., sweet, salty, savory, crunchy, creamy), and again, they did so much more for tempting than for neutral food. In contrast, participants situated neutral foods quite differently. Specifically, for neutral foods, participants much more often described visual features (e.g., green, round, small) and slightly more features related to the production, purchase, and preparation of the foods (e.g., grows on a tree, comes in bags, has to be cooked). Correlational analyses also showed that participants were more likely to describe a situated eating experience for tempting foods when they reported that they found this food very attractive and had a strong desire to eat it (see Keesman et al., 2015, for similar findings in the domain of alcohol).

From our theoretical perspective, participants retrieve situated conceptualizations of earlier experiences with a food when asked to describe its features. When they find the food very attractive, the situated conceptualization is particularly likely to contain simulations of eating the food, as this produced the earlier rewarding experiences. They then proceed to describe the content of these situated conceptualizations, listing their features via pattern completion inferences to food cues. The situated conceptualizations that participants retrieve for tempting food most likely reflect idiosyncratic rewarding eating experiences, as participants describe features of eating and enjoying the food in rich background situations.

Much empirical work further shows that situated cues associated with attractive food and eating can trigger hedonic thoughts, cravings, and eating behavior, which is consistent with our prediction that activating a situated conceptualization of a rewarding eating experience can lead to desire. Brief descriptions of eating situations involving high-calorie foods, for example, trigger hedonic thoughts about food in chronic dieters, who have trouble resisting such indulgences (Papies, Stroebe, & Aarts, 2007). Being exposed to the sight or smell of attractive food triggers cravings and facilitates overeating, again especially among participants who have difficulties regulating their eating (e.g., Fedoroff, Polivy, & Herman, 1997; Rogers & Hill, 1989). Notably, these effects are specific for the cued food (Fedoroff, Polivy, & Herman, 2003), suggesting that the desires triggered activate specific situated conceptualizations, rather than a general desire to eat.

Physiological and neuroimaging research examining responses to food cues further supports a grounded cognition perspective on desire. When exposed to attractive food cues, people respond as if they were actually eating or preparing to eat the food, reflecting simulations in neural and bodily systems. First consider how food cues trigger salivation (as originally proposed by Pavlov decades ago). Numerous studies show that exposure to attractive food triggers increased salivation in anticipation of food intake, especially in participants who have trouble regulating their eating behavior and maintaining a healthy diet (Brunstrom, Yates, & Witcomb, 2004; Ferriday & Brunstrom, 2011; Naumann, Trentowska, & Svaldi, 2013), especially for preferred foods (Rogers & Hill, 1989). From our perspective, attractive food cues activate situated conceptualizations that produce eating simulations via pattern completion inferences, thereby increasing salivation in anticipation of consumption.

Much neuroimaging research further shows that our brains respond to food cues as if we were actually eating, tasting, and enjoying the respective foods. Viewing attractive food pictures or even just reading food words activates brain areas similar to those activated by actually eating these foods, including primary and secondary taste cortices (anterior insula, frontal operculum) and reward areas (orbitofrontal cortex; e.g., Barrós-Loscertales et al., 2012; Simmons et al., 2005; van der Laan et al., 2011; see also Lopez, Wagner, & Heatherton, Chapter 7, this volume; Roefs, Houben, & Werthmann, Chapter 16, this volume). These effects are particularly pronounced for high-calorie foods and for hungry perceivers, and they correlate with individual reports of hunger and desire for food (Killgore et al., 2003; Siep et al., 2009; Wang et al., 2004). Furthermore, these effects are stronger in individuals who experience difficulty resisting high-calorie foods, such as overweight individuals and those at risk for overweight (Stice, Spoor, Ng, & Zald, 2009; Stice, Yokum, Burger, Epstein, & Small, 2011). These findings demonstrate that attractive food triggers simulations of eating the food in the same brain areas that become active when actually eating it, and may reflect the reward typically experienced.

Linguistic labels can affect these neural responses and also the associated subjective experiences. In one study, tasting a food stimulus that was labeled as "rich and delicious" increased activation in reward areas in the brain, compared to tasting the same stimulus when it was labeled "boiled vegetable water" (Grabenhorst, Rolls, & Bilderbeck, 2008). Woods and colleagues (2011) showed that tasting the same drink with labels suggesting different levels of sweetness changed neural responses in the primary taste cortex, as well as participants' experiences of the drink's sweetness. Similarly, labels suggesting that a wine was more expensive increased reward responses in the brain when tasting it, along with judged pleasantness (Plassmann, O'Doherty, Shiv, & Rangel, 2008). We suggest that such labels activate fitting situated conceptualizations and specific simulations in sensory regions in the brain, which become superimposed on the actual taste perception and thus affect experience (cf. Hansen, Olkkonen, Walter, & Gegenfurtner, 2006). Not only neural responses, but even hormonal responses to food can be modulated by food labels, as shown by a study where a milkshake that was labeled "indulgent" rather than "sensible" triggered a steep decline in the gastrointestinal peptide ghrelin after consumption, suggesting a state of physiological satiety (Crum, Corbin, Brownell, & Salovey, 2011). Again it appears that the food label and appearance trigger a specific simulation that then affects our neural and physiological responses and actual sensory and hedonic experiences.

Research on cross-modal effects during food perception and eating behavior has demonstrated that not only linguistic labels, but also cues from other modalities can affect a person's experience of eating. The color of food, for example, is a strong cue for expectations with regard to eating experiences and significantly facilitates flavor identification (Spence, Levitan, Shankar, & Zampini, 2010), presumably by serving as a cue to retrieve a fitting situated conceptualization of eating that specific food. Further, research has shown that a variety of sounds related to eating can similarly affect what we expect of a food, how much we like it, and how much we eat (for a review, see Spence & Shankar, 2010). In one study, for example, hearing the sound of bacon sizzling in a pan increased participants' perceptions of bacon flavor in a product they tasted, compared to a different sound, suggesting that the sound may have activated a simulation of bacon taste that then increased actual taste perceptions (Spence, Shankar, & Blumenthal, 2010). Such results suggest that cross-modal cues retrieve situated conceptualizations of specific eating experiences, which then lead to partial simulations of the associated tastes, which in turn strengthen actual taste experiences.

All of these findings are consistent with our grounded perspective on desire, indicating that both linguistic labels and nonlinguistic cues belong to situated memories of eating experiences. As a result, perceiving these cues can trigger simulations of eating that then influence actual eating experiences.

Desire for Alcohol

Situated conceptualizations of reward experiences also appear to play central roles in the desire for alcohol. As we will see, much research on alcohol cues and alcohol outcome expectancies demonstrates the powerful effects of such cues on desire and motivated behavior.

Drinking alcohol is in part represented in terms of beliefs about the effects of alcohol, such as becoming more sociable, relaxed, or happy when drinking. Consistent with our grounded theory of desire, alcohol expectancies can be viewed as situated memories that have been established idiosyncratically and thus vary strongly with individual experiences (see B. T. Jones, Corbin, & Fromme, 2001; Stein, Goldman, & Del Boca, 2000). Additionally, the degree to which one expects a reward experience from drinking has been shown to motivate and increase consumption (for an overview, see Reich, Below, & Goldman, 2010). Similarly, recent studies directly examining the representation of alcohol have shown that alcohol is strongly represented in terms of drinking situations, particularly their social features. In addition, the strength of this social situatedness was related to actual drinking behavior in a bar context (Keesman et al., 2015). Experimental studies have further shown that priming outcome expectancies with word cues (e.g., *confident, sociable, sexy*), leads to increased drinking, especially among heavy drinkers (Stein et al., 2000). Conversely, interventions designed to challenge such outcome expectancies have sometimes been shown to reduce drinking (e.g., having participants notice that they experience positive outcomes typically associated with alcohol, even though they consumed placebo drinks; see B. T. Jones et al., 2001).

Extensive work on the effects of alcohol cues shows that exposing participants to contextual cues for drinking (e.g., a bar environment, alcohol-related pictures, the smell of alcohol, the sight of alcoholic beverages) activates alcohol-related thoughts and approach impulses and increases the desire to drink (for reviews, see Field, Schoenmakers, & Wiers, 2008; Wiers & Stacy, 2006). In the context of drinking habits, Sheeran and colleagues (2005) demonstrated that exposing students to words related to socializing increased the accessibility of the concept of drinking and the motivation to drink, but only among habitual drinkers, presumably because these cues activated situated conceptualizations of drinking in social contexts for them. From the perspective of our theory, we interpret these findings as showing that outcome expectancies and situated alcohol cues constitute elements of situated conceptualizations for rewarding drinking experiences. Thus, exposure to these cues can activate situated conceptualizations of drinking, and via pattern completion inferences, trigger the desire to drink.

Further research in this domain similarly shows that activating situated conceptualizations of drinking alcohol can trigger pattern completion inferences that represent various consequences of drinking (in the absence of actual alcohol consumption). Mere priming with alcohol-related words among social drinkers, for example, has been shown to produce cognitive responses typically associated with alcohol, such as performing worse on cognitive tasks (Fillmore, Carscadden, & Vogel-Sprott, 1998), aggressive thoughts (Bartholow & Heinz, 2006), and judging women as more attractive (Friedman, McCarthy, Förster, & Denzler, 2005).

Furthermore, alcohol cues trigger embodied responses that suggest partial simulations of drinking experiences. Exposure to alcohol-related cues in neuroimaging studies, for example, has been shown to activate brain areas associated with reward and cravings in problematic drinkers (e.g., Myrick et al., 2004; Schacht et al., 2011). In cue-reactivity studies, addicts' physiological responses to cues that are associated with drug use (including alcohol, nicotine, and cocaine) are very similar to the effects actually produced by taking the drug, such as increased heart rate and sweat gland activity (see Carter & Tiffany, 1999, for a meta-analysis). This suggests that exposure to drug-related cues triggers embodied simulations of drug use that produce physiological changes associated with actually using the drugs. Studies using placebo designs have similarly shown that the mere expectancy of drinking alcohol can lead to physiological changes as if participants were actually drinking alcohol, such as impaired motor performance (Vuchinich & Sobell, 1978), increased male sexual arousal (Terence & Lawson, 1976), and reduced arousal during an anxiety-provoking interaction (Wilson & Abrams, 1977; for a meta-analysis, see Mckay & Schare, 1999). Across studies, the effects of expecting to drink alcohol are strongest in research settings imitating natural drinking environments, compared to lab settings (Mckay & Schare, 1999), which supports the important role of contextual cues in producing simulations of drinking experiences. Thus, being reminded of drinking or expecting to drink alcohol has the same cognitive, affective, and behavioral effects as if one were indeed drinking. Furthermore, these simulations become increasingly likely as more alcohol-related contextual cues are present, thereby increasing the likelihood of retrieving a situated conceptualization of an earlier alcohol experience.

Together, these findings support our theory that situated conceptualizations, pattern completion inferences, and simulations play central roles in the desire for alcohol. Additionally, these situated conceptualizations appear to be grounded in bodily systems, such that they can trigger compelling embodied simulations of drinking and its consequences.

Implications and Final Thoughts

Relations to Dual-Process Theories and Habits

We believe that the basic mechanisms in our theory underlie both the impulsive and reflective processes that are widely viewed as producing desire and its regulation (e.g., Hofmann, Friese, & Wiers, 2008; Metcalfe & Mischel, 1999; Strack & Deutsch, 2004), as well as the processes that lead to habitual behavior and to potential habit change (e.g., Aarts & Dijksterhuis, 2000; Ouellette & Wood, 1998). From our perspective, an impulse or a habitual response is activated when a situational cue triggers a situated conceptualization that has become well entrenched in memory. Because the situated conceptualization is highly learned, relatively little processing may be required to activate it, such that it becomes active quickly, intrusively, and/or unconsciously (cf. Moors & De Houwer, 2006). Situated conceptualizations supporting successful self-regulation may become active in equally automatic ways if they have been stored in memory from earlier behavior. When a situated conceptualization of consuming chips on the couch becomes activated, for example, this may for some people activate long-term goals that one has often pursued in such situations, such as dieting, along with associated behaviors, such as grabbing an apple or hopping on the treadmill. The activation of such strategies is especially likely if a person has successfully pursued such a long-term goal in similar situations (Fishbach et al., 2003; Papies, Stroebe,

& Aarts, 2008), so that situated conceptualizations of pursuing the diet-ing goal in tempting situations have been stored in memory and can eas-ily be retrieved as healthy habits in response to attractive food cues.

Self-regulation can further occur when the executive system searches memory for situated conceptualizations that constitute alternatives to sit-uated conceptualization activated initially as impulses or habits (cf. Bar-rett, Wilson-Mendenhall, & Barsalou's [2014] account of emotion regula-tion). When in a tempting eating situation, for example, memory may be searched for alternative ways of handling the situation. Situated concep-tualizations of alternative behaviors could have been stored, for example, from planning healthy behavior (e.g., with situation-specific implemen-tation intentions, Gollwitzer & Sheeran, 2006) or from health education, and may later be retrieved and implemented in a deliberate, effortful way. Thus, we assume that situated conceptualizations can become activated and implemented in very different manners, thereby affecting behavior either impulsively or reflectively, producing successful as well as unsuc-cessful self-regulation. Clearly, however, our accounts of habits, impulse, and regulation require further theoretical development, together with careful empirical testing.

Relations to the Elaborated Intrusion Theory of Desire

The theory that we develop here differs in important respects from Kava-nagh et al.'s (2005) elaborated intrusion theory. Most importantly, our account focuses on situated conceptualizations that originate during con-sumptive experiences, together with the pattern completion inferences and simulations that result from cuing them later. Therefore, our theory not only focuses on mechanisms underlying desire, but also on mecha-nisms that produce motivated behavior, together with the learning of these behavioral patterns. Furthermore, our account of simulation differs from Kavanagh et al.'s account of imagery in several ways. First, whereas they focus on sensory imagery, we focus more broadly on multimodal simulations that reenact not only sensory states, but also bodily states, motor behavior, settings, and various internal states, including reward, goals, emotions, and thoughts. Second, simulation in our account takes the form not only of conscious imagery, but also unconscious reenactment of perception, action, and various internal states. Third, Kavanagh et al. tend to assume that desire primarily results from conscious elaboration of associative intrusions, whereas we assume that desire can also result from automatic simulations that are not elaborated in working memory. Finally, neural mechanisms play central roles in our account, in contrast to the central role of conscious experience in Kavanagh et al.'s account. We hasten to add that both theories share the important assumption that representations of consumption can produce desire.

Learning and Individual Differences

Our grounded cognition approach to desire is essentially a learning theory of desire. As an individual has appetitive experiences, memories of these experiences are stored in memory as situated conceptualizations, constituting a form of learning. Because different individuals have different appetitive experiences, they have different learning histories, as different populations of situated conceptualizations accumulate in memory. On later occasions, different individuals may therefore respond to the same appetitive cues differently. Because appetitive cues are likely to retrieve different situated conceptualizations across different individuals, different pattern completion inferences follow, producing different simulations of craving (or not craving).

We believe that this learning account has much potential for explaining individual differences in desire and the motivated behavior that follows. Clearly, however, this account must be developed both theoretically and empirically before this potential can be realized.

Interventions to Regulate Desire Effectively

It follows from our account that one approach to intervention aims at changing the population of situated conceptualizations that controls an individual's appetitive behavior. Effortful change of behavior may therefore eventually turn into healthy habits if the new behavior is repeated sufficiently often and in a sufficiently stable context (cf. Ouellette & Wood, 1998) to establish a new population of situated conceptualizations in memory (Papies & Barsalou, 2014). As a result, the pattern completion inferences that are triggered by relevant cues will change, thereby changing desire and the motivated behavior that follows.

Another approach to changing consumptive behavior is to control the cues that activate the situated conceptualizations stored in an individual's memory, for example by changing the environment to remove or avoid such cues (see also Hofmann, Kotabe, Vohs, & Baumeister, Chapter 3, this volume). Indeed, strategies like making food less visible are effective for reducing unhealthy eating (e.g., Wansink, Painter, & Lee, 2006). However, our account predicts that a large number of very diverse cues may potentially be involved in triggering reward simulations, making this strategy difficult to put into practice. We further assume that these cues may often be difficult for an individual to identify, as situated conceptualizations typically do not reach conscious awareness. In addition, controlling one's environment in ways such as removing or avoiding relevant cues may often simply not be possible.

Controlling the cues that activate situated conceptualizations in a less far-reaching way can be achieved by goal priming. When one presents cues in a person's environment that activate situated conceptualizations associated with specific goals (e.g., situated conceptualizations of behaviors to perform when one is dieting), behaviors that can facilitate pursuit of these goals are likely to occur as pattern completion inferences, but only among those individuals who have stored relevant situated conceptualizations from previous experiences (e.g., dieters). As a result, behaviors like buying and eating high-calorie foods will be less likely to occur after such primes, compared to behaviors like ordering a healthy salad (e.g., Anschutz, Van Strien, & Engels, 2008; Papies & Hamstra, 2010; Papies et al., 2014; Papies & Veling, 2013).

Still another approach that has proven effective is to undermine the hedonic simulations that motivate appetitive behavior, for example by mindfulness (Jenkins & Tapper, 2014; Papies et al., 2012, 2015) or reappraisal (e.g., Hofmann, Deutsch, Lancaster, & Banaji, 2010). Once a person recognizes the potential harm that these simulations can do in motivating unhealthy consumption, they can learn various strategies that make them less compelling. As a result, these simulations increasingly lose their control over behavior, such that they arise and dissipate with little effect.

Conclusion

In this chapter, we have introduced a novel theoretical framework for understanding desire and motivated behavior, based on a grounded cognition perspective. We have argued that this framework allows us to understand how desire arises from well-established mechanisms of grounded conceptual processing, and we have reviewed literature from diverse areas that can be interpreted and integrated by means of this theory. Our account suggests that even though the situated and grounded character of our cognitive systems typically helps us navigate a highly complex living environment in effective ways, it also increases our susceptibility to the myriad temptations that our living environments offer, generating various forms of desire. We hope that our analysis of desire and motivated behavior, utilizing the constructs of situated conceptualization, pattern completion inference, and simulation, will increase our understanding of how desire arises, how it affects behavior, and how situated processing mechanisms can be used to modulate these effects.

ACKNOWLEDGMENTS

This work was supported by grant No. VENI-451-10-027 from the Netherlands Organization for Scientific Research. We would like to thank Mike Keesman and Michael Häfner for helpful comments on an earlier version of this chapter.

REFERENCES

Aarts, H., & Dijksterhuis, A. (2000). Habits as knowledge structures: Automaticity in goal-directed behavior. *Journal of Personality and Social Psychology, 78*, 53–63.

Adriaanse, M. A., de Ridder, D. T. D., & de Wit, J. B. F. (2009). Finding the critical cue: Implementation intentions to change one's diet work best when tailored to personally relevant reasons for unhealthy eating. *Personality and Social Psychology Bulletin, 35*(1), 60–71.

Alberts, H. J. E. M., Thewissen, R., & Raes, L. (2012). Dealing with problematic eating behaviour: The effects of a mindfulness-based intervention on eating behaviour, food cravings, dichotomous thinking and body image concern. *Appetite, 58*(3), 847–851.

Anschutz, D. J., Van Strien, T., & Engels, R. C. M. E. (2008). Exposure to slim images in mass media: Television commercials as reminders of restriction in restrained eaters. *Health Psychology, 27*(4), 401–408.

Barrett, L. F. (2006). Solving the emotion paradox: Categorization and the experience of emotion. *Personality and Social Psychology Review, 10*(1), 20–46.

Barrett, L. F. (2013). Psychological construction: The Darwinian approach to the science of emotion. *Emotion Review, 5*(4), 379–389.

Barrett, L. F., Wilson-Mendenhall, C. D., & Barsalou, L. W. (2014). A psychological construction account of emotion regulation and dysregulation: The role of situated conceptualizations. In J. J. Gross (Ed.), *The handbook of emotion regulation* (2nd ed., pp. 447–465). New York: Guilford Press.

Barrós-Loscertales, A., González, J., Pulvermüller, F., Ventura-Campos, N., Bustamante, J. C., Costumero, V., et al. (2012). Reading salt activates gustatory brain regions: fMRI evidence for semantic grounding in a novel sensory modality. *Cerebral Cortex, 22*(11), 2554–2563.

Barsalou, L. W. (1999). Perceptual symbol systems. *Behavioral and Brain Sciences, 22*, 577–660.

Barsalou, L. W. (2003). Situated simulation in the human conceptual system. *Language and Cognitive Processes, 18*, 513–562.

Barsalou, L. W. (2008). Grounded cognition. *Annual Review of Psychology, 59*(1), 617–645.

Barsalou, L. W. (2009). Simulation, situated conceptualization, and prediction. *Philosophical Transactions of the Royal Society B: Biological Sciences, 364*(1521), 1281–1289.

Barsalou, L. W. (2011). Integrating Bayesian analysis and mechanistic theories in grounded cognition. *Behavioral and Brain Sciences, 34*(4), 191–192.

Barsalou, L. W. (2012). The human conceptual system. In M. Spivey, K. McRae, & M. Joanisse (Eds.), *The Cambridge handbook of psycholinguistics* (pp. 239–258). New York: Cambridge University Press.

Barsalou, L. W. (2013). Mirroring as pattern completion inferences within situated conceptualizations. *Cortex, 49*(10), 2951–2953.

Barsalou, L. W., Niedenthal, P. M., Barbey, A. K., & Ruppert, J. A. (2003). Social embodiment. In B. H. Ross (Ed.), *The Psychology of learning and motivation* (Vol. 43, pp. 43–92). San Diego, CA: Academic Press.

Bartholow, B. D., & Heinz, A. (2006). Alcohol and aggression without consumption alcohol cues, aggressive thoughts, and hostile perception bias. *Psychological Science, 17*(1), 30–37.

Blake, C. E., Bisogni, C. A., Sobal, J., Devine, C. M., & Jastran, M. (2007). Classifying foods in contexts: How adults categorize foods for different eating settings. *Appetite, 49*(2), 500–510.

Brunstrom, J. M., Yates, H. M., & Witcomb, G. L. (2004). Dietary restraint and heightened reactivity to food. *Physiology and Behavior, 81*(1), 85–90.

Carter, B. L., & Tiffany, S. T. (1999). Meta-analysis of cue-reactivity in addiction research. *Addiction, 94*(3), 327–340.

Chater, N., Tenenbaum, J. B., & Yuille, A. (2006). Probabilistic models of cognition: Conceptual foundations. *Trends in Cognitive Sciences, 10*(7), 287–291.

Crum, A. J., Corbin, W. R., Brownell, K. D., & Salovey, P. (2011). Mind over milkshakes: Mindsets, not just nutrients, determine ghrelin response. *Health Psychology, 30*(4), 424–429.

Fedoroff, I. C., Polivy, J., & Herman, C. P. (1997). The effect of pre-exposure to food cues on the eating behavior of restrained and unrestrained eaters. *Appetite, 28*(1), 33–47.

Fedoroff, I. C., Polivy, J., & Herman, C. P. (2003). The specificity of restrained versus unrestrained eaters' responses to food cues: General desire to eat, or craving for the cued food? *Appetite, 41*(1), 7–13.

Ferriday, D., & Brunstrom, J. M. (2011). "I just can't help myself": Effects of food-cue exposure in overweight and lean individuals. *International Journal of Obesity, 35*(1), 142–149.

Field, M., Schoenmakers, T., & Wiers, R. W. (2008). Cognitive processes in alcohol binges: A review and research agenda. *Current Drug Abuse Reviews, 1*(3), 263–279.

Fillmore, M. T., Carscadden, J. L., & Vogel-Sprott, M. (1998). Alcohol, cognitive impairment and expectancies. *Journal of Studies on Alcohol, 59*(2), 174–179.

Fishbach, A., Friedman, R. S., & Kruglanski, A. W. (2003). Leading us not unto temptation: Momentary allurements elicit overriding goal activation. *Journal of Personality and Social Psychology, 84*(2), 296–309.

Friedman, R. S., McCarthy, D. M., Förster, J., & Denzler, M. (2005). Automatic effects of alcohol cues on sexual attraction. *Addiction, 100*(5), 672–681.

Goldberg, R. F., Perfetti, C. A., & Schneider, W. (2006). Perceptual knowledge retrieval activates sensory brain regions. *Journal of Neuroscience, 26*(18), 4917–4921.

Gollwitzer, P. M., & Sheeran, P. (2006). Implementation intentions and goal achievement: A meta-analysis of effects and processes. In M. P. Zanna (Ed.), *Advances in Experimental Social Psychology* (pp. 69–119). San Diego, CA: Elsevier Academic Press.

Grabenhorst, F., Rolls, E. T., & Bilderbeck, A. (2008). How cognition modulates affective responses to taste and flavor: Top-down influences on the orbitofrontal and pregenual cingulate cortices. *Cerebral Cortex, 18*(7), 1549–1559.

Hansen, T., Olkkonen, M., Walter, S., & Gegenfurtner, K. R. (2006). Memory modulates color appearance. *Nature Neuroscience, 9*(11), 1367–1368.

Hill, A. J., Magson, L. D., & Blundell, J. E. (1984). Hunger and palatability: Tracking ratings of subjective experience before, during and after the consumption of preferred and less preferred food. *Appetite, 5*(4), 361–371.

Hofmann, W., Deutsch, R., Lancaster, K., & Banaji, M. R. (2010). Cooling the heat of temptation: Mental self-control and the automatic evaluation of tempting stimuli. *European Journal of Social Psychology, 40*(1), 17–25.

Hofmann, W., Friese, M., & Wiers, R. W. (2008). Impulsive versus reflective influences on health behavior: A theoretical framework and empirical review. *Health Psychology Review, 2*(2), 111–137.

Hofmann, W., Vohs, K. D., & Baumeister, R. F. (2012). What people desire, feel conflicted about, and try to resist in everyday life. *Psychological Science, 23*(6), 582–588.

Hsu, N. S., Frankland, S. M., & Thompson-Schill, S. L. (2012). Chromaticity of color perception and object color knowledge. *Neuropsychologia, 50*(2), 327–333.

Jeannerod, M. (1995). Mental imagery in the motor context. *Neuropsychologia, 33*(11), 1419–1432.

Jenkins, K. T., & Tapper, K. (2014). Resisting chocolate temptation using a brief mindfulness strategy. *British Journal of Health Psychology, 19*(3), 509–522.

Jones, B. T., Corbin, W., & Fromme, K. (2001). A review of expectancy theory and alcohol consumption. *Addiction, 96*(1), 57–72.

Jones, M., & Love, B. C. (2011). Bayesian fundamentalism or enlightenment? On the explanatory status and theoretical contributions of Bayesian models of cognition. *Behavioral and Brain Sciences, 34*(4), 169–188.

Kavanagh, D. J., Andrade, J., & May, J. (2005). Imaginary relish and exquisite torture: The elaborated intrusion theory of desire. *Psychological Review, 112*(2), 446–467.

Keesman, M., Papies, E. K., Ostafin, B. D., Verwei, S., Häfner, M., & Aarts, H. (2015). *Situated representations of alcohol predict drinking behavior.* Manuscript in preparation.

Kellenbach, M. L., Brett, M., & Patterson, K. (2001). Large, colorful, or noisy? Attribute- and modality-specific activations during retrieval of perceptual attribute knowledge. *Cognitive, Affective, and Behavioral Neuroscience, 1*(3), 207–221.

Keller, C., & van der Horst, K. (2013). Dietary restraint, ambivalence toward eating, and the valence and content of spontaneous associations with eating. *Appetite, 62*, 150–159.

Kiefer, M., & Barsalou, L. W. (2013). Grounding the human conceptual system in perception, action, and internal states. In W. Prinz, M. Beisert, & A. Herwig (Eds.), *Action science: Foundations of an emerging discipline* (pp. 381–407). Cambridge, MA: MIT Press.

Kiefer, M., Sim, E.-J., Herrnberger, B., Grothe, J., & Hoenig, K. (2008). The sound of concepts: Four markers for a link between auditory and conceptual brain systems. *Journal of Neuroscience, 28*(47), 12224–12230.

Killgore, W. D. S., Young, A. D., Femia, L. A., Bogorodzki, P., Rogowska, J., & Yurgelun-Todd, D. A. (2003). Cortical and limbic activation during viewing of high- versus low-calorie foods. *NeuroImage, 19*(4), 1381.

Kosslyn, S. M. (1980). *Image and mind.* Cambridge, MA: Harvard University Press.

Kosslyn, S. M. (1994). *Image and brain: The resolution of the imagery debate.* Cambridge, MA: MIT Press.

Lacey, S., Stilla, R., & Sathian, K. (2012). Metaphorically feeling: Comprehending textural metaphors activates somatosensory cortex. *Brain and Language, 120*(3), 416–421.

Lebois, L. A., Wilson-Mendenhall, C. D., Simmons, W. K., Barrett, L. F., & Barsalou, L. W. (2015). *Learning emotions.* Submitted for publication.

Lench, H. C., Flores, S. A., & Bench, S. W. (2011). Discrete emotions predict changes in cognition, judgment, experience, behavior, and physiology: A meta-analysis of experimental emotion elicitations. *Psychological Bulletin, 137*(5), 834–855.

Locher, J. L., Yoels, W. C., Maurer, D., & van Ells, J. (2005). Comfort foods: An exploratory journey into the social and emotional significance of food. *Food and Foodways, 13*(4), 273–297.

Martin, A. (2001). Functional neuroimaging of semantic memory. *Handbook of Functional Neuroimaging of Cognition, 1*(3), 153–186.

Martin, A. (2007). The representation of object concepts in the brain. *Annual Review of Psychology, 58*(1), 25–45.

Mckay, D., & Schare, M. L. (1999). The effects of alcohol and alcohol expectancies on subjective reports and physiological reactivity: A meta-analysis. *Addictive Behaviors, 24*(5), 633–647.

Metcalfe, J., & Mischel, W. (1999). A hot/cool-system analysis of delay of gratification: Dynamics of willpower. *Psychological Review, 106*(1), 3–19.

Moors, A., & De Houwer, J. (2006). Automaticity: A theoretical and conceptual analysis. *Psychological Bulletin, 132*(2), 297–326.

Myrick, H., Anton, R. F., Li, X., Henderson, S., Drobes, D., Voronin, K., et al. (2004). Differential brain activity in alcoholics and social drinkers to alcohol cues: Relationship to craving. *Neuropsychopharmacology, 29*(2), 393–402.

Naumann, E., Trentowska, M., & Svaldi, J. (2013). Increased salivation to mirror exposure in women with binge eating disorder. *Appetite, 65*, 103–110.

Nederkoorn, C., Smulders, F. T. Y., & Jansen, A. (2000). Cephalic phase responses, craving and food intake in normal subjects. *Appetite, 35*(1), 45–55.

Ouellette, J. A., & Wood, W. (1998). Habit and intention in everyday life: The multiple processes by which past behavior predicts future behavior. *Psychological Bulletin, 124*(1), 54–74.

Papies, E. K. (2013). Tempting food words activate eating simulations. *Frontiers in Psychology, 4*, 838.

Papies, E. K., & Barsalou, L. W. (2014). *A grounded theory of desire and motivated behavior.* Manuscript in preparation.

Papies, E. K., Barsalou, L. W., & Custers, R. (2012). Mindful attention prevents mindless impulses. *Social Psychological and Personality Science, 3*(3), 291–299.

Papies, E. K., & Hamstra, P. (2010). Goal priming and eating behavior: Enhancing self-regulation by environmental cues. *Health Psychology, 29*(4), 384–388.

Papies, E. K., Potjes, I., Keesman, M., Schwinghammer, S., & van Koningsbruggen, G. M. (2014). Using health primes to reduce unhealthy snack purchases among overweight consumers in a grocery store. *International Journal of Obesity, 38*(4), 597–602.

Papies, E. K., Pronk, T. M., Keesman, M., & Barsalou, L. W. (2015). The benefits of simply observing: Mindful attention modulates the link between motivation and behavior. *Journal of Personality and Social Psychology, 108*(1), 148–170.

Papies, E. K., Stroebe, W., & Aarts, H. (2007). Pleasure in the mind: Restrained eating and spontaneous hedonic thoughts about food. *Journal of Experimental Social Psychology, 43*(5), 810–817.

Papies, E. K., Stroebe, W., & Aarts, H. (2008). Healthy cognition: Processes of self-regulatory success in restrained eating. *Personality and Social Psychology Bulletin, 34*(9), 1290–1300.

Papies, E. K., & Veling, H. (2013). Healthy dining: Subtle diet reminders at the point of purchase increase low-calorie food choices among both chronic and current dieters. *Appetite, 61*, 1–7.

Plassmann, H., O'Doherty, J., Shiv, B., & Rangel, A. (2008). Marketing actions can modulate neural representations of experienced pleasantness. *Proceedings of the National Academy of Sciences, 105*(3), 1050–1054.

Pulvermueller, F. (2013). Semantic embodiment, disembodiment or misembodiment? In search of meaning in modules and neuron circuits. *Brain and Language, 127*(1), 86–103.

Reich, R. R., Below, M. C., & Goldman, M. S. (2010). Explicit and implicit measures of expectancy and related alcohol cognitions: A meta-analytic comparison. *Psychology of Addictive Behaviors, 24*(1), 13–25.

Rogers, P. J., & Hill, A. J. (1989). Breakdown of dietary restraint following mere exposure to food stimuli: Interrelationships between restraint, hunger, salivation, and food intake. *Addictive Behaviors, 14*(4), 387–397.

Ross, B. H., & Murphy, G. L. (1999). Food for thought: Cross-classification and category organization in a complex real-world domain. *Cognitive Psychology, 38*(4), 495–553.

Schacht, J. P., Anton, R. F., Randall, P. K., Li, X., Henderson, S., & Myrick, H. (2011). Stability of fMRI striatal response to alcohol cues: A hierarchical linear modeling approach. *NeuroImage, 56*(1), 61–68.

Seibt, B., Häfner, M., & Deutsch, R. (2007). Prepared to eat: How immediate affective and motivational responses to food cues are influenced by food deprivation. *European Journal of Social Psychology, 37*(2), 359–379.

Sheeran, P., Aarts, H., Custers, R., Rivis, A., Webb, T. L., & Cooke, R. (2005). The goal-dependent automaticity of drinking habits. *British Journal of Social Psychology, 44*(1), 47–63.

Siep, N., Roefs, A., Roebroeck, A., Havermans, R., Bonte, M. L., & Jansen, A. (2009). Hunger is the best spice: An fMRI study of the effects of attention, hunger and calorie content on food reward processing in the amygdala and orbitofrontal cortex. *Behavioural Brain Research, 198*(1), 149–158.

Simmons, W. K., & Barsalou, L. W. (2003). The similarity-in-topography principle: Reconciling theories of conceptual deficits. *Cognitive Neuropsychology, 20*(3–6), 451–486.

Simmons, W. K., Martin, A., & Barsalou, L. W. (2005). Pictures of appetizing foods activate gustatory cortices for taste and reward. *Cerebral Cortex, 15*(10), 1602–1608.

Simpson, J. A., & Gangestad, S. W. (1992). Sociosexuality and romantic partner choice. *Journal of Personality, 60*(1), 31–51.

Spence, C., Levitan, C., Shankar, M. U., & Zampini, M. (2010). Does food color influence taste and flavor perception in humans? *Chemosensory Perception, 3*(1), 68–84.

Spence, C., & Shankar, M. U. (2010). The influence of auditory cues on the perception of, and responses to, food and drink. *Journal of Sensory Studies, 25*(3), 406–430.

Spence, C., Shankar, M. U., & Blumenthal, H. (2010). The influence of hearing on eating, drinking, and perception. In F. Bacci & D. Melcher (Eds.), *Art and the senses* (pp. 207–238). New York: Oxford University Press.

Stein, K. D., Goldman, M. S., & Del Boca, F. K. (2000). The influence of alcohol expectancy priming and mood manipulation on subsequent alcohol consumption. *Journal of Abnormal Psychology, 109*(1), 106–115.

Stice, E., Spoor, S., Ng, J., & Zald, D. H. (2009). Relation of obesity to consummatory and anticipatory food reward. *Physiology & Behavior, 97*(5), 551–560.

Stice, E., Yokum, S., Burger, K. S., Epstein, L. H., & Small, D. M. (2011). Youth at risk for obesity show greater activation of striatal and somatosensory regions to food. *Journal of Neuroscience, 31*(12), 4360–4366.

Strack, F., & Deutsch, R. (2004). Reflective and impulsive determinants of social behavior. *Personality and Social Psychology Review, 8*(3), 220–247.

Terence, G., & Lawson, D. M. (1976). Expectancies, alcohol, and sexual arousal in male social drinkers. *Journal of Abnormal Psychology, 85*(6), 587–594.

Tetley, A., Brunstrom, J., & Griffiths, P. (2009). Individual differences in food-cue reactivity: The role of BMI and everyday portion-size selections. *Appetite, 52*(3), 614–620.

Tiffany, S. T., Cox, L. S., & Elash, C. A. (2000). Effects of transdermal nicotine patches on abstinence-induced and cue-elicited craving in cigarette smokers. *Journal of Consulting and Clinical Psychology, 68*(2), 233–240.

Van der Laan, L. N., de Ridder, D. T. D., Viergever, M. A., & Smeets, P. A. M. (2011). The first taste is always with the eyes: A meta-analysis on the neural correlates of processing visual food cues. *NeuroImage, 55*(1), 296–303.

Veling, H., Aarts, H., & Papies, E. K. (2011). Using stop signals to inhibit chronic dieters' responses toward palatable foods. *Behaviour Research and Therapy, 49*(11), 771–780.

Veltkamp, M., Aarts, H., & Custers, R. (2009). Unravelling the motivational yarn: A framework for understanding the instigation of implicitly motivated behaviour resulting from deprivation and positive affect. *European Review of Social Psychology, 20*(1), 345–381.

Veltkamp, M., Custers, R., & Aarts, H. (2011). Motivating consumer behavior by subliminal conditioning in the absence of basic needs: Striking even while the iron is cold. *Journal of Consumer Psychology, 21*(1), 49–56.

Vuchinich, R. E., & Sobell, M. B. (1978). Empirical separation of physiologic and expected effects of alcohol on complex perceptual motor performance. *Psychopharmacology, 60*(1), 81–85.

Wang, G.-J., Volkow, N. D., Telang, F., Jayne, M., Ma, J., Rao, M., et al. (2004). Exposure to appetitive food stimuli markedly activates the human brain. *NeuroImage, 21*(4), 1790–1797.

Wansink, B., Cheney, M. M., & Chan, N. (2003). Exploring comfort food preferences across age and gender. *Physiology and Behavior, 79*(4–5), 739–747.

Wansink, B., Painter, J. E., & Lee, Y.-K. (2006). The office candy dish: Proximity's influence on estimated and actual consumption. *International Journal of Obesity, 30*(5), 871–875.

Wiers, R. W., & Stacy, A. W. (2006). Implicit cognition and addiction. *Current Directions in Psychological Science, 15*(6), 292–296.

Wilson, G. T., & Abrams, D. (1977). Effects of alcohol on social anxiety and physiological arousal: Cognitive versus pharmacological processes. *Cognitive Therapy and Research, 1*(3), 195–210.

Wilson-Mendenhall, C. D., Barrett, L. F., Simmons, W. K., & Barsalou, L. W. (2011). Grounding emotion in situated conceptualization. *Neuropsychologia, 49*(5), 1105–1127.

Wilson-Mendenhall, C. D., Simmons, W. K., Martin, A., & Barsalou, L. W. (2013). Contextual processing of abstract concepts reveals neural representations of nonlinguistic semantic content. *Journal of Cognitive Neuroscience, 25*(6), 920–935.

Woods, A. T., Lloyd, D. M., Kuenzel, J., Poliakoff, E., Dijksterhuis, G. B., & Thomas, A. (2011). Expected taste intensity affects response to sweet drinks in primary taste cortex: *NeuroReport, 22*(8), 365–369.

Yeh, W., & Barsalou, L. W. (2006). The situated nature of concepts. *American Journal of Psychology, 119*(3), 349–384.

CHAPTER 3

Desire and Desire Regulation

Wilhelm Hofmann
Hiroki P. Kotabe
Kathleen D. Vohs
Roy F. Baumeister

A good deal of people's waking time is, more or less directly, spent thinking about and dealing with desire. There is no question that desires are often benign, functional, and evolutionary adaptive for the individual. However, there are cases where desire stands in conflict with important (self-regulatory) goals or (moral) values. Prime examples include the ex-smoker who, upon seeing other people smoke, reexperiences a strong craving for a cigarette despite her intention to never smoke again, or two colleagues at work who cannot help feeling sexually attracted to each other despite the fact that one of them has made public vows of faith on the not-so-long-ago wedding day. And sometimes, much more trivially, the time or opportunity to fulfill a certain desire is just not "right," such as when someone feels a strong need to pee on a long bus ride and, alas, the toilet is broken. There are both individual and societal reasons for why the capacity for desire regulation is such a highly important aspect of everyday functioning.

The primary questions that we seek to answer in this chapter are: What is desire? When does it become problematic? How does desire regulation work? When and why can it go wrong? And how can it be improved? To approach issues of desire regulation, we will draw both on the literature of self-control and emotion regulation. The self-control literature is central because desires are driving forces that sometimes need to be held in check through inhibition or overriding. Self-control research has yielded a wealth of insights on how such *inhibitory* processes may work and when they may be disturbed. More recently, the field has begun to scrutinize anticipatory, preventive strategies through which people actively set the stage for later self-control successes (Fujita, 2011;

Hofmann & Kotabe, 2012), which we believe to be an essential component of desire regulation. The literature on emotion regulation is also relevant in that desires share many similarities with emotions (Hofmann & Kotabe, 2013). Therefore, we argue that an emotion-regulation perspective may yield important practical insights into how people may become more successful at regulating problematic desires. Also, the emotion-regulation literature has, since the conception of the process model of emotion regulation (Gross, 1998), always adopted a broad focus encompassing both early-stage (antecedent-focused) and late-stage (response-focused) forms of emotion regulation, which resonates with our approach in the present chapter.

Until recently, cases of desire regulation have been mainly studied under the rubric of goal conflicts (e.g., a short-term "goal" to enjoy tasty chocolate versus a long-term goal to lose weight; a short-term "goal" to enjoy sex versus a long-term goal to be faithful). While such a terminology is elegant, parsimonious, and highly general, we believe it may actually hinder a deeper understanding of the *specific* characteristics of the two opponents involved in these motivational struggles (see Hofmann & Nordgren, Introduction, this volume). That is, by framing desire as "just" another (short-term) goal, we might sacrifice a closer analysis of the specific laws that trigger and fuel desire, and the most effective strategies to tame it. By treating desire as an affective-motivational phenomenon of its own kind, however, we can begin to ask more specific questions about how desire waxes and wanes in close interaction with environmental characteristics and how it can be strategically up- or down-regulated.

What Is Desire?

Even though the term *desire* can refer to all kinds of wishes and wants, we stay with the more narrow definition of *appetitive* desires as "those motivations that propel us to approach certain stimuli in our environment and engage in activities with them that provide us with a relative gain in immediate pleasure (including relief from discomfort)" (see Hofmann & Nordgren, Introduction, this volume). Such a definition includes desires rooted in physiological need states, such as for food, alcohol, sex, or rest, or acquired through a history of reinforcement learning as in the case of drugs, media addiction, spending urges, and so forth (Hofmann & Kotabe, 2013). Moreover, we use the term *craving* to refer to desires across domains that are particularly high intensity (e.g., "drug craving," "food craving").

Desire Components

In this chapter and elsewhere (Hofmann & Kotabe, 2013), we argue that desires are much like emotions. That is, desires share many of the major hallmark characteristics of an emotion (see also Franken, 2003; Franken, Chapter 19, this volume). Like emotions, desires are multifaceted phenomena combining affective, motivational, and cognitive components.

The affective component consists of a feeling of "wanting" of varying intensity. Desires "tell" us that a given thing, person, or activity has high momentary relevance against the backdrop of our current goals, bodily need states, and learning history. We see phenomenological experience of wanting as the core emotional experience of desire. It is separable from the mixed emotional consequences that enacting versus inhibiting desires may have—including pleasure and possibly guilt from desire enactment and frustration, and possibly pride from desire nonenactment (Kotabe, Righetti, & Hofmann, 2014). In line with an influential distinction by Berridge, Robinson, and Aldridge (2009), we identify desire with wanting (incentive salience) rather than liking (desire's hedonic impact). From a neuropsychological perspective, the current consensus is that desire originates in largely subcortical neural systems that include mesolimbic dopamine projections (Berridge et al., 2009; Peciña & Berridge, 2005). Reward signals from midbrain regions are then forwarded to prefrontal regions in the brain involved in reward representation and integration, with the orbitofrontal cortex (OFC) being among the regions most consistently implicated in the conscious representation of desire (Van der Laan, de Ridder, Viergevera, & Smeetsa, 2011).

The motivational component encompasses desire's power to prepare and instigate behavior. Desiring something means wanting to *have*, *consume*, or *do* something that we expect will yield pleasure (or reduce discomfort). When we feel tempted by a lavish-looking desert, we expect its consumption to provide us with high sensual pleasure. When an alcohol addict craves a glass of whiskey, he or she may expect that doing so will reduce distress—including, ironically, distress caused by the addiction itself. Hence, desire propels us to approach and consume things through the more or less explicit promise of pleasure or relief. Although such hedonic motives may not be the only reasons why we pursue desire, they are clearly a defining feature of desire's motivational component.

Next to the affective and motivational components desire also has an important cognitive component. According to Kavanagh, Andrade, and May's (2005) elaborated intrusion theory of desire (Andrade, May, Van Dillen, & Kavanagh, Chapter 1, this volume), desire is typically accompanied by intrusive thoughts about the object of desire. Such cognitions comprise expectations about the consequences of desire enactment and the feasibility of attaining the desired object, as well as mental simulations and fantasies. These cognitions can be quite biased through processes of motivated reasoning (see also de Ridder, de Witt Huberts, & Evers, Chapter 10, this volume), with stronger desires typically leading to more biased and distorted cognitions (Kavanagh et al., 2005). Moreover, the connection between cognition and affect is most likely not a one-way street. As a person mentally elaborates a desire, its strength may in turn, increase, as it occupies even more mental resources and triggers further elaborations. Such a dynamic processing perspective may explain why desire sometimes escalates to the point where opposing mental representations such as those related to self-regulatory goals get "crowded out," that is, temporarily forgotten (Hofmann, Friese, Schmeichel, & Baddeley, 2011; Hofmann & Van Dillen, 2012; Kavanagh et al., 2005).

Sampling Desires

How often do people experience desire and what are these desires about? In a recent experience sampling project, called the Everyday Temptations Study, we set out to approach this question empirically by collecting base rate information on the prevalence of various appetitive desires in everyday life (Hofmann, Baumeister, Förster, & Vohs, 2012a; Hofmann, Vohs, & Baumeister, 2012c). We used the experience-sampling method to capture desires "where the action takes place"—that is, as people navigate their everyday environments (Csikszentmihalyi & Larsen, 1987; Mehl & Conner, 2012). More than 200 participants from Germany were equipped with smartphones for a week. On multiple random occasions each day, they received a questionnaire via these smartphones and were asked whether they were currently experiencing a desire from a list of 15 desire domains including food, nonalcoholic drinks, sleep, sex, social contact, leisure, sports, spending, media, alcohol, tobacco, and other drugs. Participants reported a current desire about 50% of the time they were signaled. Thus, desiring something seems to be a very frequent feature of everyday life.

What were these desires about? Even though our list was probably nonexhaustive, it is informative to look at the relative frequency breakdown with which various desires were experienced over the course of the day. Figure 3.1 presents this data, together with the frequency breakdown from a similar study conducted recently in the United States involving about 100 subjects (Friese & Hofmann, 2014). The most frequently reported desires were those to eat, drink, and sleep, followed by desires for leisure/rest, social contact, and media use. These frequencies were largely replicated in the United States (i.e., the correlation of percentages for the desire categories assessed in both countries was $r = .95$).

How Does Desire Influence Behavior?

Desire emerges in a relatively automatic fashion as reward-processing centers in midbrain regions (e.g., the ventral striatum) evaluate external stimuli (or mental images thereof) against the backdrop of internal need states and an individual's learning history (Hofmann, Friese, & Strack, 2009b; Hofmann & Van Dillen, 2012). This early reward processing may have the potential to trigger fast, impulsive, and habitual responses, which may

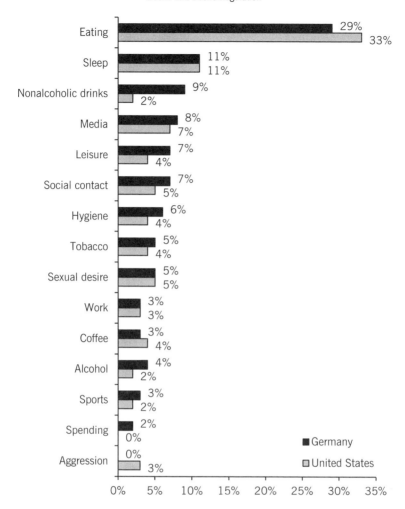

FIGURE 3.1. Desire frequencies from two experience-sampling studies conducted in Germany (Hofmann et al., 2013) and the United States (Friese & Hofmann, 2014). Spending desires were not assessed in the United States, and desires to aggress were not assessed in Germany.

even happen outside of conscious awareness (e.g., Mogenson, Jones, & Yim, 1980; Winkielman, Berridge, & Wilbarger, 2005). Such impulsive responses may be most relevant in situations where the desired stimulus is already quite close in space and time.

However, the more typical route is that desire gains access to consciousness and deeply affects our thinking and planning. As spelled out by the elaborated-intrusion theory of desire (Kavanagh et al., 2005), desire-related processing can be subject to a vicious circle of reprocessing and rumination that, in turn, increases the feeling of wanting and the motivational power of desire. As desire becomes more cognitively elaborated in working memory, so does its potential to instigate concrete action plans and behavioral intentions to consume the object of desire. Most important, elaborated desires may predispose the organism toward (sometimes problematic) consumption via two important mechanisms. First, elaborated desires may crowd out (i.e., temporarily deactivate) other representations from working memory, leading to a preoccupation with the desire at the expense of everything else, including self-regulatory goals and values (Hofmann et al., 2011; Kemps, Tiggemann, & Grigg, 2008b). Second, elaborated desires may instigate processes of motivated reasoning that license and justify indulgence (e.g., "I deserve a special treat today"; "others are having their share of cake, too"; "this is definitely going to be my last cigarette before I quit!") (de Ridder, de Witt Huberts, & Evers, Chapter 10, this volume; Hofmann & Van Dillen, 2012). In the case of problematic desire, desires can thus hijack the very mechanisms that otherwise support "reasoned" action, resulting in "passionate" behavior that people may later regret.

Sources of Conflict: What Renders Desires Problematic?

It is important to note that desires and temptations are not synonyms. That is, temptations are a special subset of desires. To say that somebody is "tempted" by something means that the person has a desire to do X on one hand *and simultaneously* has reason not to do X (Mele, 2001). Whether a person has reason not to do X will depend on whether the behavior implied by the desire *conflicts* with that person's set of endorsed self-regulatory goals, values, or otherwise activated competing motivations (Hofmann et al., 2012a). For example, the desire for sexual intimacy with a new acquaintance seems harmless unless one is already in an exclusive relationship. In modern society, it seems that intrapsychic conflict often accompanies desire because although desire is so "straightforwardly" connected to what promises immediate pleasure or relief from discomfort, its behavioral implications are often at odds with what is regarded as optimal, proper, or moral. In the Everyday Temptations Study, we found that 53.2% of desires were rated as not conflicting at all, 14.7% as mildly conflicting, 12.4% as somewhat conflicting, 10.9% as quite conflicting, and 8.8% as highly conflicting (Hofmann et al., 2012a). Thus, a nontrivial portion of desires was experienced as problematic. Accordingly, people indicated that they had attempted to resist their desire on a full 42% of occasions. They were successful about 83% of the time on average, with a lower likelihood of success for strong rather than weak desires (Hofmann et al., 2012a).

We also assessed information on the goals people reported as conflicting with their desire and proposed a taxonomy of five broad types of conflicting goals (Hofmann et al., 2012c): (1) *health-protection goals* (23% of reported goals; e.g., the goal to eat healthily, to increase one's bodily fitness, to reduce the risk of infections); (2) *abstinence/restraint goals* (9%; e.g., the goal to save money, to end a dependency, to remain faithful); (3) *achievement-related goals* (28%; e.g., academic and work-related goals); (4) *time-use goals* (29%; e.g., the goal to use one's time efficiently, to not delay things, to get things done); (5) *social goals* (11%; e.g., the goal to improve or maintain one's social recognition, to conform to moral values and beliefs). Health-protection and abstinence/restraint goals reflect people's knowledge that the unrestrained enactment of certain desires carries health risks such as coronary heart disease from consuming too many unhealthy foods, lung cancer from smoking, or premature death from sexually transmitted diseases such as HIV. Achievement-related and time-use goals reflect people's knowledge that desire enactment may get in the way of important long-term projects, academic and work goals, or sport aspirations. For instance, surfing social media too often may interfere with one's study goals, giving in to the desire to rest and relax too often may hinder progress on the latest sales report, and so forth. Finally, social goals reflect people's knowledge that desire enactment may impact one's social reputation and/or interfere with one's internalized moral values and beliefs.

According to moral foundations theory (Graham et al., 2013), morality is based on several core moral principles: care ("don't harm other people"); fairness ("don't pursue your own advantage in disproportionate ways"); loyalty ("don't betray your in-group"); authority ("don't disrespect laws, rules, and authority figures"); and sanctity ("don't do something 'impure' or 'indecent'"). Another core moral principle may be honesty ("don't manipulate the truth"; Hofmann, Wisneski, Brandt, & Skitka, 2014). Each of these principles can, to various degrees, be violated by the enactment of a given desire. Take, for example, a typical case of adultery, brought about by strong sexual desire. It may result in harm (e.g., the emotional harm felt by the partner upon finding out), fairness violations (one partner unfairly pursuing his or her self-interest), betrayal (breaking the trust of the in-group partner), subversion of moral authority (e.g., religious norms related to monogamy), degradation (doing something "impure"), and dishonesty (the lying typically involved). People may be motivated to regulate their desires to the extent that they endorse these moral principles and anticipate their desire enactment will violate them.

Although there were some prominent connections between specific desires and specific opposing goals in the database (e.g., desire for tobacco vs. reducing health damage; spending desire vs. saving expenses), desire–goal conflicts came in many different combinations (see Hofmann et al., 2012c, Supplementary Figure 2). Thus, one and the same desire can be experienced as a temptation for many different reasons. Moreover, many desires were seen as conflicting with more than just one goal.

Interestingly, the amount of conflict experienced was not only a function of the importance assigned to these goals, but also of the number of goals with which a given desire was perceived to be in conflict. This suggests that a person's motivation to regulate a certain desire increases as that desire challenges the overall configuration of goals that the person holds. Taken together, a considerable portion of human desire is experienced as conflicting, due to a large number of possible reasons. We next turn to the various ways people may deal with such problematic desires through various mechanisms and strategies of desire regulation.

How Does Desire Regulation Work?

Given that desires and cravings may sometimes be experienced as conflicting with one's set of self-regulatory goals and values, the question emerges how tempting desires can be effectively controlled. In the remainder of this chapter, we focus on three general routes through which desire may be successfully regulated (in the sense that the behavior driven by the desire is not enacted): constraining the emergence of desire, desire down-regulation, and inhibition/overriding. These three routes are illustrated in Figure 3.2 in the context of a random person, Bill, who wants to get a better grip on his frequent desire for alcohol.

Constraining the Emergence of Desire

The first route, which has been the focus of more recent self-control research, encompasses those early-stage strategies that may lead an individual to not experience desire to begin with. As humans, we can play a quite active role with regard to the types of situations and stimuli we encounter in our day-to-day lives. These preventive strategies (Hofmann & Kotabe, 2012) require considerable foresight and experience as to which situations and stimuli are more likely to trigger problematic desire than others. As people extract evaluative lessons from their past behavior (Baumeister, Vohs, DeWall, & Zhang, 2007), however, they may become increasingly better at avoiding problematic desire. In the drinking example, when arranging meetings with his best friend, Bill may learn to avoid those places that typically trigger a strong desire for alcoholic drinks (bar) and suggest meeting in places that largely prevent the desire and/or opportunity for alcohol (spa) (see Figure 3.2, illustration on the left).

Situation and Stimulus Control

One common motto of all sorts of prevention is "the sooner the better." The same applies to desire prevention. Arguably the most effective strategy to prevent desire is to avoid exposure to tempting situations or stimuli

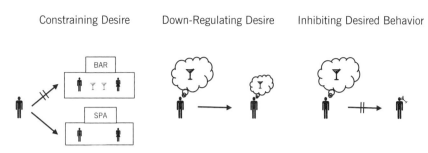

Constraining Desire   Down-Regulating Desire   Inhibiting Desired Behavior

FIGURE 3.2. Illustration of three general routes to desire regulation with a drinking example. *Constraining desire*: putting oneself into a situation that has a low (spa) rather than high (bar) potential of triggering a desire for alcohol. *Down-regulating desire*: employing mental strategies such as reappraisal or acceptance that reduce the strength of the desire for alcohol. *Inhibiting desired behavior*: employing self-control capacities (i.e., executive functions) to inhibit or override the desire to consume alcohol.

altogether via strategies of situation and stimulus control (Mahoney & Thoresen, 1972). These strategies rest on the earlier notion that external stimuli play a seminal role in the emergence of desire. As they interact with a person's learning history and current need states, such "impellers" can greatly alter the odds that people will experience temptation to begin with (Finkel, 2014; Hofmann & Van Dillen, 2012). Situation and stimulus control techniques can either be learned and applied by a person directly (e.g., keeping one's home free of unhealthy but tempting foods), or they can be imposed by public policy makers and other choice architects through so-called "nudges" (Thaler & Sunstein, 2009). The use of situation and stimulus control in public policy can be seen, for example, in "no smoking" policies at restaurants and in school cafeterias that primarily offer healthy options. Because situation and stimulus control are not always feasible (e.g., when one cannot avoid or escape a temptation-rich environment), however, these strategies clearly cannot be the sole solution.

Are some people better at anticipating problematic situations in their daily lives? One intriguing finding of the Everyday Temptations Study was that individuals high in trait self-control (TSC) showed signs of higher situation and stimulus control (rather than more effective late-stage inhibition): they reported lower average desire strength, lower average conflict, and less need to use active resistance to control desire (Hofmann et al., 2012a). We believe this pattern of findings to—at least partially—reflect the impact of preventive strategies. High-TSC individuals may be better at constraining their desire landscape in a way that reduces the need for effortful control. In support, independent raters rated the desires reported by high-TSC participants as less problematic for the "average person" than the desires reported by low-TSC participants (Hofmann et al., 2012a).

Furthermore, we believe that individuals high in TSC should be distinct from individuals with high values on what has been called the restraint bias (Nordgren, van Harreveld, & van der Pligt, 2009). The restraint bias stands for overoptimistic beliefs about one's capacity for self-control. Because of their overconfidence, people high in the restraint bias tend to overexpose themselves to tempting situations, which typically results in more frequent self-control failures (Nordgren et al., 2009; see also Ruttan & Nordgren, Chapter 11, this volume). We therefore predict that individuals high in TSC harbor more realistic impulse control beliefs than individuals high in the restraint bias. Their more realistic willpower self-assessment (and more realistic appreciation of the power of the situation) may guide high-TSC individuals in avoiding risky situations and in removing tempting stimuli from their environment when such strategies are feasible.

Early-Stage Distraction

Another, more proximal mechanism than situation and stimulus control that appears to constrain the potential for desire experience is early-stage distraction upon stimulus encounter. The underlying idea is that, sometimes, people may be so focused on a given current goal or activity (e.g., reading a very engaging novel) that tempting stimuli in their environment do not capture the amount of attention that would otherwise lead to the conscious representation (and reprocessing) of desire in working memory. Indeed, recent research has shown that cognitively demanding tasks unrelated to the temptation at hand may prevent the emergence of desire (Kemps et al., 2008a; Van Dillen, Papies, & Hofmann, 2013). For instance, Van Dillen and colleagues (Van Dillen et al., 2013, Study 1) asked participants to categorize pictures of tempting (e.g., brownies) versus nontempting (e.g., radishes) food stimuli according to spatial location while imposing either a low or high mental load during each trial of the task due to a secondary task. Participants in the low cognitive load condition made slower spatial categorizations of attractive food pictures compared to neutral food pictures. This suggests that they may have allocated more attention to tempting as compared to neutral stimuli. Participants under high cognitive load, however, were equally fast to respond to tasty and neutral food items, suggesting that they did not process the hedonic relevance of the attractive food. Accordingly, participants in the high load condition reported lower snack cravings following the categorization task. The upside is that powerful early-stage distraction may sometimes constrain or eliminate the experience of desire, which has clear potential for craving interventions (Florsheim, Heavin, Tiffany, Colvin, & Hiraoka, 2008). However, this strategy will only work to the extent that such powerful distractors can be easily found and are applied *before* strong cravings emerge, as some research suggests possible detrimental effects of distraction at later stages (Friese, Hofmann, & Wänke, 2008; Shiv & Fedorikhin, 1999). Also note that cognitive load and prior self-control exertion do not appear to be functionally equivalent, as recent work by Vohs et al. (2012) suggests that prior self-control exertion intensifies desire experiences (see also Wagner, Altman, Boswell, Kelley, & Heatherton, 2013).

Down-Regulation

The second route, implied by our view of desire as emotion, encompasses those emotion-regulatory strategies that lead to the effective *down-regulation* of desire (see also Hofmann, Koningsbruggen, Stroebe, Ramanathan, & Aarts, 2010). In this case, desire is experienced and a prepotent action tendency may be activated, but the focus of regulation is on the desire experience rather than on the prepotent action tendency. The idea is that certain regulatory strategies may be more or less effective at reducing the intensity of the experienced desire. Just as a glaring fire can be reduced in its power through the right strategy (e.g., repeatedly pouring buckets of water over it), and eventually extinguished, desire may be reduced below a critical level and eventually fade as the individual employs the right mental strategy to deal with it. This implies that there may also be dysfunctional strategies in dealing with desire (e.g., suppression).[1] In the drinking example, suppose that Bill has learned to mentally accept his desire for alcohol as a transient state (see acceptance strategy below), resulting in a decrease of desire intensity over time (Figure 3.2, middle illustration).

Reappraisal

One means of desire down-regulation can be brought about through strategies that modify how a tempting stimulus is appraised. Pioneering work by Walter Mischel on delay of gratification has shown that school-children are better able to resist immediate rewards, such as marshmallows, if they learn to cognitively reappraise these rewards in nonconsummatory ways (e.g., imagining the marshmallows as white puffy clouds) (Mischel & Baker, 1975). Recent research applying this idea in adults has demonstrated that cognitive reappraisal can have a profound impact on affective reactions to tempting stimuli. For instance, bringing people into an abstract rather than concrete mindset (Fujita & Han, 2009) or having people imagine tempting stimuli in nonconsummatory ways (Hofmann,

---

[1]Further, note that there may be certain situations where the regulatory goal of the individual consists of up-regulating desire, but the key difference is that these are typically situations in which the desire experience is "wanted" rather than "unwanted" (e.g., trying to up-regulate one's sexual desire to satisfy one's partner).

Deutsch, Lancaster, & Banaji, 2010b) appears to interfere with the early reward processing of these stimuli.

Another potential way to shape the initial, automatic appraisal of tempting stimuli is through evaluative conditioning (Hofmann, De Houwer, Perugini, Baeyens, & Crombez, 2010a). That is, pairing a tempting stimulus (e.g., alcohol) repeatedly with a negative unconditioned stimulus (e.g., a picture of a severe physical injury) can decrease desire for alcohol among problematic drinkers, as recent research has shown (Houben, Havermans, & Wiers, 2010; Van Gucht, Baeyens, Vansteenwegen, Hermans, & Beckers, 2010). A second promising method is avoidance training, in which people are trained to respond to tempting stimuli with avoidance responses (Wiers, Eberl, Rinck, Becker, & Lindenmeyer, 2011; Wiers, Rinck, Kordts, Houben, & Strack, 2010). In one intervention, inpatients with alcoholism underwent cognitive-behavioral therapy and four 15-minute training sessions to help them avoid alcohol stimuli. Compared with a control group that only received cognitive-behavioral therapy, the treatment group showed reduced cravings after the avoidance treatment as well as reduced relapse a year after treatment (Wiers et al., 2011).

Acceptance and Disidentification

Two related promising strategies high in their potential to down-regulate problematic desires are acceptance and disidentification. Both strategies are often said to be at the heart of the concept of *mindfulness*—which has been inspired by Buddhist thinking—even though additional components such as awareness may contribute to the broad phenomenon of mindfulness as well (Baer, Smith, Hopkins, Krietemeyer, & Toney, 2006). Acceptance refers to the ability to refrain from judging and controlling (i.e., suppressing) inner experiences such as desires and cravings (Forman et al., 2007; Lacaille et al., 2014). With acceptance, the individual "may be encouraged to simply observe their feelings, and accept their presence, rather than try to control or eliminate them. As such, the individual is encouraged to build up a degree of tolerance for uncomfortable feelings" (Jenkins & Tapper, 2014, p. 510). Disidentification (or "cognitive defusion") refers to the ability to mentally distance oneself from one's own thoughts and emotions by learning to view them as "transient" mental events, rather than experiencing them as statements of facts.

Accepting desires and cravings in a nonjudgmental way and seeing them as fleeting mental states instead of trying to suppress them may make it easier for people to mentally decouple themselves from the maladaptive vicious circle of reprocessing and rumination (Kavanagh et al., 2005). The overall evidence suggests that both acceptance (Alberts, Mulkens, Smeets, & Thewissen, 2010; Westbrook et al., 2013) and disidentification (Jenkins & Tapper, 2014; Lacaille et al., 2014; Moffitt, Brinkworth, Noakes, &

Mohr, 2012), as well as interventions combining the two strategies (Forman et al., 2007), may help people to better regulate their cravings and desires across a number of domains such as smoking and eating, although effects were not always consistent across studies or were dependent on moderators (e.g., Jenkins & Tapper, 2014; Moffitt et al., 2012).

Suppression

As noted above, accepting a desire may facilitate desire regulation. How does the opposite strategy fare? Is the willful suppression or negation of desire experiences an effective regulatory strategy? Most of the literature on appetitive thought suppression suggests otherwise (Barnes & Tantleff-Dunn, 2010; Erskine, 2008; Johnston, Bulik, & Anstiss, 1999; Mann & Ward, 2001). The problem with the forced suppression of desire is that, even though suppression may provide some short-term relief, it may often backfire, leading to so-called ironic rebound effects (Wegner, 1994). According to the work by Daniel Wegner, when we try to actively suppress something, attention may be redirected toward the very mental content we try to suppress. The "boomerang" effect of suppression may result in the hyper-accessibility of desire-related thoughts, and may thus, ironically, contribute to the escalation of desire by advancing the elaboration of desire-related content in working memory (Kavanagh et al., 2005).

The generally maladaptive effect of suppression leaves open the possibility that some people may suffer less (or more) from ironic rebound effects. For instance, there is some evidence that suppression may well be effective for those individuals who are particularly skilled at directing their attention in a top-down manner (Brewin & Smart, 2005). Further, the Everyday Temptations Study showed that a measure of perfectionism tapping primarily into negative, dysfunctional perfectionism was associated with stronger desire intensity in daily life (Hofmann et al., 2012a), as well as more intense feelings of conflict, and more frequent desire resistance. Although speculative, this finding could indicate that people high in dysfunctional perfectionism may become overly preoccupied with regulating their desires, making too much use of counterproductive strategies such as suppression. Such an interpretation would also be consistent with work linking dysfunctional perfectionism to an over-reliance on emotion suppression (vs. reappraisal) strategies (Bergman, Nyland, & Burns, 2007).

Inhibition and Overriding

The third route, implied by traditional self-control research, encompasses those abilities and strategies that enable the effective *inhibition* or *overriding* of the prepotent, desire-related behavior. In this case, a problematic desire is experienced, and a prepotent action tendency is activated. The focus of this (late-stage) strategy is on preventing or limiting the impact of the prepotent action tendency on actual behavior (rather than on down-regulating the desire). In the drinking example, this route would corre-spond to Bill feeling a strong urge to order a drink in a bar but preventing himself from calling out to the waiter (inhibition), or ordering a glass of water instead (overriding) (Figure 3.2, right illustration). Note that desire inhibition, due to its focus on the nonenactment of the behavior implied by the desire, is thus conceptually distinct from desire suppression, where the focus is on the suppression of the desire experience—an emotion-regulation strategy. The basic assumption is that desire processing may activate motor schemas that, unless inhibited, may be expressed in overt behavior once a certain threshold of activation is reached (Norman & Shallice, 1986; Strack & Deutsch, 2004). Inhibition implies that the indi-vidual manages to keep that prepotent action tendency from influenc-ing behavior (by deactivating it) for as long as the tempting episode lasts (i.e., until another potent stream of motivation takes precedence, or until other mechanisms lead to a disengagement from the desire). Inhibition can thus be linked to a *"do not"* self-regulatory mindset or goal. Over-riding goes one step further in that the individual attempts to replace the problematic desire-related behavior with a more acceptable substitute behavior (i.e., deactivation of the prepotent action tendency *and* selection of an alternative scheme of action). It can thus be linked to a *"do instead"* self-regulatory mindset or goal. In our example, Bill may either have a "do not" goal to not drink any alcohol, or he may have a "do instead" goal to order a nonalcoholic cocktail or beer whenever he has a strong desire for an alcoholic drink.[2]

A plethora of cognitive experimental research has linked the con-cept of inhibition and response overriding to executive functioning (for a review, see Hofmann, Schmeichel, & Baddeley, 2012b). Poor executive functioning, especially poor inhibitory control capacity (Miyake, Fried-man, Emerson, Witzki, & Howerter, 2000), has been implicated in a large number of further impulse-control problems ranging from drug (ab)use (Berkman, Falk, & Lieberman, 2011; Nigg et al., 2006) to inadequate social responding (von Hippel & Gonsalkorale, 2005) to sexual cheat-ing in romantic relationships (Pronk, Karremans, & Wigboldus, 2011). A number of studies across diverse domains have demonstrated that people low in behavioral inhibition are more strongly influenced by prepotent action tendencies than those high in inhibition (e.g., Hofmann, Friese, & Roefs, 2009a; Houben & Wiers, 2009; Nederkoorn, Houben, Hofmann, Roefs, & Jansen, 2010; Payne, 2005). Further, a range of situational fac-tors such as cognitive load (Friese et al., 2008), prior self-control exertion (Baumeister, Bratslavsky, Muraven, & Tice, 1998; Hofmann et al., 2012c;

---

[2]In this chapter, we will not discuss further a third option, which could be labelled as *moderation*, that is, the regulatory goal to satisfy a given desire only up to a certain point but no further (e.g., so-called "controlled" drinking).

Vohs & Heatherton, 2000), environmental or social stressors (Inzlicht, McKay, & Aronson, 2006), and alcohol intoxication have been linked to state reductions in inhibitory control (Hagger, Wood, Stiff, & Chatzisarantis, 2010; Lavie, Hirst, de Fockert, & Viding, 2004; Richeson et al., 2003; Schoofs, Preuss, & Wolf, 2008), as measured, for example, via performance on a Stroop task. Hence, temporary reductions in executive functioning may be one of several possible underlying mechanisms mediating the effects of these situational "risk" factors on desire regulation (Hofmann et al., 2012b).

A recent close-up analysis of more than 2,200 food desires contained in the Everyday Temptations Study serves as a good illustration of how behavioral inhibition (as measured with the Stroop task) affects everyday desire regulation in interaction with dietary restraint goals (Herman & Polivy, 1980). Among those high in dietary restraint (but not those low in dietary restraint), behavioral inhibition had a large effect on the successful inhibition of unhealthy food desires, such that those low in inhibitory control reported failing to resist unhealthy foods about three times more often than those high in inhibitory control (Hofmann, Adriaanse, Vohs, & Baumeister, 2013). Moreover, only people who were high in both dietary restraint and inhibitory control reported weight loss on average over the following 4 months whereas people high in dietary restraint but low in inhibitory control reported some weight *gain* on average. In other words, these analyses suggest that the combination of high dietary restraint and low inhibitory control is particularly problematic with regard to day-to-day food intake and long-term weight gain. Supporting the distinction between desire regulation and inhibition of desire-related behavior, inhibitory control was unrelated to the reported strength of food desires. In sum, these results suggest that inhibitory control plays an important role in determining successful versus failed inhibition of desires for tempting but unhealthy foods among people who hold a "do not" goal to abstain from such foods.

Because executive functions such as behavioral inhibition can be trained, at least to some extent (for a discussion, see Shipstead, Redick, & Engle, 2012), there is a large potential for intervention research aimed at finding ways to improve the management of unwanted desires and cravings (see also Lopez, Wagner, & Heatherton, Chapter 7, this volume). One way this might work is by training executive functions in general, hoping that people will then inhibit problematic desire-related behavior more effectively when needed. However, this strategy hinges on people's motivation to actually recruit executive functions in such situations. A second, perhaps even more promising way may be to tighten the link between desire-related cues in the environment and inhibitory processes, with the goal of making response inhibition the dominant, habitual response upon stimulus encounter. For instance, Houben, Nederkoorn, Wiers, and Jansen (2011) found that participants trained to inhibit responses toward alcohol stimuli in a modified go/no-go task showed a subsequent reduction in weekly alcohol intake, whereas those trained to react to alcohol stimuli with go-responses showed a relative increase. Similar results have been obtained in the eating domain (Houben & Jansen, 2010), and with different variations of response inhibition cueing (Veling, Aarts, & Stroebe, 2013).

Summary and Conclusion

Desire experiences are immensely common in our day-to-day lives. This is hardly surprising, as appetitive desires are deeply connected to those needs that have secured our species' survival over the millennia. New types of desires, such as those for addictive substances or those for social media, have managed to attach themselves to the basic mechanism of wanting. However, as Freud already noted so prominently (Freud, 1930, 1949), with desire comes the potential for mental conflict and the need to regulate desire in accordance with individual, social, and societal constraints on its enactment—and sometimes even its experience. We have proposed some of these reasons for conflict in more detail here, but more systematic research is clearly needed toward an exhaustive taxonomy of desire-related conflicts.

Wherever such conflict stems from, there is no denying that humans are remarkably effective desire regulators. However, this capacity is far from perfect, as a quick look into contemporary societal problems with overeating, all sorts of addictions, and sexual abuse will so readily attest. Our review of the available literature suggests that, just as with emotion regulation (Gross, 1998), effective desire regulation can take place at various stages of desire processing. Desire regulation strategies can be roughly divided into (1) those early-stage strategies that constrain desire experiences by preventing exposure to situations or stimuli that elicit desire or through early-stage distraction that prevents the emergence of desire, (2) those strategies that support the effective down-regulation of consciously experienced desire, such as reappraisal, acceptance, and disidentification, and (3) those late-stage strategies that involve the inhibition or overriding of desire-related behavior.[3]

One exciting issue for future research will be to disentangle how these general desire regulation strategies interact with each other. Our review suggests that these different strategies may not be employed to the same extent by everybody nor effective to the same extent for everybody;

---

[3]Even though we have treated down-regulation and inhibition as conceptually separate mechanisms, it is often possible, of course, for both mechanisms to be empirically associated with each other. For instance, (1) successful inhibition may lead to an eventual reduction of desire, (2) effective down-regulation may make inhibitory activity more effective, and (3) some strategies, such as mindful attention, may aid both down-regulation of desire experiences *and* the inhibition of prepotent action tendencies.

however, we still need to find out much more about how they interact with features of the person, situation, and the specific content domain of interest. Finally, as psychological insights into desire and desire regulation continue to stimulate new treatment methods and technologies, we predict that applied research is likely to make exciting progress in the years to come regarding how to help people deal with troubling desires.

REFERENCES

Alberts, H. J. E. M., Mulkens, S., Smeets, M., & Thewissen, R. (2010). Coping with food cravings. Investigating the potential of a mindfulness-based intervention. *Appetite, 55*(1), 160–163.

Baer, R. A., Smith, G. T., Hopkins, J., Krietemeyer, J., & Toney, L. (2006). Using self-report assessment methods to explore facets of mindfulness. *Assessment, 13*(1), 27–45.

Barnes, R. D., & Tantleff-Dunn, S. (2010). Food for thought: Examining the relationship between food thought suppression and weight-related outcomes. *Eating Behaviors, 11*(3), 175–179.

Baumeister, R. F., Bratslavsky, M., Muraven, M., & Tice, D. M. (1998). Ego depletion: Is the active self a limited resource? *Journal of Personality and Social Psychology, 74*, 1252–1265.

Baumeister, R. F., Vohs, K. D., DeWall, N., & Zhang, L. (2007). How emotion shapes behavior: Feedback, anticipation, and reflection, rather than direct causation. *Personality and Social Psychology Review, 11*, 167–203.

Bergman, A. J., Nyland, J. E., & Burns, L. R. (2007). Correlates with perfectionism and the utility of a dual process model. *Personality and Individual Differences, 43*(2), 389–399.

Berkman, E. T., Falk, E. B., & Lieberman, M. D. (2011). In the trenches of real-world self-control: Neural correlates of breaking the link between craving and smoking. *Psychological Science, 22*(4), 498–506.

Berridge, K. C., Robinson, T. E., & Aldridge, J. W. (2009). Dissecting components of reward: "Liking," "wanting," and learning. *Current Opinion in Pharmacology, 9*(1), 65–73.

Brewin, C. R., & Smart, L. (2005). Working memory capacity and suppression of intrusive thoughts. *Journal of Behavior Therapy and Experimental Psychiatry, 36*(1), 61–68.

Csikszentmihalyi, M., & Larsen, R. E. (1987). Validity and reliability of the experience-sampling method. *Journal of Nervous and Mental Disease, 175*, 526–536.

Erskine, J. A. K. (2008). Resistance can be futile: Investigating behavioural rebound. *Appetite, 50*(2–3), 415–421.

Finkel, E. J. (2014). The I3 Model: Metatheory, theory, and evidence. In J. M. Olson & M. P. Zanna (Eds.), *Advances in experimental social psychology* (Vol. 49, pp. 1–104). San Diego, CA: Academic Press.

Florsheim, P., Heavin, S., Tiffany, S., Colvin, P., & Hiraoka, R. (2008). An experimental test of a craving management technique for adolescents in substance-abuse treatment. *Journal of Youth and Adolescence, 37*(10), 1205–1215.

Forman, E. M., Hoffman, K. L., McGrath, K. B., Herbert, J. D., Brandsma, L. L., & Lowe, M. R. (2007). A comparison of acceptance- and control-based strategies for coping with food cravings: An analog study. *Behaviour Research and Therapy, 45*(10), 2372–2386.

Franken, I. H. (2003). Drug craving and addiction: Integrating psychological and neuropsychopharmacological approaches. *Progress in Neuropsychopharmacological Biological Psychiatry, 27*(4), 563–579.

Freud, S. (1930). *Civilization and its discontents.* London: Hogarth.

Freud, S. (1949). *New introductory lectures on psychoanalysis.* London: Hogarth. (Original work published 1933)

Friese, M., & Hofmann, W. (2014). *How state mindfulness shapes self-regulatory processes in everyday life.* Unpublished manuscript.

Friese, M., Hofmann, W., & Wänke, M. (2008). When impulses take over: Moderated predictive validity of implicit and explicit attitude measures in predicting food choice and consumption behaviour. *British Journal of Social Psychology, 47*, 397–419.

Fujita, K. (2011). On conceptualizing self-control as more than the effortful inhibition of impulses. *Personality and Social Psychology Review, 15*(4), 352–366.

Fujita, K., & Han, H. A. (2009). Moving beyond deliberative control of impulses: The effect of construal levels on evaluative associations in self-control conflicts. *Psychological Science, 20*(7), 799–804.

Graham, J., Haidt, J., Koleva, S., Motyl, M., Iyer, R., Wojcik, S. P., et al. (2013). Moral foundations theory: The pragmatic validity of moral pluralism. *Advances in Experimental Social Psychology, 47*, 55–130.

Gross, J. J. (1998). The emerging field of emotion regulation: An integrative review. *Review of General Psychology, 2*, 271–299.

Hagger, M. S., Wood, C., Stiff, C., & Chatzisarantis, N. L. (2010). Ego depletion and the strength model of self-control: A meta-analysis. *Psychological Bulletin, 136*(4), 495–525.

Herman, C. P., & Polivy, J. (1980). Restrained eating. In A. J. Stunkard (Ed.), *Obesity* (pp. 208–225). Philadelphia: Saunders.

Hofmann, W., Adriaanse, M., Vohs, K. D., & Baumeister, R. F. (2013). Dieting and the self-control of eating in everyday environments: An experience sampling study. *British Journal of Health Psychology, 19*, 523–539.

Hofmann, W., Baumeister, R. F., Förster, G., & Vohs, K. D. (2012a). Everyday temptations: An experience sampling study of desire, conflict, and self-control. *Journal of Personality and Social Psychology, 102*(6), 1318–1335.

Hofmann, W., De Houwer, J., Perugini, M., Baeyens, F., & Crombez, G. (2010a). Evaluative conditioning in humans: A meta-analysis. *Psychological Bulletin, 136*, 390–421.

Hofmann, W., Deutsch, R., Lancaster, K., & Banaji, M. R. (2010b). Cooling the heat of temptation: Mental self-control and the automatic evaluation of tempting stimuli. *European Journal of Social Psychology, 40*, 17–25.

Hofmann, W., Friese, M., & Roefs, A. (2009a). Three ways to resist temptation: The independent contributions of executive attention, inhibitory control, and affect regulation to the impulse control of eating behavior. *Journal of Experimental Social Psychology, 45*, 431–435.

Hofmann, W., Friese, M., Schmeichel, B. J., & Baddeley, A. D. (2011). Working memory and self-regulation. In K. D. Vohs & R. F. Baumeister (Eds.), *The handbook of self-regulation: Research, theory, and applications* (Vol. 2, pp. 204–226). New York: Guilford Press.

Hofmann, W., Friese, M., & Strack, F. (2009b). Impulse and self-control from a dual-systems perspective. *Perspectives on Psychological Science, 4*, 162–176.

Hofmann, W., Koningsbruggen, G. M., Stroebe, W., Ramanathan, S., & Aarts, H. (2010c). As pleasure unfolds: Hedonic responses to tempting food. *Psychological Science, 21*, 1863–1870.

Hofmann, W., & Kotabe, H. P. (2012). A general model of preventive and interventive self-control. *Social and Personality Psychology Compass, 6*, 707–722.

Hofmann, W., & Kotabe, H. P. (2013). Desire and desire regulation: Basic processes and individual differences. In J. J. Gross (Ed.), *Handbook of emotion regulation* (2nd ed., pp. 346–360). New York: Guilford Press.

Hofmann, W., Schmeichel, B. J., & Baddeley, A. D. (2012b). Executive functions and self-regulation. *Trends in Cognitive Sciences, 3*, 174–180.

Hofmann, W., & Van Dillen, L. F. (2012). Desire: The new hotspot in self-control research. *Current Directions in Psychological Science, 21*, 317–322.

Hofmann, W., Vohs, K. D., & Baumeister, R. F. (2012c). What people desire, feel conflicted about, and try to resist in everyday life. *Psychological Science, 23*(6), 582–588.

Hofmann, W., Wisneski, D. C., Brandt, M. J., & Skitka, L. J. (2014). Morality in everyday life. *Science, 345*, 1340–1343.

Houben, K., Havermans, R. C., & Wiers, R. W. (2010). Learning to dislike alcohol: Conditioning negative implicit attitudes toward alcohol and its effect on drinking behavior. *Psychopharmacology, 211*(1), 79–86.

Houben, K., & Jansen, A. (2010). Training inhibitory control: A recipe for resisting sweet temptations. *Appetite, 56*, 345–349.

Houben, K., Nederkoorn, C., Wiers, R. W., & Jansen, A. (2011). Resisting temptation: Decreasing alcohol-related affect and drinking behavior by training response inhibition. *Drug and Alcohol Dependence, 116*, 132–136.

Houben, K., & Wiers, R. W. (2009). Response inhibition moderates the relationship between implicit associations and drinking behavior. *Alcoholism: Clinical and Experimental Research, 33*, 1–8.

Inzlicht, M., McKay, L., & Aronson, J. (2006). Stigma as ego depletion: How being the target of prejudice affects self-control. *Psychological Science, 17*(3), 262–269.

Jenkins, K. T., & Tapper, K. (2014). Resisting chocolate temptation using a brief mindfulness strategy. *British Journal of Health Psychology, 19*(3), 509–522.

Johnston, L., Bulik, C. M., & Anstiss, V. (1999). Suppressing thoughts about chocolate. *International Journal of Eating Disorders, 26*(1), 21–27.

Kavanagh, D. J., Andrade, J., & May, J. (2005). Imaginary relish and exquisite torture: The elaborated intrusion theory of desire. *Psychological Review, 112*, 446–467.

Kemps, E., Tiggemann, M., & Christianson, R. (2008a). Concurrent visuo-spatial processing reduces food cravings in prescribed weight-loss dieters. *Journal of Behavior Therapy and Experimental Psychiatry, 39*(2), 177–186.

Kemps, E., Tiggemann, M., & Grigg, M. (2008b). Food cravings consume limited cognitive resources. *Journal of Experimental Psychology: Applied, 14*(3), 247–254.

Kotabe, H. P., Righetti, F., & Hofmann, W. (2014). *Affective forecasting in self-control.* Unpublished manuscript.

Lacaille, J., Ly, J., Zacchia, N., Bourkas, S., Glaser, E., & Knauper, B. (2014). The effects of three mindfulness skills on chocolate cravings. *Appetite, 76*, 101–112.

Lavie, N., Hirst, A., de Fockert, J. W., & Viding, E. (2004). Load theory of selective attention and cognitive control. *Journal of Experimental Psychology: General, 133*(3), 339–354.

Mahoney, M. J., & Thoresen, C. E. (1972). Behavioral self-control: Power to the person. *Educational Researcher, 1*(10), 5–7.

Mann, T., & Ward, A. (2001). Forbidden fruit: Does thinking about a prohibited food lead to its consumption? *International Journal of Eating Disorders, 29*(3), 319–327.

Mehl, M. R., & Conner, T. S. (Eds.). (2012). *Handbook of research methods for studying daily life*. New York: Guilford Press.

Mele, A. (2001). *Autonomous agents: From self-control to autonomy*. Oxford, UK: Oxford University Press.

Mischel, W., & Baker, N. (1975). Cognitive appraisals and transformations in delay behavior. *Journal of Personality and Social Psychology, 31*, 254–261.

Miyake, A., Friedman, N. P., Emerson, M. J., Witzki, A. H., & Howerter, A. (2000). The unity and diversity of executive functions and their contributions to complex "frontal lobe" tasks: A latent variable analysis. *Cognitive Psychology, 41*, 49–100.

Moffitt, R., Brinkworth, G., Noakes, M., & Mohr, P. (2012). A comparison of cognitive restructuring and cognitive defusion as strategies for resisting a craved food. *Psychology and Health, 27*(Suppl. 2), 74–90.

Mogenson, G. J., Jones, D. L., & Yim, C. Y. (1980). From motivation to action: Functional interface between the limbic system and the motor system. *Progress in Neurobiology, 14*(2–3), 69–97.

Nederkoorn, C., Houben, K., Hofmann, W., Roefs, A., & Jansen, A. (2010). Control yourself or just eat what you like? Weight gain over a year is predicted by an interactive effect of response inhibition and a preference for high fat foods. *Health Psychology, 29*, 389–393.

Nigg, J. T., Wong, M. M., Martel, M. M., Jester, J. M., Puttler, L. I., Glass, J. M., et al. (2006). Poor response inhibition as a predictor of problem drinking and illicit drug use in adolescents at risk for alcoholism and other substance use disorders. *Journal of the American Academy of Child and Adolescent Psychiatry, 45*(4), 468–475.

Nordgren, L. F., van Harreveld, F., & van der Pligt, J. (2009). The restraint bias: How the illusion of self-restraint promotes impulsive behavior. *Psychological Science, 20*(12), 1523–1528.

Norman, D. A., & Shallice, T. (1986). Attention to action. Willed and automatic control of behavior. In R. J. Davidson, G. E. Schwartz, & D. Shapiro (Eds.), *Consciousness and self regulation: Advances in research* (pp. 1–18). New York: Plenum Press.

Payne, B. K. (2005). Conceptualizing control in social cognition: How executive control modulates the expression of automatic stereotyping. *Journal of Personality and Social Psychology, 89*, 488–503.

Peciña, S., & Berridge, K. C. (2005). Hedonic hot spot in nucleus accumbens shell: Where do ?-opioids cause increased hedonic impact of sweetness? *Journal of Neuroscience, 25*(50), 11777–11786.

Pronk, T. M., Karremans, J. C., & Wigboldus, D. H. J. (2011). How can you resist?: Executive control helps romantically involved individuals to stay faithful. *Journal of Personality and Social Psychology, 100*(5), 827–837.

Richeson, J. A., Baird, A. A., Gordon, H. L., Heatherton, T. F., Wyland, C. L., Trawalter, S., et al. (2003). An fMRI investigation of the impact of interracial contact on executive function. *Nature Neuroscience, 6*, 1323–1328.

Schoofs, D., Preuss, D., & Wolf, O. T. (2008). Psychosocial stress induces working memory impairments in an n-back paradigm. *Psychoneuroendocrinology, 33*(5), 643–653.

Shipstead, Z., Redick, T. S., & Engle, R. W. (2012). Is working memory training effective? *Psychological Bulletin, 138*(4), 628–654.

Shiv, B., & Fedorikhin, A. (1999). Heart and mind in conflict: The interplay of affect and cognition in consumer decision making. *Journal of Consumer Research, 26*(3), 278–292.

Strack, F., & Deutsch, R. (2004). Reflective and impulsive determinants of social behavior. *Personality and Social Psychology Review, 8*(3), 220–247.

Thaler, R. H., & Sunstein, C. R. (2009). *Nudge: Improving decisions about health, wealth, and happiness.* New York: Penguin.

Van der Laan, L. N., de Ridder, D. T. D., Viergevera, M. A., & Smeetsa, P. A. M. (2011). The first taste is always with the eyes: A meta-analysis on the neural correlates of processing visual food cues. *Neuroimage, 55*, 296–303.

Van Dillen, L. F., Papies, E., & Hofmann, W. (2013). Turning a blind eye to temptation: How task load can facilitate self-regulation. *Journal of Personality and Social Psychology, 3*, 427–443.

Van Gucht, D., Baeyens, F., Vansteenwegen, D., Hermans, D., & Beckers, T. (2010). Counterconditioning reduces cue-induced craving and actual cue-elicited consumption. *Emotion, 10*(5), 688–695.

Veling, H., Aarts, H., & Stroebe, W. (2013). Using stop signals to reduce impulsive choices for palatable unhealthy foods. *British Journal of Health Psychology, 18*(2), 354–368.

Vohs, K. D., Baumeister, R. F., Mead, N. L., Hofmann, W., Ramanathan, S., & Schmeichel, B. J. (2012). *Engaging in self-control heightens urges and feelings.* Manuscript in revision.

Vohs, K. D., & Heatherton, T. F. (2000). Self-regulatory failure: A resource-depletion approach. *Psychological Science, 11*, 249–254.

von Hippel, W., & Gonsalkorale, K. (2005). "That is bloody revolting!" Inhibitory control of thoughts better left unsaid. *Psychological Science, 16*(7), 497–500.

Wagner, D. D., Altman, M., Boswell, R. G., Kelley, W. M., & Heatherton, T. F. (2013). Self-regulatory depletion enhances neural responses to rewards and impairs top-down control. *Psychological Science, 24*(11), 2262–2271.

Wegner, D. M. (1994). Ironic processes of mental control. *Psychological Review, 101*, 34–52.

Westbrook, C., Creswell, J. D., Tabibnia, G., Julson, E., Kober, H., & Tindle, H. A. (2013). Mindful attention reduces neural and self-reported cue-induced craving in smokers. *Social Cognitive and Affective Neuroscience, 8*(1), 73–84.

Wiers, R. W., Eberl, C., Rinck, M., Becker, E. S., & Lindenmeyer, J. (2011). Retraining automatic action tendencies changes alcoholic patients' approach bias for alcohol and improves treatment outcome. *Psychological Science, 22*(4), 490–497.

Wiers, R. W., Rinck, M., Kordts, R., Houben, K., & Strack, F. (2010). Retraining automatic action-tendencies to approach alcohol in hazardous drinkers. *Addiction, 105*(2), 279–287.

Winkielman, P., Berridge, K. C., & Wilbarger, J. L. (2005). Unconscious affective reactions to masked happy versus angry faces influence consumption behavior and judgments of value. *Personality and Social Psychology Bulletin, 31*, 121–135.

CHAPTER 4

Desire over Time
The Multifaceted Nature of Satiation

Joseph P. Redden

Nearly everyone experiences the phenomenon of satiation every day. For instance, a once loved song now makes us want to change the radio, a special restaurant no longer seems the obvious choice, a large piece of chocolate cake gets eaten a bit less enthusiastically, a new toy is no longer played with, skydiving becomes less exhilarating, and a new acquaintance becomes a little less exciting. These examples all illustrate the effects of satiation, which is defined here as the drop in enjoyment with repeated consumption. Of course, satiation is not an imperative— enjoyment may increase as one gains familiarity with an unknown stimulus (Zajonc, 1968) or drug addictions alter normal neural processes (Nestler & Malenka, 2004). However, these exceptions aside, it is a stylized fact that nearly everyone satiates on nearly every experience at high levels of repeated consumption. This chapter highlights this ubiquitous phenomenon, provides a framework for understanding its nature, and discusses the implications of its effects.

Because satiation occurs for virtually every experience, it follows that how much one likes something is quite dynamic and constantly changing. It is then somewhat inadequate to characterize one with a high level of desire as having an enduring trait (e.g., a chocoholic); instead, it seems more appropriate to capture only a current state of desire as a sort of snapshot within an ongoing movie. The prevailing desire state will then reflect the current level of satiation, which depends on the past quantity consumed, the variety of things previously consumed, and the time since the last consumption. Satiation ensures that current desire incorporates each of these and other factors, such that liking reflects all changes

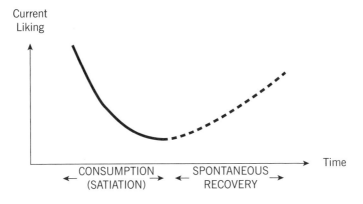

FIGURE 4.1. The consumption cycle.

with ongoing behavior over time. Thus, a full understanding of desire must incorporate the dynamics of and recovery from satiation, which are sketched in Figure 4.1 and discussed next.

The Consumption Cycle

Satiation as Decreased Liking

The notion of satiation is a deeply ingrained core concept in a number of disciplines. Introductory psychology courses generally include a unit on habituation (Thompson & Spencer, 1966), whereby an organism responds less to a stimulus with repeated exposure. Similarly, another basic process of psychology is adaptation (Helson, 1964), which is often demonstrated by having students notice how putting their hand in warm water will feel quite different depending on whether that hand was previously in either cold or hot water. In a dramatically different field of study, economic theory has a core tenet of diminishing marginal utility (Bernoulli, 1954) in which each additional dollar of wealth adds less and less to overall utility. Likewise, marketers have incorporated the well-known topic of advertising wear-out in which an ad steadily loses its effectiveness after being seen many times (Pechmann & Stewart, 1988). Finally, food scientists understand the importance of energy regulation (Benelem, 2009), whereby food is more valued and liked when one is in a state of hunger versus a state of satiety. Although these effects all span quite a broad range of domains, they all share one critical defining characteristic—a decreased response after repeated exposure. That is, there is satiation as it is defined here.

Recovery from Satiation

Upon getting satiated with a favorite experience, a simple remedy is consuming something different (i.e., variety). Although variety is an effective response to satiation in some cases, it is often not an ideal solution. First, variety requires expanding the set of less preferred options (i.e., trading down). For instance, one might become bored with a favorite restaurant and instead go to a second restaurant that is not generally liked as much. Second, variety may be absent in many situations where there is little choice. Examples include small children having food prepared by their parents, employees completing the tasks assigned by their supervisor, or news channels that all incessantly focus on the same hot news story of the day. Third, variety can work against an overall goal by increasing consumption. For example, adding variety to a four-course meal increased overall food intake by over 40% (Rolls, van Duijvenvoorde, & Rolls, 1984), presumably an undesirable outcome for many on a restrictive diet. These examples are not isolated cases, but rather they reflect the fact that variety is not an ideal response to recover from satiation.

More generally, it is widely assumed that the effects of satiation naturally dissipate over time as shown in Figure 4.1. In their seminal work on habituation, Thompson and Spencer (1966) called this process *spontaneous recovery*. For example, in one of the few studies of this process, people did not experience satiation effects when eating the same macaroni and cheese dish once a week for 5 weeks (Epstein, Carr, Cavanaugh, Paluch, & Bouton, 2011). The recovery period here of 7 days apparently provided enough time for people to recover from any past satiation. However, it should be noted that other work suggests that spontaneous recovery is not always quite so spontaneous. After hearing the chorus of their favorite song 20 times, participants seemingly showed little recovery in satiation even after 3 weeks (Galak, Redden, & Kruger, 2009). Regardless, satiation is not permanent, and people typically recover from it at some point.

The Benefits and Consequences of Satiation

The dynamic nature of desire resulting from satiation and recovery serves at least three vital purposes that each could have provided great value in our evolutionary development. First, satiation helps focus attention on changes in the environment, which are likely to be more important than constants. Here, a novel experience elicits an increased response and interest, which die off through satiation if the experience remains unchanged and poses little ongoing threat or opportunity. Second, satiation encourages variety seeking, which would have been necessary to ensure that an ancestor consumed an adequate amount of various needed nutrients. Third, satiation reduces the potential for overconsumption that could leave one less mobile and more vulnerable to predators. Regardless of these distal mechanisms, it is clear that satiation is a valuable adaptation that now extends to virtually every stimulus.

Although satiation is both necessary and important for well-being, it also presents a number of challenges for a wide range of audiences. For those focused on general happiness and well-being, satiation has been portrayed as a "hedonic treadmill" in which people must constantly find new and different experiences just to maintain a steady level of happiness (Brickman & Campbell, 1971; see also Oishi, Westgate, Tucker, & Komiya, Chapter 14, this volume). Policy makers and health workers must overcome satiation to keep people in compliance with interventions, while marketers face a similar challenge in increasing the usage and brand loyalty of their products. Finally, and perhaps of most significance, satiation poses a particular challenge for people trying to attain goals. Satiation makes it increasingly challenging to adhere to a restricted diet (e.g., eating salads for lunch every day) or a beneficial exercise regimen (e.g., going to the gym five times a week). Although people may find it particularly enjoyable when they initially start these endeavors, the inexorable march of satiation virtually guarantees that this enjoyment will be fleeting. Of course, when the activity no longer provides enjoyment, the likelihood of compliance invariably falls.

The Nature of Satiation

General Intuition

People often attribute satiation to physiological causes. For instance, after eating a large amount of food makes it less enjoyable, people often state that they "feel full" (Mook & Votaw, 1992). This view implies that food physically fills the stomach, and this distension signals to the body that the food should no longer be rewarding. The widespread acceptance of this account is reflected in aphorisms such as "his eyes were bigger than his stomach" or saying "unbuckle your belt" before a good meal. More generally, the intuitive belief is that the body provides feedback about consumption, and this feedback becomes less positive over the course of repeated consumption.

Although physiological mechanisms may contribute to satiation, they struggle to fully account for the various phenomena (McSweeney & Murphy, 2000). For instance, the food domain is where one might expect physiological explanations to be particularly appropriate, yet there are quite a few aspects this account cannot explain (see also Roefs, Houben, & Werthmann, Chapter 16, this volume). First, eating a food can decrease the liking of that food in a matter of a couple minutes (Hetherington, Rolls, & Burley, 1989), which is far too fast for any type of digestive process. Second, though a large meal can satiate one on that food, a novel food can instantly restore salivation (Epstein, Caggiula, Rodefer, Wisneiwski, & Mitchell, 1993) and seemingly eliminate effects of satiation. A common example of this is salivating over a dessert after becoming "full" from the entrée. Third, the extent of satiation is not closely linked to the caloric or macronutrient content of what has been eaten (Johnson & Vickers, 1993; Rolls, Hetherington, & Burley, 1988), indicating that a physiological inventory is not the driver of satiation. More generally, beyond the domain of food, physiological accounts would be less applicable to noningested stimuli such as art, aromas, cognitive work tasks, or social interactions (Galak et al., 2009; McSweeney & Swindell, 1999; Rolls & Rolls, 1997). The sum of this evidence makes a strong case that satiation is not just a physiological effect; in fact, it seems to be largely nonphysiological.

Specificity of Satiation

A core finding in the satiation literature is that satiation is greatest for the stimulus consumed and less for stimuli not consumed. This characteristic has been extensively studied as a phenomenon called sensory-specific satiety (Rolls, Rolls, Rowe, & Sweeney, 1981). This research paradigm involves first eating and rating liking of several samples from a range of different foods, next eating only one of those foods until choosing to stop, and then eating and rating liking for each of the sample foods again. The key finding is that liking drops much more for the food eaten in the middle step than any of the other samples. In fact, this increased drop also extends to other foods that share the same flavor (Johnson & Vickers, 1993), texture (Guinard & Brun, 1998), shape (Rolls, Rowe, & Rolls, 1982), or odor (Rolls & Rolls, 1997). These effects of sensory-specific satiety seem to peak a couple of minutes after ingestion, and subsequently diminish very little even after 60 minutes (Hetherington et al., 1989).

The core notion of sensory-specific satiety is that people satiate on a particular aspect of an experience. For food, this aspect is often flavor (Epstein et al., 1993; Johnson & Vickers, 1993), perhaps because flavor is highly salient. More generally, satiation appears to be greatest for the particular aspects garnering focal attention. For example, when eating jellybeans with labels that focused on the specific flavor (e.g., cherry or lemon) rather than the general candy type (e.g., jellybean), people satiated less quickly with the specific labels (Redden, 2008). Although everyone ate the same exact assortment of jellybeans, the more specific categorization made the experience seem less repetitive within that category. This indicates that the specificity of satiety depends on the focus of attention and the framing of an experience—a finding consistent with a nonphysiological view of satiation.

Constructed Aspect

Satiation does not simply reflect a running inventory of attributes that accumulates through consumption and depletes over time with physiological processing and forgetting (McAlister, 1982). A growing body of evidence indicates that satiation is instead largely constructed in the moment. For example, people show less satiation when they have less memory for past consumption, whether it be due to distractions that reduce encoding (Higgs & Woodward, 2009) or impairments causing amnesia (Rozin, Dow, Moscovitch, & Rajaram, 1998). In fact, merely imagining consumption can produce effects of satiation for subsequent consumption (Larson, Redden, & Elder, 2014; Morewedge, Huh, & Vosgerau, 2010). Satiation apparently arises in part from mental processes that recall and simulate past consumption.

Recent work posits that the construction of satiation entails a subjective sense of the extent of past consumption. After people viewed the same beach photo for 5 minutes, making them place themselves on a scale with altered ranges to make their level of exposure seem higher than others made that same beach photo less enjoyable on a subsequent exposure (Redden & Galak, 2013). Satiation was similarly increased by speeding up an online running clock to make it seem like less time had passed since the last consumption occasion (Galak, Redden, Yang, & Kyung, 2014). People seemingly construct satiation based on an observation of whether they have consumed the same thing repeatedly.

Insight into Satiation

Given that people often cite "being full" as the reason they stop eating (Mook & Votaw, 1992), it is perhaps not surprising that people seem to have little insight into the future course of satiation over time. People who ate yogurt every day over the course of a week expected to like it less over time, but instead actually came to like this previously unfamiliar food more (Kahneman & Snell, 1992). Likewise, people expected that having the same snack repeatedly each week would be much more satiating than it actually was (Simonson, 1990). People similarly do not realize that they could reduce their satiation by slowing down their rate of consumption (Galak, Kruger, & Loewenstein, 2013), or inserting breaks (Nelson & Meyvis, 2008; Nelson, Meyvis, & Galak, 2009); they instead chose faster consumption and no breaks in both cases.

More generally, people find it difficult to imagine how their future desire will differ from their current desire (Loewenstein & Schkade, 1999). That is, when in a "hot" state of desire, it is hard to imagine being in a "cold" state of satiation, and vice versa. As a result, people seemingly overestimate the satiating effect of consuming a favorite once again (Ratner, Kahn, & Kahneman, 1999), yet also underestimate the extent to which they will satiate on a product once they buy it and start using it in the future (Wang, Novemsky, & Dhar, 2009). In sum, people do not have an accurate insight into their future satiation, as it can easily be over- or underestimated.

Factors Influencing the Satiation Rate

Given that people apparently have little ability to predict satiation based on insight and intuition, controlled experimentation is required to identify the factors that can influence the satiation rate. It is important for people to understand how a factor affects satiation because this allows one to strategically manage desire. That is, for something one wants to consume less (e.g., chocolate ice cream), increasing the rate of satiation would contribute toward attaining the goal of improved long-term health. In contrast, for a virtue one wants to consume more (e.g., running on a treadmill), the opposing strategy of decreasing satiation would be more beneficial toward goal achievement and health. Using satiation as a means to encourage or discourage virtues and vices respectively could prove quite effective, especially given the ubiquity of chronic self-control failures due to a lack of willpower (Baumeister, 2002; Carver & Scheier, 1998). Of course, the strategic use of satiation first requires an understanding of the factors that influence the rate of satiation.

The remainder of this section discusses factors that have been shown to affect the rate of satiation (see Table 4.1). In some instances, the researchers explicitly measured enjoyment (or liking, desire, etc.) at multiple points in time so that satiation was clearly captured. However, in other cases, the only dependent measure was a behavior such as repeated choice or quantity consumed. The latter are still cited here as evidence of altering satiation because satiation likely contributed to the resulting behavior; of course, factors beyond satiation could instead be the drivers of those effects. These findings have still been included here because the behavioral data is compelling and quite relevant to important outcomes (e.g., consumer health). They also serve to underscore the opportunities and importance of measuring ongoing enjoyment to understand if satiation plays a critical role.

Accelerants of Satiation

Salient Sensory Aspect

A number of different aspects of the stimulus have been shown to influence satiation. In the domain of food, an obvious shared flavor has been found to increase sensory-specific satiety. People satiated more when two

TABLE 4.1. Factors Influencing the Satiation Rate

Effect on satiation	Factor	Examples
Accelerates	Salient sensory aspect	Guinard & Brun (1998); Inman (2001); Johnson & Vickers (1993); Raynor & Epstein (2001); Rolls et al. (1982, 1984, 1988)
	Reduced stimulus complexity	Berlyne (1971); Nicolao, Irwin, & Goodman (2009); O'Donohue & Geer (1985)
	Greater stimulus strength	Finkelstein & Fishbach (2010); O'Sullivan et al. (2010); Thompson & Spencer (1966); Galak, Kruger, & Loewenstein (2012)
	Faster consumption rate	Herrnstein (1990); Herrnstein & Prelec (1991); McAlister (1982); Nelson & Meyvis (2008); Thompson & Spencer (1966)
	Comparatively frequent consumption	Galak et al. (2014); Redden & Galak (2013); Sackett et al. (2010)
	Increased attention on consumption	Geier, Wansink, & Rozin (2012); Larson, Redden, & Elder (2014); Morewedge et al. (2010); Polivy et al. (1986); Redden & Haws (2013)
Slows	Increased variety	Heatherington et al. (2006); Raynor & Epstein (2001); Rolls et al. (1982, 1984)
	Cues of variety	Brown (1953); Galak et al. (2009); Kahn & Wansink (2004); Raghunathan & Irwin (2001); Redden (2008)
	Less encoding	Brunstrom & Mitchell (2006); Epstein et al. (2005); Higgs & Donohoe (2011); Higgs & Woodward (2009)
	Less attention to quantity consumed	Redden & Hawes (2013); Sevilla & Redden (2014); Wansink, Painter, & North (2005)

foods shared a flavor of blueberry over a creamy texture (Johnson & Vickers, 1993), and consumers tended to switch their purchases among flavors of chips more than brand (Inman, 2001). However, when eating bread, sharing the same hardness led to greater sensory-specific satiety than the flavor (Guinard & Brun, 1998). More generally, though, it seems that repeated consumption of a conscious sensory aspect leads to the greatest satiation (Raynor & Epstein, 2001). For many foods (perhaps not bread), this is likely the flavor. There is also evidence that satiation is faster for foods with a strong savory or sweet aspect (Rolls et al., 1984), and there is less satiation when the repeated aspect is a color shared by foods (Rolls et al., 1982) or a common macronutrient (Rolls et al., 1988).

Reduced Stimulus Complexity

Although this has not been widely tested, it is likely that more complex and intense experiences lead to more stimulation and less satiation (Berlyne, 1971; O'Donohue & Geer, 1985). For instance, a more complicated musical composition would satiate at a slower rate than a simple acoustic piece (Berlyne, 1971). Likewise, people adapt faster to material possessions than experiences (Nicolao, Irwin, & Goodman, 2009), perhaps because experiences are rich and constantly change with each episode.

Greater Stimulus Strength

Similar to stimulus complexity, another factor increasing the rate of satiation is stimulus strength. For instance, it is obvious that weakening a flavor to the point where it cannot be detected would likely slow satiation on that flavor. More subtle evidence has found that people show a greater drop in liking for spaghetti bolognese over five occasions when eating a lower-calorie versus the regular version (O'Sullivan, Alexander, Ferriday, & Brunstrom, 2010). Similarly, the mere perception of a change can matter, as people reported being hungrier after eating a sample simply labeled as healthy versus not (Finkelstein & Fishbach, 2010). However, it should be noted that the seminal work on habituation states that a defining characteristic is slower habituation to a stronger stimulus (Thompson & Spencer, 1966). To the extent satiation derives from habituation in a context, the stimulus strength and satiation may have a more complicated relationship.

Faster Consumption Rate

The rate of consumption would be an obvious candidate to accelerate satiation, and it does (Herrnstein, 1990; McAlister, 1982; Thompson & Spencer, 1966). Surprisingly, though, people seem largely unaware of the effect of consumption rate. People satiated less quickly to a massage prolonged by inserting breaks into it (Nelson & Meyvis, 2008; Nelson et al., 2009), even though they would choose beforehand to have no breaks. A similar lack of insight can also be seen in the rate of eating, as people left to their own devices satiate faster than those explicitly instructed to slow down (Galak et al., 2013). In a similar vein, in an effect called melioration (Herrnstein & Prelec, 1991), people tend to consume a favorite too frequently though they would benefit from slowing down their rate of consumption to allow more time for recovery from satiation.

Comparatively Frequent Consumption

There is also recent work showing that the mere perception of greater past consumption can increase the rate of satiation. In one study of this (Redden & Galak, 2013), participants were asked to indicate their frequency of seeing a beach photo using a scale in which the endpoints were designed to make them appear high or low on the scale. Participants made to respond higher on the scale (though actual usage was the same) then experienced greater satiation when seeing the same photo again. Similarly, satiation increased when people felt the experience itself seemed shorter (Sackett, Meyvis, Nelson, Converse, & Sackett, 2010) or less time had passed between consumption episodes (Galak et al., 2014) because an online clock made time appear to pass faster than reality.

Increased Attention on Consumption

A growing body of evidence indicates that the rate of satiation increases with greater monitoring of the quantity consumed. For example, people ate less of a candy when the wrappers of previously eaten pieces remained visible on the table rather than being thrown in the trash (Polivy, Herman, Hackett, & Kuleshnyk, 1986). People similarly ate fewer potato chips when there was a red chip to serve as a quantity cue every fifth chip versus every tenth chip (Geier, Wansink, & Rozin, 2012). In fact, a study focused on satiation indeed found that explicitly asking people to count the number of times they swallowed while eating a food led to a faster decline in enjoyment (Redden & Haws, 2013). This satiation from greater monitoring may even be triggered by merely thinking about consumption. People experienced greater satiation on cheese after imagining eating a cheese cube 30 times versus moving a cube (Morewedge et al., 2010), or even just rating the attractiveness of a food in an ad 60 times versus 20 times (Larson et al., 2014). These findings indicate that satiation increases as one thinks more about how much one has consumed something (even hypothetically) in the past.

Retardants of Satiation

Increased Variety

One obvious remedy for satiation is to increase variety. People indeed ate over 40% more calories when a four-course meal had a different food versus the same food for each course (Rolls et al., 1984). People also showed less decline in the liking of a food when their free eating was briefly interrupted to sample another food (Hetherington, Foster, Newman, Anderson, & Norton, 2006). The effect of variety on satiation and intake is so strong that it has often been cited as a contributing factor in the growing obesity rate (Raynor & Epstein, 2001). Variety can even affect satiation when it should be a "trivial" change that does not change the sensory experience. For example, people showed greater satiation on the color of M&M's eaten even though the color is merely cosmetic and does not alter the flavor (Rolls et al., 1982).

Cues of Variety

Beyond actual changes in variety, satiation also slows with the mere perception of greater variety and less repetition. People ate more M&M's when the large number of colors was made more evident by organizing the candies by color or varying the distribution of the colors (Kahn & Wansink, 2004), and poured more for consumption when variety was present due to quantity misperceptions (Redden & Hoch, 2009). Likewise, when nature photos were categorized more specifically (e.g., arctic wildlife, bird, beach, desert) versus more generally (animal or nature), people experienced less satiation while viewing them (Redden, 2008). Though not exactly a measure of satiation, similar differences in hedonic contrasts also depend on whether experiences are placed into a shared category (Brown, 1953; Raghunathan & Irwin, 2001).

Interestingly, people apparently need cues to fully appreciate the variety in their consumption and experience the reduced satiation it potentially brings. People given a bowl of a single candy and then a bowl of varied candy showed less satiation when eating the first candy again if first asked to reflect on the varied candy (Galak et al., 2009). It seems that satiation largely arises from thoughts about consumption of just the target stimulus, but this focus can be easily expanded by redirecting attention to appreciate the available variety.

Less Encoding

Effects of satiation that span the days between consumption occasions likely depend at least somewhat on memory. As a result, factors that inhibit encoding consumption into memory can reduce satiation. For example, distractions such as watching television during lunch led to greater intake at a later meal (Higgs & Donohoe, 2011; Higgs & Woodward, 2009), presumably because of poor encoding and less lingering satiation. Similarly, people showed less drop in salivation to pizza stimuli while completing a hard versus an easy visual memory task (Epstein, Saad, Giacomelli, & Roemmich, 2005), and they showed less drop in the desire to eat after eating snack cakes while playing a computer game (Brunstrom & Mitchell, 2006). These findings all demonstrate that the rate of satiation decreases as encoding the consumption experience becomes increasingly difficult.

Less Attention to Quantity Consumed

An emerging body of evidence identifies attention to the quantity consumed as an underlying driver of satiation. People satiate at a slower rate when left to themselves versus being instructed to monitor the quantity being consumed (Redden & Haws, 2013; Sevilla & Redden, 2014). However, there are instances when this natural monitoring system is less active and has less effect on satiation. For example, when eating soup from a bowl that refilled without their knowledge, people ate over 70% more soup yet did not indicate feeling more sated (Wansink, Painter, & North, 2005). Beyond being difficult (or nearly impossible) in some contexts, the attention to the quantity consumed can also be less active when satiation is maladaptive. When chocolate candy was available only for a limited time, people got less satiated because they paid less attention to the quantity consumed (Sevilla & Redden, 2014). These examples all indicate that satiation slows as people pay less attention to the quantity consumed.

Individual Differences in Satiation

It is clear that rates of satiation differ widely across people. For example, I satiate on sushi at a very slow rate and could likely eat it every day, but my wife would shudder at such an impoverished diet. Although there are clearly large individual differences, past research on satiation has not typically focused on them. Even so, there have been some traits that have been linked to changes in the rate of satiation.

Age

Rolls and colleagues (1991) found that people between 45 and 60 years old did not show typical sensory-specific satiety effects relative to their younger counterparts. Specifically, although older people did show signs of satiation, they were not greater for the eaten food versus other uneaten foods. This effect has also been replicated by others (Hollis & Henry, 2007).

Trait Self-Control

When measured using Tangney, Baumeister, and Boone's (2004) general trait self-control (TSC) scale, with items such as "I am good at resisting temptation," people with higher TSC satiated faster while eating an unhealthy candy bar versus a healthy snack of raisins (Redden & Haws, 2013). Here, process evidence indicated that they do this because they pay more attention to the quantity consumed when a food is unhealthy and turn off this monitoring for a healthy food not requiring vigilance. People with higher TSC also show greater evidence of spreading satiation whereby eating one food leads to greater satiation on a broader range of uneaten foods (Haws & Redden, 2013). These differences in satiation potentially help those with high TSC more consistently exert restraint (see also Harmon-Jones, Gable, & Harmon-Jones, Chapter 8, this volume).

Emotional Clarity

Satiation involves both the positive enjoyment of a liked stimulus as well as the negative feelings that can arise from repetition. People who are better able to separate these two emotions experienced less satiation when listening to instrumental music (Poor, Duhachek, & Krishnan, 2012). This suggests that people may be able to train themselves to reduce the impact of negative feelings from satiation.

Obesity

It would not be surprising to find a link between the rate of satiation and obesity given the former's effect on intake quantity. Indeed, adult women who were obese showed less reduction in salivation compared to nonobese counterparts when seeing the same food repeatedly (Epstein, Paluch, & Coleman, 1996). This effect was also replicated with children (Temple, Giacomelli, Roemmich, & Epstein, 2007), suggesting that satiation may contribute somewhat to the onset of obesity.

A Framework for Satiation

The previously cited examples illustrate the ubiquity and diversity of factors that can influence the rate of satiation. Such wide-ranging effects suggest that satiation is likely multiply determined; that is, there are multiple processes simultaneously contributing to satiation. Historically, research on satiation has generally fallen into one of two schools of thought. The first is the notion that experiences become less enjoyable as they satisfy a need, whether it be physiological hunger or cognitive boredom. The second is that satiation is largely driven by more psychological processes (e.g., adaptation, habituation) whereby nearly any stimulus loses its effectiveness in eliciting a reaction with repeated exposure. Both schools of thought envision satiation as arising from automatic low-level processes that are largely unavoidable. The simple result is that satiation increases as past consumption increases. These leading accounts of satiation both can be called "metered" approaches in that satiation directly results from the lingering effects of accumulated past consumption.

I propose here a novel taxonomy for satiation that expands beyond these metered approaches and the physiological versus psychological distinction. Specifically, it posits a homeostatic, perceptual, and reflective component that each contributes to satiation. These components taken together can readily account for the full range of satiation effects that have been found. As shown in Figure 4.2, each component is subsequently discussed in terms of potential mechanisms, stimulus types, onset delay, and core drivers.

Homeostatic Component

The homeostatic component maps largely onto a physiological account of satiation. This account proposes that the body has an internal set value (e.g., an optimal body weight), and that an internal signal indicates deviations from this internal target (Cabanac, 1971). Pleasure then reflects whether the current stimulus helps satisfy a lacking need state as indicated by the internal signal. In other words, pleasure indicates the usefulness of the stimulus to the body in reaching a desired homeostatic state of balance.

Given that repeated consumption satisfies such needs, it is invariable that satiation arises as the pleasure declines. Cabanac (1971) calls this "negative alliesthesia" to reflect the changing sensation that satiation and

	Homeostatic	Perceptual	Reflective
Potential Mechanisms	Internal set points Negative alliesthesia Hormones (e.g., leptin)	Adaptation Habituation	Memory recall inferences Metacognitions Top-down judgments
Stimulus Type	Ingested	Strong sensory aspect	Nearly all experiences
Onset Delay	Few minutes delay (depends on stimulus)	Instantaneous (interwoven with experience)	Milliseconds (linked to recall)
Core Driver	Bodily feedback	Muted response	Monitoring quantity

FIGURE 4.2. Taxonomy for components of satiation.

homeostasis bring. We can see how this component would work by imagining a person who is quite thirsty after being outside on a hot day. If she then comes inside and drinks some lemonade, the first sip is undoubtedly quite enjoyable as it quenches thirst. Of course, as she drinks more of the lemonade, she quickly moves out of a state of thirst and the enjoyment decreases in a corresponding manner.

This homeostatic account has been frequently employed to account for satiation and consumption quantities in the food domain (Benelem, 2009; Berthoud, 2004). As well, researchers have identified increasing levels of leptin during eating as a potential candidate as the internal signal for the hunger need (Kenny, 2013). Here, leptin modulates the sensitivity of the reward areas of the brain such that they are less responsive (i.e., produce less enjoyment) as increased leptin indicates greater past consumption.

Although it certainly could also apply to boredom with any task that induces cognitive fatigue and strained effort (O'Hanlon, 1981), the homeostatic component would be expected to primarily arise with ingested stimuli (e.g., food, drink). It is this physical material that the body will process to produce the internal signal to indicate a current need state. Of course, this feedback process will take time to develop, but its onset could be in a matter of minutes (perhaps 15–30 minutes for food). Regardless, the core driver of satiation here is bodily feedback about the extent to which a need state still has not been satisfied.

Perceptual Component

Beyond physiological drivers of satiation, there also exist well-known mechanisms of a more perceptual nature. The two predominant perceptual mechanisms would be adaptation and habituation. Adaptation decreases the sensory intensity of an experience as it deviates less from a point of reference (or adaptation level) that continually adjusts by incorporating recent exposures (Helson, 1964; Parducci, 1995). Similarly, yet not the same, habituation to a repeated stimulus reduces subsequent responses as people increasingly pay less attention to the stimulus (McSweeney & Swindell, 1999; Thompson & Spencer, 1966). We can clarify the distinction between these mechanisms by continuing the previous example of drinking lemonade on a hot day. The first few sips of lemonade provide great pleasure, but subsequent sips typically start to deliver less pleasure. This decline in pleasure occurs as the taste senses adjust such that lemonade and all other drinks now seem less sweet compared to the updated reference point (adaptation), and the conscious experience focuses on other more interesting aspects of the environment such as the sounds and people in the room (habituation). Of course, both mechanisms produce the key defining characteristic of satiation—a drop in enjoyment with repeated consumption.

Although other psychological mechanisms could also contribute to satiation, previous research has generally highlighted adaptation or habituation. For example, the lower satiation rate for experiences versus materials goods was linked to slower hedonic adaptation (Nicolao et al., 2009). Likewise, habituation can account for a wide range of the effects found in the satiation and motivation literatures (McSweeney & Swindell, 1999), even in the food domain, which presumably involves a larger physiological component than most other domains. Furthermore, the richly studied phenomenon of sensory-specific satiety has been tied to neural areas known to be active during habituation (O'Doherty et al., 2000). This evidence demonstrates that adaptation and habituation almost certainly contribute to the phenomenon of satiation.

The perceptual component of satiation exerts its influence nearly instantaneously. In fact, the very nature of it implies that its effects appear during the experience with which it is intertwined. As well, its contribution to satiation is likely greatest for experiences with a strong sensory aspect that potentially captures perceptual attention. This instantaneous effect and sensory focus suggest why the perceptual component likely accounts for sensory-specific satiety (O'Doherty et al., 2000), as well as a broad range of stimuli (McSweeney & Swindell, 1999). It can also easily account for why satiation decreases with distractions such as television (Higgs & Woodward, 2009) or difficult cognitive tasks (Brunstrom & Mitchell, 2006; Epstein et al., 2005) as these both impede habituation. More generally, the core notion of the perceptual account is that satiation reflects a muted response to a repeated, unchanging stimulus.

Reflective Component

The third component of satiation is more reflective in that it involves higher-order cognitions about the self and consumption. The general notion is that people reflect on their past consumption, and they feel more satiated if it seems like they have had the same thing over and over. For example, after listening to the chorus of their favorite song 20 times, people could once again enjoy their favorite song as much as ever only if they were asked to recall other musical artists heard during the intervening 3 weeks (Galak et al., 2009). This indicates that satiation is seemingly constructed in the moment partially based on judgments about past consumption.

Emerging evidence continues to provide growing support for a reflective component of satiation. Satiation decreased when people had difficulty recalling past consumption episodes of their favorite food because they inferred this indicated they had not consumed it much (Redden & Galak, 2013). Likewise, people had less lingering satiation when made to feel that more time had passed since the last consumption episode (Galak et al., 2014), or that their past consumption was less than that for other people (Redden & Galak, 2013). This reflective component also easily accounts for why increased tracking of the quantity consumed leads to greater satiation, as intermittent red potato chips (Geier et al., 2012), counting the number of swallows (Redden & Haws, 2013), or empty candy wrappers (Polivy et al., 1986) trigger reflection on the amount consumed. Beyond these and other examples, given that such reflective thoughts could apply to practically any repeated experience over any time frame, the reflective component of satiation potentially underlies a wide range of satiation phenomena. The key driver here is a reflection on the fact that one is repeatedly consuming the same thing.

Multiply Determined

This framework posits that (at least) three different components contribute to satiation. The contribution of each component will understandably vary across the context. For example, imagine a large meal at a restaurant. At the start of the meal, satiation after the first few bites is almost certainly driven by the perceptual component. As the meal progresses, and physiological feedback develops from digestion, the homeostatic component may eventually contribute more to satiation. Finally, a week after the meal, the reflective component most likely drives satiation when one thinks about eating the same entrée at that same restaurant again. Of course, we could easily see different patterns in other domains (e.g., no homeostatic component for music) or time frames (e.g., reflective component at the start if recently consumed).

Although the relevance of each component will vary across contexts, each of the multiple components likely operates in a simultaneous yet integrative fashion. That is, one might satiate from homeostatic, perceptual, and reflective processes with each contributing to an overall level of satiation. For instance, consider the finding that making the variety in a food assortment merely more salient increases intake (Kahn & Wansink, 2004). There would likely be digestive effects at some point, as well as perceptual effects that derive from less sensory-specific satiety (Rolls et al., 1982), and even reflective effects as the experience seems less repetitive (Redden, 2008). Perhaps the variety effect is so robust and strong precisely because it simultaneously taps into each component.

Furthermore, we can imagine that the components work together in other ways. To continue the food example of M&M's, one homeostatic account is that increased leptin levels reduce the sensitivity of neural reward areas (Kenny, 2013). It could also be that this reduced sensitivity in a general reward area also amplifies the perceptual and reflective components. Put another way, the three components may operate in not only an independent fashion but also an interactive fashion. This multifaceted nature of satiation perhaps explains the ubiquity of satiation and the diversity of factors that moderate the rate of satiation.

Future Directions

The previous framework has identified three components of satiation: homeostatic, perceptual, and reflective. There are potentially several other components that future research will uncover. Or, more likely, these three components will be broken down into more specific subcomponents. For instance, the perceptual component has already identified adaptation and habituation as underlying mechanisms, but there could certainly be others, such as those related to categorization (Redden, 2008). Likewise, the reflective component may rely on very different inferences during the initial onset versus recovery from satiation, or on whether there is a goal to increase consumption. Neural studies of satiation (e.g., fMRI) may prove useful in teasing out specific differences both between and within the three components.

One goal of this chapter is to highlight the dynamic, changing aspect of desire created by satiation. An important implication of this is that desire and liking cannot be captured with a snapshot at a single point in time. Instead, one must repeatedly measure desire over time to properly understand enjoyment and allow for the effects of satiation. For example, although people tend to want something more when it is scarce (Worchel, Lee, & Adewole, 1975), scarcity increased enjoyment only over time by slowing the rate of satiation (Sevilla & Redden, 2014). Therefore, one looking just at initial enjoyment would conclude that scarcity has no effect on ongoing temptation, when exactly the opposite is true. As a result of these changes over time, longitudinal studies with regular sampling will likely grow in popularity as a research tool (e.g., see Hofmann, Baumeister, Forster, & Vohs, 2011), and will potentially become a standard tool in the area of taste testing and product marketing.

An understanding of the dynamics of desire over time will also be critical for designing effective interventions. Many people with self-control problems (e.g., obesity) suffer consequences primarily because of a pattern of chronic self-control failures. One way to limit such behavior is to increase satiation on the tempting item such that resisting it becomes quite easy and natural. This chapter has identified a framework for understanding and influencing satiation that a wide range of audiences (e.g., policy makers, consumers, and marketing organizations) can potentially leverage.

Although we have learned a great deal about satiation, and evidence continues to rapidly push our understanding, there are still many puzzling aspects of satiation that have defied clear answers. For example, why would people get so satiated with having the same entrée for dinner each night, yet these same people eat the same thing for breakfast each morning? How do experts overcome satiation and stay engaged so they can build up the hours of experience needed to gain expertise? Why do children often complain of being bored and having nothing to do when they are surrounded by a myriad of video games, books, toys, foods, and so forth? Hopefully, at this point, the reader realizes that the answers may lie in the different components of satiation (especially the reflective component in these instances). Future work is needed to truly uncover why these satiation phenomena happen, as well as many others, and the framework in this chapter provides a starting base for this endeavor.

REFERENCES

Baumeister, R. F. (2002). Yielding to temptation: Self-control failure, impulsive purchasing, and consumer behavior. *Journal of Consumer Research, 28*(4), 670–676.

Benelem, B. (2009). Satiation, satiety and their effects on eating behaviour. *Nutrition Bulletin, 34*(2), 126–173.

Berlyne, D. E. (1971). *Aesthetics and psychobiology.* New York: Appleton-Century-Crofts.

Bernoulli, D. (1954). Exposition of a new theory on the measurement of risk. *Econometrica, 22*, 23–36.

Berthoud, H.-R. (2004). Mind versus metabolism in the control of food intake and energy balance. *Physiology and Behavior, 81*(5), 781–793.

Brickman, P., & Campbell, D. T. (1971). Hedonic relativism and planning the good society. In M. H. Appley (Ed.), *Adaptation-level theory* (pp. 287–302). New York: Academic Press.

Brown, D. R. (1953). Stimulus-similarity and the anchoring of subjective scales. *American Journal of Psychology, 66*, 199–214.

Brunstrom, J. M., & Mitchell, G. L. (2006). Effects of distraction on the development of satiety. *British Journal of Nutrition, 96*(4), 761–769.

Cabanac, M. (1971). Physiological role of pleasure. *Science, 173*(4002), 1103–1107.

Carver, C. S., & Scheier, M. F. (1998). *On the self-regulation of behavior.* New York: Cambridge University Press.

Epstein, L. H., Caggiula, A. R., Rodefer, J. S., Wisneiwski, L., & Mitchell, S. L. (1993). The effects of calories and taste on habituation of the human salivary response. *Addictive Behaviors, 18*(2), 179–185.

Epstein, L. H., Carr, K. A., Cavanaugh, M. D., Paluch, R. A., & Bouton, M. E. (2011). Long-term habituation to food in obese and nonobese women. *American Journal of Clinical Nutrition, 94*(2), 371–376.

Epstein, L. H., Paluch, R., & Coleman, K. J. (1996). Differences in salivation to repeated food cues in obese and nonobese women. *Psychosomatic Medicine, 58*(2), 160–164.

Epstein, L. H., Saad, F. G., Giacomelli, A. M., & Roemmich, J. N. (2005). Effects of allocation of attention on habituation to olfactory and visual food stimuli in children. *Physiology and Behavior, 84*(2), 313–319.

Finkelstein, S. R., & Fishbach, A. (2010). When healthy food makes you hungry. *Journal of Consumer Research, 37*, 357–367.

Galak, J., Kruger, J., & Loewenstein, G. (2013). Slow down! Insensitivity to rate of consumption leads to avoidable satiation. *Journal of Consumer Research, 39*(5), 993–1009.

Galak, J., Redden, J. P., & Kruger, J. (2009). Variety amnesia: Recalling past variety can accelerate recovery from satiation. *Journal of Consumer Research, 36*(4), 575–584.

Galak, J., Redden, J. P., Yang, Y., & Kyung, E. J. (2014). Feast today makes fast tomorrow? Influencing satiation through perceptions of temporal distance. *Journal of Experimental Social Psychology, 52*, 118–123.

Geier, A., Wansink, B., & Rozin, P. (2012). Red potato chips: Segmentation cues can substantially decrease food intake. *Health Psychology, 31*(3), 398–401.

Guinard, J.-X., & Brun, P. (1998). Sensory-specific satiety: Comparison of taste and texture effects. *Appetite, 31*(2), 141–157.

Haws, K. L., & Redden, J. P. (2013). In control of variety: High self-control reduces the effect of variety on food consumption. *Appetite, 69*(1), 196–203.

Helson, H. (1964). *Adaptation-level theory.* New York: Harper & Row.

Herrnstein, R. J. (1990). Behavior, reinforcement, and utility. *Psychological Science, 1*(4), 217–224.

Herrnstein, R. J., & Prelec, D. (1991). Melioration: A theory of distributed choice. *Journal of Economic Perspectives, 5*(3), 137–156.

Hetherington, M. M., Foster, R., Newman, T., Anderson, A. S., & Norton, G. (2006). Understanding variety: Tasting different foods delays satiation. *Physiology and Behavior, 87*(2), 263–271.

Hetherington, M. M., Rolls, B. J., & Burley, V. J. (1989). The time course of sensory-specific satiety. *Appetite, 12*(1), 57–68.

Higgs, S., & Donohoe, J. E. (2011). Focusing on food during lunch enhances lunch memory and decreases later snack intake. *Appetite, 57*(1), 202–206.

Higgs, S., & Woodward, M. (2009). Television watching during lunch increases afternoon snack intake of young women. *Appetite, 52*(1), 39–43.

Hofmann, W., Baumeister, R. F., Forster, G., & Vohs, K. D. (2011). Everyday temptations: An experience sampling study of desire, conflict, and self-control. *Journal of Personality and Social Psychology, 102*(6), 1318–1335.

Hollis, J. H., & Henry, C. J. K. (2007). Sensory-specific satiety and flavor amplification of foods. *Journal of Sensory Studies, 22*(4), 367–376.

Inman, J. J. (2001). The role of sensory-specific satiety in attribute-level variety seeking. *Journal of Consumer Research, 28*(1), 105–120.

Johnson, J., & Vickers, Z. (1993). Effects of flavor and macronutrient composition of food servings on liking, hunger, and subsequent intake. *Appetite, 21*(1), 25–39.

Kahn, B. E., & Wansink, B. (2004). The influence of assortment structure on perceived variety and consumption quantities. *Journal of Consumer Research, 30*(4), 519–533.

Kahneman, D., & Snell, J. (1992). Predicting a changing taste: Do people know what they will like? *Journal of Behavioral Decision Making, 5*, 187–200.

Kenny, P. J. (2013). The food addiction. *Scientific American, 309*(3), 44–49.

Larson, J. S., Redden, J. P., & Elder, R. S. (2014). Satiation from sensory simulation: Evaluating foods decreases enjoyment of similar foods. *Journal of Consumer Psychology, 24*(2), 188–194.

Loewenstein, G., & Schkade, D. (1999). Wouldn't it be nice? Predicting future feelings. In D. Kahneman, E. Diener, & N. Schwarz (Eds.), *Well-being: The foundations of hedonic psychology* (pp. 85–105). New York: Sage.

McAlister, L. (1982). A dynamic attribute satiation model of variety-seeking behavior. *Journal of Consumer Research, 9*(2), 141–149.

McSweeney, F. K., & Murphy, E. S. (2000). Criticisms of the satiety hypothesis as an explanation for within-session decreases in responding. *Journal of the Experimental Analysis of Behavior, 7*(3), 347–361.

McSweeney, F. K., & Swindell, S. (1999). General-process theories of motivation revisited: The role of habituation. *Psychological Bulletin, 125*(4), 437–457.

Mook, D. G., & Votaw, M. C. (1992). How important is hedonism? Reasons given by college students for ending a meal. *Appetite, 18*(1), 69–75.

Morewedge, C. K., Huh, Y. E., & Vosgerau, J. (2010). Thought for food: Imagined consumption reduces actual consumption. *Science, 330*(6010), 1530–1533.

Nelson, L. D., & Meyvis, T. (2008). Interrupted consumption: Disrupting adaptation to hedonic experiences. *Journal of Marketing Research, 45*(6), 654–664.

Nelson, L. D., Meyvis, T., & Galak, J. (2009). Enhancing the television-viewing experience through commercial interruptions. *Journal of Consumer Research, 36*(2), 160–172.

Nestler, E. J., & Malenka, R. C. (2004). The addicted brain. *Scientific American, 290*(3), 78–85.

Nicolao, L., Irwin, J. R., & Goodman, J. K. (2009). Happiness for sale: Do experiential purchases make consumers happier than material purchases? *Journal of Consumer Research, 36*(2), 188–198.

O'Doherty, J., Rolls, E. T., Francis, S., Bowtell, R., McGlone, F., Kobal, G., et al. (2000). Sensory-specific satiety-related olfactory activation of the human orbitofrontal cortex. *NeuroReport, 11*(2), 399–403.

O'Donohue, W. T., & Geer, J. H. (1985). The habituation of sexual arousal. *Archives of Sexual Behavior, 14*(3), 233–246.

O'Hanlon, J. F. (1981). Boredom: Practical consequences and a theory. *Acta Psychologica, 49*, 53–82.

O'Sullivan, H. L., Alexander, E., Ferriday, D., & Brunstrom, J. M. (2010). Effects of repeated exposure on liking for a reduced-energy-dense food. *American Journal of Clinical Nutrition, 91*(6), 1584–1589.

Parducci, A. (1995). *Happiness, pleasure, and judgment: The contextual theory and its applications.* Mahwah, NJ: Erlbaum.

Pechmann, C., & Stewart, D. W. (1988). Advertising repetition: A critical review of wearin and wearout. *Current Issues and Research in Advertising, 11*(1–2), 285–329.

Polivy, J., Herman, C. P., Hackett, R., & Kuleshnyk, I. (1986). The effects of self-attention and public attention on eating in restrained and unrestrained subjects. *Journal of Personality and Social Psychology, 50*(6), 1253–1260.

Poor, M., Duhachek, A., & Krishnan, S. (2012). The moderating role of emotional differentiation on satiation. *Journal of Consumer Psychology, 22*(4), 507–519.

Raghunathan, R., & Irwin, J. R. (2001). Walking the hedonic product treadmill: Default contrast and mood-based assimilation in judgments of predicted happiness with a target product. *Journal of Consumer Research, 28*(3), 355–368.

Ratner, R. K., Kahn, B. E., & Kahneman, D. (1999). Choosing less-preferred experiences for the sake of variety. *Journal of Consumer Research, 26*(1), 1–15.

Raynor, H. A., & Epstein, L. H. (2001). Dietary variety, energy regulation, and obesity. *Psychological Bulletin, 127*(3), 325–341.

Redden, J. P. (2008). Reducing satiation: The role of categorization level. *Journal of Consumer Research, 34*(5), 624–634.

Redden, J. P., & Galak, J. (2013). The subjective sense of feeling satiated. *Journal of Experimental Psychology: General, 142*(1), 209–217.

Redden, J. P., & Haws, K. L. (2013). Healthy satiation: The role of decreasing desire in effective self-control. *Journal of Consumer Research, 39*(5), 1100–1114.

Redden, J. P., & Hoch, S. J. (2009). The presence of variety reduces perceived quantity. *Journal of Consumer Research, 36*(3), 406–417.

Rolls, B. J., Hetherington, M. M., & Burley, V. J. (1988). Sensory stimulation and energy density in the development of satiety. *Physiology and Behavior, 44*(6), 727–733.

Rolls, B. J., & McDermott, T. M. (1991). Effects of age on sensory-specific satiety. *American Journal of Clinical Nutrition, 54*(6), 988–996.

Rolls, B. J., Rolls, E. T., Rowe, E. A., & Sweeney, K. (1981). Sensory specific satiety in man. *Physiology and Behavior, 27*(1), 137–142.

Rolls, B. J., Rowe, E. A., & Rolls, E. T. (1982). How sensory properties of foods affect human feeding behavior. *Physiology & Behavior, 29*(3), 409–417.

Rolls, B. J., van Duijvenvoorde, P. M., & Rolls, E. T. (1984). Pleasantness changes and food intake in a varied four-course meal. *Appetite, 5*(4), 337–348.

Rolls, E. T., & Rolls, J. H. (1997). Olfactory sensory-specific satiety in humans. *Physiology and Behavior, 61*(3), 461–473.

Rozin, P., Dow, S., Moscovitch, M., & Rajaram, S. (1998). What causes humans to begin and end a meal? A role for memory for what has been eaten, as evidenced by a study of multiple meal eating in amnesiac patients. *Psychological Science, 9*(5), 392–396.

Sackett, A. M., Meyvis, T., Nelson, L. D., Converse, B. A., & Sackett, A. L. (2010). You're having fun when time flies: The hedonic consequences of subjective time progression. *Psychological Science, 21*(1), 111–117.

Sevilla, J., & Redden, J. P. (2014). Perceived scarcity reduces the rate of satiation. *Journal of Marketing Research, 51*(2), 205–217.

Simonson, I. (1990). The effect of purchase quantity and timing on variety-seeking behavior. *Journal of Marketing Research, 27*(2), 150–162.

Tangney, J. P., Baumeister, R. F., & Boone, A. L. (2004). High self-control predicts good adjustment, less pathology, better grades, and interpersonal success. *Journal of Personality, 72*(2), 271–324.

Temple, J. L., Giacomelli, A. M., Roemmich, J. N., & Epstein, L. H. (2007). Overweight children habituate slower than non-overweight children to food. *Physiology and Behavior, 91*(2–3), 250–254.

Thompson, R. F., & Spencer, W. A. (1966). Habituation: A model phenomenon for the study of neuronal substrates of behavior. *Psychological Review, 73*(1), 16–43.

Wang, J., Novemsky, N., & Dhar, R. (2009). Anticipating adaptation to products. *Journal of Consumer Research, 36*(2), 149–159.

Wansink, B., Painter, J. E., & North, J. (2005). Bottomless bowls: Why visual cues of portion size may influence intake. *Obesity, 13*(1), 93–100.

Worchel, S., Lee, J., & Adewole, A. (1975). Effects of supply and demand on ratings of object value. *Journal of Personality and Social Psychology, 32*(5), 906–914.

Zajonc, R. B. (1968). Attitudinal effects of mere exposure. *Journal of Personality and Social Psychology, 9*(2), 1–27.

CHAPTER 5

The Measurement of Desires and Craving

Michael A. Sayette
Stephen J. Wilson

Consider the following: A study claims to show that cigarette cravings were reduced by a new medication. A review of the data reveals, however, that the participants reported fairly low (if any) desire to smoke at all measurement points throughout the study. Another study tests a medication's effect on alcohol "craving" by relying on one question concerning whether the patient would choose to drink if he were discharged from the hospital with unlimited financial resources. A third experiment asks participants to report their global cravings over the past week. Few would dispute the importance of studying craving as a means to advance understanding of addiction and the development of new interventions. Inclusion of craving as a diagnostic criterion for substance use disorders in the newly minted fifth edition of the *Diagnostic and Statistical Manual of Mental Disorders* (DSM-5; American Psychiatric Association, 2013) reinforces its significance. Expensive craving studies are routinely conducted and yet when it comes to selecting the all-important measures of craving, as illustrated in these three examples the field remains far from unified in how craving is conceived and measured. One is justified in wondering just how far we have progressed since the association between craving and addiction was debated more than a half century ago (World Health Organization, 1955).

In an attempt to address this concern, in the late 1990s we participated in an effort to raise awareness of the importance of craving assessment (Sayette et al., 2000). The present chapter aims to summarize and update many of the issues raised in that earlier article, with a focus on recent work conducted in our own laboratories. Our view is that while considerable progress has been made, important conceptual issues remain to be solved.

We believe that desires and cravings may be experienced with regard to a wide range of objects (e.g., drugs, food, sex). Because there is no single accepted measure of craving, the challenge is to select the optimal measure(s) for a particular research or clinical application. One goal of this chapter is to offer some guidelines for selecting appropriate measures of craving. We begin by summarizing definitions of craving and related conceptual issues. Next, we consider self-reported craving, which is the most popular type of assessment. Included here is a summary of measurement performance issues. Factors that influence choice of craving measures are next addressed. Finally, nonverbal measures are discussed with a focus on functional brain imaging, as this response domain represents the area of greatest development since 2000. Although our chapter also likely applies to the concept of desire more broadly and to a much wider range of domains, we will focus primarily on cigarette craving.

Conceptual Issues

Though drug craving has been defined in many ways, it typically is regarded as a desire to use a drug. With few exceptions (e.g., Tiffany, 1990), craving has been conceptualized as reflecting a drug acquisitive state motivating drug use. Below we briefly summarize six definitional issues that remain unresolved (see Sayette et al., 2000 for elaboration on the first five of these issues).

First, investigators have questioned whether craving should be viewed as a dimensional construct that can be indexed along a broad continuum of desire or instead be restricted to an experience characterized by extreme desire (Kozlowski & Wilkinson, 1987; Sayette et al., 2000). Interestingly, while the latter definition is consistent with lay and dictionary definitions that specify craving to be a strong and deep desire, researchers typically assess craving as if it can be any level of desire. This distinction is not trivial. There are many studies that include "craving" in their titles that nevertheless report data indicating that participants never came close to experiencing a strong desire (see Sayette & Tiffany, 2013; Wilson & Sayette, 2015). This point can be illustrated with data collected as part of a study (Sayette, Martin, Wertz, Shiffman, & Perrott, 2001) that we conducted using both heavy and light smokers not currently interested in quitting. Shortly after smoking cue exposure, all were offered the chance to smoke their preferred brand of cigarette (sitting in front of them) without penalty. About one-third of the total sample declined to smoke this cigarette. Despite this disinclination to smoke, these participants' mean score on a 0–100 urge scale recorded just seconds earlier was 28. This value was significantly higher than their corresponding baseline mean rating (18), and thus one could interpret this change as being a significant increase in craving. Yet these smokers (all but one of whom were either nondeprived, or light smoking tobacco chippers, or both) clearly were not experiencing an intense state of craving that would drive a decision to smoke—indeed, they apparently were uninterested in smoking a cigarette. In sum, this statistically significant increase in "craving" may be somewhat inconsequential, as these smokers seemed to have no actual desire to smoke. Accordingly, the notion that all increases in craving along a continuum starting with zero are equivalent requires further consideration. While we tend to assess craving along a dimension, our suspicion is that craving starting at the upper end of the continuum may have unique properties and particular clinical significance (Sayette & Tiffany, 2013). Importantly, though, evidence to support such a position often can be obtained while desire is being measured dimensionally.

Second, researchers differ regarding the content or scope of their definition. While most define craving as a desire (or a strong desire) for drug use, others target the intention to use a drug. Tiffany and Drobes (1991) suggest the term *craving* should encompass anticipation of a drug's reinforcing effects, intention to engage in drug use, and desire for the drug. Alternatively, views of craving that include concepts in addition to desire have been criticized for including processes that are correlated with, but conceptually distinct from, craving (Kozlowski, Pillitteri, Sweeney, Whitfield, & Grahamet, 1996).

Third, there remains debate regarding the time frame of a craving experience. Some researchers have measured craving assuming it to be fairly stable (e.g., rating craving for a particular day or week). Alternatively, craving can be viewed as a momentary state (Gawin, 1991). It has become apparent that craving vacillates over the course of a day, and ratings obtained at different times have different meanings and predictive power (Shiffman, Paty, Gnys, Kassel, & Hickcox, 1996).

Fourth, though most investigators assume individuals must be subjectively aware—or metaconscious (see Sayette, Schooler, & Reichle, 2010a)—of their state, some have suggested that craving might exist outside of conscious awareness (Berridge & Robinson, 1995). If one can crave without awareness, then nonverbal measures such as neural activation, drug seeking, and drug use behavior ought to feature at least as prominently as self-report measures in craving assessment. When craving is only measured as drug use behavior, however, one can question the utility of invoking any craving construct, conscious or otherwise (Mello, 1978).

Fifth, there remain questions concerning the extent to which craving and drug use should be associated. Some have suggested particular situations in which measures drawn from different response systems (e.g., psychophysiology, self-report, behavior) should converge (Baker, Morse, & Sherman, 1987; Sayette, Martin, Hull, Wertz, & Perrott, 2003a). Of particular interest has been the putative association between craving and relapse. Many researchers have linked craving to relapse, claiming that craving is necessary for relapse (e.g., Ludwig & Wikler, 1974). This view has been criticized on both conceptual (Tiffany, 1990) and empirical (Perkins, 2009) grounds. Most would agree that craving is not an inevitable concomitant of relapse (Baker et al., 1987; Kassel & Shiffman, 1992). Nevertheless, a recent literature review suggests that measures related to craving do in fact predict relapse and have clinical relevance (Sayette & Tiffany, 2013; see also Franken, Chapter 19, this volume). Despite this clinical relevance, limitations in the manipulation and measurement of craving (e.g., with regard to intensity) clearly have hampered understanding of the association between desire and use.

Finally, the emotional valence of a craving state requires further consideration. Traditionally, the affect associated with craving has been assumed to be negative (e.g., frustration: Tiffany, 1992). Indeed, a negative reinforcement view of addiction is that drug use may ensue in order to alleviate cravings (Niaura et al., 1988). Other investigators suggest, however, that cravings also can be associated with positive affect (Baker et al., 1987; Sayette & Hufford, 1995). Building on Baumeister, Heatherton, and Tice's (1994) assertion that people may sometimes acquiesce in their own self-regulation failures, we have suggested that at times individuals may indulge their cravings (Sayette et al., 2003b). The idea is that, in some instances (e.g., when one intends to satisfy one's craving by using the substance in the very near future), individuals may savor the craving experience, such that the craving itself is rewarding. From an economic perspective, Loewenstein (1987) has described *savoring* as the "positive utility derived from anticipation of future consumption" (p. 667). Children who hoard their Halloween candy rather than eating it, for example, may prefer savoring their candy to actually consuming it. More recently, we have examined the instances in which craving seems to evoke both positive and negative affect reactions simultaneously (Griffin & Sayette, 2008). The idea that cravings can reflect ambivalence fits with various approaches to craving (Breiner, Stritzke, & Lang, 1999; Griffin & Sayette, 2008; Kavanagh, Andrade, & May, 2005; see also van Harreveldt, Nohlen, & Schneider, Chapter 13, this volume). The expanded use of nonverbal affect measures such as facial coding, electroencephalography (EEG), and functional magnetic resonance imaging (fMRI) has begun to offer new insights into the hedonic tone of cravings.

In summary, while research has proliferated examining the clinical utility of craving, many of the same conceptual questions plaguing the field at the time of our prior review remain unresolved. To some extent, difficulty selecting appropriate measures is attributable to a failure to articulate what is meant by craving (Sayette et al., 2000). Regardless of one's definition, however, it is critical for researchers to select measures appropriate for their definition and to draw conclusions that are appropriate to the measure. The remainder of this chapter addresses a range of methodological issues associated with the assessment of drug craving.

Self-Report Measures of Craving

Nearly all conceptualizations of craving assume that drug-motivational processes can be indexed, at least in part, through self-report measures of subjective experience. These measures are popular due to their face validity, ease of construction, and ease of use. Yet self-reports of craving do not permit a *direct readout of an individual's craving state*. This interpretation of the meaning of a self-report measure, which assumes a one-to-one mapping of verbal reports to hypothetical internal states, has been described as the correspondence view of test meaning (Wiggens, 1973). Although intuitively appealing, the correspondence view rests on a number of implausible assumptions. In our prior article, we detailed a number of measurement performance issues that distinguished the many types of self-report instruments (Sayette et al., 2000). We briefly summarize them below.

Validity

The most critical concern when considering measures of craving is their validity. In a general sense, validity refers to the appropriateness of inferences made about scientific data (Cook & Campbell, 1979). The validity of a measure has been defined as the "appropriateness, meaningfulness, and usefulness of inferences" made from test scores (American Educational Research Association, American Psychological Association, & National Council on Measurement in Education, 1985). There are several types of validity that apply to different aspects of craving measurement performance, including face validity, content-related validity, criterion-related validity, convergent validity, and discriminant validity (for elaboration see Sayette et al., 2000). Especially important is *construct validity*, which refers to the adequacy and explanatory power of scientific concepts, such as craving. Construct validation involves associating multiple measures with other theoretically relevant behaviors under conditions that are believed to affect the construct (e.g., during drug abstinence or drug cue exposure). This process typically requires the amassing of data from a variety of sources and experimental contexts (Cronbach & Meehl, 1955).

   One innovative example of such cross-validation comes from recent work integrating ecological momentary assessment (EMA) and fMRI methods to study craving (Berkman, Falk, & Lieberman, 2011). In the study, fMRI was used to measure brain responses during a motor task involving the suppression of unwanted actions in a sample of smokers shortly before they attempted to quit smoking. Subsequently, EMA methods were used to assess the relationship between self-reported craving and smoking while participants attempted to quit smoking. Greater activation during the suppression of actions in several brain regions (i.e., right inferior frontal gyrus, pre-supplementary motor area, and basal ganglia) prior to cessation was associated with a weaker correlation between craving and smoking during the quit attempt. The data obtained using EMA thus offer support toward the validity and clinical relevance of the fMRI results.

In general, there is no single craving construct; there are as many craving constructs as there are craving theories. Evidence for construct validity is more likely to develop as the adequacy of craving theories increases (Sayette et al., 2000). The validity of craving measures is affected by a number of criteria. These include reliability, reactivity (obtrusiveness), specificity, sensitivity, and floor and ceiling effects.

Reliability

The reliability of a self-report measure typically refers to its ability to provide scores that are consistent and stable. Several different kinds of reliability can be measured, reflecting different sources of variance in observed scores (see Sayette et al., 2000; Wray, Gass, & Tiffany, 2014). Perhaps the most important advantage of high reliability is the relationship between reliability and validity. That is, the power to reveal the impact of any pharmacological or behavioral manipulation on craving will depend, in part, on the extent to which the measure of craving is reliable.

Reactivity

Measuring craving using a self-report assessment necessarily requires participants to reflect on their experience, which under certain conditions may influence craving itself. It is well established that self-monitoring can change the behavior being monitored (Perlmuter, Noblin, & Hakami, 1983). Self-report assessment brings craving into awareness by eliciting controlled processing that demands attentional resources (see Sayette et al., 2010a). Because many aspects of a drug-use routine may be automatized (Tiffany, 1990), such a shift in processing resulting from assessment may create or modify a conscious craving experience (Baker & Brandon, 1990). Increasing the frequency with which a measure is administered may exacerbate this problem. Generally, studies using pre- and post-manipulation designs include noncraving "control" manipulations to account for a main effect of measurement. This approach does not, however, control for *interactions* between the repeated use of a measure and a craving manipulation (Carlsmith, Ellesworth, & Aronson, 1976). A baseline urge assessment may, for example, be more likely to cue a craving for a nicotine-deprived heavy smoker than for a nondeprived light smoker. In our view, this relative lack of concern with the reactivity of craving measures remains an important challenge for the field.

Specificity

Specificity refers to the ability of a measure to capture the construct of interest without being affected by other variables. A drug craving measure with adequate specificity should be relatively insensitive to other factors, such as hunger or fatigue. In part due to the myriad conceptualizations of craving that exist, there has been little research aimed at determining the specificity of craving measures. This issue is just as problematic when considering nonverbal craving measures.

Sensitivity

Sensitivity refers to the ability of a measure to detect variation in the construct of interest. Different measures, or different items on a scale, may have different thresholds for detecting craving (see Cook & Selltiz, 1964). Thus the item "I would do almost anything for a cigarette now" may have less sensitivity than "It would be nice to smoke right now," as presumably a stronger degree of craving would be required before change would result on the former item relative to the latter one (though see Kozlowski & Wilkinson, 1987).

Ceiling and Floor Effects

Ceiling and floor effects are especially relevant to craving assessment. A ceiling effect occurs when individuals tend to report similarly high craving levels at or near the endpoint of the measurement scale despite actual differences in experienced craving. Our prior review across multiple labs revealed that under high craving conditions (e.g., heavy smokers who are nicotine deprived), ceiling effects are not uncommon (Sayette et al., 2000). A floor effect occurs when a scale is insensitive to craving, leading to scores that are uniformly low. Low levels of craving report may be an accurate depiction of a minimal craving experience (perhaps due to an ineffective manipulation) or may be due to floor effects resulting from a scale with a high sensitivity threshold.

To avoid ceiling effects, studies might include approaches such as data transformation, questionnaires containing a wide range of craving levels represented across the items, computerized adaptive testing, or magnitude estimation. As detailed elsewhere, however, none of these alternatives offers perfect solutions to ceiling effects (Sayette & Tiffany, 2013). Nevertheless, ceiling effects should not be ignored when interpreting craving data. Provocative conclusions (e.g., that heavily dependent or nicotine-deprived smokers are *less* reactive to cues than are less dependent or nondeprived smokers) should first rule out the possibility that the highest cravers simply had less room on the scale to display their full cravings.

Number of Items

Self-report questionnaires differ on a variety of dimensions. Often the decision to select one format over another has been idiosyncratic and few data are available to evaluate them. Perhaps the most discussed issue concerns the number of items on the scale (see Sayette et al., 2000, for elaboration regarding various assessment parameters that have varied on self-report instruments). Clearly reliability can be increased with the use of multi-item, relative to single-item, scales. Yet it also is likely that increasing the number of items on the self-report measure would increase the reactivity of the measure. During certain craving induction procedures, immediate responses to craving manipulations are desired (e.g., Sayette & Hufford, 1995), and especially brief ratings may reduce the chance that the time required to complete the measure will interfere with (either by increasing or decreasing) craving levels. While debate persists on this issue, it has been our experience that brief, even single-item, urge scales, which are easiest to administer in experimental research, tend to be similarly sensitive in capturing cravings as are longer scales (Wertz & Sayette, 2001). Indeed, a recent trend has been toward use of shorter craving measures when conducting laboratory craving research. For instance, a four-item version of the popular Questionnaire of Smoking Urges now is often used in studies requiring repeated assessments (e.g., Wray et al., 2014), in lieu of the original 32-item scale (Tiffany & Drobes, 1991).

Factors Affecting the Choice of Self-Report Measure

Between- versus Within-Subject Comparisons

One important issue that needs to be considered in designing measures of craving is whether one is primarily interested in between-person differences or within-person changes in craving. Within-subject designs provide inherent controls for many variables that could otherwise influence craving ratings. For example, such designs are somewhat less sensitive to the wording of items and to idiosyncratic interpretation of them by participants, as these effects are likely to hold constant across multiple administrations of the assessment. Conversely, within-subject designs are vulnerable to effects arising from repeated measurements, including the possibility that an earlier assessment actually provokes craving that is then reflected in a later assessment (see Sayette, Griffin, & Sayers, 2010b).

When an investigator is trying to characterize the craving response of different groups in a between-subject analysis, particular attention needs to be given to whether the assessment is subject to floor or ceiling effects for one group but not the other. For example, if one administers an assessment to highly dependent and nondependent drug users, the former may concentrate their ratings at the high end of the scale, such that the scale becomes insensitive to that group's experience. Parallel issues arise in within-subject designs if there is a manipulation that raises or lowers participants' craving between assessments; an assessment that was sensitive at one time may not be sensitive at the other.

Craving versus Craving Change

Many studies involve manipulating participants' craving from an initial baseline level. Investigators must determine the most meaningful index of craving following the manipulation. One approach is to adjust for base-line levels by calculating a change score or a residual score, or by using baseline scores as covariates in analyses. One rationale for obtaining (and correcting for) baseline measures is that individuals differ in the way they use and respond to the measurement scale. That is, some of the between-person variance in craving scores may be due to consistent measurement error (as distinct from either random error on each measurement occa-sion or true between-person variance). In this case, including a baseline score allows one to "norm" the relevant measures to each individual's standard (see Collins & Horn, 1991).

The distinction between changes in craving and absolute scores has important implications for interpreting experimental data. It is important to recognize a priori whether the key measure in a particular study is one of craving increase or absolute level of craving. Depending on the purpose of the study or one's conceptualization of craving, the variable of interest may differ. With respect to cigarette craving, we recently suggested that the absolute craving produced by a combination of nicotine deprivation and exposure to in vivo smoking cues has been a relatively neglected measure, overshadowed by studies focusing on change from a precue or neutral cue baseline to craving during smoking cue (Sayette & Tiffany, 2013). Part of our argument was that across multiple laboratories, it is this combined-peak provoked craving that is more clinically relevant than is the measure of increase in craving following cue exposure. Moreover, in many cases the assumptions supporting a focus on change in cravings are questionable (e.g., that a neutral cue exposure craving score captures cravings that are exclusively uncued, especially when the respondent is already in a drug-deprived state; see Sayette & Tiffany, 2013).

Recall versus Real-Time

Laboratory studies often ask participants to report their craving in real time ("How are you feeling *now*?"). Shiffman et al. (1997) found that recall of cravings prior to a lapse was inaccurate and biased, compared to recordings made at the time. When participants are instructed to *recall* their prior craving, these reports are subject to biases that can affect autobiographical recall (Hammersley, 1994; Sayette et al., 2000). Since our prior article, advances have been made in the use of ambulatory real-time assessment in the natural environment (Shiffman et al., 1997). Consequently, it is becoming less common for investigators to rely on retrospective assessment of cravings. EMA offers considerable promise. Increasingly it is apparent that cravings do not exist in a vacuum and that they are affected by a host of contextual factors (Shiffman, Stone, & Hufford, 2008; Wray, Godleski, & Tiffany, 2011). Cravings collected in one's natural environment permit an examination that embraces these contextual variables. For instance, one can observe how cues such as drinking alcohol or experiencing negative affect (as they are actually encountered in the real world) can trigger cigarette cravings (Shiffman et al., 1996, 2002). Accordingly, EMA is a particularly valuable method for shedding light on factors that provoke and modulate craving within individuals. In addition, recent work has highlighted innovative ways in which EMA can be combined with other methods (e.g., combining EMA with fMRI; Berkman et al., 2011; Wilson, Smyth, & MacLean, 2014) to study craving processes across multiple levels of analysis. On the other hand, there is no getting around the idea that monitoring one's experiences in the natural environment can and will alter the experience as it would otherwise unfold. More generally, to the extent that ecological assessments require self-report, they remain subject to other shortcomings. Even when responding in (near) real time, individuals may have difficulty accurately accessing and/or verbalizing the motives, thoughts, and emotions that underlie their behavior. In addition, individuals may be implicitly or explicitly motivated to respond inaccurately, especially when it comes to stigmatized or otherwise undesirable behaviors.

Nonverbal Measures of Craving

Nonverbal measures of craving used in research have included (1) reinforcement "proxies," (2) drug self-administration, (3) cognitive processing, (4) expressive behavior, (5) peripheral psychophysiological responding, and (6) neurobiological responding. Interpretation of these responses is a function of one's theory of craving. If self-reports of craving are viewed as the gold standard for measurement (albeit an imperfect one), then the following responses are likely viewed simply as behaviors or reactions that are related to (self-reported) craving or, as in the case of cognitive processing, an effect of craving. Accordingly, these measures would be considered less central to the assessment of craving. In contrast, if one believes that craving is a construct that is only imperfectly indexed by a variety of both self-report and nonverbal measures, then nonverbal measures play a more critical role in the assessment of craving. In this case, however, it is important that the selected measures are consistent with a particular theory of craving (e.g., Baker et al., 1987; Tiffany, 1990) and not simply responses that are correlated with reports of craving. In sum, depending on the aims of the study, these nonverbal measures may serve as craving responses, craving-related responses, or effects of craving.

Sayette et al. (2000) detailed each of these nonverbal approaches to craving assessment. In the intervening years, by far the greatest advances have been with neurobiological assessment. Accordingly, here we will only briefly cover these first five domains and will focus our attention primarily on the use of brain imaging techniques to assess craving.

Drug Reinforcement Proxies

If craving reflects a motivation to use drugs, then the extent to which anticipated drug use is perceived to be reinforcing can be used as a measure of craving. Anticipated drug reinforcement has been measured several different ways. Often they involve measurement of choice behavior leading to drug administration. Specifically, investigators have quantified the perceived reinforcement value of drugs by asking participants to choose between drug use and varying amounts of money (e.g., MacKillop et al., 2008). Presumably, the greater the value attributed to drug use, the greater the drug craving. We have found such measures to be especially sensitive to our manipulations of cigarette craving (Sayers & Sayette, 2013; Sayette et al., 2003a; Sayette, Loewenstein, Griffin, & Black, 2008). An alternative approach to assess reinforcement is to measure the amount of work a participant is willing to perform in order to receive the drug (e.g., Darredeau, Stewart, & Barrett, 2013; Rusted, Mackee, Williams, & Willner, 1998).

Drug Self-Administration

Some researchers have suggested that direct assessment of drug use may be preferable to self-report measures of craving (Perkins, 2009). Reliance on drug use behaviors is also favored by those who oppose use of any craving construct (e.g., Mello, 1978), or those testing animal models of craving. A number of forces other than drug craving, however, can affect drug use. One can experience a strong craving, but if the drug is unavailable, if one is determined to quit, or if use may extend the time in the laboratory, then drug use may not ensue. Conversely, one might use a drug in the absence of a craving (Tiffany, 1990). Several measures of drug use have been selected to infer craving in laboratory studies, including latency to initial use of the drug and drug use topography measures (Sayette et al., 2000).

Cognitive Processing

Craving has long been linked to changes in cognitive processing (Keys, Brozek, Henschel, Mickelsen, & Taylor, 1950). Over the past 25 years there has been considerable effort directed toward assessing the effects of craving on nonautomatic cognitive resources (Sayette & Hufford, 1994; Tiffany, 1990). Researchers have used a range of approaches to assess the redistribution of cognitive resources during craving. These include secondary response time tasks, working memory tasks, and cognitive performance measures suggesting that while one is craving, performance on these measures tends to deteriorate (e.g., Wilson, Sayette, Fiez, & Brough, 2007). We have found that under high craving conditions, measures of secondary response time correlates with self-reported urge (Sayette et al., 2003a).

In addition, a variety of implicit cognitive tasks have been used to index the salience of drug-related information without making individuals aware of the purpose of assessment. This salience presumably reflects a cognitive preoccupation with drug-related material. These include word stem completions, perceptual identification, categorization tasks, and color-naming variants of the Stroop task in which drug-related stimuli interfere with the ability to name the color of a presented word. With regard to smoking, we have found that interference on a smoking Stroop task on quit day predicted time to relapse, even after controlling for self-reported urges (Waters et al., 2003). More direct approaches to evaluating attentional bias involve eye tracking methods, which also have revealed that individuals tend to focus more on drug-related stimuli while craving (e.g., Field, Mogg, & Bradley, 2004). Whether these changes are manifestations of a craving construct or instead just effects of craving, they may be useful in determining addiction vulnerability. While this type of assessment has proven useful, it is not a perfect index of craving (Sayette et al., 2000). One issue in particular that must be addressed concerns the use of multitrial tasks that assess cognitive performance. Exposure to a smoking cue may not only affect cognitive processing during that trial, but may carry over and affect performance on a subsequent neutral trial (see Wilson et al., 2007). Indeed, as discussed below, such carryover effects also may be an issue for neurobiological responding (Breiter et al., 1997; Franklin et al., 2011; Gloria et al., 2009).

Expressive Behavior

Assessing facial expressive behavior is an important measure of emotional responses (Barlow, 1988). Because craving is thought to be affective in nature, an anatomically based facial coding system may prove useful for detecting craving. As with cognitive measures, depending on one's model of craving these facial signals may reflect craving-related affect or a measure of craving itself (Sayette et al., 2003a). Advantages of objective facial coding systems include the ability to unobtrusively measure immediate responses, to assess positive and negative affect independently, and to discriminate between different emotions (see Ekman & Rosenberg, 2005).

We have used the Facial Action Coding System (FACS; Ekman & Friesen, 1978) to code participants' responses to smoking cues. Depending on the experimental conditions, we have observed that self-reported craving can be linked to both positive-affect-related signals (when expecting to smoke very soon) and negative-affect-related signals (when not permitted to smoke) (Sayette & Hufford, 1995; Sayette et al., 2003b). We have also found that while craving, smokers displaying facial expressions related to emotional suppression during smoking cue exposure are more likely to subsequently increase the degree to which they value smoking a cigarette (Sayers & Sayette, 2013). Finally, FACS has revealed a link between facial expressions related to ambivalence displayed during a smoking cue exposure and clinical measures of smoking ambivalence (Griffin & Sayette, 2008). Limitations of FACS include reliance on expressions that must be visible to humans, the need for extensive coder training, and the extremely time-consuming nature of coding facial expressions, though recently there have been advances in the automated coding of FACS that may make such coding more feasible in the future (e.g., Cohn & Sayette, 2010).

An alternative measure of facial muscle activity is facial electromyography (EMG), which has been used to study craving (e.g., Elash, Tiffany, & Vrana, 1995). Facial EMG can detect even those subacute muscle movements that are not visible to the human eye. A disadvantage of facial EMG is that the ability to capture a range of discrete emotions requires use of increasing numbers of electrodes, which may interfere with a participant's natural craving experience. As with facial coding, activation of a particular muscle is not specific to craving.

Startle Reflex

The magnitude of the reflexive eye blink to startling stimuli has been shown to capture the processing of both positive (decreased startle) and negative (increased startle) emotional states (e.g., Lang, Bradley, & Cuthbert, 1990), and has been used to assess craving. Elash et al. (1995) found smoking-related imagery to increase startle responding, suggesting an increase in the processing of negative affect. Hutchison, Niaura, and Swift (1997) found smoking cue exposure to attenuate prepulse inhibition of the startle reflex, a measure thought to be associated with changes in information processing. As more data are collected, the role of startle reflex in craving assessment will be better understood.

Peripheral Psychophysiological Responding

A number of models propose that peripheral psychophysiological responses should index craving (Sayette et al., 2000). Changes in heart rate, skin temperature, blood pressure, skin conductance, and salivation have been included in craving studies, though the pattern of responding has often differed (Carter & Tiffany, 1999). These measures have been criticized for a variety of reasons (see Sayette et al., 2000). Psychophysiological systems serve functions that are independent of a motivation for drug use, and it is unclear which patterns of response ought to be related to drug craving (Niaura et al., 1988; Tiffany, 1990). It has been suggested that psychophysiological measures should be linked conceptually to craving (Zinser, Fiore, Davidson, & Baker, 1999).

Neurobiological Responding

There has been tremendous growth in the use of functional brain imaging to study responses in the human brain during the experience of craving in the last 15 years. Functional brain imaging methods, which allow for the noninvasive measurement of signals associated with neural activity, can be organized into two broad categories (Bandettini, 2009; Shibasaki, 2008). One category of methods, which involves measuring either electrical (EEG) or magnetic (magnetoencephalography) changes that directly arise from neural activity, has excellent temporal resolution but relatively poor spatial resolution (see also Harmon-Jones, Gable, & Harmon-Jones, Chapter 8, this volume). The second category of methods measures blood flow and/or metabolic rate in the brain as a proxy for neural activity; these techniques have somewhat limited temporal resolution but comparatively good spatial resolution and include fMRI, positron emission tomography (PET), single-photon emission computer tomography (SPECT), and near-infrared spectroscopy (NIRS). Of the various functional brain imaging methods, fMRI currently is the most widely used in human neuroscience research, including research on craving, because it does not require radioactive tracers (as in PET and SPECT), can be used to visualize subcortical structures (unlike NIRS), and has a reasonably good balance of temporal and spatial resolution (on the order of seconds and millimeters, respectively). More precisely, the majority of studies have used fMRI to measure a signal produced by changes in the relative concentration of oxygenated and deoxygenated blood (i.e., blood oxygen level–dependent [BOLD] fMRI; Ogawa, Lee, Kay, & Tank, 1990)—a correlate of neural activity—under conditions designed to provoke craving.

Because it allows researchers to measure patterns of neural activity related to emotional and cognitive processes as they unfold over time, fMRI provides an attractive approach to the nonverbal assessment of craving. Since fMRI data can be linked to a host of other useful sources of knowledge (e.g., nonhuman animal neuroscience research, basic human brain imaging research regarding the patterns of brain activation associated with various cognitive operations), they offer a wealth of information that may not be accessible using other types of measures, including self-report. For instance, a recent fMRI study found that neural responses to health messages designed to promote smoking cessation in a brain region called the medial prefrontal cortex predicted subsequent reductions in cigarette use above and beyond self-reported intentions to change smoking behavior (Falk, Berkman, Whalen, & Lieberman, 2011).

Research using fMRI has generated considerable data regarding patterns of brain activation associated with exposure to stimuli designed to elicit craving (Chase, Eickhoff, Laird, & Hogarth, 2011; Engelmann et al., 2012; see also Lopez, Wagner, & Heatherton, Chapter 7, this volume). With few exceptions, fMRI studies have adopted cue-reactivity procedures very similar to those used in behavioral research (Chase et al., 2011; Engelmann et al., 2012; Wilson, Sayette, & Fiez, 2004). That is, the majority have focused on differences between brain responses during passive or active processing of drug cues (e.g., simply viewing versus using coping to reduce affective reactions to drug cues, respectively) and brain responses during the presentation of control stimuli. In addition, in most cases, prior studies have incorporated multiple presentations of drug and control cues. As with the use of multiple items in self-report measures, the decision to incorporate multiple presentations of drug-related and control cues in brain imaging studies of craving is rooted in fundamental concepts from measurement and statistics (Nunnally, 1978). In particular, one (often implicit) goal of this approach is to increase statistical power by reducing measurement error, an important consideration given the relatively low signal-to-noise ratio inherent in fMRI and most brain imaging methods, more generally (Culham, 2006). Specifically, within some limit, the reliability of the estimated brain response to drug and control cues is assumed to increase as more stimuli of each type are presented and responses are averaged across events or blocks within each condition. A second assumption underlying this approach is that responses to drug and control cues do not interact with one another and, accordingly, that it is possible to subtract the response associated with control cues from the response associated with drug cues in order to identify patterns of brain activation that are in some way unique to drug-related stimuli and craving.

One potential limitation of the cue-reactivity methods often used in fMRI craving research is that in order to repeatedly present cues within the constraints of the neuroimaging environment, often in relatively rapid succession, many studies have adopted procedures and stimuli that are suboptimal for evoking robust urge states. Specifically, the majority of studies have used solely visual cues, most commonly photographic stimuli presented for a few seconds at a time (Yalachkov, Kaiser, & Naumer, 2012). Such methods have proven useful for identifying differences in the patterns of brain activity associated with drug-related and control cues (Engelmann et al., 2012). Multisensory cues, however, appear to be more effective than visual cues at revealing relationships between cue-related brain activity and self-reported urge (Yalachkov et al., 2012), perhaps in part because participants exposed to static drug pictures and related visual stimuli in brain imaging cue reactivity studies often report very modest levels of craving. This is not surprising, as behavioral research indicates that multimodal stimuli—particularly multimodal in vivo cues (e.g., the sight, smell, and touch of a lit cigarette)—provoke significantly stronger cravings and associated physiological responses than visual cues alone (e.g., Shadel, Niaura, & Abrams, 2001). The limited potency of visual cues is likely further dampened by the cramped and noisy conditions under which fMRI studies are conducted.

Thus, although often overlooked, a crucial consideration when using fMRI (and other brain imaging methods) to examine craving is the strength of urges that one seeks to provoke (see Wilson & Sayette, 2015). As above, the particular steps that are taken with respect to this issue should be guided by theory regarding the nature of craving and the specific goals of the study. For example, if one seeks only to characterize phasic neurobiological responses to discrete drug stimuli, the magnitude of subjective craving may be less central. If, on the other hand, the aim is to examine neural activity associated with a robust and enduring craving state, urge intensity is a critical factor.

More generally, it is important for investigators using fMRI and other brain imaging methods to be mindful of how well the designs they select fit with the hypothesized time course of craving responses. That is, depending on how craving is conceptualized, the rapid multiple presentation design used by many studies may or may not be a good match for the expected duration of cue-induced craving responses. Related to this point, there is evidence that both the subjective and peripheral physiological changes elicited by drug cues persist for several minutes (Heishman, Lee, Taylor, & Singleton, 2010). Accordingly, care must be taken to avoid a situation in which there is a problematic discrepancy between the temporal structure of the methods used to provoke craving and the manner in which these craving responses are likely to unfold over time. Designs that include several brief cue trials or blocks are best suited for assessing effects that are ephemeral and stimulus-locked; such methods may be suboptimal when the neurobiological responses of interest exhibit a more diffuse and protracted pattern (i.e., when they do not follow an abrupt "on and off" course).

Relatedly, if a strong craving is elicited during early trials of a multiple trial design (perhaps after the very first drug cue trial), all of the drug-related and ostensibly neutral cue trials that follow may very well occur against the backdrop of an already elevated craving state. This overlap can pose a possible methodological concern, as any interactions between the responses to discrete cues and those associated with more enduring changes in craving (in particular those resulting in a dampening of responses to drug cues and/or an increase in responses to neutral cues) have the potential to weaken sensitivity to detect neural effects of interest. For instance, as noted above, one risk is that the neural responses produced by drug cues will carry over and "contaminate" the signal measured during subsequent control trials/blocks, thereby interfering with the ability to distinguish between conditions (Franklin et al., 2011; Wilson et al., 2007). In line with this concern, there is some evidence that prior exposure to drug-associated stimuli (particularly those linked to drug delivery) may influence neurobiological responses under purportedly neutral conditions (Breiter et al., 1997; Gloria et al., 2009) although, to our knowledge, studies have yet to directly assess the nature and implications of carryover in brain imaging research. Nonetheless, the possibility of carryover effects warrants consideration in the use of fMRI and related methods to study craving.

Given concerns about possible carryover effects and our desire to provoke robust levels of craving, we have developed an fMRI-based cue exposure procedure that differs in key ways from the cue-reactivity methods used in many other studies. Our protocol involves administering in vivo smoking cues (i.e., the touch and sight of a preferred brand of cigarette). In addition, unlike cue-reactivity approaches that involve the interleaved presentation of several brief neutral and drug cue trials or blocks, our design incorporates a small number of cues, each of which is presented for a relatively extended duration. Finally, cues are administered in a fixed order (nondrug cues always preceding the cigarette cue) to avoid carryover effects that, if present, would compromise the ability to detect neural responses of interest. Similar methods have been used to provoke strong craving states in studies using PET (e.g., Brody et al., 2002; Grant et al., 1996) and, more recently, in perfusion-based fMRI studies using arterial spin labeling instead of the BOLD contrast mechanism to measure blood flow in the brain (e.g., Franklin et al., 2011, 2007).

In a series of studies, we have shown that, when paired with acute nicotine deprivation, this cue exposure protocol effectively provokes strong subjective cravings in the scanner. For instance, urge ratings averaged 74 (on a 0–100 scale) in nicotine-deprived active (i.e., nonquitting) smokers during cigarette cue exposure in our initial study using the approach (Wilson, Sayette, Delgado, & Fiez, 2005). We have used this potent craving manipulation in combination with various experimental conditions to examine the neurobiological responses associated with the appetitive motivational state that immediately precedes cigarette use (Wilson et al., 2005), as well as the modulation of this anticipatory state by treatment status (Wilson, Sayette, & Fiez, 2012), attitudes toward smoking (Wilson, Creswell, Sayette, & Fiez, 2013a), and the use of cognitive coping techniques (Wilson, Sayette, & Fiez, 2013b).

In summary, several types of nonverbal measures have been used to study craving. While they may be less vulnerable to the response biases created by self-report assessment, they are not without their own concerns (Sayette et al., 2000). As with self-report, articulation of a craving theory is needed to best interpret these nonverbal responses.

Conclusion

Craving is currently a hot construct: expensive studies ask whether new interventions can reduce craving, what craving looks like in the brain, and whether it can inform our understanding of relapse. Concomitant with this interest must be a consideration of how we define and assess the construct. For instance, must we observe a strong desire in our studies, or is even the mildest desire relevant to craving? While the initial section of the chapter identified a range of unresolved questions that persist, researchers nevertheless have made progress in the understanding of craving-related processes in the past 15 years. A wide variety of measures have been introduced to assess craving responding, whether they be viewed as measures of craving per se, as correlates of craving, or merely as effects of craving. We have found that cravings, often due to a combination of drug abstinence and cue exposure, are linked to relapse and a host of other clinically pertinent phenomena (Sayette & Tiffany, 2013). By studying brain responses during strong craving states, we have gained new insight into neurobiological and psychological processes associated with the experience and modulation of the urge to use drugs (e.g., Wilson, Sayette, & Fiez, 2012, 2013b). None of the measures discussed here is appropriate across all settings, and thus measurement selection poses a formidable challenge. Relevant issues include the anticipated potency of the craving experience, amount of time available for administering the measures, and number of times that the measure will be administered. Awareness of the limitations and strengths of different measures should lead to improved craving assessment. By systematically manipulating craving levels, putative measures of craving can be evaluated. Such efforts are required in order to provide support for the construct validity of a particular model of craving. Improved measurement is essential if we are to optimize research efforts directed at better understanding drug craving.

ACKNOWLEDGMENTS

Preparation of this chapter was supported in part by Grants No. R01 CA10605 and No. R01 CA184779 from the National Cancer Institute to Michael A. Sayette and by the Eunice Kennedy Shriver National Institute of Child Health and Human Development of the National Institutes of Health under BIRCWH award

No. K12HD055882, "Career Development Program in Women's Health Research at Penn State," to Stephen J. Wilson.

REFERENCES

American Educational Research Association, American Psychological Association, & National Council on Measurement in Education. (1985). *Standards for educational and psychological testing.* Washington, DC: American Psychological Association.

American Psychiatric Association. (2013). *Diagnostic and statistical manual of mental disorders* (5th ed.). Arlington, VA: Author.

Baker, T. B., & Brandon, T. H. (1990). Validity of self-reports in basic research. *Behavioral Assessment, 12,* 33–51.

Baker, T. B., Morse, E., & Sherman, J. E. (1987). The motivation to use drugs: A psychobiological analysis of urges. In C. Rivers (Ed.), *The Nebraska Symposium on Motivation: Alcohol use and abuse* (pp. 257–323). Lincoln: University of Nebraska Press.

Barlow, D. H. (1988). *Anxiety and its disorders.* New York: Guilford Press.

Bandettini, P. A. (2009). What's new in neuroimaging methods? *Annals of the New York Academy of Sciences, 1156,* 260–293.

Baumeister, R. F., Heatherton, T. F., & Tice, D. M. (1994). *Losing control: How and why people fail at self-regulation* (pp. 156–168). San Diego, CA: Academic Press.

Berkman, E. T., Falk, E. B., & Lieberman, M. D. (2011). In the trenches of real-world self-control: Neural correlates of breaking the link between craving and smoking. *Psychological Science, 22,* 498–506.

Berridge, K. C., & Robinson, T. E. (1995). The mind of an addicted brain: Neural sensitization of wanting versus liking. *Current Directions in Psychological Science, 4,* 71–76.

Breiner, M. J., Stritzke, W. G. K., & Lang, A. R. (1999). Approaching avoidance: A step essential to the understanding of craving. *Alcohol Research and Health, 23,* 197–206.

Breiter, H. C., Gollub, R. L., Weisskoff, R. M., Kennedy, D. N., Makris, N., Berke, J. D., et al. (1997). Acute effects of cocaine on human brain activity and emotion. *Neuron, 19,* 591–611.

Brody, A. L., Mandelkern, M. A., London, E. D., Childress, A. R., Lee, G. S., Bota, R. G., et al. (2002). Brain metabolic changes during cigarette craving. *Archives of General Psychiatry, 59*(12), 1162–1172.

Carlsmith, J. M., Ellesworth, P. C., & Aronson, E. (1976). *Methods of research in social psychology.* Reading, MA: Addison Wesley.

Carter, B. L., & Tiffany, S. T. (1999). Meta-analysis of cue reactivity in addiction research. *Addiction, 94,* 327–340.

Chase, H. W., Eickhoff, S. B., Laird, A. R., & Hogarth, L. (2011). The neural basis of drug stimulus processing and craving: An activation likelihood estimation meta-analysis. *Biological Psychiatry, 70,* 785–793.

Cohn, J. F., & Sayette, M. A. (2010). Spontaneous behavior in a small group can be measured automatically: An initial demonstration. *Behavior Research Methods, 42,*1079–1086.

Collins, L. M., & Horn, J. L. (Eds.). (1991). *Best methods for the analysis of change: Recent advances, unanswered questions, future directions.* Washington, DC: American Psychological Association.

Cook, T. D., & Campbell, D. T. (1979). *Quasi-experimentation*. Chicago: Rand-McNally.

Cook, S. W., & Selltiz, C. (1964). A multiple indicator approach to attitude measurement. *Psychological Bulletin, 62*, 36–55.

Cronbach, L. J., & Meehl, P. E. (1955). Construct validity in psychological tests. *Psychological Bulletin, 52*, 281–302.

Culham, J. C. (2006). *Functional neuroimaging: Experimental design and analysis*. Cambridge, MA: MIT Press.

Darredeau, C., Stewart, S. H., & Barrett, S. P. (2013). The effects of nicotine content information on subjective and behavioural responses to nicotine-containing and denicotinized cigarettes. *Behavioural Pharmacology, 24*, 291–297.

Ekman, P., & Friesen, W. V. (1978). *Facial Action Coding System*. Palo Alto, CA: Consulting Psychologists Press.

Ekman, P., & Rosenberg, E. L. (Eds.). (2005). *What the face reveals: Basic and applied studies of spontaneous expression using the facial action coding system* (FACS) (2nd ed.). New York: Oxford University Press.

Elash, C. A., Tiffany, S. T., & Vrana, S. R. (1995). Manipulation of smoking urges and affect through a brief-imagery procedure: Self-report, psychophysiological, and startle probe responses. *Experimental and Clinical Psychopharmacology, 3*, 156–162.

Engelmann, J. M., Versace, F., Robinson, J. D., Minnix, J. A., Lam, C. Y., Cui, Y., et al. (2012). Neural substrates of smoking cue reactivity: A meta-analysis of fMRI studies. *NeuroImage, 60*, 252–262.

Falk, E. B., Berkman, E. T., Whalen, D., & Lieberman, M. D. (2011). Neural activity during health messaging predicts reductions in smoking above and beyond self-report. *Health Psychology, 30*, 177–185.

Field, M., Mogg, K., & Bradley, B. P. (2004). Eye movements to smoking-related cues: Effects of nicotine deprivation. *Psychopharmacology, 173*, 116–123.

Franklin, T. R., Wang, Z., Suh, J. J., Hazan, R., Cruz, J., Li, Y., & Childress, A. R. (2011). Effects of varenicline on smoking cue-triggered neural and craving responses. *Archives of General Psychiatry, 68*, 516–526.

Franklin, T. R., Wang, Z., Wang, J., Sciortino, N., Harper, D., Li, Y., et al. (2007). Limbic activation to cigarette smoking cues independent of nicotine withdrawal: A perfusion fMRI study. *Neuropsychopharmacology, 32*, 2301–2309.

Gawin, F. H. (1991) Cocaine addiction: Psychology and neurophysiology. *Science, 251*, 1580–1586.

Gloria, R., Angelos, L., Schaefer, H. S., Davis, J. M., Majeskie, M., Richmond, B. S., et al. (2009). An fMRI investigation of the impact of withdrawal on regional brain activity during nicotine anticipation. *Psychophysiology, 46*, 681–693.

Grant, S., London, E. D., Newlin, D. B., Villemagne, V. L., Liu, X., Contoreggi, C., et al. (1996). Activation of memory circuits during cue-elicited cocaine craving. *Proceedings of the National Academy of Sciences of the United States of America, 93*, 12040–12045.

Griffin, K. M., & Sayette, M. A. (2008). Facial reactions to smoking cues relate to ambivalence about smoking. *Psychology of Addictive Behaviors, 22*, 551–556.

Hammersley, R. (1994). A digest of memory phenomena for addiction research. *Addiction, 89*, 283–293.

Heishman, S. J., Lee, D. C., Taylor, R. C., & Singleton, E. G. (2010). Prolonged duration of craving, mood, and autonomic responses elicited by cues and imagery in smokers: Effects of tobacco deprivation and sex. *Experimental and Clinical Psychopharmacology, 18*, 245–256.

Hutchison, K., Niaura, R., & Swift, R. (1997). The effects of high vs. low nicotine cigarettes on prepulse inhibition. *Psychophysiology, 34,* S45.

Kassel J. D., & Shiffman, S. (1992). What can hunger teach us about drug craving?: A comparative analysis of the two constructs. *Advances in Behaviour Research and Therapy, 14,*141–167.

Kavanagh, D. J., Andrade, J., & May, J. (2005). Imaginary relish and exquisite torture: The elaborated intrusion theory of desire. *Psychological Review, 112,* 446–467.

Keys, A., Brozek, J., Henschel, A., Mickelsen, O., & Taylor, H. L. (1950). *The biology of human starvation* (Vol. 2). Minneapolis: University of Minnesota Press.

Kozlowski, L. T., Pillitteri, J. L., Sweeney, C. T., Whitfield, K. E., & Graham, J. W. (1996). Asking questions about urges or cravings for cigarettes. *Psychology of Addictive Behaviors, 10,* 248–260.

Kozlowski, L. T. & Wilkinson, D. A. (1987). Use and misuse of the concept of craving by alcohol, tobacco, and drug researchers. *British Journal of Addiction, 82,* 31–36.

Lang, P. J., Bradley, M. M., & Cuthbert, B. N. (1990). Emotion, attention, and the startle reflex. *Psychological Review, 97,* 377–395.

Loewenstein, G. (1987). Anticipation and the valuation of delayed consumption. *Economic Journal, 97,* 666–684.

Ludwig, A. M., & Wikler, A. (1974). "Craving" and relapse to drink. *Quarterly Journal of Studies on Alcohol, 35,* 108–130.

MacKillop, J., Murphy, J. G., Ray, L. A., Eisenberg, D. T. A., Lisman, S. A., Lum, J. K., et al. (2008). Further validation of the cigarette purchase task for assessing the relative reinforcing efficacy of nicotine in smokers. *Experimental and Clinical Psychopharmacology, 16,* 57–65.

Mello, N. K. (1978). A semantic aspect of alcoholism. In H. D. Cappell & A. E. LeBlanc (Eds.), *Biological and behavioral approaches to drug dependence* (pp. 73–87). Toronto: Addiction Research Foundation.

Niaura, R. S., Rohsenow, D. J., Binkoff, J. A., Monti, P. M., Pedraza, M., & Abrams, D. B. (1988). Relevance of cue reactivity to understanding alcohol and smoking relapse. *Journal of Abnormal Psychology, 97,* 133–152.

Nunnally, J. C. (1978). *Psychometric theory* (2d ed.). New York: McGraw-Hill.

Ogawa, S., Lee, T. M., Kay, A. R., & Tank, D. W. (1990). Brain magnetic resonance imaging with contrast dependent on blood oxygenation. *Proceedings of the National Academy of Sciences of the United States of America, 87,* 9868–9872.

Perkins, K. A. (2009). Does smoking cue-induced craving tell us anything important about nicotine dependence? *Addiction, 104,* 1610–1616.

Perlmuter, L. C., Noblin, C. D., & Hakami, M. (1983). Reactive effects of tests for depression: theoretical and methodological considerations. *Journal of Social and Clinical Psychology, 1,* 128–139.

Rusted, J. M., Mackee, A., Williams, R., & Willner, P. (1998). Deprivation state but not nicotine content of the cigarette affects responding by smokers on a progressive ratio task. *Psychopharmacology, 140,* 411–417.

Sayers, W. M., & Sayette, M. A. (2013). Suppression on your own terms: Internally generated displays of craving suppression predict rebound effects. *Psychological Science, 24,* 1740–1746.

Sayette, M. A., Griffin, K. M., & Sayers, W. M. (2010b). Counterbalancing in smoking cue research: A critical analysis. *Nicotine and Tobacco Research, 11,* 1068–1079.

Sayette, M. A., & Hufford, M. R. (1994). Effects of cue exposure and deprivation on cognitive resources in smokers. *Journal of Abnormal Psychology, 103*, 812–818.

Sayette, M. A., & Hufford, M. R. (1995). Urge and affect: A facial coding analysis of smokers. *Experimental and Clinical Psychopharmacology, 3*, 417–423.

Sayette, M. A., Loewenstein, G., Griffin, K. M., & Black, J. (2008). Exploring the cold-to-hot empathy gap in smokers. *Psychological Science, 19*, 926–932.

Sayette, M. A., Martin, C. S., Hull, J. G., Wertz, J. M., & Perrott, M. A. (2003a). The effects of nicotine deprivation on craving response covariation in smokers. *Journal of Abnormal Psychology, 112*, 110–118.

Sayette, M. A., Martin, C. S., Wertz, J. M, Shiffman, S., & Perrott, M. A. (2001). A multidimensional analysis of cue-elicited craving in heavy smokers and tobacco chippers. *Addiction, 96*, 1419–1432.

Sayette, M. A., Schooler, J. W., & Reichle, E. D. (2010a). Out for a smoke: The impact of cigarette craving on zoning-out during reading. *Psychological Science, 21*, 26–30.

Sayette, M. A., Shiffman, S., Tiffany, S. T., Niaura, R. S., Martin, C. S., & Shadel, W. G. (2000). The measurement of drug craving. *Addiction, 95*, S189–S210.

Sayette, M. A., & Tiffany, S. T. (2013). Peak provoked craving: An alternative to smoking cue-reactivity. *Addiction, 108*, 1019–1025.

Sayette, M. A., Wertz, J. M., Martin, C. S., Cohn, J. F., Perrott, M. A., & Hobel, J. (2003b). Effects of smoking opportunity on cue-elicited urge: A facial coding analysis. *Experimental and Clinical Psychopharmacology, 11*, 218–227.

Shadel, W. G., Niaura, R., & Abrams, D. B. (2001). Effect of different cue stimulus delivery channels on craving reactivity: Comparing *in vivo* and video cues in regular cigarette smokers. *Journal of Behavior Therapy and Experimental Psychiatry, 32*, 203–209.

Shibasaki, H. (2008). Human brain mapping: Hemodynamic response and electrophysiology. *Clinical Neurophysiology, 119*, 731–743.

Shiffman, S., Gwaltney, C. J., Balabanis, M., Liu, K. S., Paty, J. A., Kassel, J. D., et al. (2002). Immediate antecedents of cigarette smoking: An analysis from ecological momentary assessment. *Journal of Abnormal Psychology, 111*, 531–545.

Shiffman, S., Hufford, M., Hickox, M., Paty, J. A., Gnys, M., & Kassel, J. (1997). Remember that?: A comparison of real-time versus retrospective recall of smoking lapses. *Journal of Consulting and Clinical Psychology, 65*, 292–300.

Shiffman, S., Paty, J. A., Gnys, M., Kassel, J. D., & Hickcox, M. (1996). First lapses to smoking: Within-subjects analyses of real-time reports. *Journal of Consulting and Clinical Psychology, 64*, 366–379.

Shiffman, S., Stone, A. A., & Hufford, M. (2008). Ecological momentary assessment. *Annual Review of Clinical Psychology, 4*, 1–32.

Tiffany, S. T. (1990). A cognitive model of drug urges and drug-use behavior: Role of automatic and nonautomatic processes. *Psychological Review, 97*, 147–168.

Tiffany, S. T. (1992). A critique of contemporary urge and craving research: Methodological, psychometric, and theoretical issues. *Advances in Behaviour Research and Therapy, 14*, 123–139.

Tiffany, S. T., & Drobes, D. J. (1991). The development and initial validation of a questionnaire on smoking urges. *British Journal of Addiction, 86*, 1467–1476.

Waters, A. J., Shiffman, S., Sayette, M. A., Paty, J., Gwaltney, C., & Balabanis, M. (2003). Attentional bias predicts outcome in smoking cessation. *Health Psychology, 22*, 378–387.

Wertz, J. M., & Sayette, M. A. (2001). Effects of smoking opportunity on attentional bias in smokers. *Psychology of Addictive Behaviors, 15*, 268–271.

Wiggens, J. S. (1973). *Personality and prediction: Principles of personality assessment.* Reading, MA: Addison-Wesley.

Wilson, S. J., Creswell, K. G., Sayette, M. A., & Fiez, J. A. (2013a). Ambivalence about smoking and cue-elicited neural activity in quitting-motivated smokers faced with an opportunity to smoke. *Addictive Behaviors, 38,* 1541–1549.

Wilson, S. J., & Sayette, M. A. (2015). Neuroimaging craving: Urge intensity matters. *Addiction, 110,* 195–203.

Wilson, S. J., Sayette, M. A., Delgado, M. R., & Fiez, J. A. (2005). Instructed smoking expectancy modulates cue-elicited neural activity: A preliminary study. *Nicotine and Tobacco Research, 7,* 637–645.

Wilson, S. J., Sayette, M. A., & Fiez, J. A. (2004). Prefrontal responses to drug cues: A neurocognitive analysis. *Nature Neuroscience, 7,* 211–214.

Wilson, S. J., Sayette, M. A., & Fiez, J. A. (2012). Quitting-unmotivated and quitting-motivated cigarette smokers exhibit different patterns of cue-elicited brain activation when anticipating an opportunity to smoke. *Journal of Abnormal Psychology, 121,* 198–211.

Wilson, S. J., Sayette, M. A., & Fiez, J. A. (2013b). Neural correlates of self-focused and other-focused strategies for coping with cigarette cue exposure. *Psychology of Addictive Behaviors, 27,* 466–476.

Wilson, S. J., Sayette, M. A., Fiez, J. A., & Brough, E. (2007). Carry-over effects of smoking cue exposure on working memory performance. *Nicotine and Tobacco Research, 9,* 613–619.

Wilson, S. J., Smyth, J. M., & MacLean, R. R. (2014). Integrating ecological momentary assessment and functional brain imaging methods: New avenues for studying and treating tobacco dependence. *Nicotine and Tobacco Research, 16*(2), S102–S110.

World Health Organization. (1955). The Craving for Alcohol: A symposium by members of the WHO Expert Committees on Mental Health and on Alcohol. *Quarterly Journal of Studies on Alcohol, 16*(3), 3–66.

Wray, J. M., Gass, J. C., & Tiffany, S. T. (2014). The reliability and correlates of cue-specific craving in nondaily smokers. *Drug and Alcohol Dependence, 134,* 304–308.

Wray, J. M., Godleski, S. A., & Tiffany, S. T. (2011). Cue-reactivity in the natural environment of cigarette smokers: The impact of photographic and *in vivo* smoking stimuli. *Psychology of Addictive Behaviors, 25,* 733–737.

Yalachkov, Y., Kaiser, J., & Naumer, M. J. (2012). Functional neuroimaging studies in addiction: Multisensory drug stimuli and neural cue reactivity. *Neuroscience and Biobehavioral Reviews, 36,* 825–835.

Zinser, M. C., Fiore, M. C., Davidson, R. J., & Baker, T. B. (1999). Manipulating smoking motivation: Impact on an electrophysiological index of approach motivation. *Journal of Abnormal Psychology, 108,* 240–254.

PART II

Neuroscience of Desire and Desire Regulation

CHAPTER 6

Motivation and Pleasure in the Brain

Morten L. Kringelbach
Kent C. Berridge

The pursuit of pleasure is ubiquitous throughout the animal kingdom, suggesting that pleasure is a fundamental principle of brain function that facilitates the survival of species and individuals. It helps us make decisions optimizing the allocation of brain resources for efficient behavior. Much progress has been made over the last 15 years in mapping the functional neuroanatomy and neurochemistry of pleasure in mammals, which has at least three major subcomponents: wanting, liking, and learning. This has brought clarity to earlier research that had confounded the complex psychological components of pleasure, especially the difference between wanting and liking and their intricate interplay over time in the pleasure cycles. The new science of pleasure and motivation can help us understand affective disorders including depression and addiction—and may help to improve subjective well-being.

Over 60 years ago, the young scientists James Olds and Peter Milner made a most remarkable discovery of what appeared at the time to be a brain pleasure center: rats would repeatedly press a lever to receive tiny jolts of electricity delivered through electrodes implanted deep within their brains—even up to 2,000 times per hour (Olds, 1956; Olds & Milner, 1954). The discovery was a surprise, as the scientists intended to probe brain areas of punishment. But one of the electrodes accidentally was misplaced in a different site in the brain, revealing the existence of the reward circuit.

These so-called "pleasure electrodes" were so powerful that rats would sometimes pursue them over other rewards such as food. Eventually electrode pursuit could even result in gradual starvation, at least under extreme conditions when all of the rat's foraging efforts needed to be devoted to food in order to survive (Berridge & Valenstein, 1991).

Under more lenient conditions, rats ate enough to thrive but then spent much of their time pressing excessively for the brain electrode reward. Almost immediately other scientists reproduced these effects, and made similar findings in higher primates and humans (Heath, 1972; Sem-Jacobsen, 1976; Valenstein, 1973).

Further research in the next decade demonstrated that brain dopamine is one of the main chemicals conveying neural signals in these regions (Yokel & Wise, 1975). Dopamine was found to be important to the electrode reward effects and also to many addictive drugs. In the minds of many scientists and the general public, dopamine consequently became known as the brain's chief "pleasure chemical" (Hoebel, Rada, Mark, & Pothos, 1999; Shizgal, 1999; Wise & Bozarth, 1985).

The discovery of pleasure electrodes and dopamine seemed to solve the question of how pleasure is produced in a brain, and even for some to promise an easy fix to unhappiness. Writers began to envisage brave new worlds where electrical brain stimulation and drugs could induce bliss. In the 1960s, therapists began implanting electrodes into the brains of human patients suffering from depression or other psychological disorders (Heath, 1972).

Yet, the early "pleasure electrodes" did not lead to a breakthrough in the treatment of mental illness, and may even have misled scientists about how pleasure comes about in the brain. In fact, subsequent research suggests that brain dopamine and most "pleasure electrodes" do not produce actual pleasure sensations at all (Berridge & Kringelbach, 2008). Instead, these produce only a form of "wanting" or motivation to obtain the electrode stimulation or another reward. The true pleasure generators in the brain are much more restricted and rather fragile (Kringelbach & Berridge, 2012; Berridge & Kringelbach, 2013).

This new view of pleasure has come from careful scientific analyses of the brain networks involved in reward for humans and animals. Pleasure-generating systems turn out to be more complex than earlier thought. This new understanding of the pleasures of the brain may also offer insights into the complexities of happiness, which may, someday, hopefully lead to better ways to enhance the quality of life (Berridge & Kringelbach, 2011).

The Basic Pleasures of Life

Pleasure is at the heart of many human experiences, and the capacity for pleasure is important for healthy well-being. Conversely, a lack of pleasure, anhedonia, is a major component in mental illnesses such as depression and anxiety (see also Treadway, Chapter 15, this volume). Treatments of mood disorders will benefit if brain mechanisms of pleasure can be understood. But more than that, a better understanding of pleasure and reward is essential to understanding fundamental biological principles of how reward works. All animals including humans have to survive and procreate, and reward is the common currency that makes this happen. Pleasure can be thought of as evolution's boldest trick for sustaining and nourishing interest in the things most important to survival (Kringelbach, 2005, 2009).

Seen in this light, food and sex are important fundamental pleasures, and in social species such as humans, there is in addition a strong motivation to interact with other conspecifics, perhaps most importantly when bringing up children to reproductive age, which ensures the survival of the species (Parsons, Stark, Young, Stein, & Kringelbach, 2013; Parsons, Young, Murray, Stein, & Kringelbach, 2010). So the social and cultural pleasures are as much a part of the human hedonic repertoire as basic pleasures.

But how does one measure something as seemingly subjective as pleasure? We can ask people to give pleasure ratings of how they feel, but subjective ratings may not always fully capture underlying pleasure reactions. Further, it may be difficult to see how any form of pleasure can measured in other animals, where the causal role of particular brain systems can best be studied.

One window into such unspoken pleasures can be found by observing how parents decide whether their newborn baby likes a sweet taste or dislikes a bitter taste by watching affective facial expressions (Steiner, 1973). Tasty food pleasures can elicit related facial reactions in other animals too, from apes to rodents, which are evolutionarily homologous and similar in brain mechanisms to expressions of humans (Steiner, Glaser, Hawilo, & Berridge, 2001). Rats and mice will, for example, lick their lips contentedly when given sweet tastes, while aversive tastes will lead to gapes, head shakes, and frantic wiping of the mouth. By measuring the numbers of facial expressions elicited by a taste, we have a good measure of its hedonic impact or how much it is *liked*, which can then be linked to brain activity (Figure 6.1, left panel).

Hedonic Hotspots: Pleasure Generators

Using these behavioral tools combined with precise targeting of specific brain regions has allowed for a much more refined understanding of how particular brain systems generate pleasure from sensations. In a set of experiments on the neural causation of pleasure, we have found "hedonic hotspots" deep below the cortex in the rat brain (Peciña & Berridge, 2005) (Figure 6.1, left panel). These brain sites are capable of amplifying a sensory pleasure to make it more "liked" when neurons in the hotspot are neurochemically stimulated. In this way, a palatable sweet taste becomes even nicer.

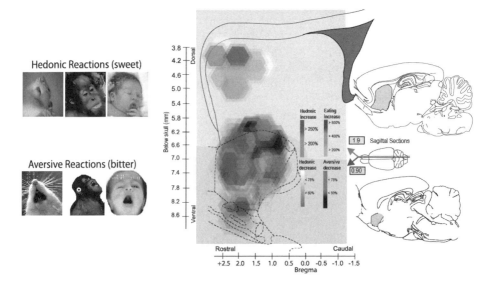

FIGURE 6.1. Hedonic reactions for studying hedonic and motivational hotspots. On the left are shown the positive and negative hedonic reactions to taste found in humans and other animals. On the right are shown details of the hedonic hotspot for pleasure generation in the nucleus accumbens (sagittal view of medial shell and of neostriatum). This is a causation map: colors reflect hedonic or motivation consequences (on "liking" reactions or on food intake) of mu opioid agonist microinjections at each site. Red/orange symbols in the rostrodorsal hotspot show sites that caused doubling or higher levels of hedonic "liking" reactions to sucrose taste. By comparison, at caudal sites the same opioid microinjections only suppressed aversive "disgust" reactions to bitter quinine (purple; e.g., suppressed gapes) or bivalently suppressed both "liking" and "disgust" reactions (blue). Green sites denote increases in motivation "wanting" to eat without any hedonic change in either "liking" or disgust (enhanced motivation also extended through all red/purple/blue sites in the nucleus accumbens). Adapted from Richard, Castro, Difeliceantonio, Robinson, and Berridge (2013) and based on data from Peciña and Berridge (2005). Copyright 2013 by Morten L. Kringelbach and Kent C. Berridge. Adapted by permission. (Purchasers can download a color version of this figure from *www.guilford.com/p/hofmann2.*)

    One pleasure-amplifying hotspot is in the nucleus accumbens, a major structure within brain reward circuits, particularly in its subregion near the center of the brain called the medial shell. Another hotspot lies within the main output target of the nucleus accumbens, called the ventral pallidum, which lies even deeper and near the bottom of the forebrain. Each hotspot is tiny, being only a cubic millimeter in volume in the brains of rats and presumably about a cubic centimeter in a human brain. Each hotspot constitutes only one-tenth to one-third of its brain structure, indicating tight localization of pleasure-generating circuits.

Within the small brain hotspots, taste pleasure is amplified by neurochemical stimulation via several neurotransmitters related to addictive drugs or to natural appetite states. For example, pleasure "liking" is enhanced when hotspots are stimulated by opioid neurotransmitters such as enkephalins or endorphins, which are the brain's natural version of the drugs heroin or morphine. Another pleasure-enhancing neurotransmitter is anandamide, a natural brain version of the psychoactive ingredient in marijuana. Yet another may be orexin, which is released by the brain during hunger and by acting in a hotspot helps to make food taste better.

Elevations of pleasure seem to require unanimous activation of an entire network of hotspots together, and defection by any single hotspot can prevent the hedonic enhancement. The stringency of a network requirement may make intense pleasures relatively rare.

From this evidence, it is clear that actual reward pleasure lies in active processes of the brain and mind as a reaction to a stimulus, rather than any physical stimulus itself. Pleasure is thus never merely a sensation, but rather something that the brain adds to sensations and experiences.

Return to Dopamine, False-Pleasure Electrodes, and Addictive "Wanting"

As mentioned earlier, dopamine has been the most famous reward-associated neurochemical for over half a century (Hoebel et al., 1999; Shizgal, 1999; Wise & Bozarth, 1985). But recent findings indicate dopamine does not actually generate pleasure after all, as mentioned above, but instead contributes something subtle to reward, more related to motivation than to pleasure (Berridge, 2007).

This also means that pleasure fluctuates with brain state, and naturally with hunger or fullness, and thus often occurs in short-term cycles with phases of expectation, consummation, and satiety (see Figure 6.2). In short, although reward was long thought to be a unitary process, it actually contains at least three major psychological components, each with distinguishable neurobiological mechanisms: *Liking* is the actual pleasure component or hedonic impact of a reward, which can be generated in the hedonic hotspots. *Wanting* is the motivation for reward, often triggered by reminders or by thinking about the reward, which can be changed by modulating dopamine. Both contribute to *learning*, which help form the associations, representations, and predictions about future rewards based on past experiences (see also Papies & Barsalou, Chapter 2, this volume). These components are linked to one another in the pleasure cycle.

In recent years many experiments by labs including ours have shown that manipulations of brain dopamine levels cause changes in "wanting" for a reward rather than "liking" for that reward. One example is gene-manipulated mutant mice that have extra-high levels of dopamine in

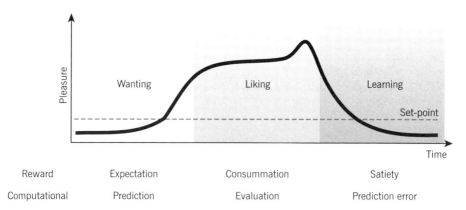

FIGURE 6.2. Pleasure cycles. The brain needs to optimize resource allocation for survival, and individuals are limited in the number of concurrent behaviors they can engage in. Survival depends on engagement with rewards and typically follows a cyclical time course common to many everyday moments of positive affect. Within this pleasure cycle rewards act as motivational magnets to initiate, sustain, and switch states. Typically, rewarding moments go through a phase of expectation or wanting for a reward, which sometimes leads to a phase of consummation or liking of the reward, which can have a peak level of pleasure (e.g., encountering a loved one, a tasty meal, sexual orgasm, a drug rush, winning a gambling bet). This can be followed by a satiety or learning phase, where one learns and updates predictions for the reward. (Purchasers can download a color version of this figure from *www.guilford.com/p/hofmann2*.)

their brain, via selective disruption of the molecular vacuum cleaner that normally sucks dopamine out of a synapse (the dopamine transporter molecule) (Robinson, Sandstrom, Denenberg, & Palmiter, 2005). The high-dopamine mice do "want" sweet rewards more and try to get to the reward much more quickly than normal rodents, but their pleasure-elicited facial expressions of "liking" sweetness never increase and are actually lower than normal.

Similar enhancement of "wanting" without "liking" is caused by directly stimulating dopamine release in the nucleus accumbens of rats via a painless microinjection of amphetamine (Tindell, Berridge, Zhang, Peciña, & Aldridge, 2005; Wyvell & Berridge, 2000). The elevated dopamine makes cues for a sweet reward trigger intense pulses of motivation to obtain, but when they actually taste the sugary treat it is no more pleasant than normal. Conversely, rats that have lost nearly all their brain dopamine fail to "want" any rewards at all and will voluntarily starve to death unless nursed and passively nourished. Yet the dopamine-free rats that refuse to eat have completely normal "liking" for any taste put in their mouth. Likewise, in humans, brain levels of dopamine appear to more closely track people's ratings of wanting for a tasty food or an addictive drug such as cocaine than to track their liking ratings for the same reward (Evans et al., 2006; Leyton et al., 2002; see also Franken, Chapter 19, this volume).

Given this new knowledge, it now seems clear that "pleasure electrodes" might not be so pleasurable as originally assumed, but perhaps also instead linked to the psychological process of "wanting" that can occur without "liking." Indeed, the original electrodes that rats worked to activate turned on brain dopamine and, if given freely, often motivated avid eating during the stimulation. But food tastes do not become more pleasant during brain electrode stimulation that makes a rat eat, unlike during a hotspot opioid stimulation or during natural hunger. Instead, the rats show more "disliking" facial reactions to sugar taste during the stimulation as though the electrode had made sweetness become bitter or disgusting—even though the same electrode makes them consume large quantities of food whenever turned on.

Similarly in humans, classic brain electrode stimulation sometimes made people thirstily want to drink fluids—or strongly wish to engage in sex —as well as to press thousands of times on their buttons that activated the electrode (Heath, 1972). Yet exclamations of pleasure were typically not produced by electrode stimulations, and many reports of the experience were often dominated more by undercurrents of anxiety than by any pleasurable sensation.

In the past decade, new techniques of deep brain stimulation deliver pulses of stimulation programmed by computer to electrodes implanted in brain structures related to reward, in conditions ranging from depression or obsessive–compulsive disorder (OCD) to Parkinson's disease (Kringelbach, Green, & Aziz, 2011; Kringelbach, Jenkinson, Owen, & Aziz, 2007b). Sometimes the stimulation has led to side effects where the patients have experienced manic mood episodes characterized by nearly compulsive energetic motivation to shop or engage in hobbies, become romantically attracted to nearby strangers, or fall into fits of mirthful laughter (Kringelbach, Green, Owen, Schweder, & Aziz, 2010). Yet these states are not necessarily pleasant. The energetic motivation can become dominated by anxiety and hostility, or even paranoia, and the electrode-evoked laughter can become so unpleasant that the patient asks for help to make it stop. All of these conditions may reflect activation of dopamine-related brain systems of "wanting" that simply by pass the generators of pleasure "liking" (Berridge & Valenstein, 1991). In our view, it still remains unknown whether any of Olds and Milner's electrodes indicated true pleasure (Figure 6.2).

Something similar may happen in the brains of some drug addicts. Intense "wanting" may be triggered by drug-related cues, and the vulnerability to such urges may last a long time, creating an enduring risk of relapse (see also Franken, Chapter 19, this volume). The reason is that addictive drugs not only activate brain dopamine systems, but in some people the drugs also may permanently change those systems. The change is neural sensitization, which leaves the brain's mesolimbic systems hyperreactive to addictive drugs and associated cues in a way that may generate intense "wanting." This neural change, called incentive sensitization, may well last years (Robinson & Berridge, 1993, 2001). Persisting long after detox is finished and withdrawal feelings have gone away, incentive sensitization would leave the person vulnerable to cue-triggered urges to take the drug again despite sincere wishes not to do so, especially at moments of stress or in other states that stimulate reactivity of brain dopamine systems. Such elevated "wanting" could persist even if tolerance left the addict no longer "liking" the drug as much as before.

Manipulating Hedonic Valence in the Brain

Positive (desire) and negative (dread) emotions can be controlled via hedonic mechanisms. Recent studies have demonstrated existence of an *affective keyboard mechanism* in the medial shell of the nucleus accumbens for generating intense dread versus desire. This *accumbens keyboard* has a remarkable anatomical orderliness in the arrangement of valence generators (Figure 6.3). Intense dread–desire motivations can be induced with localized disruptions, arranged by valence along a rostrocaudal gradient in the shell (Richard & Berridge, 2011, 2013). Just as a musical keyboard generates many different notes according to key location, the affective keyboard can generate many mixtures of desire versus fear, each mixture triggered at a different anatomical location.

Furthermore, although anatomical location biases the valence of desire versus dread released by the keyboard, valence at many sites can be *retuned* by context and psychological factors. The presence of a stressfully overstimulating sensory environment such as bright lights and loud music (e.g., Iggy Pop) remaps the accumbens bivalent keyboard by expanding the fear-generating zone while shrinking the desire-generating zone (Reynolds & Berridge, 2008). Conversely, a comfortable and quiet homelike ambience remaps in opposite direction, expanding desire and shrinking fear. Such psychological top-down remapping can retune a single site in the nucleus accumbens so that it releases opposite motivations in different situations, reversing its mode of operation.

The switch in operating mode may involve recruiting different neurobiological components. Fear generation demands endogenous dopamine activity at D_1 and D_2 receptors simultaneously within a "key" site (implicating roles for both a "direct" output path to the tegmentum and an "indirect" path to the ventral pallidum and hypothalamus), whereas positive desire generation by the same site requires only its D_1 dopamine signal (potentially indicating a more dominant role for neurons of its "direct" path to the ventral tegmentum).

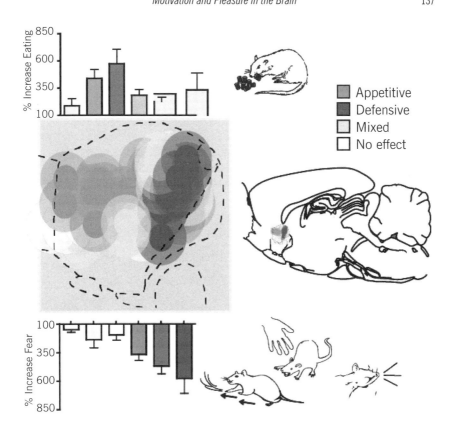

FIGURE 6.3. Affective keyboard for intense desire and dread in the nucleus accumbens. The keyboard pattern of intense motivated behaviors is revealed in the consequences of drug microinjections at various rostrocaudal sites in the medial shell. Microinjections of drugs that relatively inhibit accumbens neurons via amino acid neurotransmitters (e.g., a GABA agonist or a glutamate antagonist) may in turn disinhibit or release motivation-generating circuits in downstream target structures. Rostral green sites released stimulation of eating by up to 600% (desire only). Caudal red sites released purely increased fearful reactions at levels up to 600% over normal (dread only; escape attempts, distress calls, defensive bite attempts; spontaneous anti-predator treading/burying). Yellow sites released both desire and dread in the same rats during the same 1-hour test. Just as a keyboard has many notes, the bars shown in the figure reflect the many graded mixtures of affective desire–dread released as microinjection sites move rostrocaudal location in medial shell (appetitive desire to eat at top; fearful dread reactions at bottom). Adapted from Berridge and Kringelbach (2013) and based on data from Richard and Berridge (2011, 2013). Copyright 2013 by Kringelbach and Berridge. Adapted by permission. (Purchasers can download a color version of this figure from *www.guilford.com/p/hofmann2.*)

Neurochemical signals similarly switch the operating modes of an accumbens microdomain to generate different affects and motivations. For example, in the rostral nucleus accumbens hotspot, opioid stimulation generates intense "liking" plus "wanting" for reward, while microinjection of dopamine or glutamate-related drugs generates "wanting" alone. Conversely, in a caudal nucleus accumbens shell key, microinjections inducing opioid or dopamine stimulation generate "wanting," whereas glutamate AMPA blockade instead generates fear, and GABA signals add disgust to the fear. Thus, a variety of intense affective states can be created by changing the manipulation of a single site.

Of Mice and Men: From Pleasure Causes to Pleasure Codes

While findings from brain studies of rodents have contributed enormously to our fundamental understanding of how pleasure is generated, it is also clear that the brain of a rodent is not much larger than a human opposable thumb. How well do these important findings of animal pleasure relate to human pleasure—and in particular to those perhaps unique higher-order pleasures such as friends and loved ones, or money, culture, music, and dance?

Evolutionary forces have been busy since humans and rats shared a common ancestor 100 million years ago. In terms of brain changes, the perhaps most significant change has happened in the rapid proportional expansion of the prefrontal cortex, while similar increases have not taken place in the overall amount of, for example, gray matter in the rest of the brain (Rakic, 2009).

Modern neuroimaging techniques have allowed us to probe the brain substrate of human pleasure, even though brain scanners are not particularly friendly environments for inducing much pleasure. Yet, with some ingenuity studies have managed to look at changes in brain activity related to both fundamental pleasures such as food (Kringelbach, O'Doherty, Rolls, & Andrews, 2003; Rolls, Kringelbach, & de Araujo, 2003; Small et al., 2003; Small, Zatorre, Dagher, Evans, & Jones-Gotman, 2001) and sex (Georgiadis et al., 2006; Georgiadis & Kringelbach, 2012), and to higher-order pleasures such as music (Gebauer, Kringelbach, & Vuust, 2012; Salimpoor, Benovoy, Larcher, Dagher, & Zatorre, 2011; Salimpoor et al., 2013) and money (O'Doherty, Kringelbach, Rolls, Hornak, & Andrews, 2001).

Human brains notice, remember, think about, and plan for pleasure, beyond causing the pleasant feeling at the moment. All of this can be considered a form of pleasure coding in the brain, for which the expanded prefrontal cortex plays especially important roles. We have shown that hedonic coding especially occurs in a specific part of the lower prefrontal cortex, the orbitofrontal cortex (OFC), hanging right above the eyes

(Kringelbach, 2005) (Figure 6.4). Particularly, a region located in the *mid-anterior subregion* of OFC (roughly around 1 cubic centimeter in size) shows neuroimaging activity tightly correlated with the subjective pleasantness of a nice sensation, such as the taste of chocolate milk or of tomato juice (Kringelbach et al., 2003).

These tasty sensations do not simply cause activity in the OFC in the same way all the time, but rather vary in activity according to just how pleasant the taste is at the moment. Taste pleasantness is modulated by selective satiety, or what can be called the dessert stomach phenomenon. Why do we always seem to have room for dessert even when we feel

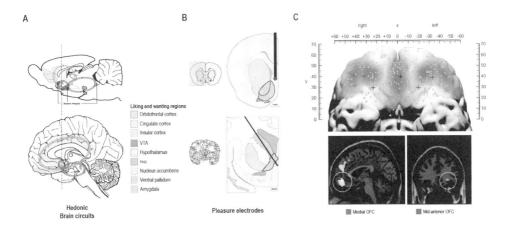

FIGURE 6.4. Brain pleasure networks, "pleasure electrodes," and the orbitofrontal cortex. (A) Pleasure is processed in hedonic networks, where hedonic causation has been identified in rodents as arising from interlinked subcortical hedonic hotspots, such as in the nucleus accumbens and ventral pallidum, where neural activation may increase "liking" expressions to sweetness. Similar pleasure coding and incentive salience networks have also been identified in humans. (B) The so-called "pleasure" electrodes in rodents and humans were unlikely to have elicited much true pleasure, but perhaps only incentive salience or desire. (C) Subjective pleasure is faithfully coded by orbitofrontal cortex (OFC) activations in people. Sensory pleasures appear to be most faithfully represented by a mid-anterior OFC site (orange). Pleasant sensations are also coded by activation in a medial strip of the OFC (green), but the medial strip may not as faithfully track changes in pleasure as the orange mid-anterior site. Smaller symbols show results of a large meta-analysis of 267 orbital areas, which indicated that a medial subregion of the OFC monitored learning and memory of reward values (green area and round blue dots), whereas a lateral orbitofrontal subregion monitored punishers (purple and orange triangles) (Kringelbach & Rolls, 2004). Independently, posterior subregions of the OFC represented complex or abstract reinforcers (such as money), whereas anterior subregions represented sensory rewards such as taste. (Purchasers can download a color version of this figure from *www.guilford.com/p/hofmann2.*)

completely full from the main course? In part, it is because the dessert is the only part of the meal that we haven't tasted yet. From an evolutionary perspective, this has the clear advantage of helping to obtain a sufficiently wide variety of nutrients.

Selective satiety is not just good for restaurants but is useful for studying reward representation in the brain, because it provides a way of altering the affective value of a stimulus without modifying the taste's physical attributes. As a result, any differences in brain activity can be attributed to the change in the impact of the reward, or the reward value. The important finding is that when people drink a large amount of tomato juice to satiety, their mid-anterior site in the orbitofrontal brain immediately afterwards stops activating to this taste, and they simultaneously report the tomato taste as no longer pleasant, whereas they still like and have activity to the taste of chocolate milk. The converse was true when people drank too much chocolate milk. These selective changes in *liking* for tomato or chocolate tastes due to satiety effects are strong evidence that the mid-anterior site of the OFC tracks the pleasure of a sensation, and not any simpler psychological or physical feature.

Similar orbitofrontal coding of pleasure has also been found for sexual orgasm, in a study by Janniko Georgiadis of the University of Groningen in the Netherlands. Sexual pleasure was examined in women who were either having real sexual orgasms or instead only faking an orgasm and its expressions, as in the movie *When Harry Met Sally* (Georgiadis et al., 2006b; Georgiadis & Kringelbach, 2012; Georgiadis, Kringelbach, & Pfaus, 2012). In short, the pleasure of diverse rewards may be coded by the OFC (Kringelbach, 2005).

Other regions of the cortex also have been implicated in coding pleasure, though the evidence for selective hedonic coding is not yet quite as convincing as for the mid-anterior site of the OFC. Those regions include a more medial strip of OFC located in the middle of the prefrontal lobe, parts of the anterior cingulate cortex, slightly higher in the central front of the brain, and a site in the insular cortex that sits deep inside the lateral surface of the prefrontal lobe. These results have implicated a network of key brain regions involved in pleasure and reward (Figure 6.4). Activity is found in this pleasure network for a whole range of basic sensory pleasures such as food, sex, or addictive drugs (Völlm et al., 2004), and higher-order pleasures including money, music, empathy, and even compassion (Kringelbach & Berridge, 2010; Kringelbach & Phillips, 2014).

The very existence of a brain pleasure network raises some interesting and challenging questions for understanding how a sense of well-being comes about. Taken together, the current evidence from animals and humans would suggest that the subcortical hotspot regions are perhaps most important for generating core processes of pleasure, while cortical regions may be more linked to coding and interfacing pleasure with cognition and conscious appraisal. It is also clear that fine-grained neural dynamics and oscillations within the pleasure system are important and interact closely with the brain's so-called resting state networks (Zhang & Raichle, 2010).

Recently, the combination of brain imaging with therapeutic deep brain stimulation in patients has shown some interesting results for relief from suffering. For example, we found that some forms of chronic pain can be relieved with deep brain stimulation, which is experienced as pleasurable by the patient (Kringelbach, Pereira, Green, Owen, & Aziz, 2009). Simultaneous MEG (magnetoencephalography) scanning showed activity in brain regions including the mid-anterior OFC (Kringelbach et al., 2007a). Stimulation of specific parts of the pleasure system for treating severe depression is also being investigated by others (Mayberg et al., 2005), although the long-term efficacy of such treatments still remains an open question (Lozano et al., 2012).

Desire for a Science of Well-Being?

At a deeper level, how might understanding brain pleasure networks apply to more general questions of human well-being or happiness? Pleasure has traditionally been thought of as providing one part of happiness, though there has been debate about its relative contribution (see also Oishi, Westgate, Tucker, & Komiya, Chapter 14, this volume). Since Aristotle, for example, well-being or happiness has often been thought to consist of at least two ingredients: hedonia (pleasure or positive affect) and eudaimonia (cognitive appraisals of meaning and life satisfaction). While some progress has been made in understanding brain hedonics, as shown in this chapter, it is important not to overinterpret our findings. In particular, hardly anything is known about how brain systems relate to the eudemonia component of happiness. Therefore science has not yet made substantial progress toward understanding the functional neuroscience of broader feelings of well-being or happiness.

Still, we can imagine several possible ways to relate happiness to particular hedonic psychological processes discussed above. For example, one way to conceive of hedonic happiness is as "liking" without "wanting." That is, a state of pleasure without disruptive desires, a state of contentment. Another possibility is that moderate "wanting," matched to positive "liking," facilitates engagement with the world. A little incentive salience may add zest to the perception of life and perhaps even promote the construction of meaning, just as in some patients therapeutic deep brain stimulation may help lift the veil of depression by making life events more appealing. However, too much "wanting" can readily spiral into maladaptive patterns such as addiction, and is a direct route to great unhappiness (see also Oishi, Westgate, Tucker, & Komiya, Chapter 14, this volume).

Finally, all might agree that happiness springs not from any single component but from the interplay of higher pleasures, positive appraisals of life meaning, and social connectedness, all combined and merged by interaction between the brain's networks of pleasure and meaningfulness. Achieving the right hedonic balance in such ways may be crucial to keep one not just free of distress—but even to achieve a degree of bliss.

REFERENCES

Berridge, K. C. (2007). The debate over dopamine's role in reward: The case for incentive salience. *Psychopharmacology, 191*, 391–431.

Berridge, K. C., & Kringelbach, M. L. (2008). Affective neuroscience of pleasure: Reward in humans and animals. *Psychopharmacology, 199*, 457–480.

Berridge, K. C., & Kringelbach, M. L. (2011). Building a neuroscience of pleasure and well-being. *Psychology of Well-Being: Theory, Research and Practice, 1*(1), 1–3.

Berridge, K. C., & Kringelbach, M. L. (2013). Neuroscience of affect: Brain mechanisms of pleasure and displeasure. *Current Opinion in Neurobiology, 23*, 294–303.

Berridge, K. C., & Valenstein, E. S. (1991). What psychological process mediates feeding evoked by electrical stimulation of the lateral hypothalamus? *Behavioral Neuroscience, 105*, 3–14.

Evans, A. H., Pavese, N., Lawrence, A. D., Tai, Y. F., Appel, S., Doder, M., et al. (2006). Compulsive drug use linked to sensitized ventral striatal dopamine transmission. *Annals of Neurology, 59*, 852–858.

Gebauer, L., Kringelbach, M. L., & Vuust, P. (2012). Ever-changing cycles of musical pleasure: The role of dopamine and anticipation. *Psychomusicology, Music, Mind and Brain, 22*, 152–167.

Georgiadis, J. R., Kortekaas, R., Kuipers, R., Nieuwenburg, A., Pruim, J., Reinders, A. A., et al. (2006). Regional cerebral blood flow changes associated with clitorally induced orgasm in healthy women. *European Journal of Neuroscience, 24*, 3305–3316.

Georgiadis, J. R., & Kringelbach, M. L. (2012). The human sexual response cycle: Brain imaging evidence linking sex to other pleasures. *Progress in Neurobiology, 98*, 49–81.

Georgiadis, J. R., Kringelbach, M. L., & Pfaus, J. G. (2012). Sex for fun: A synthesis of human and animal neurobiology. *Nature Reviews Urology, 9*, 486–498.

Heath, R. G. (1972). Pleasure and brain activity in man: Deep and surface electroencephalograms during orgasm. *Journal of Nervous and Mental Disease, 154*, 3–18.

Hoebel, B. G., Rada, P. V., Mark, G. P., & Pothos, E. N. (1999). Neural systems for reinforcement and inhibition of behavior: Relevance to eating, addiction, and depression. In D. Kahneman, E. Diener, & N. Schwarz (Eds.), *Well-being: The foundations of hedonic psychology* (pp. 558–572). New York: Russell Sage Foundation.

Kringelbach, M. L. (2005). The orbitofrontal cortex: Linking reward to hedonic experience. *Nature Reviews Neuroscience, 6*, 691–702.

Kringelbach, M. L. (2009). *The pleasure center: Trust your animal instincts.* New York: Oxford University Press.

Kringelbach, M. L., & Berridge, K. C. (2010). *Pleasures of the brain*. New York: Oxford University Press.

Kringelbach, M. L., & Berridge, K. C. (2012). A joyful mind. *Scientific American, 307*, 40–45.

Kringelbach, M. L., Green, A. L., & Aziz, T. Z. (2011). Balancing the brain: Resting state networks and deep brain stimulation. *Frontiers of Integrative Neuroscience, 5*, 8.

Kringelbach, M. L., Green, A. L., Owen, S. L. F., Schweder, P. M., & Aziz, T. Z. (2010). Sing the mind electric: Principles of deep brain stimulation. *European Journal of Neuroscience, 32*, 1070–1079.

Kringelbach, M. L., Jenkinson, N., Green, A. L., Owen, S. L. F., Hansen, P. C., Cornelissen, P. L., et al. (2007a). Deep brain stimulation for chronic pain investigated with magnetoencephalography. *NeuroReport, 18*, 223–228.

Kringelbach, M. L., Jenkinson, N., Owen, S. L. F., & Aziz, T. Z. (2007b). Translational principles of deep brain stimulation. *Nature Reviews Neuroscience, 8*, 623–635.

Kringelbach, M. L., O'Doherty, J., Rolls, E. T., & Andrews, C. (2003). Activation of the human orbitofrontal cortex to a liquid food stimulus is correlated with its subjective pleasantness. *Cerebral Cortex, 13*, 1064–1071.

Kringelbach, M. L., Pereira, E. A. C., Green, A. L., Owen, S. L. F., & Aziz, T. Z. (2009). Deep brain stimulation for chronic pain. *Journal of Pain Management, 3*, 301–314.

Kringelbach, M. L., & Phillips, H. (2014). *Emotion: Pleasure and pain in the brain*. Oxford, UK: Oxford University Press.

Kringelbach, M. L., & Rolls, E. T. (2004). The functional neuroanatomy of the human orbitofrontal cortex: Evidence from neuroimaging and neuropsychology. *Progress in Neurobiology, 72*, 341–372.

Leyton, M., Boileau, I., Benkelfat, C., Diksic, M., Baker, G., & Dagher, A. (2002). Amphetamine-induced increases in extracellular dopamine, drug wanting, and novelty seeking: A PET/[11C]raclopride study in healthy men. *Neuropsychopharmacology, 27*, 1027–1035.

Lozano, A. M., Giacobbe, P., Hamani, C., Rizvi, S. J., Kennedy, S. H., Kolivakis, T. T., et al. (2012). A multicenter pilot study of subcallosal cingulate area deep brain stimulation for treatment-resistant depression. *Journal of Neurosurgery, 116*, 315–322.

Mayberg, H. S., Lozano, A. M., Voon, V., McNeely, H. E., Seminowicz, D., Hamani, C., et al. (2005). Deep brain stimulation for treatment-resistant depression. *Neuron, 45*, 651–660.

O'Doherty, J., Kringelbach, M. L., Rolls, E. T., Hornak, J., & Andrews, C. (2001). Abstract reward and punishment representations in the human orbitofrontal cortex. *Nature Neuroscience, 4*, 95–102.

Olds, J. (1956). Pleasure centers in the brain. *Scientific American, 195*, 105–116.

Olds, J., & Milner, P. (1954). Positive reinforcement produced by electrical stimulation of the septal area and other regions of rat brain. *Journal of Comparative and Physiological Psychology, 47*, 419–427.

Parsons, C. E., Stark, E. A., Young, K. S., Stein, A., & Kringelbach, M. L. (2013). Understanding the human parental brain: A critical role of the orbitofrontal cortex. *Social Neuroscience, 8*, 525–543.

Parsons, C. E., Young, K. S., Murray, L., Stein, A., & Kringelbach, M. L. (2010). The functional neuroanatomy of the evolving parent–infant relationship. *Progress in Neurobiology, 91*, 220–241.

Peciña, S., & Berridge, K. C. (2005). Hedonic hot spot in nucleus accumbens shell: Where do mu-opioids cause increased hedonic impact of sweetness? *Journal of Neuroscience, 25*, 11777–11786.

Rakic, P. (2009). Evolution of the neocortex: A perspective from developmental biology. *Nature Reviews Neuroscience, 10*, 724–735.

Reynolds, S. M., & Berridge, K. C. (2008). Emotional environments retune the valence of appetitive versus fearful functions in nucleus accumbens. *Nature Neuroscience, 11*, 423–425.

Richard, J. M., & Berridge, K. C. (2011). Nucleus accumbens dopamine/glutamate interaction switches modes to generate desire versus dread: D1 alone for appetitive eating but D1 and D2 together for fear. *Journal of Neuroscience, 31*, 12866–12879.

Richard, J. M., & Berridge, K. C. (2013). Prefrontal cortex modulates desire and dread generated by nucleus accumbens glutamate disruption. *Biological Psychiatry, 73*, 360–370.

Richard, J. M., Castro, D. C., Difeliceantonio, A. G., Robinson, M. J., & Berridge, K. C. (2013). Mapping brain circuits of reward and motivation: In the footsteps of Ann Kelley. *Neuroscience and Biobehavioral Reviews, 37*, 1919–1931.

Robinson, S., Sandstrom, S. M., Denenberg, V. H., & Palmiter, R. D. (2005). Distinguishing whether dopamine regulates liking, wanting, and/or learning about rewards. *Behavioral Neuroscience, 119*, 5–15.

Robinson, T. E., & Berridge, K. C. (1993). The neural basis of drug craving: An incentive-sensitization theory of addiction. *Brain Research Reviews, 18*, 247–291.

Robinson, T. E., & Berridge, K. C. (2001). Incentive-sensitization and addiction. *Addiction, 96*, 103–114.

Rolls, E. T., Kringelbach, M. L., & de Araujo, I. E. T. (2003). Different representations of pleasant and unpleasant odors in the human brain. *European Journal of Neuroscience, 18*, 695–703.

Salimpoor, V. N., Benovoy, M., Larcher, K., Dagher, A., & Zatorre, R. J. (2011). Anatomically distinct dopamine release during anticipation and experience of peak emotion to music. *Nature Neuroscience, 14*, 257–262.

Salimpoor, V. N., van den Bosch, I., Kovacevic, N., McIntosh, A. R., Dagher, A., & Zatorre, R. J. (2013). Interactions between the nucleus accumbens and auditory cortices predict music reward value. *Science, 340*, 216–219.

Sem-Jacobsen, C. W. (1976). Electrical stimulation and self-stimulation with chronic implanted electrodes: Interpretation and pitfalls of results. In A. Wauquier & E. T. Rolls (Eds.), *Brain-stimulation reward* (pp. 505–520). Amsterdam: Elsevier-North Holland.

Shizgal, P. (1999). On the neural computation of utility: Implications from studies of brain stimulation reward. In D. Kahneman, E. Diener, & N. Schwarz (Eds.), *Well-being: The foundations of hedonic psychology* (pp. 500–524). New York: Russell Sage Foundation.

Small, D. M., Gregory, M. D., Mak, Y. E., Gitelman, D., Mesulam, M. M., & Parrish, T. (2003). Dissociation of neural representation of intensity and affective valuation in human gustation. *Neuron, 39*, 701–711.

Small, D. M., Zatorre, R. J., Dagher, A., Evans, A. C., & Jones-Gotman, M. (2001). Changes in brain activity related to eating chocolate: From pleasure to aversion. *Brain, 124*, 1720–1733.

Steiner, J. E. (1973). The gustofacial response: Observation on normal and anencephalic newborn infants. *Symposium on Oral Sensation and Perception, 4,* 254–278.

Steiner, J. E., Glaser, D., Hawilo, M. E., & Berridge, K. C. (2001). Comparative expression of hedonic impact: Affective reactions to taste by human infants and other primates. *Neuroscience and Biobehavioral Reviews, 25,* 53–74.

Tindell, A. J., Berridge, K. C., Zhang, J., Peciña, S., & Aldridge, J. W. (2005). Ventral pallidal neurons code incentive motivation: Amplification by mesolimbic sensitization and amphetamine. *European Journal of Neuroscience, 22,* 2617–2634.

Valenstein, E. S. (1973). *Brain control: A critical examination of brain stimulation and psychosurgery.* London: Wiley-Interscience.

Völlm, B. A., de Araujo, I. E. T., Cowen, P. J., Rolls, E. T., Kringelbach, M. L., Smith, K. A., et al. (2004). Methamphetamine activates reward circuitry in drug naïve human subjects. *Neuropsychopharmacology, 29,* 1715–1722.

Wise, R. A., & Bozarth, M. A. (1985). Brain mechanisms of drug reward and euphoria. *Psychiatric Medicine, 3,* 445–460.

Wyvell, C. L., & Berridge, K. C. (2000). Intra-accumbens amphetamine increases the conditioned incentive salience of sucrose reward: Enhancement of reward "wanting" without enhanced "liking" or response reinforcement. *Journal of Neuroscience, 20,* 8122–8130.

Yokel, R. A., & Wise, R. A. (1975). Increased lever pressing for amphetamine after pimozide in rats: Implications for a dopamine theory of reward. *Science, 187,* 547–549.

Zhang, D., & Raichle, M. E. (2010). Disease and the brain's dark energy. *Nature Reviews Neurology, 6,* 15–28.

CHAPTER 7

Neuroscience of Desire Regulation

Richard B. Lopez
Dylan D. Wagner
Todd F. Heatherton

> I keep a close watch on this heart of mine,
> I keep my eyes wide open all the time,
> I keep the ends out for the tie that binds,
> Because you're mine, I walk the line.
> —JOHNNY CASH,[1] "I Walk the Line"

This excerpt well captures human beings' marked ability to monitor and control behavior in the service of aspirations and goals beneficial to health and well-being. For Cash, that goal was presumably the long-term commitment to June that caused him to "walk the line." For other individuals, it may be restricting food intake to maintain a slender figure, or faithfully attending support group meetings to remain sober and accountable to others who wish to do the same. Regardless of one's motivation to "walk the line," these lyrics show that the jukebox continues to deliver insights into human behavior (Pennebaker et al., 1979). They also raise questions about the situations in which these valued goals may fade from view and flee the mind: when an especially intense desire takes hold and pushes our thoughts and behavior to satisfy an immediate, gratifying impulse. Psychologists and neuroscientists have begun to uncover how and why we fail to "walk the line"—when we stagger away from it and experience self-control failure. To this end, researchers in the social brain sciences have identified neural mechanisms associated with how desire is

---

represented and guides behavior on the one hand, as well as those that support the regulation of desire on the other.

In this chapter, we review these mechanisms in turn. Specifically, we will first consider how the brain processes reward and promotes reward-seeking behaviors, and then discuss how other brain systems can be recruited to curb desires and reduce the likelihood of acting upon impulses. Along the way, we will also incorporate theoretical models of desire and desire regulation that we believe the brain sciences are well equipped to validate. The chapter concludes with the most recent threads of neuroscience research that extend the literature and address key questions such as: What are the situations in which individuals are most likely to give in to desires (especially unfavorable and/or harmful ones)? Are brain systems amenable to training programs so that people can improve their capacity to effectively exert control over their desires? Although the neuroscience of desire and desire regulation is in its infancy, the field is beginning to address these issues head on, with increasing theoretical and methodological vigor.

Neural Mechanisms of Desire: How the Brain Processes Reward

Although the human experience of desire, in its various forms and intensities, is universal, the underlying mechanisms that give rise to it and its effects on behavior are not thoroughly understood. If anything, the emphasis to date has largely been on the human capacity to control desires, but recently there has been a galvanizing shift toward parsing out the psychological and neural components of desire (Hofmann & Van Dillen, 2012; see Part 1 in this volume). Without a doubt, there are many neural processes that work in concert to engender and shape our desires. For example, brain systems associated with memory formation (e.g., the hippocampus) form a functional loop with midbrain dopaminergic neurons when novel, rewarding stimuli are encoded and entered into long-term memory (Lisman & Grace, 2005). Of course, desiring a stimulus, whether it be a highly craved food item, sexual partner, or drug of abuse, necessitates retrieval of sensory and conceptual representations from memory. We do not downplay the importance of these other brain regions and networks, but for the purposes of this chapter we are going to focus on the mesolimbic dopamine pathway (MDP).

The MDP has been repeatedly shown in both human and animal work to be the critical brain system that undergirds reward processing (see also Kringelbach & Berridge, Chapter 6, this volume). Haber and Knutson (2010) review the functional neuroanatomy of the reward circuit in both humans and primates, identifying both cortical and subcortical regions in the MDP (Haber & Knutson, 2009). These regions include neurons in the ventral tegmental area (VTA), a midbrain structure that sends dopaminergic projections to the nucleus accumbens, a cluster of neurons in the ventral striatum (VS). The VS has reciprocal connections with a set of cortical regions, including the ventromedial prefrontal cortex (VMPFC), orbitofrontal cortex (OFC), and anterior cingulate cortex (ACC) (see Figure 3 in Haber & Knutson, 2009).

How does the well-defined neural architecture of the MDP support the process of learning to desire rewarding things in the first place? And which computational and psychological mechanisms facilitate this process? In the past several decades there has been an impressive surge of research confronting these questions. Neuroscientists have implemented a wide array of tools to link brain function associated with reward representations in the MDP to motivated behaviors in which stimuli are desired and readily sought after. One line of work has discovered the initial, core computations the brain carries out when an organism is faced with a stimulus that acquires reward value. In a particularly impactful and seminal paper, Schultz, Dayan, and Montague (1997) offer a set of empirical findings that support a learning-based model of reward processing in which dopamine neurons in the VTA demonstrate firing patterns indicative of a prediction error signal (Schultz et al., 1997). This prediction error is characterized by a discrepancy between what an organism expects to happen in a given context and what actually happens. For example, when an animal receives an unexpected reward, there is a burst of activity in VTA dopamine neurons at the time of reward receipt. However, once a neutral cue (e.g., a tone) becomes a conditioned stimulus that reliably predicts the reward, those neurons show a temporal shift in their firing and will fire sooner, in response to the cue and no longer to the reward itself. The fundamental learning computation to predict reward from cues is essential for navigating daily life. For without such a learning process in place, the world we experience would be a "great blooming, buzzing confusion" (James, 1890/1950). Moreover, from an evolutionary perspective this mechanism has adaptive value; for instance, one might imagine its usefulness in helping our foraging ancestors discriminate between safe and toxic food sources, or learn physical cues signalling health and fertility in a potential mate.

Fast-forward many thousands of years to our modern, 21st-century existence in which our species is bombarded with more sensory cues—many in tantalizing high definition—than we have ever encountered before (e.g., multiple streams of increasingly accessible digital media). How does the MDP, plus its attendant learning mechanism that can anticipate and discriminate rewards, fare in this cue onslaught and affect subsequent behavior? One line of thinking proposes that the reward component that the MDP primarily supports is incentive salience, a process by which reward-predicting stimuli (cues) acquire motivational value and mobilize approach behaviors toward the reward (Berridge & Robinson, 1998, 2003; Kringelbach & Berridge, 2009). Incentive salience is often characterized by "wanting," a subconscious motivational state that does not necessarily entail subjective desire but can still drive behavior (e.g., Winkielman, Berridge, & Wilbarger, 2005). Additional brain regions, such as the VMPFC and OFC, need to be recruited so that "wanting" breaks into conscious awareness and becomes explicit desire (Kringelbach & Berridge, 2009).

Whether desire arises from implicit "wanting" and leads to compulsive behavior in an automatic fashion, or from an explicit, goal-driven state (cf. Hofmann & Van Dillen, 2012), the MDP remains the key actor in how the brain engenders desire in response to rewarding stimuli. Accordingly, many researchers in the social brain sciences are focusing their investigations on reward processing in the MDP during functional magnetic resonance imaging (fMRI), a method that provides measures of task-evoked, regional blood-flow dynamics throughout the brain.[2] This non-invasive "peeking" into the human brain as it represents and responds to rewarding stimuli presents a great opportunity for neuroscientists and psychologists to examine implicit processes that underlie desire (see also Sayette & Wilson, Chapter 5, this volume). This is especially true given that people are often unaware of the extent to which cues activate goals, desires, and behaviors (Bargh & Morsella, 2008), particularly compulsive behaviors (Stacy & Wiers, 2010). Cues can even activate implicit cognitive processes that predict substance use (Rooke, Hine, & Thorsteinsson, 2008; Tiffany, 1990).

Some of the earliest imaging work on reward processing observed striatal activity in response to monetary incentives, specifically cues that predict delivery of a cash reward (Knutson, Westdorp, Kaiser, & Hommer, 2000), suggesting that the striatum represents the value of a desired, rewarding stimulus. Other research groups have also found this value-based coding in the striatum by having participants complete a variety of monetary-based decision-making tasks (Delgado, Nystrom, Fissell, Noll, & Fiez, 2000; Hsu, Bhatt, Adolphs, Tranel, & Camerer, 2005). Given this MDP activity in response to monetary rewards and preferred choices, social brain scientists proceeded to ask how the brain encodes the value of *appetitive* cues, such as high caloric foods and drugs of abuse. To address this question, they turned to addiction research and adapted cue-reactivity paradigms, which have consistently produced strong effects across different drug domains (Carter & Tiffany, 1999; see also Sayette & Wilson, Chapter 5, this volume). The original cue-reactivity tasks exposed participants to sensory cues of a desired, sometimes forbidden substance (e.g., alcohol cues shown to alcoholics seeking treatment),

---

[2]Although the dopaminergic prediction error mechanism described above occurs at the level of neurons, the blood-oxygenation-level-dependent signal acquired during fMRI serves as a reliable proxy for neuron-level firing patterns (Logothetis, Pauls, Augath, Trinath, & Oeltermann, 2001).

and then measured concomitant changes in self-reported craving and physiological responses.

Our lab has developed a cue-reactivity paradigm (Demos, Kelley, & Heatherton, 2011) that reliably elicits reward-related activity in the MDP (particularly VS and OFC). To ensure that activity in these regions reflects implicit (incidental) reward processing, we ask participants to make simple perceptual judgments about the images (e.g., whether the depicted scene takes place indoors or outdoors, or whether people are present in the image or not). Therefore, participants are naive to the true task and are unlikely to generate or elaborate a conscious desire in response to the cues they view.

One of the first studies our lab conducted implementing the paradigm tested whether reward is coded in a domain-specific manner and whether individual differences in reward activity predicted future behavior (Demos, Heatherton, & Kelley, 2012). During an fMRI session, participants viewed images from multiple reward categories, namely the eating and sexual domains, and completed the task as described above. Findings supported a domain-specific account of rewarding processing in the MDP. Specifically, there was a positive relationship between food-cue-specific activity in the VS and subsequent weight gain 6 months following the scan. There was also a positive relationship between cue reactivity to erotic images and dyadic sexual desire scores. Critically, these effects followed a double dissociation: food cue activity was correlated only with weight gain and not sexual desire scores, while the reverse was true for erotic cue activity. A key implication of this study is that higher sensitivity of the MDP (indexed by greater VS activation) can drive future behaviors in which there is a strong desire to obtain a reward. Of note, participants in this study showed marked variability in both their food and sexual cue reactivity (see scatter plots in Figure 2 of Demos et al., 2012). This variability may reflect differential tuning of participants' reward processing in the MDP, with genetic factors and previous experience with a given reward or reward domain likely dictating the tuning.

This MDP tuning is even more pronounced in drug-using populations. Frequently, individuals who struggle with addiction engage in compulsive drug-seeking behaviors marked by implicit desire ("wanting"). Social brain scientists have sought to identify neural correlates of this distinctive MDP tuning in special populations. One initial study compared non-alcohol-dependent controls and alcohol-dependent participants exhibited higher VS activation in response to alcohol cues (Heinz et al., 2004). A similar effect was observed in smokers responding to appetitive smoking cues (David et al., 2005), and remarkably, cocaine users show VS activation to subliminally presented (33 milliseconds) cocaine cues (Childress et al., 2008). These studies reveal that MDP tuning in these different populations affects reward processing of choice substances, providing a reliable brain-based marker of these groups' impulsive "wanting" behaviors.

More recent fMRI studies have identified additional brain systems that may stimulate implicit desire and reward-seeking behaviors in these populations. For example, Wagner, Cin, Sargent, Kelley, and Heatherton (2011) showed smokers and nonsmokers naturalistic film clips, some of which depicted people smoking, and interrogated spontaneous activation patterns in response to smoking scenes in particular. They found that smokers recruited regions in the action observation network (Buccino et al., 2004; Hamilton & Grafton, 2006) more so than their nonsmoking counterparts (Wagner et al., 2011). Although participants were in the scanner during the study and unable to perform any movements, the observed activity may represent precursor motor representations that increase the likelihood of engaging in the depicted smoking behavior. In this way, Wagner and colleagues' finding highlights the role of the action observation network, corroborating William James's original hypothesizing of the tight links between imagining actions and executing them (James, 1950/1890). This line of work also illustrates the multifaceted nature of how desire is instantiated in the brain, for in addition to a core system (the MDP) that represents the salience and value of tempting stimuli, other sets of regions are called upon to prepare motor movements to obtain the coveted object (after all, Eve did have to reach for the apple). As we already alluded to before, collectively these brain mechanisms allowed for our evolutionary development and survival as a species. However, in our modern, cue-saturated lives, unhealthy eating choices abound, drugs (legal and illegal) become easy to abuse, and a quick hook-up with a stranger is only a few mouse clicks or smartphone taps away. Assuming we uphold goals of temperance and restraint (at least in some domains), we're tasked with navigating through this thicket of temptation. Thankfully, there are neural mechanisms of desire regulation that offer us some hope as we "walk the line." Let us turn to these steadying mechanisms.

Neural Mechanisms of Desire Regulation

There has been no shortage of theorizing in psychology on how human beings regulate the push and pull of desire and impulses. Across many models, there is the common trope of desire mobilizing behavior to satisfy an impulse, and self-control as a restraining force to blunt desire and inhibit behavior (Baumeister & Heatherton, 1996; Hoch & Loewenstein, 1991; Hofmann, Friese, & Strack, 2009; Kruglanski et al., 2012; Metcalfe & Mischel, 1999; see also Hofmann, Kotabe, Vohs, & Baumeister, Chapter 3, this volume). In the past decade or so, social neuroscientists have seized the opportunity to test these models by exploring neural correlates of desire regulation and self-control processes. Some of the earliest studies focused on people's capacity to actively control emotional responses to affective stimuli. These studies identified regions in the prefrontal cortex (PFC), specifically the dorsolateral and ventrolateral PFC, that people recruit when consciously changing their emotional reactivity (Ochsner et al., 2004; Ochsner, Bunge, Gross, & Gabrieli, 2002; Wager, Davidson, Hughes, Lindquist, & Ochsner, 2008).

Inspired by this line of work, other social brain scientists wondered whether these same prefrontal systems might also be involved in the control of appetitive behaviors—when the target of regulation is not a negative emotion, but a desire for a rewarding stimulus. In a recent review (Heatherton & Wagner, 2011), we argue that prefrontal systems are recruited in a domain-general manner, but that the subcortical target of regulation will vary based on an individual's goals and regulatory context.[3] Specifically, the PFC will suppress activity in the amygdala in contexts that call for control of affective reactions, whereas it will inhibit activity in the MDP (e.g., the VS) to regulate appetitive behavior. In either case, activity in the PFC and subcortical systems interacts in the throes of an intense emotion or temptation will dictate self-control outcomes (see Figure 7.1; Heatherton & Wagner, 2011). Our balance model predicts that self-control failure is especially likely whenever activity in subcortical systems becomes unchecked and unregulated by the PFC.

The extent to which prefrontal systems are utilized in the service of a regulatory goal is a critical question for studying desire control. In a short time, the tools of brain imaging have made promising inroads. Hare and colleagues (2009) conducted one of the first studies to tackle this question. Dieters completed a food decision-making task during an fMRI scan, while brain activity was measured as the dieters made their choices, one of which was honored at the end of the study. The main finding was that the dorsolateral PFC modulates activity in the VMPFC, a region in the MDP hypothesized to encode the value of appetitive food stimuli. One example of this modulation effect was a negative relationship between activity in the dorsolateral PFC and VMPFC (see Figure 3C in Hare et al., 2009) in response to appealing food items during trials in which participants exerted self-control (i.e., opted not to eat the depicted food).

Another important region in the PFC that neuroscientists have focused on in desire regulation research is the inferior frontal gyrus, or

---

[3]Although rewarding and emotional stimuli are primarily processed in subcortical systems, there are cortical regions that also encode affective and appetitive aspects of stimuli, so "subcortical target" is a bit of a misnomer. Since our 2011 review, cited above, subsequent work has identified regulatory mechanisms between PFC systems and cortical sites associated with evaluative processing, such as the OFC (Wagner, Altman, Boswell, Kelley, & Heatherton, 2013) and VMPFC (Hare, Camerer, & Rangel, 2009).

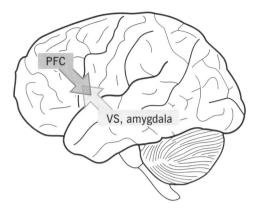

FIGURE 7.1. Schematic depiction of the balance model of self-regulation. Interactions between subcortical systems related to affect and reward (ventral striatum [VS] and amygdala, respectively) and the PFC are thought to govern behavioral outcomes.

ventrolateral PFC more generally (IFG/VLPFC). Activity in this region was observed in early cognitive neuroscience work as a robust correlate of stopping prepotent motor responses in the context of response inhibition tasks (Aron, Robbins, & Poldrack, 2004). In a more recent review (Aron, Robbins, & Poldrack, 2014), the authors highlight the role of IFG/VLPFC in impulse control disorders, citing work showing that impaired IFG/VLPFC functioning characterized illicit drug use in a large sample of adolescents (Whelan et al., 2012). This implicates IFG/VLPFC in the successful regulation of desires for rewarding stimuli. Indeed, Kober and colleagues (2010) found that smokers recruited a set of regions in the PFC (including IFG/VLPFC; see their Table S1) when employing cognitive strategies aimed at reducing their craving for cigarettes. They also found a statistical relationship between PFC and VS (assessed via mediation analysis) that supported successful control of craving (Kober et al., 2010).

With this mounting evidence, social neuroscientists have set out to establish ecological validity of the IFG/VLPFC's regulatory functions. To do so, they have taken the "brain-as-predictor" approach (Berkman & Falk, 2013) linking activity in the IFG/VLPFC with daily self-control dilemmas requiring successful desire regulation. One of the first demonstrations of this link was in the smoking domain (Berkman, Falk, & Lieberman, 2011). Heavy cigarette smokers in smoking-cessation programs completed a go/no-go response inhibition task (Casey et al., 1997) while undergoing an fMRI scan and then reported on their daily smoking behaviors for several weeks after the scanning session. Berkman and others found that those smokers who showed higher IFG/VLPFC activity during inhibitory (no-go) trials smoked less in their daily lives, even in the face of high levels of prior craving (see Figure 4 in Berkman et al., 2011). Another important finding was that those smokers with greater amygdala activation during inhibitory trials (likely an index of the strength of the prepotent response to be inhibited) were more likely to succumb to strong desires to smoke. The findings in this study support our balance model of self-regulation (Heatherton & Wagner, 2011), and demonstrate that IFG/VLPFC activity is not merely a correlate of lab-based performance on a response inhibition. Rather, this activity seems to reflect an individual's self-control capacity in the face of strong everyday desires.

In a more recent study we found a similar effect with predicting real-world eating behaviors (Lopez, Hofmann, Wagner, Kelley, & Heatherton, 2014). Participants first completed an fMRI session, during which they completed the cue-reactivity paradigm described above and a go/no-go task, and then reported on their daily eating behaviors 1 week after the scan. Higher cue reactivity in the VS predicted stronger food desires, greater likelihood of giving in to those desires, and more food eaten, while greater IFG/VLPFC activity associated with response inhibition in the go/no-go task facilitated successful resistance to desires (i.e., reduced likelihood of giving in to a desire; see Figure 1 in Lopez et al., 2014).

We have only scratched the surface of understanding how our prefrontal systems serve as our better angels in regulating desires and guiding our behaviors. And despite the extraordinary opportunity modern brain imaging affords to view the live workings of the human brain, new questions outpace any answers. This is especially true of questions pertaining to higher-order cognitive processes that entail flexible control of impulses and behaviors across (or even within) individuals. We now consider the most recent studies and new theorizing in the neuroscience of desire regulation that we hope will push the frontier of knowledge further.

Latest Research Developments in the Neuroscience of Desire Regulation

Given that neuroscience has localized both desire-generating brain systems (i.e., the MDP) and desire-regulating ones (e.g., the IFG/VLPFC), researchers can now finely probe psychological processes and interrogate accompanying patterns of activity in these systems. The two methodological approaches that follow from this idea are: (1) manipulating processes of interest and measuring subsequent neural activity, and (2) measuring naturally occurring variability in those processes, and noting any associated changes in neural activity. In short, the first is the traditional experimental approach that contextually constrains which neural mechanisms may be engaged and to what extent, while the second is an individual differences approach. With regard to the first approach, we would expect brain mechanisms of desire to be engaged and/or exaggerated in specific contexts, such as those in which people's self-control capacity is somehow compromised, allowing reward-related activity in the MDP to have free reign.

This scenario hits close to home in the chronic dieting population, a group that is prone to experience self-control failure in the eating domain despite repeated efforts to curb intake (Heatherton, Polivy, & Herman, 1991; Herman & Mack, 1975; see also Roefs, Houben, & Werthmann, Chapter 16, this volume). Under neutral conditions, dieters are generally successful in restraining their eating, and in fact show little reward activity in the VS (cf. Figure 3 in Demos et al., 2011). However, situational triggers such as negative distress (e.g., Heatherton et al., 1991; Heatherton, Striepe, & Wittenberg, 1998), dietary violations (Heatherton & Baumeister, 1991), and self-regulatory depletion (Vohs & Heatherton, 2000) can throw the rider off the horse, sending the horse down the road of failure.

These triggers were originally identified behaviorally and often led to increased levels of desire and consumption. But it remains unclear how the brain gives rise to such effects. A line of work conducted in our lab has studied all three triggers while dieters underwent fMRI scans and completed the cue-reactivity paradigm, as described above. Consistent patterns of amplified reward activity in the MDP (VS and/or OFC) in response to food cues when dieters were distressed (Wagner, Boswell, Kelley, & Heatherton, 2012), when their diets were broken by a milkshake preload (Demos et al., 2011), and when their self-regulatory capacity was diminished (Wagner et al., 2013).

Another sphere of research in our lab, corresponding to the individual differences approach, has investigated the link between intersubject variability in reward processing and self-control and real-world self-control outcomes. Our study on the neural predictors of giving in to daily temptations to eat (Lopez et al., 2014) and the Demos et al. (2012) study predicting long-term weight gain suggest that sensitivity of the brain's reward systems (i.e., the VS) to food cues predisposes people to succumb to desires to eat on a daily basis, which, over time, may translate to patterns of overeating and weight gain. There is much to be explored with the individual differences approach. One new dimension of this uncharted territory is the self-relevance of tempting stimuli and how these stimuli are represented in the brain, giving rise to subjective desire. One recent study by Giuliani, Mann, Tomiyama, and Berkman (2014) measured brain activity as participants regulated their desires for personally craved stimuli, identifying a set of prefrontal regions specific to regulation of those stimuli (versus noncraved stimuli), including the DLPFC and IFG/VLPFC.

Another rapidly developing research platform seeks to determine whether brain systems that underlie regulation of desire are amenable to training, and if so which systems should be the targets of training programs. With our balance model in view, one can make two reasonable suggestions: (1) given that self-control failure is more likely when desires and impulses, mediated by reward processing systems, dominate and govern behavior, these systems should be the targets of training regimens with the goal of dampening responsivity to rewarding stimuli; (2) conversely, since activity in prefrontal systems seems to represent one's capacity to regulate and override desires, these systems should also be the focus of training programs. With regards to the first approach, the empirical support is scarce at best, but there are some hints that it may be tractable. A new study by Gross and associates (2014) provides compelling evidence that higher-order value computations in the medial PFC may be carried out in a common value space, regardless of the object or domain whose value is computed (Gross et al., 2014). As the authors argue, this raises the possibility that the value of different stimuli and behaviors is exchangeable. If that is the case, then a self-control training program could target this region of PFC, which has reciprocal connections with subcortical reward systems in the MDP, as we showed earlier. Such a program could decrease the value of previously desired stimuli (a savory food item) and increase the value of a self-relevant goal to diet and exercise regularly. A demonstration of medial PFC modulation by Schonberg and colleagues (2014) offers the possibility that evaluative processing may indeed be plastic and changed via relatively simple, cue-based interventions.

The second suggestion has increasing support from neuroimaging studies. In one study, participants showed changes in recruitment of prefrontal regions following inhibitory control training, with some regions' activity increasing in the post- versus pretraining comparison and others decreasing their activity (Berkman, Kahn, & Merchant, 2014). This pattern of regions increasing and decreasing activity may represent different aspects that promote efficiency in the context of response inhibition (i.e., proactive versus reactive control). Follow-up studies should consider how these aspects might translate into effective self-control in daily life, and the extent to which changes in prefrontal systems have domain-general versus domain-specific effects (e.g., whether motor control training via a go/no-go task can positively impact self-control outcomes in the eating domain). Another recent study showed decreased DLPFC recruitment following a 1- hour training session that caused participants to alter their food preferences (Schonberg, Bakkour, Hover, Mumford, & Poldrack, 2013). This suggests that although there is strong evidence that prefrontal systems support self-control, inhibitory processes carried out by these systems might become automatized (indexed by less activity) and lead to successful desire regulation. To conclude, the jury is still out with regard to which brain systems should be the targets of training procedures, and neuroscientists will need to consider how the magnitude and direction of changes in PFC activation patterns meaningfully track with behavioral outcomes.

Conclusion

In this chapter, we teased apart neural mechanisms that generate desire and prompt us to pursue tempting stimuli. We saw that the core reward-processing system is the MDP, with both subcortical (VS) and cortical (VMPFC, OFC) regions as key players. We next reviewed prefrontal systems that interact with the MDP to keep desire in check and control behavior in a domain-general fashion. Lastly, we surveyed the interesting but wild terrain of the latest desire regulation research. Currently, there are more questions than answers, but the neuroscience of desire regulation is well positioned to address those questions. Social brain scientists are beginning to leverage more sophisticated brain imaging modalities, including measures of structural and functional connectivity, as well as multivariate techniques to analyze patterns of neural activity within and across regions. We are hopeful that the next several decades will be an exciting and quickly evolving period for the field, as our understanding of the brain's role in generating and controlling desires will come into greater and greater focus.

REFERENCES

Aron, A. R., Robbins, T. W., & Poldrack, R. A. (2004). Inhibition and the right inferior frontal cortex. *Trends in Cognitive Sciences, 8*(4), 170–177.

Aron, A. R., Robbins, T. W., & Poldrack, R. A. (2014). Inhibition and the right inferior frontal cortex: one decade on. *Trends in Cognitive Sciences, 18*(4), 177–185.

Bargh, J. A., & Morsella, E. (2008). The unconscious mind. *Perspectives on Psychological Science, 3*(1), 73–79.

Baumeister, R. F., & Heatherton, T. F. (1996). Self-regulation failure: An overview. *Psychological Inquiry, 7*(1), 1–15.

Berkman, E. T., & Falk, E. B. (2013). Beyond brain mapping: Using neural measures to predict real-world outcomes. *Current Directions in Psychological Science, 22*(1), 45–50.

Berkman, E. T., Falk, E. B., & Lieberman, M. D. (2011). In the trenches of real-world self-control: Neural correlates of breaking the link between craving and smoking. *Psychological Science, 22*(4), 498–506.

Berkman, E. T., Kahn, L. E., & Merchant, J. S. (2014). Training-induced changes in inhibitory control network activity. *Journal of Neuroscience, 34*(1), 149–157.

Berridge, K. C., & Robinson, T. E. (1998). What is the role of dopamine in reward: hedonic impact, reward learning, or incentive salience? *Brain Research Reviews, 28*(3), 309–369.

Berridge, K. C., & Robinson, T. E. (2003). Parsing reward. *Trends in Neurosciences, 26*(9), 507–513.

Buccino, G., Vogt, S., Ritzl, A., Fink, G. R., Zilles, K., Freund, H.-J., et al. (2004). Neural circuits underlying imitation learning of hand actions: An event-related fMRI study. *Neuron, 42*(2), 323–334.

Carter, B. L., & Tiffany, S. T. (1999). Meta-analysis of cue-reactivity in addiction research. *Addiction, 94*(3), 327–340.

Casey, B. J., Trainor, R. J., Orendi, J. L., Schubert, A. B., Nystrom, L. E., Giedd, J. N., et al. (1997). A developmental functional MRI study of prefrontal activation during performance of a go-no-go task. *Journal of Cognitive Neuroscience, 9*(6), 835–847.

Childress, A. R., Ehrman, R. N., Wang, Z., Li, Y., Sciortino, N., Hakun, J., et al. (2008). Prelude to passion: Limbic activation by "unseen" drug and sexual cues. *PLoS One, 3*(1), e1506.

David, S. P., Munafò, M. R., Johansen-Berg, H., Smith, S. M., Rogers, R. D., Matthews, et al. (2005). Ventral striatum/nucleus accumbens activation to smoking-related pictorial cues in smokers and nonsmokers: A functional magnetic resonance imaging study. *Biological Psychiatry, 58*(6), 488–494.

Delgado, M. R., Nystrom, L. E., Fissell, C., Noll, D. C., & Fiez, J. A. (2000). Tracking the hemodynamic responses to reward and punishment in the striatum. *Journal of Neurophysiology, 84*(6), 3072–3077.

Demos, K. E., Heatherton, T. F., & Kelley, W. M. (2012). Individual differences in nucleus accumbens activity to food and sexual images predict weight gain and sexual behavior. *Journal of Neuroscience, 32*(16), 5549–5552.

Demos, K. E., Kelley, W. M., & Heatherton, T. F. (2011). Dietary restraint violations influence reward responses in nucleus accumbens and amygdala. *Journal of Cognitive Neuroscience, 23*(8), 1952–1963.

Giuliani, N. R., Mann, T., Tomiyama, A. J., & Berkman, E. T. (2014). Neural systems underlying the reappraisal of personally craved foods. *Journal of Cognitive Neuroscience, 26*(7), 1390–1402.

Gross, J., Woelbert, E., Zimmermann, J., Okamoto-Barth, S., Riedl, A., & Goebel, R. (2014). Value signals in the prefrontal cortex predict individual preferences across reward categories. *Journal of Neuroscience, 34*(22), 7580–7586.

Haber, S. N., & Knutson, B. (2010). The reward circuit: Linking primate anatomy and human imaging. *Neuropsychopharmacology, 35*(1), 4–26.

Hamilton, A. F. de C., & Grafton, S. T. (2006). Goal Representation in Human Anterior Intraparietal Sulcus. *Journal of Neuroscience, 26*(4), 1133–1137.

Hare, T. A., Camerer, C. F., & Rangel, A. (2009). Self-control in decision-making involves modulation of the vmPFC valuation system. *Science, 324*(5927), 646–648.

Heatherton, T. F., & Baumeister, R. F. (1991). Binge eating as escape from self-awareness. *Psychological Bulletin, 110*(1), 86–108.

Heatherton, T. F., Polivy, J., & Herman, C. P. (1991). Restraint, weight loss, and variability of body weight. *Journal of Abnormal Psychology, 100*(1), 78–83.

Heatherton, T. F., Striepe, M., & Wittenberg, L. (1998). Emotional distress and disinhibited eating: The role of self. *Personality and Social Psychology Bulletin, 24*(3), 301–313.

Heatherton, T. F., & Wagner, D. D. (2011). Cognitive neuroscience of self-regulation failure. *Trends in Cognitive Sciences, 15*(3), 132–139.

Heinz, A., Siessmeier, T., Wrase, J., Hermann, D., Klein, S., Grüsser-Sinopoli, S. M., et al. (2004). Correlation between dopamine d2 receptors in the ventral striatum and central processing of alcohol cues and craving. *American Journal of Psychiatry, 161*(10), 1783–1789.

Herman, C. P., & Mack, D. (1975). Restrained and unrestrained eating. *Journal of Personality, 43*(4), 647–660.

Hoch, S. J., & Loewenstein, G. F. (1991). Time-inconsistent preferences and consumer self-control. *Journal of Consumer Research, 17*(4), 492–507.

Hofmann, W., Friese, M., & Strack, F. (2009). Impulse and self-control from a dual-systems perspective. *Perspectives on Psychological Science, 4*(2), 162–176.

Hofmann, W., & Van Dillen, L. (2012). Desire: The new hot spot in self-control research. *Current Directions in Psychological Science, 21*, 317–322.

Hsu, M., Bhatt, M., Adolphs, R., Tranel, D., & Camerer, C. F. (2005). Neural systems responding to degrees of uncertainty in human decision-making. *Science, 310*(5754), 1680–1683.

James, W. (1950). *The principles of psychology.* New York: Dover.

Knutson, B., Westdorp, A., Kaiser, E., & Hommer, D. (2000). FMRI visualization of brain activity during a monetary incentive delay task. *NeuroImage, 12*(1), 20–27.

Kober, H., Mende-Siedlecki, P., Kross, E. F., Weber, J., Mischel, W., Hart, C. L., et al. (2010). Prefrontal–striatal pathway underlies cognitive regulation of craving. *Proceedings of the National Academy of Sciences, 107*(33), 14811–14816.

Kringelbach, M. L., & Berridge, K. C. (2009). Towards a functional neuroanatomy of pleasure and happiness. *Trends in Cognitive Sciences, 13*(11), 479–487.

Kruglanski, A. W., Bélanger, J. J., Chen, X., Köpetz, C., Pierro, A., & Mannetti, L. (2012). The energetics of motivated cognition: A force-field analysis. *Psychological Review, 119*(1), 1–20.

Lisman, J. E., & Grace, A. A. (2005). The hippocampal-VTA loop: Controlling the entry of information into long-term memory. *Neuron, 46*(5), 703–713.

Logothetis, N. K., Pauls, J., Augath, M., Trinath, T., & Oeltermann, A. (2001). Neurophysiological investigation of the basis of the fMRI signal. *Nature, 412*(6843), 150–157.

Lopez, R. B., Hofmann, W., Wagner, D. D., Kelley, W. M., & Heatherton, T. F. (2014). Neural predictors of giving in to temptation in daily life. *Psychological Science, 25*(7), 1337–1344.

Metcalfe, J., & Mischel, W. (1999). A hot/cool-system analysis of delay of gratification: Dynamics of willpower. *Psychological Review, 106*(1), 3–19.

Ochsner, K. N., Bunge, S. A., Gross, J. J., & Gabrieli, J. D. E. (2002). Rethinking feelings: An fMRI study of the cognitive regulation of emotion. *Journal of Cognitive Neuroscience, 14*(8), 1215–1229.

Ochsner, K. N., Ray, R. D., Cooper, J. C., Robertson, E. R., Chopra, S., Gabrieli, J. D. E., et al. (2004). For better or for worse: Neural systems supporting the cognitive down- and up-regulation of negative emotion. *NeuroImage, 23*(2), 483–499.

Pennebaker, J. W., Dyer, M. A., Caulkins, R. S., Litowitz, D. L., Ackreman, P. L., Anderson, D. B., et al. (1979). Don't the girls get prettier at closing time: A country and western application to psychology. *Personality and Social Psychology Bulletin, 5*(1), 122–125.

Rooke, S. E., Hine, D. W., & Thorsteinsson, E. B. (2008). Implicit cognition and substance use: A meta-analysis. *Addictive Behaviors, 33*(10), 1314–1328.

Schonberg, T., Bakkour, A., Hover, A. M., Mumford, J. A., Nagar, L., Perez, J., et al. (2014). Changing value through cued approach: An automatic mechanism of behavior change. *Nature Neuroscience, 17*(4), 625–630.

Schonberg, T., Bakkour, A., Hover, A. M., Mumford, J. A., & Poldrack, R. A. (2013). Influencing food choices by training: Evidence for modulation of frontoparietal control signals. *Journal of Cognitive Neuroscience, 26*(2), 247–268.

Schultz, W., Dayan, P., & Montague, P. R. (1997). A neural substrate of prediction and reward. *Science, 275*(5306), 1593–1599.

Stacy, A. W., & Wiers, R. W. (2010). Implicit cognition and addiction: A tool for explaining paradoxical behavior. *Annual Review of Clinical Psychology, 6*, 551–575

Tiffany, S. T. (1990). A cognitive model of drug urges and drug-use behavior: Role of automatic and nonautomatic processes. *Psychological Review, 97*(2), 147–168.

Vohs, K. D., & Heatherton, T. F. (2000). Self-regulatory failure: A resource-depletion approach. *Psychological Science, 11*(3), 249–254.

Wager, T. D., Davidson, M. L., Hughes, B. L., Lindquist, M. A., & Ochsner, K. N. (2008). Prefrontal–subcortical pathways mediating successful emotion regulation. *Neuron, 59*(6), 1037–1050.

Wagner, D. D., Altman, M., Boswell, R. G., Kelley, W. M., & Heatherton, T. F. (2013). Self-regulatory depletion enhances neural responses to rewards and impairs top-down control. *Psychological Science, 24*(11), 2262–2271.

Wagner, D. D., Boswell, R. G., Kelley, W. M., & Heatherton, T. F. (2012). Inducing negative affect increases the reward value of appetizing foods in dieters. *Journal of Cognitive Neuroscience, 24*(7), 1625–1633.

Wagner, D. D., Cin, S. D., Sargent, J. D., Kelley, W. M., & Heatherton, T. F. (2011). Spontaneous action representation in smokers when watching movie characters smoke. *Journal of Neuroscience, 31*(3), 894–898.

Whelan, R., Conrod, P. J., Poline, J.-B., Lourdusamy, A., Banaschewski, T., Barker, G. J., et al. (2012). Adolescent impulsivity phenotypes characterized by distinct brain networks. *Nature Neuroscience, 15*(6), 920–925.

Winkielman, P., Berridge, K. C., & Wilbarger, J. L. (2005). Unconscious affective reactions to masked happy versus angry faces influence consumption behavior and judgments of value. *Personality and Social Psychology Bulletin, 31*(1), 121–135.

CHAPTER 8

Individual Differences in Desire and Approach Motivation

Eddie Harmon-Jones
Philip A. Gable
Cindy Harmon-Jones

In this chapter, we approach the empirical study of individual differences in desire from the perspective of approach motivation. We define approach motivation as simply *the urge to go toward* (Harmon-Jones, Harmon-Jones, & Price, 2013), and we believe many variations of desire fit this definition. By our definition, which is based on decades of experimental, clinical, and neurological research, approach motivation (desire) does not require a stimulus or goal; it is not necessarily toward a positive outcome; and it is not necessarily experienced as a positive state. Evidence presented below will clarify why this is so.

By defining *desire* as fundamentally an approach-motivated state, we seek to distinguish the term from the more commonly used discrete emotion of desire, which is usually assumed to be an affective state positive in valence and associated with positive outcomes (e.g., desire for a delicious dessert or attractive individual). We believe this subjectively positive affective state is only one way through which desire can manifest. As the chapter unfolds, we hope it becomes clear why we prefer an empirically based definition of approach motivation, and how this definition relates to a broader understanding of desire.

In this chapter, we review research on individual differences in approach motivation and how they relate to electrophysiological indices and influence cognitive and emotive responses. We focus primarily on the most widely used measure of individual differences in approach motivation, the behavioral activation system (BAS) sensitivity scale developed by Carver and White (1994). This questionnaire was based on the original version of Gray's (1990) reinforcement sensitivity theory. Carver and White's (1994) BIS/BAS questionnaire is designed to assess individual differences in BAS sensitivity as well as behavioral inhibition system (BIS) sensitivity.

The scale consists of 20 items, and responses to the items are expressed on 4-point scales (1 = strongly disagree, 4 = strongly agree). It is comprised of three BAS subscales and one BIS subscale. The BAS subscales are Reward-Responsiveness, which contains "items that focus on positive responses to the occurrence of anticipation of reward" (Carver & White, 1994, p. 322); Drive, which contains "items pertaining to the persistent pursuit of desired goals" (Carver & White, 1994, p. 322); and Fun-Seeking, which contains "items reflecting both a desire for new rewards and a willingness to approach a potentially rewarding event on the spur of the moment" (Carver & White, 1994, p. 322). As these examples show, all three BAS subscales clearly relate to individual differences in desire. BAS-Total, which is calculated as the sum of all BAS items, is widely used in research, though the subscales are used as well. The BIS subscale contains "items referencing reactions to the anticipation of punishment" (Carver & White, 1994, p. 322). Because the BIS scale was based on the original version of reinforcement sensitivity theory, it measures punishment sensitivity.

Individual Differences in Approach Motivation: The Case of the BAS

Motivational direction—the urge to move toward or approach versus the urge to move away or withdraw—is a fundamental motivational property of living organisms. One major theory concerned with motivational direction is the reinforcement sensitivity theory of Jeffrey Gray (1970). The theory proposed a BAS and a BIS. Originally, the theory proposed that the BAS was sensitive to signals of conditioned reward (stimuli associated with innate rewards), nonpunishment, and escape from punishment. Consequently, the BAS was proposed to cause movement toward goals, and to be involved in generating anticipatory positive affect. BAS sensitivity was also proposed to be associated with personality characteristics related to optimism, reward responsiveness, and impulsiveness, all of which are varieties of desire. These broad personality characteristics in turn relate to clinical problems such as addictive behaviors, high-risk impulsive behaviors, and mania. A low level of BAS sensitivity (deficiency of desire) was proposed to incline individuals toward unipolar depression. Research has supported these propositions (Nusslock, Shackman, Harmon-Jones, Alloy, Coan, et al., 2011; see also Treadway, Chapter 15, this volume).

It may seem odd to conceive of anger as a relating to desire; however, evidence suggests that this is the case (see also Denson, Schofield, & Fabianssohn, Chapter 18, this volume). State anger is associated with a behavioral urge to approach, and aggress against, the anger-evoking stimulus. Similarly, trait anger is associated with the BAS.

Although Gray positioned the BAS in positive affect terms, research has suggested that individual differences in BAS are positively related to anger, a negative affect. This relationship occurs even though items on the BAS questionnaire all measure responses to rewarding situations, such as "When I get something I want I feel excited and energized." Thus, no semantic overlap occurs between the BAS items and items on trait anger measures. Despite this, several studies have found that scores on Carver and White's (1994) BAS scale correlate positively with self-reported anger and/or aggression, at both trait (Cooper, Gomez, & Buck, 2008; Harmon-Jones, 2003; Smits & Kuppens, 2005) and state levels (Carver, 2004).

If individual differences in BAS predispose one toward more anger, would situational influences that prime positive approach motivation also trigger more angry responses, particularly for individuals who score high in BAS? This idea was tested by having participants listen to an ostensible pilot radio broadcast that had been found to reliably evoke anger in previous experiments (Harmon-Jones, Harmon-Jones, Abramson, & Peterson, 2009b). After participants listened to this broadcast, they completed one of three questionnaires that were used to manipulate their mindsets: positive high approach (steps to obtain a desired goal), positive low approach (a positive event happened without the participant's action), or neutral (an ordinary day). Then they completed a questionnaire assessing their attitudes toward the speaker in the broadcast and how likely it was that they would recommend other radio jobs for the speaker. Responses to this questionnaire were considered aggressive inclinations because the participants were told their responses would be given to the radio station. Individual differences in BAS sensitivity interacted with the mindset manipulation to predict aggressive inclinations. Specifically, individuals who scored higher in BAS and who completed the high approach mindset manipulation were the least likely to like the speaker and recommend the speaker for future jobs (Harmon-Jones & Peterson, 2008).

Desire may relate to anger because when approach motivation is activated and goals are blocked, anger results (Carver & Harmon-Jones, 2009). However, we believe that this explanation does not account for all instances of anger being associated with approach motivation. For example, it does not easily explain the individual differences evidence reviewed previously, nor does it account for evidence linking approach motivation to angry states that occurred prior to the evocation of approach motivation or were unrelated to a given approach motivation (Harmon-Jones et al., 2013). We also believe it would fail to account for other instances of angry approach that result from changes in neurochemical processes (Hortensius, Schutter, & Harmon-Jones, 2012) or bodily expressions (Harmon-Jones & Peterson, 2009). In other words, anger may be associated with desire because of the stimulus (goal frustration) or because of the response association (approach motivation is anger's primary behavioral expression). The research linking anger with approach motivation suggests that approach motivation is not necessarily experienced as a positive affective state.

The Psychophysiology of Desire

According to reinforcement sensitivity theory, individual differences in the sensitivity of the BAS should relate to reward sensitivity and responses. Below, we review research that examined associations between individual differences in BAS and emotive psychophysiological responses. One primary advantage of testing these associations using psychophysiological responses instead of self-report measures is that the observed associations will not be due to overlap in semantic meaning or participants' implicit theories, because psychophysiological responses related to emotion processes are unlikely to be influenced by semantic meaning.

Asymmetric Frontal Cortical Activity

Individual differences in BAS have been examined in relationship with asymmetric frontal cortical activity. The impetus for testing the association of the BAS with this variable was that activity in the left and right frontal cortical regions is involved in the experience and expression of positive affect/approach motivation and negative affect/withdrawal motivation, respectively (e.g., Goldstein, 1939). Research from the 1930s, as well as more recent research, revealed that individuals who had experienced lesions to their left frontal cortex were likely to show depressive symptoms, whereas individuals who had experienced lesions to their right frontal cortex were likely to show manic symptoms (Gainotti, 1972; Robinson & Price, 1982). This human research fits well with research from a variety of nonhuman animal species in showing hemispheric asymmetries underlying appetitive and avoidant behaviors (for review, see Vallortigara & Rogers, 2005).

In humans, these asymmetric activations are specific to the frontal cortex. In most of the research on individual differences, asymmetric activity in right versus left frontal cortical areas is usually assessed by electroencephalographic (EEG) recordings. More specifically, alpha frequency band activity is derived from the EEG. It is the band of choice because it is abundant in the EEG and it is inversely related to regional brain activity using hemodynamic measures (Cook, O'Hara, Uijtdehaage, Mandelkern, & Leuchter, 1998) and behavioral tasks (Davidson, Chapman, Chapman, & Henriques, 1990). Often, difference scores are used, consistent with the early lesion research that suggests that asymmetry may be the critical variable, with one hemisphere inhibiting the other, particularly in emotive processes.

Two studies from 1997 found that individual differences in BAS related to greater left than right frontal activity at resting baseline (Harmon-Jones & Allen, 1997; Sutton & Davidson, 1997). One study also found that individual differences in BIS related to greater right than left frontal activity (Sutton & Davidson, 1997), but the other study found a nonsignificant relationship between BIS and asymmetrical frontal activity (Harmon-Jones & Allen, 1997). More recent studies have replicated the BAS result, and the BIS result is often null (Amodio, Master, Yee, & Taylor, 2008; Coan & Allen, 2003).

The tendency toward rash action during extreme positive emotional states, or positive urgency, has been shown to be an important trait predictor in a number of substance abuse problems and psychopathologies. For example, when individuals are in states of strong desire, they may have a tendency to act more impulsively. Recent research found that greater positive urgency was associated with greater relative left frontal EEG activity at baseline (Mechin & Gable, 2014).

Impulsivity is the tendency to engage in rapid, unplanned actions without considering potential consequences, and is likely related to high BAS/high trait desire. Much past work has linked impulsivity with alcohol use. But what is it about impulsivity that leads to alcohol use? Mechin and Gable (2014) examined whether approach motivation—assessed through greater left than right frontal asymmetry—might be one mechanism that moderates the link between alcohol and impulsivity. If approach motivation moderates this link, then individual differences in trait impulsivity should predict greater left frontal activity to alcohol pictures but not to neutral pictures. Participants completed measures of trait impulsivity. Then, they viewed pictures of alcoholic beverages and neutral (rock) pictures while EEG activity was recorded. Results revealed that greater trait impulsivity predicted greater left frontal asymmetry during alcohol pictures but not during neutral pictures. These results demonstrate that individual differences in trait impulsivity potentiate the effects of alcohol cues on asymmetrical frontal cortical activity. More broadly, results suggest that individual differences in impulsivity may enhance approach motivation toward alcohol cues, suggesting that approach motivation may moderate the relationship between impulsivity and alcohol use. Gable, Mechin, Hicks, and Adams (2015) extended these findings by demonstrating that greater left frontal activity in a resting state predicted greater positive urgency, a trait measure of rash action. These results suggest that approach motivation may underlie some facets of impulsivity, even in the absence of appetitive stimuli.

Similarly, bipolar disorder, which has been found to be directly associated with BAS sensitivity scores (Alloy et al., 2006; Meyer, Johnson, & Carver, 1999), relates to greater relative left frontal cortical activity at resting baseline when individuals are in a manic episode (Kano, Nakamura, Matsuoka, Iida, & Nakajima, 1992). Moreover, individuals with bipolar proneness and clinical levels of bipolar disorder evidence even greater relative left frontal activity than nonbipolar individuals during angering events (Harmon-Jones et al., 2002) and during extremely difficult tasks that offer the promise of reward (Harmon-Jones et al., 2008). Finally, individuals with less severe forms of bipolar disorder (i.e., cyclothymia, bipolar II) who have elevated relative left frontal cortical activity at resting baseline are more likely to convert to a more severe form of bipolar disorder (bipolar I) in subsequent years (Nusslock et al., 2012).

Individual differences in BAS have also been related with neural excitability of the left and right primary motor cortex as assessed by transcranial magnetic stimulation (TMS; Schutter, de Weijer, Meuwese, Morgan, & van Honk, 2008). Cortical responses obtained from the motor cortex are strongly correlated with prefrontal cortex activity (Kähkönen, Komssi, Wilenius, & Ilmoniemi, 2005). Thus, this TMS methodology informs research on asymmetric frontal cortical activity. To measure neural excitability of left and right primary motor cortex, TMS of increasing intensity is applied over the primary motor cortex, and thumb twitches are measured. The lowest TMS pulse intensity that causes a thumb twitch is the motor threshold. The motor threshold is a product of the excitability of axonal fibers of corticospinal neurons and interneurons that influence the output cells in the motor cortex (Moll et al., 1999). Consistent with the predictions of Schutter et al. (2008), individuals with higher BAS scores (relative to BIS scores) had greater left over right motor cortical excitability as measured by this TMS method.

The above results illustrate that individuals can differ in approach motivation even at rest, suggesting that approach motivation or desire does not need a stimulus or goal.

Affective Modulated Startle Eyeblink Responses

Another widely used measure in emotive psychophysiology is the startle eyeblink reflex. It is assessed from the electromyographic (EMG) response of the orbicularis oculi muscle (underneath the eye) to a startling noise. Research dating back to the late 1980s has revealed that the magnitude of the startle eyeblink reflex is influenced by motivationally significant stimuli. In a typical experiment using this measure, individuals view photographs that vary in affective pleasantness and arousal (e.g., erotica, wind sailing, severed hand, snakes, household objects), as bursts of 95 to 100 dB white noise are presented intermittently during photograph presentation (Vrana, Spence, & Lang, 1988).

The startle eyeblink is a defensive response generated by amygdala neurons. The startle eyeblink is smaller when evoked during the midst of viewing arousing pleasant photographs and larger when evoked during the midst of viewing arousing unpleasant photographs (Lang, 1995). This pattern of responses is likely due to response matching, whereby the appetitive motivation caused by desire-evoking photographs subtracts from the defensive motivation evoked by the startle noise, and the defensive/avoidant motivation caused by the arousing unpleasant photographs adds to the defensive motivation evoked by the startle noise.

Individual differences in BAS sensitivity relate to startle eyeblink responses when viewing affective pictures (Hawk & Kowmas, 2003). In particular, as compared to individuals scoring low in BAS, individuals scoring high in BAS respond more to desire-arousing pleasant stimuli such as erotica or appetizing foods (i.e., they have smaller startle eyeblinks). Other research has revealed that individual differences in approach emotions (i.e., enjoyment, surprise, and anger) relate to the same pattern of startle responses (Amodio & Harmon-Jones, 2011).

Event-Related Potentials to Startle Probes

Other research has related individual differences in BAS to asymmetrical frontal event-related potentials (ERPs) to emotive stimuli (Peterson, Gable, & Harmon-Jones, 2008). ERPs are electrical brain responses that are assessed with and extracted from the ongoing EEG. They are often measured by averaging the responses to discrete events, and the components or waveforms are often named according to their electrical polarity and timing or number. For example, the N1 is a negative-going wave that peaks approximately 100 msec after event onset and is associated with selective attention (Hillyard, Hink, Schwent, & Picton, 1973). The P3 is a positive-going wave that peaks approximately 300 msec after event onset and is related to updating of working memory (Donchin & Coles, 1988). Larger N1s have been found to occur to startle probes presented during negative affective stimuli, presumably because of enhanced selective attention during such states. In contrast, smaller P3s have been found to occur to startle probes during both positive and negative affective stimuli, presumably because greater working memory processes are activated by both types of motivationally significant stimuli (Cuthbert, Schupp, Bradley, McManis, & Lang, 1998).

Given the body of research suggesting that asymmetrical frontal cortical activity is involved in emotive processes, research examined asymmetrical frontal N1 and P3 amplitudes in relation to the BAS (Peterson et al., 2008). It was found that individuals scoring higher in BAS sensitivity had smaller left frontal P3 amplitudes to startle probes during positive stimuli (but not neutral stimuli), suggesting that these individuals dedicated more working memory processes to desirable stimuli.

ERPs to Affective Pictures

The previous study examined ERPs to startle noise probes presented during the midst of affective picture viewing, to follow up on research by Cuthbert et al. (1998). In more recent research using many more affective pictures (which is necessary to obtain reliable ERPs to complex stimuli like pictures), ERPs beginning at picture onset were examined and related to individual differences in BAS (Gable & Harmon-Jones, 2012). In particular, the N1 was examined, as it is one of the earliest ERPs influenced by the motivational significance of stimuli (Keil, Müller, Gruber, Wienbruch, Stolarova, et al., 2001; Foti, Hajcak, & Dien, 2009). The fact that motivationally significant stimuli cause an increase in the amplitude of the N1 is likely due to the early allocation of attention to such stimuli (Keil et al., 2001).

In the study on individual differences in BAS and N1 amplitudes to appetitive pictures, participants viewed appetitive (delicious desserts) and neutral (rock) pictures (Gable & Harmon-Jones, 2012). Consistent with past research, N1 amplitudes were larger to appetitive pictures than to neutral pictures. Moreover, higher BAS scores were related to larger N1 amplitudes to appetitive pictures but not to neutral pictures.

Another ERP component that is larger to motivationally significant stimuli is the late positive potential (LPP; Foti, Hajcak, & Dien, 2009). The LPP begins approximately 300 msec after stimulus onset and lasts for several hundred miliseconds (Gable & Adams, 2013; Gable, Adams, & Proudfit, 2014). Consistent with research suggesting that anger is an approach-oriented emotion (Carver & Harmon-Jones, 2009), research has found that individual differences in BAS were correlated with larger LPPs to anger pictures but not to neutral pictures. In addition, individual differences in BAS correlated with greater relative left frontal activity to anger pictures (Gable & Poole, 2012). These results suggest that trait desire relates to two neurophysiological responses of anger.

Functional Magnetic Resonance Imaging

Functional magnetic resonance imaging (fMRI) measures changes in blood oxygenation and blood flow responses associated with metabolic activity that are required by certain populations of neurons (Johnstone, Kim, & Whalen, 2009). Studies assessing fMRI during reward-type tasks have linked certain patterns of neural activation such as ventral striatum and orbitofrontal activation with individual differences in BAS. In one study, compared to individuals who scored low in BAS, individuals who scored high in BAS evidenced more ventral striatum activation during the receipt of a reward and more medial orbitofrontal activation during both the receipt and omission of a reward (Simon et al., 2010).

Following from research that has found that individuals high in BAS have more frequent and intense food cravings and are more likely to be overweight or have excessive food intake disorders (Franken & Muris, 2005), another study examined fMRI responses to pictures of appetizing foods (e.g., chocolate cake, pizza; Beaver et al., 2006). In response to appetizing food pictures, individuals who scored higher in BAS evidenced greater activation in a fronto–striatal–amygdala–midbrain network, a network previously implicated in reward processing. They also evidenced with greater left anterolateral orbitofrontal cortical activation in response to appetizing foods, consistent with the previously reviewed research on asymmetrical frontal cortical activity and approach motivation.

Consistent with research linking the BAS to anger, other studies have found that individual differences in BAS predict activation in neural regions involved in aggression when the individuals view facial expressions of anger. In particular, higher BAS Drive scores were associated with more amygdala activation and less ventral anterior cingulate and ventral striatal activation to facial expressions of anger compared to sad and neutral expressions (Beaver, Lawrence, Passamonti, & Calder, 2008).

The Effects of Approach Motivation on Cognitive Scope

Affective states differ in motivational intensity. That is, positive and negative affective states can range from low to high in motivational intensity. With positive affective states in particular, some are low in approach motivational intensity (e.g., joy after watching a funny film), whereas others are high in motivational intensity (e.g., enthusiasm while approaching a desirable object).

Research conducted over the last several years has revealed that motivational intensity influences cognitive scope (Harmon-Jones, Gable, & Price, 2013). For example, positive affective states low in approach motivational intensity broaden cognitive scope, whereas positive affective states high in approach motivational intensity narrow it. These associations of cognitive scope with motivational intensity may be functional for the organism. With low-approach-oriented positive affective states, a broadened cognitive scope may assist the organism with discovering new goals, as low approach positive states typically occur following goal acquisition. With high-approach-oriented positive affective states, a narrowed cognitive scope may assist organisms in shutting out irrelevant cognitions as they go toward and attempt to obtain the desired objects.

Consistent with these ideas, Easterbrook (1959) proposed that emotional arousal causes a reduction in the "range of cue utilization." However, Easterbrook referred to drive as "a dimension of emotional arousal or general covert excitement, the innate response to a state of biological deprivation or noxious stimulation. . . . The emotional arousal is greater in neurotic than in normal subjects" (p. 184). Thus Easterbrook viewed this state as negative. However, emotional arousal can be positive or negative, and arousal may reflect motivational intensity.

Several experiments have revealed that low approach positive affect broadens cognitive scope (Gable & Harmon-Jones, 2008, Study 1; Gable & Harmon-Jones, 2011, Studies 1–2; Price & Harmon-Jones, 2010), but high approach positive affect narrows cognitive scope (Gable & Harmon-Jones, 2008, Studies 2–4; Gable & Harmon-Jones, 2010; Gable & Harmon-Jones,

2011, Studies 1–2; E. Harmon-Jones & Gable, 2009; Price & Harmon-Jones, 2010).

In line with the present chapter's focus on individual differences in desire, research has found that individual differences in BAS correlate with more attentional narrowing following the evocation of high approach positive affect (Gable & Harmon-Jones, 2008, Study 3). In this study, the appetitive stimuli were photographs of desserts or cute baby animals, and attentional scope with measured with Navon's (1977) letters task. Similar relationships between trait BAS and attentional narrowing after anger-inducing photographs have also been observed (Gable, Poole, & Harmon-Jones, in press).

Subsequent studies have revealed that photographs of alcohol also narrow attention, particularly for individuals who possess a strong desire to consume alcohol (Hicks, Friedman, Gable, & Davis, 2012). Additional research has found that greater left frontal activity to alcohol pictures predicts even more narrowed attention after alcohol images are primed (Gable, Mechin, & Browning, 2014). Alcohol cues narrow attentional scope for individuals who are motivated to consume alcohol and who are high in approach motivation, suggesting a nonpharmacological means by which alcohol produces a narrow mindset. Alcohol cues may contribute to cognitive and behavioral deficits, as well as drinking behaviors, in part because they lead to the inability to process a broad range of information in the environment. Together, these results suggest that trait desire may cause greater "virtual" alcohol myopia.

Resolving Motivational Conflict: Cognitive Dissonance Reduction

The self-control of desire can be analyzed through the lens of the action-based model of cognitive dissonance, which has prompted research examining individual differences in BAS (Harmon-Jones, Schmeichel, Inzlicht, & Harmon-Jones, 2011). Before reviewing this individual differences research, however, we review cognitive dissonance theory and its action-based model (Harmon-Jones, Amodio, & Harmon-Jones, 2009a), which we believe may shed further light on the self-control of desire.

Cognitive dissonance theory originally predicted that when a person has two or more elements of knowledge (cognitions) that are relevant to but inconsistent with each other, discomfort or dissonance results (Festinger, 1957). Dissonance was hypothesized to motivate individuals to decrease the inconsistency between cognitions.

The action-based model of dissonance was proposed to address why individuals experience dissonance and are motivated to reduce it. The action-based model assumes that the cognitions that cause dissonance are those with action or motivational implications. When these cognitions are in conflict with one another, dissonance is aroused, because these conflicting motivational impulses are likely to interfere with effective action (Harmon-Jones et al., 2009a). This type of conflict has been found to activate the anterior cingulate cortex (ACC), a neural region that has been found to be involved in negative affective responses to the detection of basic cognitive conflicts (Hajcak & Foti, 2008), as well as the conflicts aroused by typical dissonance manipulations (van Veen, Krug, Schooler, & Carter, 2009). When the conflict occurs (i.e., dissonance is aroused), dissonance reduction often occurs. According to the action-based model, dissonance reduction, which often involves a change in cognitions, helps organisms behave effectively. Thus the action-based model views the dissonance reduction process as an approach-motivated process that is aimed at translating one behavioral intention or motivational impulse into effective, often goal-directed, action. Dissonance reduction is often an adaptive process (Harmon-Jones et al., 2009a) that is present in a number of species (Egan, Bloom, & Santos, 2010).

This model can be applied to our understanding of self-control dilemmas. Imagine a person who needs to lose weight. He has dissonance because of his conflicting desires. He craves fattening food but also yearns to lose weight. Dissonance likely fluctuates often for this individual, and after a particularly enjoyable meal, he may experience an intense bout of dissonance because his recent behavior conflicts with his strong desire to lose weight. He may reduce it by downplaying the importance of weight loss. On the other hand, he may reduce the dissonance by doubling his exercise the day after and by fasting. The theory of dissonance predicts that he will reduce dissonance in the direction of *the cognition that is most resistant to change*. Which cognition is most resistant to change may fluctuate often in a person's day. The difficulty for researchers (or anyone wanting to predict behavior) is to know which cognition is most resistant to change in a given situation.

Most researchers studying dissonance in the lab have viewed behavioral commitments or decisions created in the lab as the cognition most resistant to change (Beauvois & Joule, 1999; Brehm & Cohen, 1962). Indeed, recent behavioral commitments or decisions (e.g., eating fattening food) are often the cognitions most resistant to change, but they may not always be, as preexisting beliefs, attitudes, or other motivations may trump the recent decision, as the previous example as well as some research illustrates (Scheier & Carver, 1980).

When individuals make a decision or behavioral commitment, they are often prepared to follow through with the commitment (Beckmann & Irle, 1985; Gollwitzer, 1990; Harmon-Jones & Harmon-Jones, 2002; Kuhl, 1984). This stage has been called an action-oriented state, or implemental mindset; it is where intentions are created to enact behaviors associated with a desired goal (Gollwitzer & Sheeran, 2006). The action-based model posits that during this stage individuals are approach motivated to behave in accord with the commitment.

Experiments have supported this prediction by revealing that immediately after dissonance-arousing behavioral commitments, individuals have greater relative left frontal cortical activity (Harmon-Jones, Gerd-jikov, & Harmon-Jones, 2008; Harmon-Jones et al., 2011). Moreover, when individuals engage in more action-oriented processing following a dissonance-arousing commitment, they evidence greater relative left frontal cortical activity and more attitude change in line with the commitment (Harmon-Jones, Harmon-Jones, Fearn, Sigelman, & Johnson, 2008). In addition, the greater relative left frontal activity is correlated with more attitude change in line with the commitment (Harmon-Jones et al., 2008). Finally, manipulated decreases in relative left frontal activity decrease the amount of attitude change individuals demonstrate (Harmon-Jones et al., 2008). Taken together, these results suggest that immediately after individuals make dissonance-arousing behavioral commitments, they are more approach motivated and this increased approach motivation then causes more attitude change in support of the recent behavioral commitment.

Other research has revealed that individual differences in desire (BAS) relate to this dissonance-related attitude change (Harmon-Jones et al., 2011). In one study, trait BAS was correlated with more spreading of alternatives (more liking for the chosen over the rejected decision alternative) after individuals made a difficult decision. In another study, trait BAS was correlated with attitudes being more consistent with a recent behavioral commitment (induced compliance or perceived high choice to engage in counterattitudinal behavior). These studies suggest that individuals who score high in trait approach motivation show more dissonance reduction, as predicted by the action-based model.

The evidence linking approach motivation and cognitive dissonance reveals that approach motivation (desire) does not require a stimulus or goal and it is not necessarily experienced as a positive state.

Summary and Conclusion

Individual differences in desire have been found to influence a number of variables related to emotive responding. For example, BAS sensitivity influences how individuals respond to positively and negatively valenced approach-related events, measured physiologically and behaviorally. Also, BAS sensitivity influences cognitive dissonance reduction, suggesting that it may influence how individuals respond to self-control dilemmas.

Most of the reviewed research has gone beyond the "zero-variable" theorizing that concerned Wicklund (1990), whereby personality researchers simply associate behavioral responses with self-reports of those same behaviors. Instead, most of the reviewed research on individual differences in approach motivation concerns variables that are not obviously linked with the individual differences measures used. For example, questionnaire items often used to assess trait approach motivation focus on positive reactions to rewards, but research has demonstrated that trait approach motivation relates to a variety of anger-related responses. Similarly, individual differences in approach motivation relate to cognitive dissonance reduction, an emotive cognitive process that is also unrelated to items on the questionnaires assessing trait approach motivation.

In addition, the reviewed research demonstrates it is also important to examine how contextual variables interact with individual differences in approach motivation to influence responses. For instance, trait approach motivation has been found to interact with situationally aroused approach motivation to influence attentional scope (Gable & Harmon-Jones, 2008) and aggressive inclinations after anger was aroused (Harmon-Jones & Peterson, 2008). We hope this review assists in advancing theory and research on approach motivation and desire.

REFERENCES

Alloy, L. B., Abramson, L. Y., Walshaw, P. D., Cogswell, A., Smith, J. M., Neeren, A. M., et al. (2006). Behavioral approach system (BAS) sensitivity and bipolar spectrum disorders: A retrospective and concurrent behavioral high-risk design. *Motivation and Emotion, 30*, 143–155.

Amodio, D. M., & Harmon-Jones, E. (2011). Trait emotions and affective modulation of the startle eyeblink: On the unique relationship of trait anger. *Emotion, 11*, 47–51.

Amodio, D. M., Master, S. L., Yee, C. M., & Taylor, S. E. (2008). Neurocognitive components of the behavioral inhibition and activation systems: Implications for theories of self-regulation. *Psychophysiology, 45*, 11–19.

Beaver, J. D., Lawrence, A. D., Passamonti, L., & Calder, A. J. (2008). Appetitive motivation predicts the neural response to facial signals of aggression. *Journal of Neuroscience, 28*, 2719 –2725.

Beaver, J. D., Lawrence, A. D., van Ditzhuijzen, J., Davis, M. H., Woods, A., & Calder, A. J. (2006). Individual differences in reward drive predict neural responses to images of food. *Journal of Neuroscience, 26*, 5160–5166.

Beauvois, J. L., & Joule, R. V. (1999). A radical point of view on dissonance theory. In E. Harmon-Jones & J. Mills (Eds.), *Cognitive dissonance: Progress on a pivotal theory in social psychology* (pp. 43–70). Washington, DC: American Psychological Association.

Beckmann, J., & Irle, M. (1985). Dissonance and action control. In J. Kuhl & J. Beckmann (Eds.), *Action control: From cognition to behavior* (pp. 129–150). Berlin: Springer-Verlag.

Brehm, J. W., & Cohen, A. R. (1962). *Explorations in cognitive dissonance.* New York: Wiley.

Carver, C. S. (2004). Negative affects deriving from the behavioral approach system. *Emotion, 4*, 3–22.

Carver, C. S., & Harmon-Jones, E. (2009). Anger is an approach-related affect: Evidence and implications. *Psychological Bulletin, 135*, 183–204.

Carver, C. S., & White, T. L. (1994). Behavioral inhibition, behavioral activation, and affective responses to impending reward and punishment: The BIS/BAS scales. *Journal of Personality and Social Psychology, 67*, 319–333.

Coan, J. A., & Allen, J. J. B. (2003). Frontal EEG asymmetry and the behavioral activation and inhibition systems. *Psychophysiology, 40*, 106–114.

Cook, I. A., O'Hara, R., Uijtdehaage, S. H. J., Mandelkern, M., & Leuchter, A. F.

(1998). Assessing the accuracy of topographic EEG mapping for determining local brain function. *Electroencephalography and Clinical Neurophysiology, 107,* 408–414.

Cooper, A., Gomez, R., & Buck, E. (2008). The relationship between the BIS and BAS, anger, and responses to anger. *Personality and Individual Differences, 44,* 403–413.

Cuthbert, B. N., Schupp, H. T., Bradley, M. M., McManis, M., & Lang, P. J. (1998). Probing affective pictures: Attended startle and tone probes. *Psychophysiology, 35,* 344–347.

Davidson, R. J., Chapman, J. P., Chapman, L. J., & Henriques, J. B. (1990). Asymmetric brain electrical activity discriminates between psychometrically matched verbal and spatial cognitive tasks. *Psychophysiology, 27,* 528–543.

Donchin, E., & Coles, M. G. H. (1988). Is the P300 component a manifestation of context updating? *Behavioral and Brain Sciences, 11,* 355–72.

Easterbrook, J. A. (1959). The effect of emotion on cue utilization and the organization of behavior. *Psychological Review, 66,* 183–201.

Egan, L., Bloom, P., & Santos, L. R. (2010). Choice-induced preferences in the absence of choice: Evidence from a blind two choice paradigm with young children and capuchin monkeys. *Journal of Experimental Social Psychology, 46,* 204–207.

Festinger, L. (1957). *A theory of cognitive dissonance.* Evanston, IL: Row, Peterson, & Co.

Foti, D., Hajcak, D., & Dien, J. (2009). Differentiating neural responses to emotional pictures: Evidence from temporal-spatial PCA. *Psychophysiology, 46,* 521–530.

Franken, I. H. A., & Muris, P. (2005). Individual differences in reward sensitivity are related to food craving and relative body weight in healthy women. *Appetite, 45,* 198–201.

Gable, P. A., & Adams, D. L. (2013). Nonaffective motivation modulates the sustained LPP (1,000–2,000 ms). *Psychophysiology, 50*(12), 1251–1254.

Gable, P. A., Adams, D. L., & Proudfit, G. H. (2014). Transient tasks and enduring emotions: The impacts of affective content, task relevance, and picture duration on the sustained late positive potential. *Cognitive, Affective, and Behavioral Neuroscience, 14*(3), 1–10.

Gable, P. A., & Harmon-Jones, E. (2008). Approach-motivated positive affect reduces breadth of attention. *Psychological Science, 19,* 476–482.

Gable, P. A., & Harmon-Jones, E. (2010). The effect of low vs. high approach-motivated positive affect on memory for peripherally vs. centrally presented information. *Emotion, 10,* 599–603.

Gable, P. A., & Harmon-Jones, E. (2011). Attentional consequences of pre-goal and post-goal positive affects. *Emotion, 11,* 1358–1367.

Gable, P. A., & Harmon-Jones, E. (2012). Trait behavioral approach sensitivity (BAS) relates to early (< 150 ms) electrocortical responses to appetitive stimuli. *Social Cognitive Affective Neuroscience, 8,* 795–798.

Gable, P. A., Mechin, N. C., & Browning, L. E. (2014). *Neural correlates of virtual alcohol myopia.* Manuscript in preparation.

Gable, P. A., Mechin, N., Hicks, J., & Adams, D. L. (2015). Supervisory control system and frontal asymmetry: Neurophysiological traits of emotion-based impulsivity. *Social Cognitive and Affective Neuroscience.*

Gable, P. A., & Poole, B. D. (2012). Influence of trait behavioral inhibition and behavioral approach motivation systems on the LPP and frontal asymmetry to anger pictures. *Social Cognitive and Affective Neuroscience, 9,* 182–190.

Gable, P. A., Poole, B. D., Harmon-Jones, E. (in press). Anger perceptually and conceptually narrows cognitive scope. *Journal of Personality and Social Psychology.*

Gainotti, G. (1972). Emotional behavior and hemispheric side of the lesion. *Cortex, 8*(1), 41–55.

Goldstein, K. (1939). *The organism: An holistic approach to biology, derived from pathological data in man.* New York: American Book.

Gollwitzer, P. M. (1990). Action phases and mind-sets. In E. T. Higgins & R. M. Sorrentino (Eds.), *Handbook of motivation and cognition: Foundations of social behavior* (Vol. 2, pp. 53–92). New York: Guilford Press.

Gollwitzer, P. M., & Sheeran, P. (2006). Implementation intentions and goal achievement: A meta-analysis of effects and processes. In M. P. Zanna (Ed.), *Advances in experimental social psychology* (Vol. 38, pp. 69–119). San Diego, CA: Elsevier Academic Press.

Gray, J. A. (1970). The psychophysiological basis of introversion-extraversion. *Behaviour Research and Therapy, 8,* 249–266.

Gray, J. A. (1990). Brain systems that mediate both emotion and cognition. *Cognition and Emotion, 4*(3), 269–288.

Hajcak, G., & Foti, D. (2008). Errors are aversive: Defensive motivation and the error-related negativity. *Psychological Science, 19,* 103–108.

Harmon-Jones, C., Schmeichel, B. J., Inzlicht, M., & Harmon-Jones, E. (2011). Trait approach motivation relates to dissonance reduction. *Social Psychological and Personality Science, 2,* 21–28.

Harmon-Jones, E. (2003). Anger and the behavioral approach system. *Personality and Individual Differences, 35,* 995–1005.

Harmon-Jones, E., Abramson, L. Y., Nusslock, R., Sigelman, J. D., Urosevic, S., Turonie, L., et al. (2008). Effect of bipolar disorder on left frontal cortical responses to goals differing in valence and task difficulty. *Biological Psychiatry, 63,* 693–698.

Harmon-Jones, E., Abramson, L. Y., Sigelman, J., Bohlig, A., Hogan, M. E., & Harmon-Jones, C. (2002). Proneness to hypomania/mania or depression and asymmetrical frontal cortical responses to an anger-evoking event. *Journal of Personality and Social Psychology, 82,* 610–618.

Harmon-Jones, E., & Allen, J. J. B. (1997). Behavioral activation sensitivity and resting frontal EEG asymmetry: Covariation of putative indicators related to risk for mood disorders. *Journal of Abnormal Psychology, 106,* 159–163.

Harmon-Jones, E., Amodio, D. M., & Harmon-Jones, C. (2009a). Action-based model of dissonance: A review, integration, and expansion of conceptions of cognitive conflict. In M. P. Zanna (Ed.), *Advances in Experimental Social Psychology, 41,* 119–166. San Diego, CA: Academic Press.

Harmon-Jones, E., & Gable, P. A. (2009). Neural activity underlying the effect of approach-motivated positive affect on narrowed attention. *Psychological Science, 20,* 406–409.

Harmon-Jones, E., Gable, P. A., & Price, T. (2013). Does negative affect always narrow and positive affect always broaden the mind?: Considering the influence of motivational intensity on cognitive scope. *Current Directions in Psychological Science, 22,* 301–307.

Harmon-Jones, E., Gerdjikov, T., & Harmon-Jones, C. (2008). The effect of induced compliance on relative left frontal cortical activity: A test of the action-based model of dissonance. *European Journal of Social Psychology, 38,* 35–45.

Harmon-Jones, E., & Harmon-Jones, C. (2002). Testing the action-based model of cognitive dissonance: The effect of action-orientation on post-decisional attitudes. *Personality and Social Psychology Bulletin, 28,* 711–723.

Harmon-Jones, E., Harmon-Jones, C., Abramson, L. Y., & Peterson, C. K. (2009b). PANAS positive activation is associated with anger. *Emotion, 9,* 183–196.

Harmon-Jones, E., Harmon-Jones, C., Fearn, M., Sigelman, J. D., & Johnson, P. (2008). Action orientation, relative left frontal cortical activation, and spreading of alternatives: A test of the action-based model of dissonance. *Journal of Personality and Social Psychology, 94,* 1–15.

Harmon-Jones, E., Harmon-Jones, C., & Price, T. F. (2013). What is approach motivation? *Emotion Review, 5,* 291–295.

Harmon-Jones, E., & Peterson, C. K. (2008). Effect of trait and state approach motivation on aggressive inclinations. *Journal of Research in Personality, 42,* 1381–1385.

Harmon-Jones, E., & Peterson, C. K. (2009). Supine body position reduces neural response to anger evocation. *Psychological Science, 20,* 1209–1210.

Hawk, L. W., & Kowmas, A. D. (2003). Affective modulation and prepulse inhibition of startle among undergraduates high and low in behavioral inhibition and approach. *Psychophysiology, 40,* 131–138.

Hicks, J. A., Friedman, R. S., Gable, P. A., & Davis, W. E. (2012). Interactive effects of approach motivational intensity and alcohol cues on the scope of perceptual attention. *Addiction, 107,* 1074–1080.

Hillyard, S. A., Hink, R. F., Schwent, V. L., & Picton, T. W. (1973). Electrical signs of selective attention in the human brain. *Science, 182,* 177–180.

Hortensius, R., Schutter, D. J. L. G., & Harmon-Jones, E. (2012). When anger leads to aggression: Induction of relative left frontal cortical activity with transcranial direct current stimulation increases the anger-aggression relationship. *Social Cognitive Affective Neuroscience, 7,* 342–347.

Johnstone, T., Kim, M. J., & Whalen, P. J. (2009). Functional magnetic resonance imaging in the affective and social neurosciences. In E. Harmon-Jones & J. S. Beer (Eds.), *Methods in social neuroscience* (pp. 313–336). New York: Guilford Press.

Kähkönen, S., Komssi, S., Wilenius, J., & Ilmoniemi, R. J. (2005). Prefrontal TMS produces smaller EEG responses than motor-cortex TMS: Implications for rTMS treatment in depression. *Psychopharmacology, 181,* 16–20.

Kano, K., Nakamura, M., Matsuoka, T., Iida, H., & Nakajima, T. (1992). The topographical features of EEGs in patients with affective disorders. *Electroencephalography and Clinical Neurophysiology, 83,* 124–129.

Keil, A., Müller, M. M., Gruber, T., Wienbruch, C., Stolarova, M., & Elbert, T. (2001). Effects of emotional arousal in the cerebral hemispheres: a study of oscillatory brain activity and event-related potentials. *Clinical Neurophysiology, 112*(11), 2057–2068.

Kuhl, J. (1984). Volitional aspects of achievement motivation and learned helplessness: Toward a comprehensive theory of action-control. In B. A. Maher (Ed.), *Progress in experimental personality research* (Vol. 13, pp. 99–171). New York: Academic Press.

Lang, P. J. (1995). The emotion probe: Studies of motivation and attention. *American Psychologist, 50,* 372–385.

Mechin, N., Gable, P. A., & Hicks, J. A. (2014). *Impulsivity enhances left-frontal activation to alcohol cues.* Manuscript in preparation.

Meyer, B., Johnson, S. L., & Carver, C. S. (1999). Exploring behavioural activation and inhibition sensitivities among college students at risk for bipolar spectrum symptomatology. *Journal of Psychopathology and Behavioral Assessment, 21,* 275–292.

Moll, G. H., Heinrich, H., Wischer, S., Tergau, F., Paulus, W., & Rothenberger, A. (1999). Motor system excitability in healthy children: Developmental aspects from transcranial magnetic stimulation. *Electroencephalography and Clinical Neurophysiology, 51*, 243–249.

Navon, D. (1977). Forest before trees: The precedence of global features in visual perception. *Cognitive Psychology, 9*, 353–383.

Nusslock, R., Harmon-Jones, E., Alloy, L. B., Urosevic, S., Goldstein, K. E., & Abramson, L. Y. (2012). Elevated left mid-frontal cortical activity prospectively predicts conversion to bipolar I disorder. *Journal of Abnormal Psychology, 121*, 592–601.

Nusslock, R., Shackman, A. J., Harmon-Jones, E., Alloy, L. B., Coan, J. A., & Abramson, L. Y. (2011). Cognitive vulnerability and frontal brain asymmetry: Common predictors of first prospective depressive episode. *Journal of Abnormal Psychology, 120*, 497–503.

Peterson, C. K., Gable, P., & Harmon-Jones, E. (2008). Asymmetrical frontal ERPs, emotion, and behavioral approach/inhibition sensitivity. *Social Neuroscience, 3*, 113–124.

Price, T. F., & Harmon-Jones, E. (2010). The effect of embodied emotive states on cognitive categorization. *Emotion, 10*, 934–938.

Robinson, R. G., & Price, T. R. (1982). Post-stroke depressive disorders: A follow-up study of 103 patients. *Stroke, 13*, 635–641.

Scheier, M. F., & Carver, C. S. (1980). Private and public self-attention, resistance to change, and dissonance reduction. *Journal of Personality and Social Psychology, 39*(3), 390–405.

Schutter, D. J., de Weijer, A. D., Meuwese, J. D., Morgan, B., & van Honk, J. (2008). Interrelations between motivational stance, cortical excitability, and the frontal electroencephalogram asymmetry of emotion: A transcranial magnetic stimulation study. *Human Brain Mapping, 29*, 574–80.

Simon, J. J., Walther, S., Fiebach, C. J., Friederich, C. J., Stippich, C., Weisbrod, M., et al. (2010). Neural reward processing is modulated by approach- and avoidance-related personality traits. *NeuroImage, 49*, 1868–1874.

Smits, D. J., & Kuppens, P. (2005). The relations between anger, coping with anger, and aggression, and the BIS/BAS system. *Personality and Individual Differences, 39*(4), 783–793.

Sutton, S. K., & Davidson, R. J. (1997). Prefrontal brain asymmetry: A biological substrate of the behavioral approach and inhibition systems. *Psychological Science, 8*, 204–210.

Vallortigara, G., & Rogers, L. J. (2005). Survival with an asymmetrical brain: Advantages and disadvantages of cerebral lateralization. *Behavioral and Brain Sciences, 28*, 575–633.

van Veen, V., Krug, M. K., Schooler, J. W., & Carter, C. S. (2009). Neural activity predicts attitude change in cognitive dissonance. *Nature Neuroscience, 12*, 1469–1474.

Vrana, S. R., Spence, E. L., & Lang, P. J. (1988). The startle probe response: A new measure of emotion? *Journal of Abnormal Psychology, 97*, 487–491.

Wicklund, R. A. (1990). *Zero-variable theories and the psychology of the explainer.* New York: Springer-Verlag.

CHAPTER 9

Developmental Changes in Reward Sensitivity and Cognitive Control across Adolescence

Implications for Desire

Adriana Galván

Adolescence is characterized by significant changes in behavioral, physiological, and neurobiological systems. There is a marked increase in reward-seeking and approach behaviors that is relevant for understanding desire and urges as individuals transition into adolescence. Historical notions of the adolescent have focused on the significant hormonal changes that occur at puberty. However, new research using cutting-edge technology to visualize the healthy human brain presents a more nuanced picture of adolescence. Tools such as structural and functional magnetic resonance imaging (sMRI and fMRI) have informed our understanding of how the brain functions across the lifespan.

This chapter will review the current research from cognitive neuroscience illustrating how development of brain regions previously implicated in desire, such as reward regions, may contribute to intriguing behavioral shifts observed during this critical developmental window. The chapter first defines the developmental period of adolescence and describes contemporary conceptual frameworks used to interpret research findings on adolescence. This section is followed by a review of the neurobiology of reward processing and development of regions implicated in reward. Then, neuroimaging studies that examine reward processing, cognitive control, and interactions between regions implicated in each during adolescence are described in greater detail. Finally, the chapter closes with a discussion about the potential interactions between developing brain regions and pubertal hormones in producing reward behaviors and desires in adolescents.

What Is Adolescence?

Despite the recent explosion of research on the adolescent brain, there is yet to be a standard definition of this period of life. Age, pubertal status, and characteristic behaviors are all indicators of adolescence, yet none of these factors alone characterizes who an adolescent is. Adolescence is not synonymous with puberty, although the two are undeniably related. Instead, the term *adolescence* also captures the behavioral changes, swings in mood states, and awareness of self that occur during this time, in addition to biological maturation. Hall coined the phrase "storm and stress" (Hall, 1904) in reference to the conflict with parents, mood disruptions, and risky behavior commonly associated with adolescence. Scholars now broadly define adolescence as a "transitional" period in life between childhood and adulthood (e.g., Steinberg, 2008) that generally begins at the onset of puberty and ends when individuals attain independence from caregivers.

Current Frameworks
of Adolescent Behavior and Brain Development

The advent of neuroimaging methods has provided researchers with the opportunity to uncover the neural changes that confer characteristic adolescent behaviors. Based on neurobiological rodent models and adult imaging studies, several conceptual models of these behaviors have been developed to provide a framework for generating and testing hypotheses. Most of these frameworks are variations of opponent-process or dual-process models that distinguish between a fast, automatic, unconscious way of processing information and a slow, deliberative, conscious, and advanced way of processing (Chick & Reyna, 2011; Evans, 2008).

Specific to neurobiological development, similar theories have been described: a subcortical versus cortical system (Casey, Getz, & Galván, 2008), an early-emerging "bottom-up" system that expresses exaggerated reactivity to motivational stimuli and later-maturing "top-down" cognitive control system (Casey & Jones, 2010), and a socioemotional versus regulatory system (Steinberg, 2008). Another well-known model of adolescent motivated behavior, the triadic model (Ernst & Fudge, 2009), comprises three neural nodes, each holding functional control over distinct cognitive constructs: approach (striatum), avoidance (amygdala), and behavioral regulation (prefrontal cortex [PFC]). Involvement of these systems depends on the context in which the motivated behavior occurs.

Although there is strong support from empirical studies for these models, they are nonetheless under constant refinement. New empirical evidence and reassessment of the implications of these models help fine-tune how the field conceptualizes adolescent behavior and the role that changing neural systems play in normative development. A few recent papers have begun to ask how contextual factors (Galván, 2012a; Somerville & Casey, 2010) and neural network approaches (Pfeifer & Allen, 2012) can further advance these models. Additionally, considering how these adolescent brain changes may help confer adaptive advantages during this transitional developmental windows is important (Crone & Dahl, 2012). It is clear that no one model will completely explain adolescent behavior, but these models may set the stage for understanding the role that changing neurobiological systems play in development.

Reward and Approach Behaviors

The psychological state of desire, of strongly wanting to have something or wishing for something to occur, is represented in mesolimbic motivational neurocircuitry (see also Kringelbach & Berridge, Chapter 6, this volume; Lopez, Wagner, & Heatherton, Chapter 7, this volume). This network, including the striatum, ventral tegmental area (VTA), amygdala, thalamus, hippocampus, and other limbic and cortical areas (Cacioppo, Bianchi-Demicheli, Frum, Pfaus, & Lewis, 2012), has also been heavily linked to reward processing and undergoes dynamic changes across the transition to adolescence. This section briefly reviews the basic neuroscience of reward processing (more detailed descriptions are found in other chapters) and then focuses on the unique developmental changes that occur in this network during adolescence.

A reward, any stimulus that an organism finds appetitive, elicits increased approach behavior. The neural regions that govern these behaviors share a few characteristics. First, they are rich in the neurotransmitter dopamine and bidirectionally communicate with one another, comprising what is known as the "reward system." Second, these systems are conserved across age, organisms, and species. Third, adolescence marks a pivotal time in reward processing, when individuals of all species exhibit increased behavioral motivation to obtain rewards and greater arousal in response to rewards (Galván, 2013).

Reward Neurocircuitry

Dopamine is a neurotransmitter that detects, responds to, and learns from rewarding events (Schultz, Dayan, & Montague, 1997). Dopamine neurons fire vigorously in response to rewards (Roitman, Wheeler, Wightman, & Carelli, 2008), social interactions (Robinson, Heien, & Wightman, 2002), and unexpected events or stimuli (Takahashi et al., 2009).

At the center of the reward network is the cortico-ventral basal ganglia circuit (Haber, 2011), which includes the ventral striatum (VS), the anterior cingulate cortex (ACC), the orbitofrontal cortex (OFC), and the ventral pallidum and midbrain. Additionally, auxiliary structures, including the dorsolateral PFC, amygdala, hippocampus, thalamus, habenula, and regions in the brainstem, help regulate reward neurocircuitry (Haber & Knutson, 2010).

The VS is the striatal region that has been most strongly implicated in reward. It includes the nucleus accumbens and the broad continuity between the caudate nucleus and putamen (Heimer et al., 1999). Most input to the VS is from the OFC, insular cortex, cingulate cortex, and amygdala (Haber, 2011). Together, this complex network facilitates the coordinated effort that is required for an organism to predict, evaluate, and respond to a reward. Within the basal ganglia there is a division of labor in which specific regions uniquely underlie different aspects of reward processing, including evaluation of reward value, anticipation of reward, predictability, and risk. The ACC and orbitofrontal regions mostly mediate value and the choice between short- and long-term gains (Haber, 2011). Cells in the VS and ventral pallidum respond to anticipation of reward and reward detection. Reward prediction signals are generated, in part, from the midbrain dopamine cells. Additionally, reward-responsive activation is found throughout the striatum and substantia nigra pars compacta (Haber, 2011). Together, the frontal regions that mediate reward, motivation, and affect regulation project primarily to the rostral striatum, including the nucleus accumbens, the medial caudate nucleus, and the medial and ventral rostral putamen (Haber, 2011).

Ontogeny of the Dopamine System

Extant research shows that there is a peak in reward- and sensation-seeking behaviors (Steinberg et al., 2009), sensitivity to monetary incentives (Smith, Xiao, & Bechara, 2011) and social rewards (Chein, Albert, O'Brien, Uckert, & Steinberg, 2011), and even greater reactivity to sweet substances in mid-adolescence (Post & Kemper, 1993; Galván & McGlennen, 2013) compared to older and younger individuals. Many mammalian species show similar patterns of reward-related behavior as humans, providing strong evidence for conservation of reward processing across evolution (Spear, 2011b). Studies in juvenile rats show an inverted U-shaped developmental trajectory in the domains of reward and novelty seeking (Douglas, Varlinskaya, & Spear, 2003), risk taking, social interactions (Douglas, Varlinskaya, & Spear, 2004), and consummatory behavior (Friemel, Spanagel, & Schneider, 2010; Spear, 2011a). They also demonstrate enhanced behavioral interest to novelty (Douglas et al., 2003) and social peers (Varlinskaya & Spear, 2008) compared to adult rats. The increased proclivity toward drugs in human adolescents versus adults is also observed in rats (e.g., Brenhouse & Andersen, 2008) and nonhuman primates (Nelson et al., 2009). Thus, researchers have leveraged this conservation across species to learn more about the ontogeny of the dopamine system and reward-related behaviors in humans by understanding the system in animal models.

Additionally, rodent models have shown that the mesocorticolimbic dopamine system undergoes significant changes during adolescence. In the striatum, dopamine levels increase during adolescence (Andersen, Dumont, & Teicher, 1997), and dopamine molecules (D_1 and D_2 receptors) that facilitate dopamine transmission in the VS increase from preadolescence to adolescence (e.g., Andersen et al., 1997). In fact, dopamine receptor binding of D_1 and D_2 receptors peaks in adolescence at levels that are about 30–45% greater than those seen in adulthood (Tarazi, Tomasini, & Baldessarini, 1999; Teicher et al., 1995). Others have demonstrated that striatal slices from adolescent rat brains were more sensitive to substances that act on dopamine, such as cocaine, than those of adults (Bolanos, Glatt, & Jackson, 1998). These neurochemical and structural changes seem to have functional significance; functional studies show that compared to adults, the adolescent rat brain releases more dopamine under rewarding conditions (Laviola, Pasucci, & Pieretti, 2001) despite reduced dopamine release in basal conditions (Andersen & Gazzara, 1993; Stamford, 1989), and it exhibits longer sustained dopamine release following a social interaction (Robinson, Zitzman, Smith, & Spear, 2011). Adolescent rodents also exhibit greater sensitivity to social rewards, as demonstrated in a recent study showing that they consume greater amounts of alcohol in the presence, rather than the absence, of peers (Logue, Chein, Gould, Holliday, & Steinberg, 2014).

A similar pattern of dopaminergic reorganization during adolescence is observed in the PFC, albeit with a more protracted elimination period (Andersen, Thompson, Rutstein, Hostetter, & Teicher, 2000). Neurons in the PFC express higher levels of D_1 receptors (Brenhouse, Sonntag, & Andersen, 2008) and activity (McCutcheon & Marinelli, 2009) during adolescence than in older or younger rodents. Together, these data suggest that during adolescence, changes in dopamine neurochemistry may alter reward sensitivity and approach behaviors.

Neuroimaging Studies of Brain Development

Although it is not possible to examine the dopamine system at the neurochemical level in humans, magnetic resonance imaging (MRI) and fMRI allow researchers to peer into the healthy, developing brain. These noninvasive tools yield clear and detailed pictures of the brain for the study of anatomical and functional changes. While MRI is used to examine the anatomy of the brain, fMRI is used to study the brain "in motion."

Structural MRI Studies

Structural MRI studies are used to characterize size, shape, and location of anatomical structures in the brain. They have provided significant knowledge about neurodevelopmental changes and have greatly advanced the dual-process models of adolescent neurobiology. Although the overall total size of the brain remains relatively stable after approximately age 6, various regions of the brain continue to exhibit subtle but significant changes in the size and structure of gray matter (neuronal cell bodies) and in their connections with other brain regions via white matter (connective tracts). The brain regions that show the greatest anatomical changes are in the PFC and striatum (Sowell, Thompson, Holmes, Jernigan, & Toga, 1999). In a longitudinal sample of 387 children, adolescents, and young adults, Giedd and colleagues found robust sex differences in developmental trajectories of several brain regions (in Lenroot et al., 2007). Specifically, the frontal lobe peaked at age 9.5 and 10.5 for females and males, respectively, while the caudate nucleus peaked at age 8.5 in females and 10.5 in males (Lenroot et al., 2007). A more recent longitudinal study in a sample of 9- to 23-year-olds shows remarkably similar results, reporting that the size of the striatum peaks in adolescence and then decreases into the early 20s (Urošević, Collins, Muetzel, Lim, & Luciana, 2012). Moreover, this nonlinear developmental pattern in the striatum paralleled measures of the behavioral approach system, with increased reward sensitivity from early to late adolescence and evidence for decline in the early 20s (Urošević et al., 2012). As discussed in the next section, these structural changes appear to be functionally meaningful and may contribute to reward and approach behaviors.

Functional MRI Studies

Regulatory Circuitry

With fMRI, participants perform a computerized task designed to assess the behavior of interest (e.g., reward processing or cognitive control) while undergoing a brain scan. In the first fMRI study in youth, Casey and colleagues (1997) observed that improvements in cognitive control across development are associated with changes in frontal cortex functioning. Since that seminal study, numerous research groups have replicated the finding (e.g., Luna et al., 2001; Bunge, Dudukovic, Thomason, Vaidya, & Gabrieli, 2002), and it is now widely accepted that delayed functional development of the PFC contributes to limitations in self-control and behavioral regulation in young participants (Casey & Caudle, 2013). Interestingly, several recent studies have demonstrated that the relatively unstable nature of the PFC in adolescents renders it more susceptible to emotional or arousing information than in adults. In a recent study, Somerville, Hare, and Casey (2011) examined cognitive control in the face of emotional cues (positive or negative emotional facial expressions). Child, adolescent, and adult participants performed a standard go/no-go task in which they were asked to press a button every time a particular cue (e.g., a neutral face) appeared on the computer screen and to inhibit pressing the button every time another type of cue (e.g., a happy, attractive face) appeared on the screen. Remarkably, the adolescent group exhibited a failure in self-control when attempting to exert cognitive control (button inhibition) in the presence of a happy face; this diminished ability was not observed in children or adults (Somerville et al., 2011). Neurobiologically, the authors found that the ability to self-control showed a monotonic increase with age in the ventrolateral PFC. In contrast, the ability to suppress a response to emotional faces revealed a different pattern of brain activity. Specifically, diminished behavioral performance by adolescents in regulating self-control to positive emotional faces was paralleled by enhanced activity in the VS (Somerville et al., 2011). These findings suggest an exaggerated ventral-striatal representation of emotional cues in adolescents that may serve to "hijack" a less fully mature PFC control response. Thus, adolescents' decisions and actions are not due solely to a less mature PFC, but rather to a tension within neural circuitry involving the VS, implicated in reward processing, and the PFC, implicated in control processing (Casey & Caudle, 2013).

However, asserting that all adolescents lack self-control due to an immature PFC is an oversimplification. Some youth exhibit this phenotype to a lesser or greater extent, highlighting the importance of considering the role of individual differences in behavior and brain development (see also Harmon-Jones, Gable, & Harmon-Jones, Chapter 8, this volume). One of the most innovative studies to examine this question was recently published after 40 years of data collection. In the original study, a cohort of 4-year-old preschoolers were assessed on their *delay-of-gratification*, the ability to resist the temptation of an immediate reward in favor of a large reward. Specifically, Walter Mischel and colleagues examined whether children would choose a small reward (one marshmallow) immediately or a larger reward (two marshmallows) after a short temporal delay. Children's behavior fell into two categories: (1) limited self-control in children who ate the treat almost immediately (low delayers) or (2) greater self-control in children who waited for some instructed amount of time in an attempt to gain two treats (high delayers). In a recent longitudinal study on the same sample of individuals (now in their 40s), Mischel collaborated with BJ Casey to examine the stability of individual differences in self-control. They found that individuals who had more difficulty delaying gratification at age 4 continued to show reduced self-control 40 years later (Casey et al., 2011). These findings highlight individual differences in self-control that are independent of age and can persist throughout the lifespan.

Motivational Circuitry

Relevant to any neurobiological discussion of desire is the role that motivational circuitry plays in the mental representation of desire. The first reward fMRI studies addressed simple questions about reward processing: Are there neurofunctional changes in reward circuitry across development? Is the adolescent brain hyposensitive or hypersensitive to reward? Two proposed hypotheses were equally intriguing: one suggested that a relative deficit in the activity of reward circuitry in adolescents compared to adults leads youth to seek out rewards and risks (Blum, Braverman, Holder, Lubar, Monastra, et al., 2000). In this view, it is reasoned that adolescents may generally attain less positive feelings from rewarding stimuli, which drives them to pursue rewards that increase activity in dopamine-related circuitry (Spear, 2000). An alternative hypothesis is that greater activation of the VS dopamine circuit underlies adolescent reward-related behavior (Chambers, Taylor, & Potenza, 2003). This theory posits that adolescent behavior is driven by reward-related appetitive systems and is consonant with dual-systems theories and the triadic model.

The majority of studies on reward processing across development have found support for enhanced reward sensitivity in striatal regions in adolescents compared to children and adults (but see Bjork et al., 2004; Bjork, Smith, Chen, & Hommer, 2010). Data from own our work suggest nonlinear patterns of striatal functional development. In an fMRI study, children, adolescents, and adults performed a youth-friendly reward task in which three cues were each associated with three reward values that ranged from least desirable (small reward) to most desirable (large reward) (Galván et al., 2006). All exhibited robust activation in the VS to reward of any size early on in the experiment. However, by the end of the experiment adolescents showed the overall greatest activation to the most desirable reward, while adults showed the least. Particularly interesting is that these neural patterns of activation paralleled the behavioral differences observed between age groups. In the beginning of the experiment, none of the groups showed differences in reaction time to the three reward types. However, by the end of the experiment, adults had learned to discriminate between them, as evidenced by faster reaction time to the most desirable reward and slowest reaction time to the least desirable reward. Adolescents became significantly slower to the least desirable reward, and children continued to show no differences in reaction between the three reward types. From this study we concluded that neural discrimination of reward value is paralleled by changes in behavior and that adolescents show heightened VS sensitivity to reward compared to children and adults (Galván et al., 2006). Similar results have been reported by other laboratories using a variety of tasks with monetary and social rewards (Chein et al., 2011; Cohen et al., 2010; Ernst et al., 2005; Geier, Terwilliger, Teslovich, Velanova, & Luna, 2010; Jarcho et al., 2012). A recent longitudinal study found that hyperactivation in motivational circuitry persists through the late adolescent years and into early adulthood (Lamm et al., 2014), underscoring the protracted development of the reward system.

Monetary earnings are the most common stimulus researchers use to stimulate the reward system, which has led some researchers to ask whether it is possible that adolescents exhibit hyperactivation to reward because the adolescent brain attributes greater value to available rewards since adolescents typically have less experience and/or access to a regular income. Three recent studies suggest that this is not the case. First, fMRI studies in which participants were awarded points rather than money reported the same adolescent phenomenon (van Leijenhorst et al., 2010). Second, in a recent study from our own group we used a primary reward instead of monetary reward task to assess reward sensitivity. Participants passively received appetitive (sugar water) and aversive (salt water) drops of liquid while undergoing fMRI (Galván & McGlennen, 2013). Adolescent participants not only found the appetitive liquid more pleasurable and the aversive liquid less pleasurable than adults, they also showed enhanced engagement of the VS to both types of liquid, suggesting that both primary and secondary rewards elicit greater striatal activation in teens versus adults (Galván & McGlennen, 2013). Third, monetary income is not predictive of striatal reactivity in response to reward, and when matched for motivation in receiving monetary reward, adolescents still show hyperactivation in reward circuitry compared to adults (Barkley-Levenson & Galván, 2014). Collectively, these studies lend support for the hypothesis that disproportionately increased activation of the VS motivational circuit characterizes adolescent neurodevelopment (Chambers et al., 2003) and is not due to developmental differences in reward valuation or motivation.

Fronto-Striatal Communication

The studies reviewed above underscore the important role that both regulatory and motivational circuitry play in adolescent reward processing. Specifically, these studies suggest that reward systems have significant influence over behavior and that there seems to be a developmental tug of war in which the inclination to seek out rewards and desires competes with an immature system that is unable to inhibit those inclinations. Until recently, most studies did not explicitly examine these systems in conjunction in adolescents. However, a few noteworthy studies examined the integration of cognitive control and reward-related processes by implementing tasks that examine behavioral regulation in the face of rewarding information. Using an antisaccade task as a measure of inhibitory control, a series of studies have shown that adolescents show improved cognitive control when they were rewarded for doing so (e.g., Geier et al., 2010). In a clever manipulation, Luna and colleagues presented participants with a simple cognitive task (Luna et al., 2001) in which good inhibitory control yielded monetary reward. During anticipation of reward on the rewarded trials, participants showed increased activation in the VS and medial frontal gyrus compared to adults, despite equitable task performance between groups (Geier et al., 2010). This increased activation is thought to contribute to significant improvements in accuracy in adolescents (Geier et al., 2010). Across a range of regions, including the putamen, VS, and parietal cortex, adolescents exhibited increased activation compared to children and adults in the rewarded trials (Padmanabhan et al., 2011). Collectively, these results suggest that younger participants have the ability to perform as well as adults when provided with an incentive to do so. Importantly, they suggest that reward may act to *enhance* or *improve* behavioral regulation in youth.

Functional Connectivity Studies

In recent years there has been an uptick in the use of functional connectivity methods, which allow examination of how individual brain regions work together during reward processing (Marreiros, Kiebel, & Friston, 2008). Effective connectivity takes the analyses one step further, providing information about causality by modeling the influence of one brain region on another (Friston, Harrison, & Penny, 2003). This type of analysis can provide new insight into functional organization of the brain by empirically testing conceptual theories about reward-driven behavior in adolescents. For instance, effective connectivity can help disentangle whether adolescents exhibit greater reward-seeking behavior than adults because signals from the VS exert robust influence over cognitive control regions or because the PFC has limited regulatory influence over reward neurocircuitry. The answer is likely a combination of both scenarios.

Using effective connectivity, Cho and colleagues (2013) examined reward processing using a reward task in a group of adolescents and adults. They found that both groups elicited activation in the VS, thalamus, and insula, with robust thalamic influence on the insula and VS, as well as insula influence on the VS. Furthermore, adolescents demonstrated significant connectivity from the VS to the thalamus (Cho et al., 2012). Interestingly, there were no statistically significant differences in connectivity modulation between adolescents and adults, which the authors speculate may be due to high individual variability among the sample (Cho et al., 2012). Nonetheless, this study suggests that the thalamus and insula provide the VS with signals about motivation, given their respective roles in identifying and responding to rewarding stimuli in the environment.

Results from a delay discounting study, in which participants are tested on their ability to wait for a larger reward in favor of a smaller immediate reward, suggest that enhanced age-related coupling between the ventromedial PFC and the VS accounts for reduced discounting across development (Christakou, Brammer, & Rubia, 2011). The authors speculate that this enhanced relationship between regulatory and affective systems helps the participants make more rational decisions.

Together, these studies have laid a strong foundation and provided a rationale for using functional connectivity approaches to study neural networks implicated in reward processing across development. These initial studies have already begun to fill in the empirical gaps of current conceptual frameworks by supporting the notion that progressive strengthening of functional connections between frontal and subcortical regions contributes to age-related increases in reward-related regulation. Similar to the burst in knowledge about the developing brain that arose when fMRI was first used to study children and adolescents (Casey et al., 1997), functional connectivity studies will yield important new insights and generate novel ways to conceptualize the development of neural networks.

Puberty-Related Changes in the Brain

The literature reviewed thus far presents strong evidence that neurobiological development is critically implicated in behavioral shifts during adolescence. However, the field continues to appreciate the important role of puberty. The metamorphosis that occurs as individuals become sexually mature generates three primary changes in the young adolescent that are critical for reproduction and maturation: (1) a reawakening of hormones that trigger the development of secondary sex characteristics, (2) significant changes in size and body structure, and (3) notable changes in behavior. The reader is directed to an excellent review by Sisk and Foster (2004) for greater detail about the biological and physical changes that accompany puberty, which typically occurs between ages 9–13 for girls and 10–14 for boys. This section will focus on the significance and function of behavioral changes that emerge, particularly as they might relate to expressions of (sexual) desire.

Puberty is initiated by the activation of the hypothalamic–pituitary–gonadal axis via gonadotropin-releasing hormone (GnRH) secretion, which triggers increased release of other pubertal hormones and culminates in sexual maturation (Sisk & Foster, 2004). These hormones also launch sexually dimorphic trajectories in brain development and play a role in reorganizing reward circuitry that supports social behaviors relevant to mate selection and the act of mating (Sisk & Zehr, 2005). In other words, changes in specific neural networks help orient the pubertal adolescent toward greater desire of sexual partners. As reviewed in a recent model, three core systems are reorganized during puberty that drive orientation toward social-emotional information processing (Scherf, Behrmann, & Dahl, 2012). Although not explicitly stated within the model, it could be argued that this reorganization also contributes to, and is necessary for, increased sensory processing that enhances desire of potential sexual partners.

The first neural network is involved in processing basic attention and visual orientation; it includes the inferior occipital cortex ("occipital face area" [OFA]; Gauthier et al., 2000), the posterior fusiform gyrus ("fusiform face area" [FFA]; Kanwisher, McDermott, & Chun, 1997), the superior temporal sulcus (STS; Hoffman & Haxby, 2000), and auxillary visuoperceptual regions of visual cortex (Scherf et al., 2012). Research in this network has shown significant changes in these regions across the pubertal transition. For instance, when presented with images of faces, adolescents (11- to 14-year-olds) exhibit robust activation of the fusiform face area that is similar to FFA activation in adults and is notably absent in children (5- to 8-year-olds) (Scherf, Bermann, Humphreys, & Luna, 2007). This result has been replicated and extended in other recent studies (Golarai et al., 2007), indicating that the core face-processing regions continue to exhibit ongoing development in adolescence.

The second neural network is critically involved in "mentalizing," the ability to understand the mental state of oneself and of others. This network includes the medial prefrontal cortex (mPFC), temporoparietal junction (TPJ), anterior temporal cortex, and cingulate gyrus. Together, these regions help individuals "mentalize" or understand the mental state, thoughts, and feelings of other people. This ability is critical for normative and successful social interaction and significantly increases during adolescence (Burnett, Sebastian, Cohen Kadosh, & Blakemore, 2011). As shown by fMRI work, during self-reflection adolescents demonstrate greater activation than adults in this neural network, which is paralleled by more accurate self-appraisals than adults (Pfeifer et al., 2009); related research suggests that adolescents exhibit greater activation in the mPFC, a classic mentalizing region, than adults do when judging emotional responses others may have to social emotions such as embarrassment and guilt (Burnett, Bird, Moll, Frith, & Blakemore, 2009).

The third network is important for emotion processing and includes the amygdala, insula, and striatum. These regions are the core limbic circuitry that supports emotion discrimination, affect, and threat (Adolphs, 2010) and undergoes significant maturation from childhood through adolescence (Giedd, Blumenthal, Jeffries, Castellanos, Liu, et al., 1999), which supports maturation of emotion processing. For example, explicit memory for emotional expression improves from late childhood through adolescence (Pine et al., 2004), particularly for fear, anger, and disgust (Herba, Landau, Russell, Ecker, & Phillips, 2006; Thomas, de Bellis, Graham, & LaBar, 2007). Also, the ability to match a visual image of a facial expression with a verbal label for the expression develops into early adolescence, particularly for the expressions of fear, disgust, and anger (Durand, Gallay, Seigneuric, Robichon, & Baudouin, 2007). Finally, using emotional faces as stimuli, researchers have described a U-shaped pattern of functional development in the amygdala with increasing activation through adolescence (Baird et al., 1999; Hare et al., 2008) and an age-related decline in activation from adolescence to adulthood (Guyer et al., 2008). There is also evidence of a qualitative shift in amygdala function from late childhood to adulthood such that children show greater activation to neutral faces while adults show greater activation to fearful faces (Thomas et al., 2001).

In terms of reward processing and pubertal hormones, the few published studies in this area have yielded mixed results. Forbes and colleagues (2010) report that plasma testosterone levels are positively related to caudate activity during reward anticipation in boys and negatively related to caudate activity during reward outcome in both sexes (Forbes et al., 2010). However, Op de Macks and colleagues (2011) found that testosterone levels correlated positively with striatal activation in both boys and girls. Although these initial studies do suggest an association between puberty, hormonal changes, and reward sensitivity in adolescence, the discrepant results underscore the need for more empirical studies in this area (Ladouceur, 2012; Goddings, Burnett Heyes, Bird, Viner, & Blakemore, 2012).

Collectively, these data suggest that the hormonal changes that occur during puberty are the impetus for behavioral increases in motivation related to social information processing and desire (Blakemore, Burnett, & Dahl, 2010; Graber, Nichols, & Brooks-Gunn, 2010; Nelson, Liebenluft, McClure, & Pine, 2005). However, much more research in this area is necessary.

Summary

The past two decades have been an exhilarating time for developmental cognitive neuroscience. The field has learned a great deal about the developing brain because of the increased sophistication of neuroimaging tools. The ability to probe the developing brain has enabled significant progress in understanding characteristic behaviors, such as increases in reward sensitivity, motivation to pursue desires, and increased passion, that emerge as children become adolescents. While the collective efforts of laboratories all around the world have led to significant strides in uncovering the dynamic nature of brain structure and function across childhood and adolescence, the field is well positioned and technologically equipped to make even greater advances. Studies that address the role of context, developmental history, peers, and hormones in reward and approach behaviors across development will undoubtedly provide a more holistic view of the developing brain.

REFERENCES

Adolphs, R. (2010). What does the amygdala contribute to social cognition? *Annals of the New York Academy of Sciences, 1191,* 42–61.

Andersen, S., Dumont, N., & Teicher, M. (1997). Developmental differences in dopamine synthesis inhibition by (±)-7-OH-DPAT. *Naunyn-Schmiedebergs Archives of Pharmacology, 356,* 173–181.

Andersen, S., & Gazzara, R. (1993). The ontogeny of apomorphine-induced alterations of neostriatal dopamine release: effects of spontaneous release. *Journal of Neurochemistry, 61*, 2247–2255.

Andersen, S., Thompson, A., Rutstein, M., Hostetter, J., & Teicher, M. (2000). Dopamine receptor pruning in prefrontal cortex during the periadolescent period in rats. *Synapse, 37*, 167–169.

Baird, A. A., Gruber, S. A., Fein, D. A., Maas, L. C., Steingard, R. J., Renshaw, P. F., et al. (1999). Functional magnetic resonance imaging of facial affect recognition in children and adolescents. *Journal of the American Academy of Child and Adolescent Psychiatry, 38*(2), 195–199.

Barkley-Levenson, E., & Galván, A. (2014). Neural representation of expected value in the adolescent brain. *Proceedings of the National Academy of Science, 111*(4), 1646–1651.

Bjork, J., Knutson, B., Fong, G., Caggiano, D., Bennett, S., & Hommer, D. (2004). Incentive-elicited brain activation in adolescents: Similarities and differences from young adults. *Journal of Neuroscience, 24*(8), 1793–1802.

Bjork, J., Smith, A., Chen, G., & Hommer, D. (2010). Adolescents, adults and rewards: Comparing motivational neurocircuitry recruitment using fMRI. *PLoS One, 5*, e11440.

Blakemore, S.-J., Burnett, S., & Dahl, R. E. (2010). The role of puberty in the developing adolescent brain. *Human Brain Mapping, 31*, 926–933.

Blum, K., Braverman, E., Holder, J., Lubar, J., Monastra, V., Miller, D., et al. (2000). Reward deficiency syndrome: A biogenetic model for the diagnosis and treatment of impulsive, addictive and compulsive behaviors. *Journal of Psychoactive Drugs, 2*, 1–112.

Bolanos, C., Glatt, S., & Jackson, D. (1998). Subsensitivity to dopaminergic drugs in periadolescent rats: A behavioral and neurochemical analysis. *Developmental Brain Research, 111*, 25–33.

Brenhouse, H., & Andersen, S. (2008). Delayed extinction and stronger reinstatement of cocaine conditioned place preference in adolescent rats, compared to adults. *Behavioral Neuroscience, 122*, 460–465.

Brenhouse, H., Sonntag, K., & Andersen, S. (2008). Transient D₁ dopamine receptor expression on prefrontal cortex projection neurons: Relationship to enhanced motivational salience of drug cues in adolescence. *Journal of Neuroscience, 28*, 2375–2382.

Bunge, S. A., Dudukovic, N. M., Thomason, M. E., Vaidya, C. J., & Gabrieli, J. D. (2002). Immature frontal lobe contributions to cognitive control in children: Evidence from fMRI. *Neuron, 33*(22), 301–311.

Burnett, S., Bird, G., Moll, J., Frith, C., & Blakemore, S. J. (2009). Development during adolescence of the neural processing of social emotion. *Journal of Cognitive Neuroscience, 21*(9), 1736–1750.

Burnett, S., Sebastian, C., Cohen Kadosh, K., & Blakemore, S. J. (2011). The social brain in adolescence: Evidence from functional magnetic resonance imaging and behavioural studies. *Neuroscience and Biobehavioral Reviews, 35*(8), 1654–1664.

Cacioppo, S., Bianchi-Demicheli, F., Frum, C., Pfaus, J. G., & Lewis, J. W. (2012). The common neural bases between sexual desire and love: A multilevel kernal density fMRI analysis. *Journal of Sexual Medicine, 9*(4), 1048–1054.

Casey, B., & Caudle, K. (2013). The teenage brain: Self control. *Current Directions in Psychological Science, 22*, 82–87.

Casey, B., Getz, S., & Galván, A. (2008). The adolescent brain. *Developmental Review, 28*(1), 62–77.

Casey, B., & Jones, R. (2010). Neurobiology of the adolescent brain and behavior: Implications for substance use disorders. *Journal of the American Academy of Child and Adolescent Psychiatry, 49,* 1189–1201.

Casey, B., Somerville, L. H., Gotlib, I. H., Ayduk, O., Franklin, N. T., Askren, M. K., et al. (2011). Behavioral and neural correlates of delay of gratification 40 years later. *Proceedings of the National Academy of Sciences, 108*(36), 14998–15003.

Casey, B., Trainor, R. J., Orendi, J. L., Schubert, A. B., Nystrom, L. E., Giedd, J. N., et al., (1997). A developmental functional MRI study of prefrontal activation during performance of a Go-No-Go task. *Journal of Cognitive Neuroscience, 9,* 835–847.

Chambers, R., Taylor, J., & Potenza, M. (2003). Developmental neurocircuitry of motivation in adolescence: A critical period of addiction vulnerability. *American Journal of Psychiatry, 160,* 1041–1052.

Chein, J., Albert, D., O'Brien, L., Uckert, K., & Steinberg, L. (2011). Peers increase adolescent risk taking by enhancing activity in the brain's reward circuitry. *Developmental Science, 14,* F1–F10.

Chick, C., & Reyna, V. (2011). A fuzzy-trace theory of adolescent risk taking: Beyond self-control and sensation seeking. In V. Reyna, S. Chapman, M. Dougherty, & J. Confrey (Eds.), *The adolescent brain: Learning, reasoning, and decision making* (pp. 379–428). Washington, DC: American Psychological Association.

Cho, Y., Fromm, S., Guyer, A., Detloff, A., Pine, D., Fudge, J., et al. (2012). Nucleus accumbens, thalamus and insula connectivity during incentive anticipation in typical adults and adolescents. *NeuroImage, 66C,* 508–521.

Christakou, A., Brammer, M., & Rubia, A. (2011). Maturation of limbic cortico-striatal activation and connectivity associated with developmental changes in temporal discounting. *NeuroImage, 54,* 1344–1354.

Cohen, J. R., Asarnow, R. F., Sabb, F. W., Bilder, R. M., Bookheimer, S. Y., Knowlton, B. J., et al. (2010). A unique adolescent response to reward prediction errors. *Nature Neuroscience, 13*(6), 669–671.

Crone, E., & Dahl, R. (2012). Understanding adolescence as a period of social-affective engagement and goal flexibility. *Nature Reviews Neuroscience, 13,* 636–650.

Douglas, L., Varlinskaya, E., & Spear, L. (2003). Novel-object place conditioning in adolescent and adult male and female rats: Effects of social isolation. *Physiology and Behavior, 80,* 317–325.

Douglas, L., Varlinskaya, E., & Spear, L. (2004). Rewarding properties of social interactions in adolescent and adult male and female rats: Impact of social versus isolate housing of subjects and partners. *Developmental Psychobiology, 45,* 153–162

Durand, K., Gallay, M., Seigneuric, A., Robichon, F., & Baudouin, J. Y. (2007). The development of facial emotion recognition: The role of configural information. *Journal of Experimental Child Psychology, 97*(1), 14–27.

Ernst, M., & Fudge, J. (2009). A developmental neurobiological model of motivated behavior: Anatomy, connectivity and ontogeny of the triadic nodes. *Neuroscience Biobehavioral Reviews, 33,* 367–382.

Ernst, M., Nelson, E., Jazbec, S., McClure, E., Monk, C. S., Leibenluft, E., et al. (2005). Amygdala and nucleus accumbens in responses to receipt and omission of gains in adults and adolescents. *NeuroImage, 25,* 1279–1291.

Evans, J. (2008). Dual-processing accounts of reasoning, judgment, and social cognition. *Annual Review of Psychology, 59*, 255–278.

Forbes, E., Ryan, N., Phillips, M., Manuck, S., Worthman, C., Moyles, D., et al., (2010). Healthy adolescents' neural response to reward: Associations with puberty, positive affect, and depressive symptoms. *Journal of the American Academy of Child and Adolescent Psychiatry, 49*, 162–172.

Friemel, C., Spanagel, R., & Schneider, M. (2010). Reward sensitivity for a palatable food reward peaks during pubertal developmental in rats. *Frontiers in Behavioral Neuroscience, 4*, 1–10.

Friston, K., Harrison, L., & Penny, W. (2003). Dynamic causal modelling. *NeuroImage, 19*, 1273–1302.

Galván, A. (2012). Judgment and decision-making in adolescence. In V. Reynda, S. Chapman, M. Dougherty, & J. Confrey (Eds.), *The adolescent brain: Learning, reasoning, and decision making* (pp. 267–289). Washington, DC: American Psychological Association.

Galván, A. (2013). The teenage brain: Sensitivity to rewards. *Current Directions in Psychological Science, 22*, 88–93.

Galván, A., Hare, T., Parra, C., Penn, J., Voss, H., Glover, G., et al. (2006). Earlier development of the accumbens relative to orbitofrontal cortex might underlie risk-taking behavior in adolescents. *Journal of Neuroscience, 26*(25), 6885–6892.

Galván, A., & McGlennen, K. (2013). Enhanced striatal sensitivity to aversive reinforcement in adolescents versus adults. *Journal of Cognitive Neuroscience, 25*, 284–296.

Galván, A., Van Leijenhorst, L., & McGlennen, K. (2012). Considerations for imaging the adolescent brain. *Developmental Cognitive Neuroscience, 2*(3), 293–302.

Gauthier, I., Tarr, M. J., Moylan, J., Skudlarski, P., Gore, J. C., & Anderson, A. W. (2000). The fusiform "face area" is part of a network that processes faces at the individual level. *Journal of Cognitive Neuroscience, 12*, 495–504.

Geier, C., Terwilliger, R., Teslovich, T., Velanova, K., & Luna, B. (2010). Immaturities in reward processing and its influence on inhibitory control in adolescence. *Cerebral Cortex, 20*, 1613–1629.

Giedd, J. N., Blumenthal, J., Jeffries, N. O., Castellanos, F. X., Liu, H., Zijdenbos, A., et al. (1999). Brain development during childhood and adolescence: A longitudinal MRI study. *Nature Neuroscience, 2*(10), 861–863.

Goddings, A., Burnett Heyes, S., Bird, G., Viner, R., & Blakemore, S. (2012). The relationship between puberty and social emotion processing. *Developmental Science, 15*, 801–811.

Golarai, G., Ghahremani, D. G., Whitfield-Gabrieli, S., Reiss, A., Eberhardt, J. L., Gabrieli, J. D., et al. (2007). Differential development of high-level visual cortex correlates with category-specific recognition memory. *Nature Neuroscience, 10*(4), 512–522.

Graber, J., Nichols, T., & Brooks-Gunn, J. (2010). Putting pubertal timing in developmental context: Implications for prevention. *Developmental Psychobiology, 52*, 254–262.

Guyer, A. E., Monk, C. S., McClure-Tone, E. B., Nelson, E. E., Roberson-Nay, R., Adler, A. D., et al. (2008). A developmental examination of amygdala response to facial expressions. *Journal of Cognitive Neuroscience, 20*(9), 1565–1582.

Haber, S. (2011). Neuroanatomy of reward: A view from the ventral striatum. In J. Gottfried (Ed.), *Neurobiology of sensation and reward*. Boca Raton, FL: CRC Press.

Haber, S., & Knutson, B. (2010). The reward circuit: Linking primate anatomy and human imaging. *Neuropsychopharmacology, 35,* 4–26.

Hall, G. (1904). *Adolescence: Its psychology and its relation to physiology, anthropology, sociology, sex, crime, religion, and education* (Vols. 1 and 2). Englewood Cliffs, NJ: Prentice-Hall.

Hare, T. A., Tottenham, N., Galván, A., Voss, H. U., Glover, G. H., & Casey, B. J. (2008). Biological substrates of emotional reactivity and regulation in adolescence during an emotional go-nogo task. *Biological Psychiatry, 63*(10), 927–934.

Heimer, L., De Olmos, J., Alheid, G., Person, J., Sakamoto, N., Shinoda, K., et al. (1999). The human basal forebrain. Part II. In F. Bloom, A. Bjorkland, & T. Hokfelt (Eds.), *Handbook of chemical neuroanatomy* (pp. 57–226). Amsterdam: Elsevier.

Herba, C., Landau, C., Russell, T., Ecker, C., & Phillips, M. (2006). The development of emotion-processing in children: Effects of age, emotion, and intensity. *Journal of Child of Psychology and Psychiatry, 11,* 1098–1106.

Hoffman, E. A., & Haxby, J. V. (2000). Distinct representations of eye gaze and identity in the distributed human neural system for face perception. *Nature Neuroscience, 3*(1), 80–84.

Jarcho, J., Benson, B., Plate, R., Guyer, A., Detloff, A., Pine, D., et al. (2012). Developmental effects of decision-making on sensitivity to reward: An fMRI study. *Developmental Cognitive Neuroscience, 2,* 437–447.

Kanwisher, N., McDermott, J., & Chun, M. M. (1997). The fusiform face area: A module in human extrastriate cortex specialized for face perception. *Journal of Neuroscience, 17*(11), 4302–4311.

Ladouceur, C. (2012). Neural systems supporting cognitive-affective interactions in adolescence: The role of puberty and implications for affective disorders. *Frontiers in Integrative Neuroscience, 6,* 65.

Lamm, C., Benson, B. E., Guyer, A. E., Perez-Edgar, K., Fox, N. A., Pine, D. S., et al. (2014). Longitudinal study of striatal activation to reward and loss anticipation from mid-adolescence into late adolescence/early adulthood. *Brain and Cognition, 89,* 51–60.

Laviola, G., Pasucci, T., & Pieretti, S. (2001). Striatal dopamine sensitization to D-amphetamine in periadolescent but not in adult rats. *Pharmacology Biochemistry and Behavior, 68,* 115–124.

Lenroot, R., Gogtay, N., Greenstein, D., Wells, E., Wallace, G., Clasen, L., et al. (2007). Sexual dimorphism of brain developmental trajectories during childhood and adolescence. *NeuroImage, 36,* 1065–1073.

Logue, S., Chein, J., Gould, T., Holliday, E., & Steinberg, L. (2014). Adolescent mice, unlike adults, consume more alcohol in the presence of peers than alone. *Developmental Science, 17*(1), 79–85.

Luna, B., Thulborn, K. R., Munoz, D. P., Merriam, E. P., Garver, K. E., Minshew, N. J., et al. (2001). Maturation of widely distributed brain function subserves cognitive development. *NeuroImage, 13*(5), 786–793.

Marreiros, A., Kiebel, S., & Friston, K. (2008). Dynamic causal modelling for fMRI: A two-state model. *NeuroImage, 39,* 269–278.

McCutcheon, J., & Marinelli, M. (2009). Technical spotlight: Age matters. *European Journal of Neuroscience, 29,* 997–1014.

Nelson, E., Herman, K., Barrett, C., Noble, P., Wojteczko, K., Chisholm, K., et al. (2009). Adverse rearing experiences enhance responding to both aversive and rewarding stimuli in juvenile rhesus monkeys. *Biological Psychiatry, 66,* 702–704.

Nelson, E., Liebenluft, E., McClure, E., & Pine, D. S. (2005). The social re-orientation of adolescence: A neuroscience perspective on the process and its relation to psychopathology. *Psychological Medicine, 35*, 163–174.

Op de Macks, Z., Gunther Moor, B., Overgaauw, S., Guroglu, B., Dahl, R., & Crone, E. (2011). Testosterone levels correspond with increased ventral striatum activation in response to monetary rewards in adolescents. *Developmental Cognitive Neuroscience, 1*, 506–516.

Padmanabhan, A., Geier, G. F., Ordaz, S. J., Teslovich, T., & Luna, B. (2011). Developmental changes in brain function underlying the influence of reward processing in inhibitory control. *Developmental Cognitive Neuroscience, 1*, 517–529.

Pfeifer, J., & Allen, N. (2012). Arrested development?: Reconsidering dual-systems models of brain function in adolescence and disorders. *Trends in Cognitive Sciences, 16*, 322–329.

Pfeifer, J. H., Masten, C. L., Borofsky, L. A., Dapretto, M., Fuligni, A. J., & Lieberman, M. D. (2009). Neural correlates of direct and reflected self-appraisals in adolescents and adults: When social perspective-taking informs self-perception. *Child Development, 80*(4), 1016–1038.

Pine, D. S., Lissek, S., Klein, R. G., Mannuszza, S., Moulton, J. L., Guardino, M., et al. (2004). Face-memory and emotion: Association with major depression in children and adolescents. *Journal of Child Psychology and Psychiatry, 45*, 1199–1208.

Post, G., & Kemper, H. (1993). Nutritional intake and biological maturation during adolescence: The Amsterdam growth and health longitudinal study. *European Journal of Clinical Nutrition, 47*, 400–408.

Robinson, D., Heien, M., & Wightman, R. (2002). Frequency of dopamine concentration transients increases in dorsal and ventral striatum of male rats during introduction of conspecifics. *Journal of Neuroscience, 22*, 10477–10486.

Robinson, D., Zitzman, D., Smith, K., & Spear, L. (2011). Fast dopamine release events in the nucleus accumbens of early adolescent rats. *Neuroscience, 176*, 296–307.

Roitman, M., Wheeler, R., Wightman, R., & Carelli, R. (2008). Real-time chemical responses in the nucleus accumbens differentiate rewarding and aversive stimuli. *Nature Neuroscience, 11*, 1376–1377.

Scherf, K. S., Behrmann, M., & Dahl, R. E. (2012). Facing changes and changing faces in adolescence: A new model for investigating adolescent-specific interactions between pubertal, brain and behavioral development. *Developmental Cognitive Neurocience, 2*(2), 199–219.

Scherf, K. S., Bermann, M., Humphreys, K., & Luna, B. (2007). Visual category-selectivity for faces, places, and objects emerges along different developmental trajectories. *Developmental Science, 10*(4), F15–F30.

Schultz, W., Dayan, P., & Montague, P. R. (1997). A neural substrate of prediction and reward. *Science, 275*, 1593–1599.

Sisk, C., & Foster, D. (2004). The neural basis of puberty and adolescence. *Nature Neuroscience, 7*, 1040–1047.

Sisk, C., & Zehr, J. L. (2005). Pubertal hormones organize the adolescent brain and behavior. *Frontiers in Neuroendocrinology, 26*(3–4), 163–174.

Smith, D., Xiao, L., & Bechara, A. (2011). Decision making in children and adolescents: Impaired Iowa Gambling Task performance in early adolescence. *Developmental Psychology, 48*(4), 1180–1187.

Somerville, L., & Casey, B. (2010). Developmental neurobiology of cognitive control and motivational systems. *Current Opinion in Neurobiology, 20*(2), 236–241.

196

Somerville, L., Hare, T., & Casey, B. (2011). Frontostriatal maturation predicts cognitive control failure to appetitive cues in adolescents. *Journal of Cognitive Neuroscience, 23*, 2123–2134.

Sowell, E., Thompson, P., Holmes, C., Jernigan, T., & Toga, A. (1999). In vivo evidence for post-adolescent brain maturation in frontal and striatal regions. *Nature Neuroscience, 2*, 859–861.

Spear, L. (2000). The adolescent brain and age-related behavioral manifestations. *Neuroscience and Biobehavioral Reviews, 24*(4), 417–463.

Spear, L. (2011a). Rewards, aversions and affect in adolescence: Emerging convergences across laboratory animal and human data. *Developmental Cognitive Neuroscience, 1*, 390–403.

Spear, L. (2011b). Rewards, aversions and affect in adolescence: Emerging convergences across laboratory animal and human data. *Developmental Cognitive Neuroscience, 1*, 392–400.

Stamford, J. (1989). Development and ageing of the rat nigrostriatal dopamine system studied with fast cyclic voltammetry. *Journal of Neurochemistry, 52*, 1582–1589.

Steinberg, L. (2008). A social neuroscience perspective on adolescent risk-taking. *Developmental Review, 28*, 78–106.

Steinberg, L., Graham, S., O'Brien, L., Woolard, J., Cauffman, E., & Banich, M. (2009). Age differences in future orientation and delay discounting. *Child Development, 80*, 28–44.

Takahashi, Y., Roesch, M., Stalnaker, T., Haney, R., Calu, D., Taylor, A., et al. (2009). The orbitofrontal cortex and ventral tegmental area are necessary for learning from unexpected outcomes. *Neuron, 62*, 269–280.

Tarazi, F., Tomasini, E., & Baldessarini, R. (1999). Postnatal development of dopamine D1-like receptors in rat cortical and striatolimbic brain regions: An autoradiographic study. *Developmental Neuroscience, 21*, 43–49.

Teicher, M., Andersen, S., & Hostetter, Jr., J. (1995). Evidence for dopamine receptor pruning between adolescence and adulthood in striatum but not nucleus accumbens. *Developmental Brain Research, 89*, 167–172.

Thomas, K. M., Drevets, W. C., Whalen, P. J., Eccard, C. H., Dahl, R. E., Ryan, N. D., et al. (2001). Amygdala response to facial expressions in children and adults. *Biological Psychiatry, 49*(4), 309–316.

Thomas, L. A., de Bellis, M. D., Graham, R., & LaBar, K. (2007). Development of emotional facial recognition in late childhood and adolescence. *Developmental Science, 10*, 547–558.

Urošević, S., Collins, P., Muetzel, R., Lim, K., & Luciana, M. (2012). Longitudinal changes in behavioral approach system sensitivity and brain structures involved in reward processing during adolescence. *Developmental Psychology, 48*, 1488–1500.

van Leijenhorst, L., Zanolie, K., van Meel, C., Westenberg, P., Rombouts, S., & Crone, E. (2010). What motivates the adolescent?: Brain regions mediating reward sensitivity across adolescents. *Cerebral Cortex, 20*(1), 61–69.

Varlinskaya, E., & Spear, L. (2008). Social interactions in adolescent and adult Sprague-Dawley rats: Impact of social deprivation and test context familiarity. *Behavioral Brain Research, 188*, 398–405.

PART III

Desire, Judgment, and Decision Making

CHAPTER 10

License to Sin

Reasoning Processes in Desire

Denise T. D. de Ridder
Jessie C. de Witt Huberts
Catharine Evers

Alarmingly high prevalence rates of obesity, addiction, financial debt, and divorce are what we have to show for our life of plenty. In a world where abundance has replaced scarcity as the source of many contemporary societal problems, the question of why people so often fail to act in accordance with their objectives, values, and intentions has become more relevant than ever. Despite their best intentions not to, dieters overeat, smokers continue to smoke, consumers overspend, and partners break their vows. To understand this puzzling phenomenon, such behavior is often explained in terms of desires taking over our rational considerations. As captured by common descriptions, it is generally assumed that dieters *succumb* to tempting cupcakes, smokers *give in* to nicotine cravings, consumers *cave in* to the special offer, and we *fall for* someone else's charms.

In line with this widespread view, psychological research investigating how we can best navigate through a world designed to appeal to our desires has predominantly focused on rational and deliberate processes as the antidote to the detrimental effect of our desires. To counter the 24-hour shopping opportunities, the advertisements luring us on every page, screen, and street corner, and the tasty, cheap, and easy food choices tempting us wherever we go, we have to keep a cool head, weigh our options, and make a wise decision. However, everyday examples suggest that thinking before acting may not always have the hypothesized effect: instead of protecting us from enacting our desires, reasoning processes may actually stimulate it. Take, for example, Sally, Mark, and Marcy, who are at a wedding party. Sally is mesmerized by the wedding cake but is in doubt as she is on a weight-loss diet that does not allow such tasty but unhealthy delicacies. Mark is getting increasingly nervous about the speech he is about to give, not sure if his jokes are indeed funny. The nerves make him crave nicotine, but a cigarette is off limits since he quit smoking 6 weeks ago. Marcy has been sipping soda water all night. As she sees her friends enjoying their drinks, she regrets her offer to be the designated driver. When the cake is cut, Sally decides that she will have a piece: it is a celebratory occasion after all. Mark also caves in and asks his friend for a cigarette, telling himself that he is allowed to have cigarettes in emergencies, and, according to Mark, this is one. Finally, when everybody raises their glass for the toast, Marcy also falls off the wagon and has a glass of champagne, reasoning that having just one glass won't interfere with her ability to drive.

Whereas most contemporary self-regulation theories would explain failure to act in accordance with one's long-term goals as the result of our impulses taking precedence over reflective considerations, the above examples suggest that people often fail to follow through on their long-term goals not merely because of being overwhelmed by desire, but rather because they generate reasons for giving in to their desires. Therefore, we postulate that through reliance on justifications to set aside long-term goals, reflective processes can play a substantial role in failing to resist desires. To clarify, we acknowledge the basic premise of self-regulation theories that reasoned processes and impulsive processes dynamically interact. However, we disagree with another important proposition in these theories: that impulses dictate behavior unless they are down-regulated by reflective processes. Rather, we put forward the novel idea that impulses may direct our reflective processes toward justifying indulgence. While this notion has a familiar appeal to many of us, surprisingly, the role of reflective processes—in particular, justification processes—has been afforded hardly any attention as an explanation for self-regulation failure. Instead, research on self-regulation failure has, to date, mainly focused on the relative strength of impulses for the gratification of immediate desires as an explanation for abandoning long-term goals. In the present chapter we present a theoretical analysis and empirical review of justification processes in self-regulation failure, exploring more deeply the observation that failure is not solely the consequence of impulsive factors, but that reflective processes can contribute as well. We first give a short overview of the conventional frameworks of self-regulation and specify the role of reasoning processes in them. In the following section, we review the empirical evidence for justification processes in self-regulation and kindred phenomena, followed by an analysis of potential mechanisms that fuel the effect. Finally, we discuss important issues raised by this novel perspective and sketch directions for future research.

Self-Regulation: Resisting Desire

At the heart of self-regulation lies the ability to transcend immediate temptations in the service of long-term goals. Thus, self-regulation dilemmas typically involve a conflict between incompatible motivations, where on the one hand hedonic attraction pulls us toward indulgence, while on the other hand our long-term goals dictate that we should resist the hedonic urge (e.g., Hofmann, Friese, & Strack, 2009). The conflict between opposing motivational forces that encompass a self-regulatory dilemma is not new, but has captured the imagination of scholars for centuries, often being described in epic terms, as a conflict between the passions and reason, the heart and mind, or emotions versus rationality. The metaphor of a horse and a rider is often used to describe this delicate interplay, where the horse symbolizes the impulsive system guided by stimulus control that has to be reined by a reflective rider. This duality is still evident in contemporary conceptualizations of self-regulation, such as the hot versus cool systems (Metcalfe & Mischel, 1999), visceral versus rational decision making (Loewenstein, 1996), and impulsive versus reflective systems (Strack & Deutsch, 2004).

Drawing on the dual-process and dual-system theories that have dominated research in social psychology the past two decades, these models contend that self-regulation is determined by two systems, a hot, impulsive, and emotional system and a cold, reflective, and rational system. Although the models differ in their specific contentions, in general they assume that tempting stimuli elicit automatic affective reactions in the impulsive system that, unless counteracted by more deliberative processes stemming from the reflective system, will lead to self-regulation failure. Importantly, whereas impulsive processes are assumed to operate in an effortless manner (e.g., Strack & Deutsch, 2004), in order for one to act in accordance with one's goals and shield those goals against interfering impulsive influences, the reflective system requires cognitive and motivational resources. As a result, if there is not sufficient cognitive and motivational capacity available, processes in the reflective system will be undermined, allowing for impulsive reactions to dictate behavior.

In line with these assumptions, the past two decades of research on self-regulation have documented how impairments of the reflective system result in self-regulation failure. For example, research on resource depletion suggests that the ability to effectively self-regulate relies on a limited resource that is depleted by effortful attempts at self-regulation. Consequently, prior acts of self-control will deplete self-regulatory resources and undermine subsequent attempts at self-regulation (Muraven & Baumeister, 2000). Such states of resource depletion caused by an initial act of self-control (e.g., resisting the impulse to eat cookies) have been linked to overeating, impulsive spending, and excessive alcohol consumption (e.g., Vohs & Faber, 2007). Beyond self-control resources, operations within the reflective system also rely on sufficient cognitive capacity. Situational factors burdening our cognitive capabilities, such as cognitive load (Ward & Mann, 2000) or emotional distress (Witkiewitz & Villaroel, 2009), increase the likelihood of self-regulation failure.

Conversely, by explaining self-regulation failure as resulting from the impairment of the reflective system, these models assume that when the reflective system has sufficient capacity or resources, people will make a reasoned and rational decision and act in line with their objectives and self-interest. This assumption is based on the rational ideal where reasoning and deliberation transcend our feelings and impulses, and rationality is assumed to be the end product of reasoning and logical thought. However, this rationalist framework has been called into question in other areas of psychology. In domains such as judgment and decision making, investigators have become increasingly aware of the limits of reasoning (e.g., Shafir, Simonson, & Tversky, 1993).

A growing body of research not only suggests that violations of rationality are accounted for by the cognitive constraints of decision makers but has also revealed that even at full capacity processes in the reflective system are prone to bias. In sharp contrast to the classical view that reasoning about possible options and weighing up their pros and cons is the most reliable way to arrive at sound decisions, a whole line of research argues that the best decisions are made in split seconds (Dijksterhuis & Nordgren, 2006) and that emotions are crucial for effective decision making (Damasio, 1994). Sometimes reasoning can even lead to poor decisions or outcomes not in line with our objectives and interests, with studies reporting that in comparison with spontaneous decisions, encouraging participants to deliberate and analyze their reasons before making a decision reduced the quality of that decision, both in terms of objective utility (e.g., Wilson & Schooler, 1991) and subjective satisfaction (e.g., Wilson et al., 1993).

Yet, while in other domains it is increasingly acknowledged that the impact of reasoning on judgment is often mediated through emotional and motivational mechanisms, to date this notion has been largely ignored in both the self-regulation literature and in dual-process theories. While dual-process models of self-regulation generally assume that the purpose of the reflective system is to constrain hedonic tendencies coming from the impulsive system, such a conceptualization fails to take into account that reasoning itself is vulnerable to our motivations and desires. Acknowledging the limits of reason puts the assumption that reflective processes exclusively stimulate behavior that is in line with our long-term goals in another perspective. Instead, these findings raise the possibility that in some cases the reflective system, rather than correcting our impulsive tendencies, will justify them. Thus, by looking for supporting arguments that allow one to set aside long-term goals, the reflective system can play a substantial role in self-regulation failure. Integrating these insights from judgment and decision making with self-regulation, we propose a justification-based mechanism of self-regulation failure. Specifically, by seeking or construing arguments that allow one to set aside long-term goals, we postulate that people sometimes indulge through reason rather than being overwhelmed by desire.

A Justification-Based Account of Self-Regulation Failure

More than ever, people in Western industrialized society are confronted with conflicting motivational pressures. People hold goals to be thin, athletic, productive, or successful but are continuously faced with temptations threatening these goals. Sally, for example, experiences a conflict between what she wants at that moment (the wedding cake) and what she should do to reach her long-term aims (skip the cake and go for the crudités instead). She could resolve this conflict by attempting to resist her urge to indulge in the cake, an effortful process that leads to effective self-regulation. Alternatively, she could resolve the motivational conflict by creating or activating justifications that allow her to indulge in the chocolate cake (for a related dissonance-based account, see also Harmon-Jones, Gable, & Harmon-Jones, Chapter 8, this volume). Thus, justification processes, which by their slow, analytical, and strategic nature would be considered a product of the reflective system in the traditional dual-process model distinction, can contribute to self-regulation failure.

By justification we mean the act of making excuses for one's discrepant behavior before actual enactment, such that the prospective failure is made acceptable for oneself. In other words, when experiencing a self-regulation dilemma between immediate impulses and long-term intentions, people resolve the conflict by developing and employing justifications that allow violations of the goal they endorse. After all, wanting to do something is a prerequisite but not sufficient for action; "one must also feel licensed to do it" (Miller & Effron, 2010, p. 115). Thus, in self-regulation conflicts where one's desire to act on one's impulses is in conflict with one's desire to achieve a long-term goal, justifications can trigger action by liberating people to act on their short-term motivations (see also Bitterly, Mislavsky, Dai, & Milkman, Chapter 12, this volume). In the present account, the involvement of a self-regulation dilemma is crucial to trigger justification processes. Without desires arising from our impulsive system that interfere with our long-term goals, justification processes are unnecessary. After all, if Sally disliked chocolate, it is unlikely she would be tempted by the chocolate-decorated wedding cake, removing the need for justifications. Likewise, if Sally did not have a long-term weight-loss goal, she would have no reason to try to resist the urge elicited by the prospect of tasting the delicious-looking wedding cake, making the need for justifications obsolete.

Evidence of justifications as a facilitator of behavior originates in judgment and decision-making literature, indicating that people are more likely to choose the option that they can justify (Shafir et al., 1993). As the need to choose often creates conflict, decision makers seek and construct reasons in order to resolve the conflict and justify their choice (e.g., Kivetz, 1999; Simonson, 1989). As the typical self-regulation dilemma of gratifying immediate desires versus the pursuit of long-term benefits by definition entails a conflict between opposing goals, justification processes seem particularly relevant for understanding self-regulation failure. Applying these principles to the context of self-regulation, one would assume that a justification-based mechanism will favor behavior in line with our intentions simply because corresponding with our long-term goals should be a compelling justification. However, as noted by Shafir et al. (1993), having a reason seems to be more important than the quality of the reason. That is, decisions are based on the mere availability of reasons; the nature and the quality of the reason tend to be disregarded: people appear to prefer "shallow but nice sounding" justifications (Simonson, 1989, p. 170). Moreover, people seem to focus on justifications that are consistent with their initial attitude to justify how they feel, constructing reasons for their present feelings (e.g., Mercier & Sperber, 2011). Thus, a justification-based mechanism would predict that when confronted with a typical self-regulation dilemma where people might be more inclined to pursue the hedonic option, people will be motivated to seek or construct justifications that will allow them to justify it. This implies that when people find themselves in a situation where they are tempted by something they know they really should not do, they might be successful in constraining themselves, unless they find a reason, any reason, to give in. As such our capacity to reason can become a liability when it comes to self-regulation failure.

Isolated illustrations of justifications facilitating behavior that is not in line with one's explicit standards come from a variety of fields, such as health behavior, moral behavior, and consumer choice. Yet these various empirical demonstrations have never been assembled to substantiate a justification-based account of self-regulation failure. In the following section we aggregate evidence for a justification-based mechanism. This includes work that was not explicitly conducted within this framework but that nevertheless seems to capture the phenomenon that we sometimes rely on justifications to allow ourselves a forbidden pleasure.

Empirical Evidence
for Justification Processes in Self-Regulation Failure

The role of justifications was first studied in the context of moral behavior where justifications could lead one to violate one's moral principles, for example, by exhibiting prejudiced, sexist, or selfish behavior (Merritt, Effron, & Monin, 2010). For example, Monin and Miller (2001)

showed that choosing an African American—who was the most quali-
fied applicant—for a hypothetical job increased the likelihood that
participants would describe a subsequent job as better suited for white
applicants, compared to participants who, based on similar descriptions,
initially chose a white applicant as best suited for the job. This and similar
findings were attributed to the fact that people whose past behavior (e.g.,
acting in a nonprejudiced way) provided them with some kind of "moral
credential" that licensed them to subsequently behave in a way that violated these principles. To describe this phenomenon, Monin and Miller
(2001) employed the term *moral self-licensing*.

Further evidence for a justification-based mechanism underlying behavior discrepant with one's long-term goals comes from studies
on consumer choice. As many purchasing decisions are tinged with a
conflict between hedonic and functional considerations, such as spending on luxuries versus saving up or spending on necessary items, they
often encompass a typical self-regulation dilemma of choosing between
immediate gratification and long-term considerations. As in general the
purchase or consumption of such luxury goods is harder to justify than
the consumption of utilitarian products, having a justification should
increase the likelihood of indulging in luxury consumption. Indeed, a
number of studies have demonstrated the facilitating role of justifications
on consumer indulgence (Khan & Dhar, 2006; Kivetz & Zheng, 2006; see
also Dholakia, Chapter 20, this volume). Typically, participants in these
studies were presented with a justification after which, allegedly in the
context of another study, they could choose between a utilitarian and
a luxury item. These studies consistently demonstrated that providing
participants with a justification (e.g., effort, excellence feedback, or contributing to charity) increased choice of a luxury product (e.g., designer
jeans, indulgent chocolate cake) over a utilitarian product (e.g., vacuum
cleaner, healthy fruit salad) compared to participants not provided with
a justification. Having a justification not only increases preference for
hedonic over functional choice but also increases hedonic consumption,
such as eating unhealthy snacks (De Witt Huberts, Evers, & De Ridder,
2012), suggesting that justification processes also play an important role
in self-regulatory processes that are under the influence of visceral drives
(e.g., hunger) and that involve actively regulating one's desires rather
than choosing.

Having established that justifications play a role in self-regulation
failure, the question arises as to what kinds of justifications people rely
on to allow themselves an otherwise forbidden pleasure. A review of the
empirical evidence reveals the following list of common justifications.
We would like to note that the categorizations are ours, and limited only
to the justifications that have actually been studied. As the justifications
people rely on may be idiosyncratically determined and influenced by
situational factors, the list of justifications may be more exhaustive in

reality. For instance, recent work by Hofmann and colleagues (Hofmann, Baumeister, Förster, & Vohs, 2012) shows that the presence of other people who are indulging decreased the willingness to resist temptations, suggesting that using other people as an example may serve as a justification as well. Nevertheless, focus group studies and the recent evidence for self-generated justifications indicate that the justifications that participants came up with were mostly related to one of the categories outlined below (e.g., De Witt Huberts, Evers, & De Ridder, 2014d; Taylor, Webb, & Sheeran, 2014; Xu & Schwarz, 2009).

Altruistic and Laudable Acts

In a series of studies by Khan and Dhar (2006), imagining oneself having contributed to a charitable cause, such as teaching children in a homeless center or improving the environment, increased choice of a luxury product (designer jeans) over a utilitarian product (vacuum cleaner) compared to people who did not have to think of benevolent deeds (Study 1). In the same series of studies, participants who imagined having donated a part of their tax refunds to a charity were more likely to subsequently choose a pair of luxurious, expensive sunglasses over a pair of practical, less expensive sunglasses (Study 2). Likewise, when participants were asked to indicate their willingness to help a foreign student with understanding a lecture, they were less likely to donate the money they earned by participating to a local charity and preferred to keep it for themselves, as compared to participants in the control condition, who did an unrelated task before being asked to donate money to charity (Study 3). In another study by Mukhopadhyay and Johar (2009) it was found that if participants thought they were contributing to charity by buying a chocolate bar, they preferred chocolate cake over fruit salad in a subsequent choice task (Study 3). What is particularly notable is that in most studies in this context participants did not actually have to perform the behavior. Even imagining laudable behavior in a vignette study or intending to help produced these results (Khan & Dhar, 2006).

Effort and Achievement

In a review of the role of justifications in self-control failure, Kivetz and Zheng (2006) concluded that the most common justifications entailed either hard work or excellence feedback, suggesting that effort and achievement can serve as a justification to allow oneself a forbidden pleasure. This phenomenon can presumably be traced back to the puritanical idea that one is entitled to the good life only after hard work (Weber, 1958), which is also reflected in findings from qualitative studies where people indicate to only allow themselves a pleasure when they feel they earned it (Xu & Schwarz, 2009). Empirical evidence for this notion comes from a line of studies by Kivetz and Zheng (2006) demonstrating that justifications such as having exerted (relatively) more effort in an unrelated task or received excellence feedback on an unrelated performance task steered participants' preference toward the more indulgent options in subsequent choices, such as favoring lowbrow over highbrow movies (Study 1b), compared to participants who did not use these justifications. Similar results were obtained in a study from our lab that demonstrated that not actual effort but perceived effort increased hedonic consumption in a subsequent indulgent taste test (De Witt Huberts et al., 2012). Participants had to complete a noninvolving task on the computer. In the effort condition, participants were told halfway through that they had to do the task again (thus doing the task for 2×5 minutes); in the control condition, participants received no such instruction (and thus completed the task as if it were a single task of 10 minutes), thereby manipulating perceived effort while keeping actual effort constant. Participants who were led to believe that they had completed two tasks consumed on average 130 calories more in a time span of 10 minutes than participants who actually performed the same task but thought they had only completed a single task.

Prior Restraint

Prior restraint can also justify subsequent indulgent choice. Mukhopadhyay and Johar (2009) asked participants to remember an instance where they had seen a product on sale that they had not intended to buy and either ended up buying it or had resisted buying it. Those who had to remind themselves of a prior instance where they had exercised restraint by not buying an attractive product tended to prefer the chocolate cake over the healthier fruit salad in a subsequent choice task, their prior restraint presumably serving as a justification for their indulgent choice. Along the same lines, Mukhopadhay, Sengtupta, and Ramanathan (2008) asked participants to recall an instance of past behavior where they either had succumbed to or had resisted a food-related temptation. Participants who were instructed to think of prior resistance ate more cookies in a subsequent taste test than participants who recalled having succumbed. Similarly, dieters who were instructed to reflect on prior foregone indulgence expressed weaker intentions of pursuing their weight-loss goals and a week later indicated they had actually done less and intended to do less to pursue their weight-loss goals compared to dieters who did not reflect on prior restraint (Effron, Monin, & Miller, 2012).

Prior Success or Failure

A justification related to prior restraint is perceived goal progress. As many self-regulation dilemmas often involve trade-offs between two opposing goals, progress toward one goal often implies moving away from the other goal. A series of studies in the context of the goal progress model (Fishbach & Dhar, 2005) demonstrated that actual or perceived goal progress in one domain led to more indulgence in the opposing domain (e.g., losing weight vs. choosing a hedonic snack; studying vs. going out with friends). Conversely, although not explicitly studied in a justification context, having failed to attain one's goal could also serve as a justification to abandon it even further. Notorious in this regard is the "what the hell effect" in restrained eaters. Numerous studies demonstrated that restrained eaters, people who have the goal of restricting food intake to reach a certain weight do not show a physiologically normal compensation effect after consuming a preload (Herman & Mack, 1975). Having broken their diet by consuming a milk shake apparently serves as a reason to completely abandon their diet for the day. This abstinence violation effect, as it is also called, has been found within other self-regulation domains as well, such as in people with alcohol dependence who are abstinent (Collins & Lapp, 1991) and smokers (Shiffman et al., 1996).

Future Choices and Intentions

Another type of frequently studied justification consists of future choices and intentions. For example, in a study by Khan and Dhar (2007) participants had to choose between a relatively healthy or indulgent snack. Whereas the choice was framed as a single-choice opportunity for half of the participants, the other half of the participants were informed that they would have the possibility of choosing between the two snacks again in the following week. Participants believing that they could choose again next week were more likely to favor the indulgent option in the present choice. Merely knowing that one would have the option to choose again at a later time presumably justified people to act indulgently, as the possibility to act in line with one's intentions in the future served as a justification to break their rules in the present. A related demonstration of how future plans and choices can endanger current self-regulation is the evidence that forming particular justifications about undoing the negative effect of an indulgent behavior can bring about that indulgent behavior. In other words, when confronted with the wedding cake, Sally may form compensatory intentions such as "I will go exercising tomorrow," which will allow her to violate her dieting rules now and indulge in the cake. Indeed, a study by Kronick and Knäuper (2010) revealed that participants who were instructed to make plans to exercise later that day consumed more M&Ms in a subsequent taste test than participants who had not been asked to make such plans. Another compelling example is the finding that restrained eaters who plan to start a weight-loss diet will use that future intention as justification to indulge in the soon-to-be-forbidden food while they still can (Urbszat, Herman, & Polivy, 2002).

Negative Emotional Events

That negative emotional events and the ensuing negative affect can also serve as justification to temporarily abandon self-regulatory goals was demonstrated in our lab (De Witt Huberts, Evers, & De Ridder, 2014b). In three studies a negative affective state was induced in participants by showing them aversive pictures. The duration of exposure to the negative pictures was manipulated such that one group was highly aware of having seen the pictures whereas the other group was only minimally aware. Only participants who were highly aware of having seen the negative pictures, and thus could use the negative affective triggers as justification, consumed more hedonic snack foods in a subsequent taste test. Importantly, the increase in hedonic consumption could not be attributed to differences in negative affect, as both groups reported feeling equally negative but differed only in the extent to which they were aware of the cause of their negative feelings (as witnessed by being able to name details of the aversive pictures they had seen).

Similar findings have been observed in the context of emotional moral events, demonstrating that feeling wronged leads to more selfish behavior (Zitek, Jordan, Monin, & Leach, 2010). Participants who were instructed to recall an occasion in which they were treated unfairly were more likely to refuse to help the experimenter with a supplementary task than participants who had to recall a time when they were bored (Study 1; Zitek et al., 2010). Likewise, when participants lost a computer game due to an unfair reason (a glitch in the program), they requested a more unfair money allocation in a future task than did participants who lost the game for a fair reason (Study 3; Zitek et al., 2010).

Summary

The most intriguing observation that emerges from the overview of empirically studied justifications is the ease with which justification can propel self-regulation failure. Merely reading about a potential justification in vignette studies, imagining a laudable act or effort, both goal achievement and failure, and considering or intending to pursue the long-term goal again can make people digress from their long-term goal. Moreover justifications can be related to the goal they violate and be, in a sense, "rational" or logical, such as justifications that involve undoing the negative effects of the indulgent behavior or perceived goal progress, but justifications can also be unrelated to the behavior that is being justified, and thereby appear to be rather arbitrary. What the various justifications that have been studied to date have in common, however, is that they seem to entail some kind of entitlement. It can be concluded that people do not seem to be very critical of the reasons they apply to violate their intentions. This apparent susceptibility to relying on justifications indicates how easily justification processes can become maladaptive, underlining their importance as an explanation for self-regulation failure.

It seems that, although appearing under different names, in the past decade quite a bit of evidence has been gathered that points toward a facilitative role for justifications in norm-violating behavior, luxury choice, and indulgent behavior, suggesting that an underlying justification-based mechanism should be taken into account when explaining self-regulatory failure across various behavioral domains.

Underlying Mechanisms of Justification-Based Self-Regulation Failure

In this section we will review several potential mechanisms by which justifications disturb self-regulation. Besides several studies investigating the mediating effect of a reinforced self-concept in justification-based self-regulation failure (Khan & Dhar, 2006; Mukhopadhyay & Johar, 2009), to our knowledge there are hardly any other studies that have directly tested the underlying mechanism. Therefore, in addition to the evidence for a reinforced self-concept, we propose several other potential underlying processes, borrowing from major psychological theories explaining human motivation, including cognitive dissonance, anticipated affect, and motivated reasoning.

Prefactual Cognitive Dissonance

Marcy's decision to have a glass of champagne despite her strong intentions and full awareness of the possible negative consequences is, although seemingly mundane, actually more counterintuitive than one might expect. After all, behaving in ways that run counter to one's wishes, intentions, or principles violates a fundamental human need to see oneself as a rational and consistent person. Yet, one of the most robust findings within psychological research is that personal inconsistency is uncomfortable and threatening (Festinger, 1957). Cognitive dissonance in its purest sense cannot account for the findings reviewed above, as the outlined evidence concerned the use of justifications before an actual transgression happens, while cognitive dissonance is concerned with the justifications that people may use to rationalize self-gratification ex-post facto (Festinger, 1957). However, a justification-based mechanism does seem to fit with the broader set of psychological theories that focus on the need for cognitive consistency and its implications. We suggest that analogous to the reliance on justifications to resolve cognitive dissonance caused by behavior in the past, it is possible that justifications might help people to resolve a conflict evoked by prospective behavior.

Human beings have the unique ability to imagine the consequences of their behavior in advance. This prefactual thinking allows people to investigate the different consequences, and potentially experience disso-nance between one's cognitions and the (future) behavior that one is con-templating. From this point of view it could be argued that the conflict Sally experiences when she is tempted by the instant pleasure of the cake while being fully aware of how guilt ridden and inadequate she might feel after eating it is similar to the cognitive dissonance she might experience after actually having succumbed to the cake. It should be noted, how-ever, that our attempt to fit the principles of a justification-based account of self-regulation failure into the framework of cognitive dissonance research remains speculative, as Festinger himself contended that cog-nitive dissonance could only be evoked by prior behavior, while others did consider prefactual cognitive dissonance to be a possibility (Brown-stein, 2003). Thus, while the discomfort induced by a self-regulation dilemma beforehand, and the actual cognitive dissonance experienced afterwards, might be phenomenally different and not count as cognitive dissonance in the classical sense, the processes remain similar in that both accounts imply that the person must experience some kind of con-flict and that this conflict is resolved by means of a justification (see Harmon-Jones, Gable, & Harmon-Jones, Chapter 8, this volume). In the case of justification-induced self-regulation failure, this process occurs beforehand, and thereby the justification is responsible for generating the behavior, whereas in the classical cognitive dissonance paradigm the conflict takes place after the transgression has become a reality, and jus-tifications are generated by the transgressive behavior.

Anticipated Affect

Closely related to, and potentially overlapping with, the prefactual cogni-tive dissonance account as an explanation for justification-induced self-regulation failure is the literature on anticipated affect. Regret and guilt are powerful forces in motivating and giving direction to behavior because people are motivated to prevent regret and guilt from happening (Simon-son, 1992). Much of the conflict experienced in self-regulation dilem-mas stems from concern about the anticipated negative consequences of a choice: Mark would not experience discord if he did not anticipate that having a cigarette would make him feel guilty afterwards. That avoiding these negative consequences is a powerful motivator of human behav-ior is evidenced by the finding that anticipated regret plays a substantial role in self-regulation, preventing people from abandoning their good intentions (Abraham & Sheeran, 2003). Similarly, work by Giner-Sorolla (2001) indicates that self-conscious emotions such as guilt and regret can boost self-regulation in self-regulatory dilemmas. For Mark, knowing that he will feel like a failure after smoking is presumably the main moti-vator to refrain from smoking. Thus, many, if not most, self-regulation conflicts involve a form of anticipated regret or guilt. This anticipated negative affect, and thereby potentially its reinforcing effect on effective self-regulation, might be countered by means of justifications.

Research has shown that justifiable decisions lead to less regret than unjustifiable decisions (Connolly & Zeelenberg, 2002). If anticipated regret leads people to engage in thoughtful decision making, using a justification, even though faulty, could give people the impression of having made a careful decision, thereby alleviating regret or guilt about one's behavior (Reb & Connolly, 2010). The anticipated regret and guilt evoked by self-regulation conflicts stimulates the seeking and construction of justifications to avoid these anticipated negative feelings. The effect of anticipated guilt was investigated in a study by Khan and Dhar (2007). After half of the participants were provided with a justification (future choice), all participants had to indicate the degree of guilt they would feel after eating the healthy option (yogurt) and the unhealthy option (cookie) before actually choosing between these products. Participants who had a justification anticipated less guilt in choosing the cookie than participants who did not have a justification. The reduced anticipated affect mediated the effect of justifications on indulgent choice. Thus, having a justification before a choice decreases the anticipated guilt related to the indulgent choice, thereby stimulating the indulgent choice.

Related evidence in support of this assumption comes from the series of studies conducted by Kivetz and Zheng (2006). They found that the effect of justifications was particularly strong in people who were dispositionally more prone to feelings of guilt. Moreover, in a subsequent study guilt was experimentally manipulated by asking participants to remember either two or eight occasions in the past week when they had failed to resist temptation. It was assumed that remembering two instances of self-regulation failure would be relatively easy, thereby conveying the impression that they often failed at self-regulation attempts and inducing relatively high levels of guilt. Having to remember eight examples of self-regulation failure within the last week was assumed to be difficult for participants, conveying the impression that they were relatively successful in sticking to their intentions, and leading to lower levels of guilt. Results indeed indicated that participants experiencing high levels of guilt were more likely to rely on a justification to allow oneself a subsequent indulgence than participants who experienced low levels of guilt. This finding is not in line with the common finding that people who experience guilt are more likely to exert self-control (Giner-Sorolla, 2001). It thus seems that justifications may undo the protective role of self-conscious emotions such as guilt and regret.

Motivated Reasoning

While it was long assumed that rationality was the end product of our capacity to reason, and thus would lead to actions that are in our own best (long-term) interest, it has been acknowledged for some time now that purely rational modes of reasoning can lead to suboptimal outcomes. In fact, research has demonstrated that reason itself is not completely rational. Instead our reasoning is biased by our motivations. According to Kunda's account of motivated reasoning (1990), people construct seemingly rational justifications for their desired beliefs. Consequently, the information search is biased in favor of information that is consistent with the desired conclusions. This allows people to draw a conclusion they desire while maintaining an illusion of objectivity.

Taking up a motivated reasoning account in the context of self-regulation failure would predict that when confronted with a tempting option, people will be naturally motivated to choose the hedonic alternative (Okada, 2005) and are consequently motivated to find reasons that justify such a choice. Thus, when Sally is tempted by the forbidden cake she justifies her feelings by coming up with arguments in favor of having the cake (e.g., "This is an exceptional occasion, so I am not really breaking my diet"). Thus, the reliance on justifications in self-regulation failure seems to be a classic example of motivated reasoning, where justifications are tinged by desire rather than objective rational formulations. After all, if the reasoning process were to be truly objective, Sally would be able to apply equally, if not more, compelling justifications for not eating the cake that fit with her intentions and beliefs (e.g., "It is bad for my weight-loss regime") and would thereby be the more justifiable option from a rational perspective. Consistent with a motivated reasoning account, it seems that when people are motivated to arrive at a certain conclusion, such as having the cake, then even trivial and irrational reasons can increase the justifiability of a decision. Thus, ironically, the evidence for motivationally constructed justifications suggests that in our attempts to appear rational we become irrational.

While use of a motivated reasoning account to explain a justification-based pathway to self-regulation failure is promising, it has never been experimentally tested in the context of self-regulation. However, findings from our lab do provide initial support for a motivated reasoning account by demonstrating that the justifiability of a forbidden pleasure is determined by its temptation strength (De Witt Huberts, Evers, & De Ridder, 2014c). Ostensibly as part of the market introduction of a new snack, participants were asked to rate how tempted they were by a new type of chocolate bar. Afterwards, supposedly to determine the marketing strategy for the product, participants had to indicate the reasons that would allow them to indulge in that particular food temptation. Results across two studies indicated that the degree of temptation (i.e., how attractive, yet forbidden the product was; Kroese, Evers, & De Ridder, 2011) determined the number of reasons participants applied or construed to allow themselves the forbidden treat. In both studies the justifications referring to visceral factors that could be used as a reason to consume the product, such as appetite and hunger, were not included, thus purely measuring justifications rather than a biological necessity to consume the hedonic product. Although the degree of temptation was not manipulated, with the study instead relying on idiosyncratically determined temptation, these results do fit the concept of motivated reasoning.

Further experimental evidence comes from a recent study by Effron, Monin, and Miller (2012) revealing that participants exaggerated prior dietary restraint, thereby creating a justification, when they expected to eat cookies but not when they expected to merely see the cookies. Another experimental study demonstrated that a smoking-urge manipulation resulted in the generation of more positive and less negative characteristics of smoking in smokers with a desire to smoke (Sayette & Hufford, 1997). These findings suggest that the extent to which one feels tempted by a product determines the number of reasons one applies and construes in order to justify its consumption. While motivated reasoning is not rational in itself, it does seem to allow us to maintain a rational self-concept while behaving irrationally. Although this may in fact be an illusion, as our reasons are trivial or irrational, the goal we may aim to achieve by applying justifications—retaining a self-concept as a reasonable person—may successfully be achieved by such a process.

Reinforced Self-Concept

In extension of the idea that justifications are construed in order to maintain an illusion of rationality, it has been argued that justifications exert their influence by counteracting the detrimental consequences of self-regulation failure to our self-concept. This premise is considered to be the underlying mechanism of moral licensing for which Monin and Miller (2001) introduced the concept of moral credentials. Monin and Miller maintained that licensing effects in stereotyping behavior arise because a prior act has protected the individual's self-perception. That is, once people viewed themselves as nonsexist or nonracist individuals because of a prior statement or endorsement, they felt freer to stereotype others. Relating this notion to self-regulation, a justification, which mostly involves something laudable about the self, such as effort or a charitable deed, functions as a kind of credential that then serves as a license to choose an option that would otherwise create negative attributions for the self, such as acting against one's intentions. Indirect evidence for such a mechanism comes from a study by Mukhopadhyay and Johar (2009) demonstrating that resisting temptation causes positive self-conscious emotions such as pride.

Evidence for this mechanism was directly tested in the context of consumer research. As the purchase of luxuries is difficult to justify and induces guilt (Okada, 2005), it is considered to produce negative self-attributions. Having chosen a virtuous option beforehand can help establish credentials that in turn can serve as a justification to choose an option that otherwise would harm one's self-concept. Khan and Dhar (2006) directly tested whether an initial benevolent choice boosted self-concept, buffering an individual against negative attributions associated with the second, indulgent, choice. After half the participants were provided with a justification (signing up for community service), all the participants had to provide self-assessments on four positive personality traits (e.g., compassionate, sympathetic). As expected, those who had committed to an altruistic act rated themselves significantly more positively on the four attributes than participants without such a justification. This boost in self-concept mediated the effect of the justification on willingness to choose an indulgent item. However, providing participants with an external reason to perform the community service (for instance, having to do community service for having committed a driving violation) attenuated the facilitating effect on indulgent choice. Presumably doing community service as punishment reversed the positive impact on self-concept. A reinforced self-concept might explain the results from studies where one did not actually need to perform a benevolent act for a justification effect to occur. If merely thinking about, intending, or planning a charitable act can lead to a more positive self-concept, then there is no need to execute one's optimistic plans in order to reap the benefits that enable one to indulge without negative consequences.

However, findings from another series of studies by Mukhopadhyay and Johar (2009) suggest that a boost in self-concept is not necessary for prior laudable acts or decisions to bring about indulgent behavior. In their studies self-esteem was measured directly after the initial decision that was supposed to act as a justification (refraining from or giving in to an impulsive purchase). In contrast to the findings by Khan and Dhar (2006), no difference in self-esteem was found between participants who did exercise restraint in the prior decision and the participants who had failed to exercise restraint. They did find, however, that participants who had exercised shopping restraint in the first decision were more likely to choose the indulgent option afterwards, demonstrating the justification effect. Interestingly however, reminding participants of their self-esteem before the second choice also increased indulgence afterwards, even in participants without a justification. These findings thus suggest that both reminding one of one's self-concept without prior restraint, and thus without a justification, and restraining oneself without actually boosting self-esteem, could produce justification effects. The authors therefore concluded that a boost in self-concept is sufficient, but not necessary, to instigate indulgent choice (Mukhopadhyay & Johar, 2009). While these findings may at first glance not be in line with the findings by Khan and Dhar (2006), they do not necessarily contradict each other. The justifications used in the studies by Khan and Dhar involved commitment to an altruistic act, which could have generated a stronger boost in self-concept than refraining from an indulgent purchase, as used by Mukhopadhyay and Johar (2009). While more research is needed to determine the effect of specific justifications on self-concept and the role of self-concept in self-regulation failure, the above findings suggest that there may be multiple pathways for justifications to instigate self-regulation failure.

Summary

Although we have discussed several potential mechanisms that could explain a justification-based route to self-regulation failure, we would like to note that this list is by no means exhaustive. Other factors not reviewed here could account for the effect of justifications on self-regulation failure. Moreover as studies directly investigating the underlying mechanisms remain scarce, leaving only indirect evidence for the proposed mechanisms, our review highlights the need for more future research into the underlying mechanisms of justification-induced self-regulation failure. What's more, the many similarities and overlap between the various explanations suggest that a justification-based route to self-regulation failure is more likely to be determined in multiple ways. Which of these mechanisms ultimately determines the effect on self-regulation failure may to a great extent be determined by the circumstances. For example, a strengthened self-concept is more likely to explain the underlying mechanism when the justification involves some altruistic deed, which touches a key aspect of the self, rather than an ephemeral justification such as not buying something. Also it is likely that in order for motivated reasoning processes to be instigated, one must feel a strong desire for a certain option, and thus already have been exposed to a temptation. Finally, individual differences such as guilt proneness could affect whether a justification-based route is determined by anticipated or experienced affect.

Conclusions and Implications

Notwithstanding the many questions that remain about the factors and mechanisms determining a justification-based pathway, the findings reviewed and analyzed in the present chapter reveal that justification processes have been underappreciated as an explanation for self-regulation failure. The reviewed findings not only demonstrate that a justification-based pathway is an important and common route to self-regulation failure in many behavioral domains, but also reveal how easily inclined people are to rely on justifications. Therefore, to capture the full scope of processes underlying self-regulation failure, it is crucial to put such a reflective route to goal derailment on the map.

Acknowledging a justification-based account as an explanation for self-regulation failure has important conceptual implications for self-regulation. First, the novel route outlined in this chapter suggests that self-regulation failure is not by default the result of the impulsive system taking precedence over the reflective system as has often been inferred. Instead the reviewed evidence indicates that even when people have the resources and capacity to act in accordance with long-term goals, they may not always do so when there is a justification to act not in accordance with goals. This novel view suggests that impulses may interfere with the motivation to recruit reflective processes for resisting temptations that may threaten long-term goals. Secondly, by suggesting that reflective processes in themselves are a potential liability for self-regulation, a justification-based account questions the general assumption of self-regulation models that the reflective system serves to correct mistakes in the impulsive system. Thus, whereas dual-system approaches to self-regulation suggest that strong impulses directly instigate indulgent behavior unless counteracted by reflective processes, our novel approach emphasizes that the competition between impulses and reflective processes takes place at a cognitive level in such a way that impulses may activate reasoning processes that license giving in. Put differently, our approach states that impulses indirectly affect indulgent behavior through deliberate reasoning about behavioral options rather than dictating behavior directly. Below we discuss the implications of these insights for classic models of self-regulation, for self-regulation in general and for future research on self-regulation.

Implications for Classic Models of Self-Regulation

A first implication of a justification-based account for classic interpretations of self-regulation failure is that self-defeating behavior is not necessarily always the result of a breakdown in personal control. Initial evidence suggests that even causes of self-regulation failure generally labelled as impulsive, such as negative affect, may not only impact behavior directly but also exert their influence via a justification-based route. In fact, states that are typically classified as impulsive may be particularly suitable for justifying behavior that otherwise would be off limits. As the accountability for behavior is typically discounted when it is perceived to be under the influence of strong impulses (Pizarro, Uhlmann, & Salovey, 2003), "impulsive" reasons for self-regulation failure, such as being in an emotional state or feeling depleted after prior self-control efforts, may be particularly plausible and thereby functional justifications that reduce judgments of responsibility for one's behavior. As a result, such "impulsive" reasons may offer an ideal compromise that allows us to indulge in a forbidden treat without bearing the negative consequences that this behavior could engender (e.g., a damaged self-image). Thus, these "impulsive" reasons can generate self-regulation failure in a deliberate manner by serving as justifications.

This new understanding also has implications for the interpretation of past findings. For example, to date self-regulation failure after prior effort or restraint has been attributed to the depletion of limited self-control resources (Muraven & Baumeister, 2000). However, in light of the present findings, failure in these cases may not always be the consequence of resource depletion, but can also be accounted for by justification processes. Therefore, beyond actual effort or restraint, it is relevant to take people's perceptions of prior effort and restraint into consideration, as the latter may make people feel entitled to indulge, leading to self-regulation failure through justification rather than depletion. Taking this one step further, it could even be speculated that justification processes moderate the impact of resource depletion on behavior, so that feelings of entitlement determine when previous efforts at self-control undermine subsequent attempts at self-control. This speculation is supported by recent findings suggesting that top-down processes, such as perceived resource depletion (Clarkson, Hirt, Jia, & Alexander, 2010) or lay theories about willpower as a limited resource (Job, Dweck, & Walton, 2010), modulate the effect of resource depletion. Recently it has also been suggested that resource depletion could be explained by a justification mechanism (Inzlicht & Schmeichel, 2012). Therefore, it is important to acknowledge that, in addition to ego depletion as proposed by the limited-resource model, self-regulation failure after initial self-control attempts can be also accounted for by other processes. Along the same lines, other conventionally impulsive determinants of self-regulation failure may operate via a justification-based mechanism. For example, self-regulation failure under emotional distress may not always be the result of emotional forces rendering us powerless over our behavior. Instead, the emotional experience may be strategically employed as a justification to indulge. With these insights, a justification-based account provides a valuable addition to the emphasis on impulsive processes in the literature on self-regulation failure, indicating that in order to improve our understanding of self-regulation failure, it is crucial to acknowledge that similar cues may lead to similar outcomes via different pathways.

Secondly, by demonstrating that reasoning processes can contribute to self-regulation failure, the justification-based account has implications for many models of self-regulation that are geared toward promoting goal-directed behavior, as they are based on the assumption that reasoning is guided solely by abstract principles. For example, most expectancy value theories and models of goal striving, such as the theory of planned behavior (Ajzen, 1991), assume that an individual's behavior is the result of a logical and rational reasoning process where people systematically weigh the options and outcomes. These models fail to consider, however, that reasoning does not happen in a vacuum. As the present findings make clear, reasoning does not yield stable norms or standards that transcend our desires, but is in itself vulnerable to more immediate motivations, thereby turning our reasoning faculties into a potential liability for effective self-regulation. In this light, it could be speculated that in contrast to what is generally assumed—for example the advice to think before you act. The advice may not always be beneficial for self-regulation. Instead, the current account suggests that leaving room for consideration and elaboration could allow for maladaptive justification processes to occur, leading to self-regulatory failure.

By showing two fundamental assumptions of self-regulation models in a different light, the evidence for a justification-based pathway of self-regulation suggests that classic models of self-regulation may have painted an incomplete picture, putting too much emphasis on impulsive explanations for self-regulation failure and on reflective processes to overcome desire.

A justification-based account also has implications for self-regulation on a broader level. The finding that the reflective system sometimes actively contributes to rather than prevents indulgence goes against the common conception that desires are unwanted forces that are passively experienced. Instead we seem to actively deal with our desires, sometimes accommodating them—leading to self-regulation failure—and sometimes resisting them, resulting in self-regulatory success. This is not to suggest that justification-induced self-regulation failure is exclusively the result of top-down processes. Relying on reasons to indulge is unlikely to be a premeditated act of deliberate self-sabotage. Contradicting such a purely rational top-down process, for example, is the recent finding that a justification in itself—a theoretical reason for allowing oneself to behave against one's intentions—does not influence self-regulatory processes unless a self-regulation conflict is salient (De Witt Huberts et al., 2012). Two studies demonstrated that after being exposed to a justification in a priming task, restrained eaters, relative to unrestrained eaters, reacted faster to words designating indulgence and exposed an attentional bias toward hedonic products. Crucially such a sensitization to hedonic cues after exposure to justifications was observed only in restrained eaters. Presumably the internalized conflict between wanting to and not being allowed to indulge makes restrained eaters particularly reactive to justifications, which allow them to temporarily reconcile their conflicting motivations. Unrestrained eaters, on the other hand, do not experience a self-regulation dilemma when wanting to eat tasty but unhealthy treats and thus do not need to rely on justifications for such indulgent behavior. This, in general, in the absence of temptation and thus of a self-regulation conflict, purely rational norms or rules are unlikely to lead to goal violations. Instead, competing motivations are required before justification processes come into play.

The requisite involvement of an active self-regulation dilemma also differentiates justification processes from a priori rules and decisions that allow one to indulge. If anything, establishing rules or reasons before one feels the push and pull of conflicting motivational forces may prevent a self-regulation dilemma from arising in the first place. So, if Sally had told herself before going to the wedding that the wedding party would be an allowable exception and that she could to eat whatever she wanted, being offered the chocolate cake would not invoke a self-regulation dilemma. In this sense, the involvement of an active self, even in self-regulation failure, provides a more complete outlook on human self-regulation abilities than the view currently endorsed in models of self-regulation. Whereas the latter suggests that at some point self-regulation abilities are limited, a justification-based pathway suggests that we still have the capacity to self-regulate. A reflective pathway to self-regulation failure may thereby be more amenable to change, and therefore create opportunities for interventions that target self-regulation failure by, for example, strengthening motivation for self-regulation. After all, if people are able but reluctant to self-regulate, supporting them by encouraging them to consider their motivation might prevent them from seeking justifications for giving up on important goals.

Taking this one step further, it could even be argued that relying on justifications to indulge, albeit responsible for self-regulation failure in the short-term, may be adaptive in the long-term. After all, in a world filled with temptations, people cannot resist all the time. Relying on justifications to indulge may be the most constructive way to deal with the ubiquitous temptation that surrounds people, as it would allow them to satisfy their hedonic needs once in a while, while retaining a sense of control. Indulging through reason may give them a vital sense of self-efficacy, enabling them to resist subsequent temptations. In other words, rather than being at the mercy of fixed, unchangeable processes, justifications allow people to feel in charge of their behavior and to take responsibility for their actions.

Future Directions

As this is among the first attempts to integrate the findings from various disciplines to substantiate a justification-based account of self-regulation failure, it gives rise to many new questions (De Witt Huberts, Evers, & De Ridder, 2014a). First of all, the present findings warrant empirical attention to the understanding of justification processes. Of major concern in this regard is insight into when the reflective system is mobilized to resist, and when to indulge in a desire. Presumably timing is of prime importance. When reflective processes are occupied with temptations before confrontation, desires may not be activated and may consequently not exert their detrimental impact on reasoning processes, leaving our reasoning processes free to support long-term goal pursuit. However, when a desire is already activated and one has sufficient reasoning capacity, the desire is likely to take control over reason, fostering justification that facilitates enactment of our desires. Other important conditions may determine whether reflective processes lead to self-regulation success or to self-regulation failure. One can imagine that the strength of temptation plays an important role in deciding to recruit reasoning processes to justify indulgence (Kroese et al., 2011), or the extent to which someone is truly committed to a long-term goal. Also, individual differences relating to, for example, (narcissistic) entitlement may prove relevant moderators in deciding whether to indulge when a justification is present. These conditions should be investigated in future research to learn more about when someone is most vulnerable to relying on justifications.

From a methodological perspective, this new conceptualization of self-regulation failure calls for new measures that can determine the various underlying processes of self-regulation success and failure. The new findings no longer allow us to equate the result with the process, such that the underlying process (impulsive vs. reflective) can be inferred by the outcome (failure vs. success). In other words, the involvement of reflective processes in self-regulation failure, in addition to the involvement of impulsive processes in self-regulatory success, suggests that research on self-regulation should now endeavor to uncover distinguishing hallmarks of the underlying process. This is especially needed considering the evidence that similar cues (e.g., negative emotions, prior restraint) can elicit self-control failure via different pathways.

It appears that explanations for the self-defeating behavior of Sally, Mark, and Marcy may have concentrated too much on the impulsive system being responsible for self-regulatory failure and the reflective system producing success. The present analysis shows that moving beyond this dualistic explanation may provide a better understanding of how desires influence our behavior. A more comprehensive view of self-regulation may contribute to interventions that enable us to deal with our desires more effectively.

REFERENCES

Abraham, C., & Sheeran, P. (2003). Acting on intentions: The role of anticipated regret. *British Journal of Social Psychology, 42*, 495–511.

Ajzen, I. (1991). The theory of planned behavior. *Organizational Behavior and Human Decision Processes, 50*, 179–211.

Brownstein, A. L. (2003). Biased predecision processing. *Psychological Bulletin, 129*, 545–568.

Clarkson, J., Hirt, E., Jia, L., & Alexander, M. (2010). When perception is more than reality: The effects of perceived versus actual resource depletion on self-regulatory behaviour. *Journal of Personality and Social Psychology, 98*, 29–46.

Collins, L. R., & Lapp, W. M. (1991). Restraint and attributions: Evidence of the abstinence violation effect in alcohol consumption. *Cognitive Therapy and Research, 15*, 69–84.

Connolly, T., & Zeelenberg, M. (2002). Regret in decision making. *Current Directions in Psychological Science, 11,* 212–220.

Damasio, A. R. (1994). *Descartes' error: Emotion, reason and the human brain.* New York: Putnam and Sons.

De Witt Huberts, J. C., Evers, C., & De Ridder, D. T. D. (2012). License to sin: Self-licensing as a mechanism underlying hedonic consumption. *European Journal of Social Psychology, 42,* 490–496.

De Witt Huberts, J. C., Evers, C., & De Ridder, D. T. D. (2014a). "Because I am worth it": A theoretical framework and empirical review of a justification-based account of self-regulation failure." *Personality and Social Psychology Review, 18*(2), 119–138.

De Witt Huberts, J. C., Evers, C., & De Ridder, D. T. D. (2014b). *Emotional license: Negative emotions as justification for self-regulation failure.* Manuscript under review.

De Witt Huberts, J. C., Evers, C., & De Ridder, D. T. D. (2014c). Thinking before sinning: Reasoning processes in hedonic consumption. *Frontiers in Psychology, 5,* 1268.

Dijksterhuis, A., & Nordgren, L. F. (2006). A theory of unconscious thought. *Perspectives on Psychological Science, 1,* 95–109.

Effron, D. A., Monin, B., & Miller, D. T. (2012). The unhealthy road not taken: Licensing indulgence by exaggerating counterfactual sins. *Journal of Experimental Social Psychology, 49*(3), 573–578.

Fishbach, A., & Dhar, R. (2005). Goals as excuses or guides: The liberating effect of perceived goal progress on choice. *Journal of Consumer Research, 32,* 370–377.

Festinger, L. (1957). *A theory of cognitive dissonance.* Stanford, CA: Stanford University Press.

Giner-Sorolla, R. (2001). Guilty pleasures and grim necessities: Affective attitudes in dilemmas of self-control. *Journal of Personality and Social Psychology, 80,* 206–221.

Herman, C. P., & Mack, D. (1975). Restrained and unrestrained eating. *Journal of Personality, 43,* 647–660.

Hofmann, W., Baumeister, R. F., Förster, G., & Vohs, K. D. (2012). Everyday temptations: An experience sampling study of desire, conflict, and self-control. *Journal of Personality and Social Psychology, 102,* 1318–1335.

Hofmann, W., Friese, M., & Strack, F. (2009). Impulse and self-control from a dual-systems perspective. *Perspectives on Psychological Science, 4,* 162–176.

Inzlicht, M., & Schmeichel, B. J. (2012). What is ego-depletion?: Toward a mechanistic revision of the resource model of self-control. *Perspectives on Psychological Science, 7,* 450–463.

Job, V., Dweck, C., & Walton, G. (2010). Ego depletion: Is it all in your head? Implicit theories about willpower affect self-regulation. *Psychological Science, 21,* 1686–1693.

Khan, U., & Dhar, R. (2006). Licensing effect in consumer choice. *Journal of Marketing Research, 153,* 259–266.

Khan, U., & Dhar, R. (2007). Where there is a way, is there a will?: The effect of future choices on self-control. *Journal of Experimental Psychology: General, 136,* 277–288.

Kivetz, R. (1999). Advances in research on mental accounting and reason-based choice. *Marketing Letters, 10,* 249–266.

Kivetz, R., & Zheng, Y. (2006). Determinants of justification and self-control. *Journal of Experimental Psychology: General, 135,* 572–587.

Kroese, F. M., Evers, C., & De Ridder, D. T. D. (2011). Tricky treats: Paradoxical effects of temptation strength on self-regulation processes. *European Journal of Social Psychology, 41*, 281–288.

Kronick I., & Knäuper, B. (2010). Temptations elicit compensatory intentions. *Appetite, 54*, 398–401.

Kunda, Z. (1990). The case for motivated reasoning. *Psychological Bulletin, 108*, 480–498.

Loewenstein, G. F. (1996). Out of control: Visceral influences on behavior. *Organizational Behavior and Human Decision Processes, 65*, 272–292.

Mercier, H., & Sperber, D. (2011). Why do humans reason?: Arguments for an argumentative theory. *Behavioral and Brain Sciences, 34*, 57–111.

Merritt, A., Effron, D. A., & Monin, B. (2010). Moral self-licensing: When being good frees us to be bad. *Social and Personality Psychology Compass, 4/5*, 344–357.

Metcalfe, J., & Mischel, W. (1999). A hot/cool-system analysis of delay of gratification: Dynamics of willpower. *Psychological Review, 106*, 3–19.

Miller, D. T., & Effron, D. A. (2010). Psychological license: When it is needed and how it functions. *Advances in Experimental Social Psychology, 43*, 115–155.

Monin, B., & Miller, D. T. (2001). Moral credentials and the expression of prejudice. *Journal of Personality and Social Psychology, 81*, 33–43.

Mukhopadhyay, A., & Johar, G. V. (2009). Indulgence as self-reward for prior shopping restraint: A justification-based mechanism. *Journal of Consumer Psychology, 19*, 334–345.

Mukhopadhyay, A., Sengupta, J., & Ramanathan, S. (2008). Recalling past temptations: An information-processing perspective on the dynamics of self-control. *Journal of Consumer Research, 35*, 445–453.

Muraven, M., & Baumeister, R. F. (2000). Self-regulation and depletion of limited resources: Does self-control resemble a muscle? *Psychological Bulletin, 126*, 247–259.

Okada, E. M. (2005). Justification effects on consumer choice of hedonic and utilitarian goods. *Journal of Marketing Research, 152*, 43–53.

Pizarro, D., Uhlmann, E., & Salovey, P. (2003). Asymmetry in judgements of moral blame and praise: The role of perceived metadesires. *Psychological Science, 14*, 267–272.

Reb, J., & Connolly, T. (2010). The effects of action, normality, and decision carefulness on anticipated regret: Evidence for a broad mediating role of decision justifiability. *Cognition and Emotion, 24*, 1405–1420.

Sayette, M. A., & Hufford, M. R. (1997). Effect of smoking urge on generation of smoking-related information. *Journal of Applied Social Psychology, 27*, 1395–1405.

Shafir, E., Simonson, I., & Tversky, A. (1993). Reason-based choice. *Cognition, 49*, 11–36.

Shiffman, S., Hickcox, M., Paty, J., Gnys, M., Kassel, J. D., & Richards, T. J. (1996). Progression from a smoking lapse to relapse: Prediction from abstinence violation effects, nicotine dependency and lapse characteristics. *Journal of Consulting and Clinical Psychology, 64*, 993–1002.

Simonson, I. (1989). Choice based on reasons: The case of attraction and compromise effects. *Journal of Consumer Research, 16*, 158–174.

Simonson, I. (1992). The influence of anticipating regret and responsibility on purchase decisions. *Journal of Consumer Research, 19*, 105–118.

Strack, F., & Deutsch, R. (2004). Reflective and impulsive determinants of social behaviour. *Personality and Social Psychology Review, 8*, 220–247.

Taylor, C., Webb, T. L., & Sheeran, P. (2014). "I deserve a treat!": Justifications for indulgence undermine the translation of intentions into action. *British Journal of Social Psychology, 53*(3), 501–520.

Urbszat , D., Herman, C. P., & Polivy, J. (2002). Eat, drink, and be merry, for tomorrow we diet: Effects of anticipated deprivation on food intake in restrained and unrestrained eaters. *Journal of Abnormal Psychology, 111*, 396–401.

Vohs, K. D., & Faber, R. J. (2007). Spent resources: Self-regulatory resource availability affects impulse buying. *Journal of Consumer Research, 33*, 537–547.

Ward, A., & Mann, T. (2000). Don't mind if I do: Disinhibited eating under cognitive load. *Journal of Personality and Social Psychology, 78*, 753–763.

Weber, M. (1958). *The Protestant ethic and the spirit of capitalism*. New York: Scribner's Press.

Wilson, T. D., & Schooler, J. W. (1991). Thinking too much: Introspection can reduce the quality of preferences and decisions. *Journal of Personality and Social Psychology, 60*, 181–192.

Wilson, T., Lisle, D., Schooler, J., Hodges, S. D., Klaaren, K. J., & LaFleur, S. J. (1993). Introspecting about reasons can reduce post-choice satisfaction. *Personality and Social Psychology Bulletin, 19*, 331–339.

Witkiewitz, K., & Villaroel, N. A. (2009). Dynamic association between negative affect and alcohol lapses following alcohol treatment. *Journal of Consulting and Clinical psychology, 77*, 633–644.

Xu, J., & Schwarz, N. (2009). Do we really need a reason to indulge? *Journal of Marketing Research, 46*, 25–36.

Zitek, E. M., Jordan, A. H., Monin, B., & Leach, F. R. (2010). Victim entitlement to behave selfishly. *Journal of Personality and Social Psychology, 98*, 245–255.

CHAPTER 11

Perceptions of Desire
A Hot–Cold Empathy Gap Perspective

Rachel L. Ruttan
Loran F. Nordgren

Desire is a frequent subject for television shows, pop music, and everyday conversations. It is desire's profound influence on human behavior that captures our attention. Desires can radically transform our thoughts, preferences, and actions. Conceptually, desire involves the conscious experience of wanting a certain object, person, or activity that will bring pleasure or relief from displeasure (Hofmann & Van Dillen, 2012). Functionally, desire provides the motivational impetus to engage in adaptive, goal-relevant behavior. Yet desire is perhaps best known for acting as a countervailing force to people's self-control efforts. Unrestrained desire contributes to a variety of well-known negative behavioral outcomes, such as obesity, infidelity, and aggression.

Despite the profound changes to behavior that desire routinely produces, it seems that people have remarkably little insight into the influence desire has on their preferences and behavior. More specifically, people have tremendous difficulty imagining how they (or others) will behave in a state of desire that is different from what they are currently experiencing. When we are in an emotionally neutral or "cold" state, we have little appreciation for how we (and others) will behave when in an emotional or "hot" state. And when gripped by desire, we underestimate the extent to which the transient hot state, and not long-term dispositional preferences, is impacting our behavior. These "hot–cold empathy gaps," as this phenomenon is known, have significant implications for how we perceive, evaluate, and make decisions surrounding desire.

To get a sense for why empathy gaps matter, consider the findings of a large-scale survey on adolescents' attitudes toward smoking. The survey found that the large majority of adolescent smokers did not intend to become long-term smokers. Specifically, only 15% of occasional smokers (those who smoked less than once a day) and only 30% of frequent smokers (those who smoked a pack a day) predicted they would be smoking in 5 years. But when the authors followed up with the same sample 5 years later, they found that 43% of the occasional smokers and over 70% of the frequent smokers were still smoking (Lynch & Bonnie, 1994).

These findings suggest that the young smokers believed they could experiment with smoking without forming a long-term habit. Yet, most of these smokers were wrong, which suggests that they neglected the power that cigarette craving would wield over their behavior. We contend that the beliefs these smokers held are a specific example of a much broader error in how people think about desire; namely, that people tend to underestimate how much desire (and affect more generally) will influence their attitudes, preference, and behavior.

We begin our discussion by formally defining the hot–cold empathy gap. We next describe research demonstrating empathy gaps in a variety of domains relevant to desire. We then turn to behavioral implications of the empathy gap, focusing, for example, on how the empathy gap might compromise people's self-control efforts. We then consider the implications of the empathy gap for social judgments and behavior. We conclude with limitations, lingering questions, and opportunities for future empathy gap research.

Defining the Empathy Gap

The idea of a hot–cold empathy gap was first developed by George Loewenstein (1996). People experience empathy gaps when predicting their responses to affective states that differ from their current state (Loewenstein, 1996, 2000; Loewenstein, O'Donaghue, & Rabin, 2003; Loewenstein & Schkade, 1999; Van Boven & Lowenstein, 2005; Van Boven, Loewenstein, Dunning, & Nordgren, 2013). Because we "project" our current affective state onto past and future decisions, the hot–cold empathy gap can be thought of as a form of *projection bias* (Loewenstein et al., 2003). Empathy gaps arise when we (wrongly) assume that our current preferences and behavior will be more similar to past or future behavioral propensities than it actually was or will be.

There are two basic types of empathy gaps: *cold-to-hot empathy gaps* and *hot-to-cold empathy gaps*. Cold-to-hot empathy gaps occur when someone who is not affectively aroused (i.e., in a cold state) attempts to predict the thoughts or behaviors of someone (either themselves or someone else) in a hot state. An example would be a satiated dieter predicting the impact hunger will have on her dietary choices. The cold-to-hot empathy gap prediction is that the satiated dieter will underestimate the impact hunger will have on her preferences and behavior and will overestimate her ability to resist tempting foods when hungry again.

A similar case occurs when making predictions in the opposite direction. The hot-to-cold empathy gap occurs when someone in a hot, affectively charged state predicts how she or another person will think and act while in a cold state. A familiar example of a hot-to-cold empathy gap involves anger-induced aggression. Angry people generally do not appreciate the extent to which their judgment and behavior are being driven by their momentary state of anger. Angry people (erroneously) believe that their decision to, say, send an angry e-mail to their boss will continue to seem like a good decision, even once the anger dissipates. Another classic example is overshopping for groceries on an empty stomach (Nisbett & Kanouse, 1969; Read & van Leeuwen, 1998).

The implications of hot-to-cold empathy gaps are somewhat different from those of cold-to-hot gaps. Whereas cold-to-hot gaps cause people to mispredict their own behavior because they underappreciate the motivational impact of hot states, the main impact of hot-to-cold empathy gaps is that someone who is gripped by affect fails to recognize that his or her current preferences and motivation won't persist once the hot state dissipates. Interestingly, cold–hot and hot–cold have similarly strong effects. In one demonstration, hungry participants were found to overbid 20 cents for a snack they would eat later when they were full, and full participants underbid 19 cents for a snack they would later eat when hungry (Fisher & Rangel, 2014).

In addition to the cold-to-hot versus hot-to-cold distinction, empathy gaps can also be categorized by whether they occur prospectively or retrospectively, and whether the judgments being made involve one's own behavior (intrapersonal empathy gaps) or concern someone else (interpersonal empathy gaps). Prospective empathy gaps occur when people attempt to estimate their thoughts and behaviors in response to future affective states that differ from their current state. A familiar case occurs when a person who is currently satiated attempts to estimate his future success at resisting tempting foods. By contrast, retrospective empathy gaps occur when people attempt to imagine thoughts or behaviors that occurred during past hot states. For example, struggling to make sense of one's regrettable behavior "the morning after" a night of drinking often involves retrospective empathy gaps.

Intrapersonal empathy gaps involve judgments about one's own past or future behavior. Reflecting on one's own ability to resist the "urge to splurge" on consumer goods would be an example of an intrapersonal empathy gap, whereas wondering whether your cousin with the spending problem will be able to control himself on your upcoming shopping trip would represent an interpersonal empathy gap. Although the nature of intra- and interpersonal empathy gaps are nearly identical, they often have quite different implications. Intrapersonal empathy gaps are usually concerned with how accurately one predicts one's own future preferences or behavior, whereas interpersonal empathy gaps often involve evaluating other people's affect-driven behavior (such as lashing out in anger).

Explanations for the Empathy Gap

Research has yet to identify a definitive explanation for why people experience empathy gaps. This is likely because there is no one simple mechanism, but rather a number of factors that produce empathy gap effects. One likely reason why empathy gaps emerge is the comprehensive and largely unconscious influence affect has on behavior (Berridge & Winkielman, 2003; Winkielman & Berridge, 2004; Zajonc, 2000). Affect profoundly influences behavior, such that nearly every category of psychological functioning—cognition, attention, physiology, perception, and memory—comes under the influence of affect. For example, affect can increase the mental accessibility of affect-relevant information, divert attention away from non-affect-relevant information, and focus visual attention on affect-relevant cues (Fox, Russo, & Dutton, 2002; Derryberry & Tucker, 1994). But because much of this influence happens outside of conscious awareness (Bechara, Damasio, Kimball, & Damasio, 1997; Winkielman & Berridge, 2004), people have great difficulty appreciating the full magnitude of affect's influence. People do have *some* understanding of how affect transforms their (and others') behavior—for example, people generally understand that hunger motivates food consumption and that fear can undermine courageous intentions—but they fail to appreciate the extent of the influence.

Another likely contributing factor is our constrained memory for affective experiences (Robinson & Clore, 2002; Loewenstein, 1996; Nordgren, van der Pligt, & van Harreveld, 2006). Though people can recall the situation that led to an affective state (e.g., "I was hungry because I hadn't eaten all day") and can recall the relative strength of the affective state (e.g., "that was the most hungry I have ever been"), they cannot freely bring forth the feeling of the affect itself (e.g., reexperiencing the prior hunger) (Loewenstein, 1996; Robinson & Clore, 2002). This inability to mentally simulate other states in effect leaves us trapped in our current affective state.

Our constrained memories for affect help to explain why empathy gaps are so difficult to overcome. Once they are no longer experiencing a given desire, people will be unable to relive their original emotional reactions, and may instead believe that their current feelings toward the event reflect how they have always felt and reacted (e.g., Eibach, Libby, & Gilovich, 2003).

Hot–Cold Empathy Gaps and Desire

Although empathy gap effects have been observed for moods and emotions, most of the research on empathy gaps has been carried out in the context of desire. In this section we will look at evidence for and the implications of empathy gaps in the context of drug craving, hunger, sexual arousal, and pain. In addition, we suggest how two additional desires—consumer desires and aggression—can be understood through an empathy gap lens.

Drug Craving

Drug craving is a principal cause of drug addiction (Killen & Fortmann, 1997; Shiffman et al., 1997). Consequently, all manner of judgments and decisions related to drug use benefit from an accurate understanding of drug craving's capacity to influence behavior. Yet, there is ample empirical evidence that people experience empathy gaps for drug craving. One study testing empathy gaps for cigarette craving asked smokers who were randomly assigned to either be satiated or actively craving cigarettes to rate their willingness to pay for a cigarette in the future (Sayette, Loewenstein, Griffin, & Black, 2008). A follow-up session then assessed their actual willingness to pay, thereby establishing the accuracy of their initial assessments. The results support a cold-to-hot empathy gap account: satiated smokers underestimated their willingness to pay for a cigarette during the second session.

In a similar study, heroin addicts who received buprenorphine (BUP), a drug similar to methadone, made real choices between getting an extra dose of BUP or various amounts of money (e.g., $10 vs. an extra dose), which they would receive when they came in for treatment 5 days later (Giordano et al., 2004). Like the participants in the cigarette smoker study, the heroin addicts made this choice when they were actively craving (right before receiving their scheduled dose of BUP) or when satiated (right after receiving a dose). Although one's current, momentary state of craving is logically irrelevant to the value one should place on an opiate 5 days later, participants who were currently experiencing craving valued the extra dose of BUP 5 days later at an average value of $60, whereas the average valuation for satiated participants was $35.

Both of these studies highlight two important features of empathy gaps. First, empathy gaps emerge quickly. Although the heroin addicts and cigarette smokers in the satiated condition made their decisions only moments after receiving the drug they were addicted to, both groups had already discounted the power of drug craving. Second, past experience does not appear to diminish the magnitude of the empathy gap. Participants in both studies were seasoned users with considerable experience with the drug, and with making tradeoffs between drugs and money. Moreover, in the study with heroin addicts, participants made eight different decisions over a span of 3 weeks, four in a craving state (before treatment) and four in a noncraving state, but there was no evidence of convergence between the two types of decision over the course of the study.

These findings help to address two important issues in addiction research. The first is why, despite widespread knowledge of their addictive properties, people experiment with drugs in the first place. If even experienced drug addicts continue to underestimate the motivational force of cravings, then clearly inexperienced users, or those contemplating whether to begin drug use, can have little understanding of craving and addiction. Importantly, this finding suggests that information-based approaches to drug education that stress the addictive and harmful nature of drug use may be largely ineffective.

Second, that past experience does not diminish empathy gaps might help to explain why recovered addicts—who have managed to overcome powerful withdrawal cravings in the past—often suddenly relapse after long periods of sobriety. The findings above suggest that recovered addicts will quickly lose their appreciation for the power of drug craving once their withdrawal symptoms fade. This is a critical point because all recovered addicts must gauge how much temptation they can safely tolerate without relapse, yet the inability to appreciate the power of drug craving may lead people to overexpose themselves to temptation (Nordgren, van Harreveld, & van der Pligt, 2009). This is a point to which we return when discussing the behavioral implications of the empathy gap.

Hunger

Hunger is a motivational state that encourages food consumption, particularly for high-calorie foods (Rolls, 1999). In addition to its direct motivational effects, hunger also distorts cognitive processes such as attention, goal accessibility, and reasoning in ways that promote impulsive eating (Nordgren & Chou, 2011). For these reasons, hunger has a substantial impact on dietary choice and represents one of the principal impediments to weight loss.

Yet it appears that people generally underestimate the influence that hunger has on their behavior. This error expresses itself in two ways. First, when people are hungry, they fail to appreciate the extent to which hunger is driving their decisions. For example, Nisbett and Kanouse (1969) asked people as they entered a grocery store to report their current hunger state and asked them to predict how much food they would purchase. Assessing shoppers in the checkout line revealed that hungry shoppers bought more food than planned, which suggests they failed to anticipate hunger's influence on their choices. In a similar study, hungry participants were asked to predict how much they would want to eat a slice of chocolate cake *after* first eating a large meal. Consistent with the hot-to-cold empathy gap, hungry participants believed that they would still want the chocolate cake on a full stomach far more than they in fact did after they ate a large meal (Gilbert, Gill, & Wilson, 2002).

Second, people who are satiated tend to underestimate their desire for food when hungry. For example, Read and Van Leeuwen (1998) had either hungry or satiated participants choose between a healthy or unhealthy snack (i.e., fruit and junk food) to be consumed 1 week later. Critically, participants were told that the meal would be consumed at a time when they were hungry and they should therefore consider what they would want to eat when hungry. When participants arrived 1 week later, they had the opportunity to change their previous choice. In line with the cold-to-hot empathy gap prediction, participants who were in a state of satiation during the initial decision were more likely to switch their food selection (from health to unhealthy).

More direct evidence for hunger-based empathy gaps comes from research on dieting. In one experiment, a group of dieters were given a hunger state manipulation (hungry vs. satiated) and were then asked to (1) indicate how much control they had over their food cravings and (2) identify how much food-related temptation they could safely allow in their environment. The results showed that satiated dieters believed they had more control over future hunger cravings compared to hungry dieters. And satiated dieters, consequently, were more willing to expose themselves to tempting food (Nordgren et al., 2009).

In a related study, experienced dieters were asked to indicate their confidence in their ability to lose weight and their weight-loss goals for the following week (Nordgren, van der Pligt, & van Harreveld, 2008). Compared to hungry participants, satiated dieters were significantly more confident in their ability to lose weight, and intended to lose more pounds. In line with a cold-to-hot empathy gap prediction, the satiated dieters were also less realistic, as they dramatically overestimated how much weight they would lose.

Sexual Desire

In 2008, Empelen and Kok surveyed 400 Dutch high school students about their sexual practices, including intentions to engage in safe sex, beliefs about the importance of safe sex, and actual condom use. Remarkably, intentions and beliefs about the importance of safe sex had *no relationship* with actual condom use. Many of the teens reported that they often engaged in risky behavior despite their intentions to practice safe sex. This finding is suggestive of the kinds of cold-to-hot empathy gaps seen in other domains—the teens intended to practice safe sex but underappreciated the power of sexual desire in the "heat of the moment."

Although fewer studies have examined this issue, there is some evidence that people experience empathy gaps for sexual arousal. For example, Loewenstein, Nagin, and Paternoster (1997) investigated the role of the empathy gap in predictions of sexual aggression. In this study, male undergraduates were randomly assigned to view sexually arousing (e.g., full-page nudes from *Playboy* magazine) or nonarousing photographs (e.g., photographs from fashion magazines). All participants then completed a vivid first-person dating scenario in which their date asked them to stop their sexual advances. Participants in the arousal condition reported significantly higher likelihoods of behaving in a sexually aggressive manner compared with nonaroused subjects.

Ariely and Loewenstein (2006) extended these findings by examining the effects of sexual arousal on three different aspects of sexually relevant judgment and choice. In this study, aroused or nonaroused male undergraduates answered questions regarding the sexual appeal of a wide range of stimuli (e.g., an obese woman, an underage girl, a 60-year-old woman, a man, an animal); willingness to engage in morally questionable behavior to obtain sex (e.g., encouraging a date to drink, lying about loving her); and willingness to engage in unprotected sex. As predicted, participants in the arousal condition found a wider range of stimuli to be attractive, were more likely to engage in morally dubious actions to obtain sex, and predicted being less likely to engage in safe sex. These findings again support the notion that nonaroused people are less able to imagine what they might do when experiencing sexual desire.

Pain

Some of the strongest evidence for empathy gaps comes from research on pain perception. In one study, Read and Loewenstein (1999) asked participants about their willingness to endure pain for money. In one condition, participants were allowed to experience a sample of the pain moments before they made their decision. A second condition experienced the sample of pain 1 week prior but made their decision pain-free. A third group made their decision without ever having experienced the sample of pain. They found that those who experienced pain while making their decision demanded more compensation than those who did not. In a later experiment, Nordgren and colleagues (2006) used a painful ice-water manipulation to hinder participants' performance on a memory test. Later, they asked participants to indicate how the pain and various other factors (e.g., skill) had affected their performance. Crucially, some participants were again exposed to the painful ice water while they made their attributions, whereas others made their attributions pain free. Nordgren and colleagues found evidence for a *retrospective cold-to-hot empathy gap*. Participants who made their attributions in a cold state (i.e., pain free) underestimated the influence pain had had on their performance. Only participants who made their attributions while experiencing pain accurately assessed its influence.

Understanding and accurately anticipating pain is an important—if not central—consideration for many medical decisions. Yet, patients seem to underestimate the severity of the pain associated with upcoming medical procedures. For example, one study found that the majority of pregnant women who intended to give birth without anesthesia reversed their decision once they went into labor, suggesting that they had initially underestimated the intensity of the pain of childbirth

(Christensen-Szalanski, 1984). Intrapersonal empathy gaps for pain will similarly affect a range of medical practices, such as elective surgeries, where patients must weigh the benefits of the surgery against the discomfort of the procedure.

Empathy gaps may also play a pivotal role in end-of-life care. Chochinov (1999) measured the daily experience of cancer patients receiving end-of-life care. Patients' daily reports of their will to live fluctuated dramatically, and their will to live was strongly correlated with their momentary pain ratings. In other words, patients' desire to live was heavily grounded in their momentary experience (how much pain are they enduring right now) rather than their average level of health and well-being. The shifting nature of patients' will to live creates considerable challenges for decisions around when life-support measures should be terminated.

In addition to intrapersonal empathy gaps for pain, interpersonal empathy gaps present a major challenge to patients' pain management. The medical literature has consistently found that physicians underestimate the severity of their patients' pain (Hodgkins, Albert, & Daltroy, 1985; Marquié et al., 2003; Pasero & McCaffery, 2001), and there is close to a consensus that, at least until recently, the medical community has tended to systematically undermedicate for pain. For example, Bernabei et al. (1998) examined the treatment of pain for cancer patients living in nursing homes. They found that nearly 40% of residents complained of daily pain, and nearly 30% of patients did not receive any pain-reducing medication.

Additional Domains

Thus far, we have examined the evidence for empathy gaps in the domain of drug craving, hunger, sexual desire, and pain. There is no theoretical reason to suspect that empathy gaps are restricted to these four states of desire. We believe that all forms of desire can be understood through an empathy gap lens. Here we briefly examine two types of desire covered in this volume: consumer desire and aggression.

Consumer Desire

Consumer desire can be defined as the urge to acquire material goods (Dholakia, Chapter 20, this volume). There is some evidence to suggest that people mispredict the motivational force consumer desire has on their behavior. For example, people have been found to underestimate the extent to which they will succumb to monetary temptation (Banaji, Bazerman, & Chugh, 2003; Epley & Dunning, 2000). In one study, 84% of participants in a prisoner's dilemma game predicted that they would cooperate with their counterpart rather than defect, but when faced with the dilemma, only 61% actually did cooperate (Epley & Dunning, 2000). The decision to defect ensured participants' own gains, at a cost to the other participant. It is possible that when participants made predictions in a cold state, they underestimated the extent to which their desire to obtain money would undermine the goal to behave in a cooperative manner.

Research also points to the existence of empathy gaps in impulsive buying. Individuals who engage in chronic impulsive buying show higher rates of depression and experience reductions in self-esteem following impulsive buying episodes (Black, 2007; Hassay & Smith, 1996). One explanation for these findings is that once an individual no longer experiences the desire (e.g., after a purchase has been made), the consumer can no longer appreciate the motivational force of the desire to acquire, and instead makes negative dispositional explanations for his or her impulsive buying (e.g., recklessness).

Aggression

Aggression is another desire that seems to conform to empathy gap predictions. When harmed, individuals often feel the desire to respond in kind, retaliating in a tit-for-tat manner (see Denson, Schofield, & Fabiansson, Chapter 18, this volume). Rather than being calculated acts of revenge, however, many acts of aggression are described as "crimes of passion"—a result of uncontrollable anger following a transgression. The classic idea of a crime of passion conjures up the image of a partner catching his or her loved one in flagrante delicto with another person. In a passionate rage, the harmed partner then aggresses against the partner and his or her lover.

There is reason to suspect that such acts of aggression reflect an empathy gap. First, the anger associated with aggression is undeniably an affectively charged hot state (e.g., Loewenstein, 1996). Moreover, the desire to aggress creates such a strong motivation to harm the other party that people are willing to enact harm even when it comes at a cost to the self (e.g., Fehr & Gächter, 2002; Xiao & Houser, 2005). It is possible that these desires to aggress result from a hot-to-cold empathy gap, such that people project their current levels of anger onto the future, creating the impression that they will always experience hostility toward the other party. Believing that the anger will never end may reduce the odds that people want to protect the relationship by not lashing out. In support of this idea, research has found that attempts to reconcile are much more successful when made after the victim has had time to "cool off" (e.g., Grimm & Mengel, 2011).

The cold-to-hot empathy gap also holds interesting implications for aggression. For example, people in a cold state (e.g., before a romantic relationship dissolves) might underestimate the intensity of their desire to behave aggressively in the future. In this vein, people may fail to put safeguards into place, such as prenuptial agreements, which could help prevent the destructive behaviors that often characterize relational disagreements.

Implications for Behavior

There is robust support for the notion that desires tend to hijack motivation, increasing the appeal of food, drugs, sex, material goods, and aggression. Although desires are an adaptive feature of the human body—people should eat when hungry and seek water when dehydrated—their influence on behavior can ultimately undermine individuals' goals and intentions. The hot–cold empathy gap has several important implications for how people manage and evaluate the self-control process.

Managing Temptation

Many self-control endeavors, such as smoking cessation, weight loss, or sexual fidelity, require people to manage temptation. In particular, people must gauge how much temptation they can safely tolerate. The cold-to-hot empathy gap predicts that people will generally overestimate their ability to handle desire-laden temptation. Recent research supports this prediction. In one line of research, Nordgren and colleagues (2009) found that people tend to demonstrate a *restraint bias*, such that they generally overestimate their capacity for impulse control, and this illusion of self-restraint leads people to overexpose themselves to temptation. To illustrate, in one field study involving recovered smokers, the authors asked the ex-smokers to estimate how much control they had over their cigarette cravings and how much cigarette-related temptation they could tolerate without relapse. Smoking status was assessed 4 months later. The results revealed that smokers who believed that they could control their cigarette cravings reported exposing themselves to greater smoking temptation, and that those who exposed themselves to more temptation were more likely to relapse.

The notion of a restraint bias has numerous implications for self-control efforts, particularly for structured interventions. For one thing, the findings above provide empirical support for Alcoholics Anonymous (AA) and other recovery programs that stress the recovered addict's continued powerlessness. In AA, for instance, it is often said that "the farther away one is from one's last drink, the closer one is to the next one" (Seeburger, 1993, p. 152).

At first glance, the AA model seems puzzling. A dominant view in psychology is that self-efficacy (i.e., beliefs about one's ability to reach goals) is vital for self-control (Bandura, 1977), and many addiction researchers advocate boosting self-efficacy (Baer, Holt, & Lichtenstein,

1986). Yet the Nordgren et al. (2009) findings suggest that unrealistic perceptions of control over desire can actually hinder self-control efforts, and that creating more realistic perceptions of control might help people manage temptation more effectively.

Goal Setting

The hot–cold empathy gap also plays an important role in (undermining) goal setting, as illustrated by an experiment in which experienced dieters indicated their confidence in their ability to lose weight and their weight-loss goals for the following week (Nordgren et al., 2007). Dieters' confidence in their ability to lose weight fluctuated dramatically as a function of their immediate hunger state. Satiated dieters reported more confidence in their ability to lose weight compared to hungry dieters, and levels of confidence, in turn, predicted how much weight the dieters intended to lose in the following week.

Research has routinely linked inconsistent or poorly defined goals with self-control failure (Baumeister & Heatherton, 1996). Setting stable, well-defined goals allows for clear decision rules (e.g., I don't eat after 9:00 P.M.). Stable standards also allow for better preparation and planning. It is much easier to develop a weight-loss program when the goal is clear and consistent (e.g., lose 5 pounds in 30 days) than if the goal is poorly defined and inconsistent. Empathy gaps, therefore, can undermine weight-loss efforts by creating constantly shifting weight-loss targets.

Implications for Social Judgment

We often have to make judgments about other people's responses to desire: Should I threaten to leave him if he does not quit using? Why did she cheat? Should the drug user go to jail? When attempting to answer questions like these, people often demonstrate interpersonal empathy gaps, underestimating the power that desires wield over *others'* behaviors.

One important implication of these interpersonal empathy gaps is the stigmatization of impulsive behaviors. When an individual fails to regulate his or her desires, people tend to generate negative attributions like self-indulgence, weak willpower, and even immorality (e.g., Crisp & Gelder, 2000; Crocker & Major, 1989). The stigma associated with impulsivity is particularly noticeable in the case of obesity: compared to their normal-weight counterparts, obese women and men earned 24% and 19% less in the workplace, respectively (Maranto & Stenoien, 2000), and 54% have reported weight stigma from colleagues (Puhl & Brownell, 2006). These inequities are thought to arise from the widespread negative stereotypes that overweight and obese persons are impulsive, lazy, and lacking in self-discipline (Puhl & Latner, 2007).

In a recent paper, Nordgren et al. (2007) hypothesized that people stigmatize impulsive behavior precisely because they fail to appreciate the influence affect has on behavior—a cold-to-hot empathy gap effect. Because people underestimate the motivational force of cravings for sex, drugs, food, and so forth, they perceive these impulses to be readily controllable. Anyone who then acts on their (ostensibly) controllable impulses is therefore blameworthy. In line with this reasoning, the researchers found that participants who were in a cold state (e.g., not hungry) made less favorable evaluations of a related impulsive behavior (impulsive eating) than did participants who were in a hot state (e.g., hungry).

Nordgren et al.'s results suggest that empathy gaps exacerbate negative social evaluations because those in a cold state possess insufficient affective experience (e.g., the absence of hunger). Recent research examined whether even harsher social evaluations may result from *prior* experience with affect-laden experiences (e.g., prior dieting experience). To illustrate, imagine someone who made a vow to his family to quit smoking, but is caught impulsively sneaking cigarettes. Who would be more prone to stigmatize his behavior: his sister who previously quit smoking (and has prior experience with cravings) or his wife who has no experience with smoking (and has no experience with cravings)? Although both individuals are in a cold state (i.e., not experiencing cravings), only the sister possesses the knowledge that she managed to endure the cravings in order to quit smoking. Her knowledge of successfully quitting (i.e., "I did it"), combined with a constrained memory for affective experiences (i.e., "I can't recall how difficult it was"), may lead the sister to more negatively evaluate the impulsive behavior (i.e., "Why can't you do it, too?").

In a series of studies, Ruttan, McDonnell, and Nordgren (2015) found support for this prediction, demonstrating that people with prior experience with a given affectively charged event (e.g., bullying) more harshly evaluated another person's impulsive behavior in response to that event (e.g., lashing out in anger). This effect was driven by the tendency for those with prior experience to view the event as less difficult to overcome. The authors further found that people failed to anticipate this psychological consequence of prior experience, instead believing that individuals with prior experience would be less likely than those with no experience to stigmatize impulsive behaviors. These findings present a paradox, such that when struggling to manage a difficult emotional event, the people we seek out for advice or comfort may be the least likely to provide it.

Contemporary and Future Questions

The empathy gap perspective offers a number of avenues for future research. We believe particularly pressing directions for research include explorations of the moderators and contextual factors that influence this effect, and of factors that might serve to combat the negative effects of the empathy gap on judgments and behaviors.

Moderators and Contextual Influences

Researchers have just begun to explore moderators of interpersonal empathy gaps. Interpersonal empathy gaps are thought to stem from *egocentric projection*, such that when attempting to predict others' preferences, attitudes, or behaviors, people first use their own affective experience as a starting point and then adjust these self-predictions to accommodate perceived differences between themselves and others (Epley, Keysar, Van Boven, & Gilovich, 2004; Van Boven & Loewenstein, 2003). From this perspective, people may not be as prone to project affective states onto others who are dissimilar to themselves, as self-predictions seem less informative when predicting the actions of dissimilar others (cf., Ames, 2004).

Recent research by O'Brien and Ellsworth (2012) found support for this idea. Participants read about a politically active student who got lost hiking without food, water, or extra clothes, and were asked whether the student would find the hunger, thirst, or cold most unpleasant. Participants made these assessments while inside a university building or outside during a cold winter day. When participants read about a hiker who shared their political orientation, the interpersonal empathy gap emerged: cold participants thought the hiker would be more bothered by the cold than did participants who completed the study indoors. By contrast, when the hiker did not share participants' political orientation, no significant differences emerged between cold conditions. Ostensibly, participants' own emotional states seemed less informative in estimating the feelings of a politically dissimilar other.

Another potential moderator of empathy gaps may be cultural context. Compared to individualistic cultures, people from collectivist cultures tend to incorporate close others into their self-concepts (Markus & Kitayama, 1991). These individuals place less emphasis on autonomy and agency and are more likely to be cognizant of the contexts in which actions are embedded (Heine, Lehman, Markkus, & Kitayama, 1999). In this vein, individuals from collectivist cultures may place less weight on their self-predictions, and may instead recognize that others have mental states different from their own (Wu & Keysar, 2007). Future research may therefore explore whether cultural context moderates empathy gap effects.

Moreover, although most research on interpersonal empathy gaps focused on specific individuals as the target of social judgments, people also regularly predict and evaluate the behavior of groups of individuals and organizations. It remains unclear whether people will demonstrate interpersonal empathy gaps when evaluating larger groups. For one, people tend to use different sets of information when predicting the behavior of groups (e.g., "what percentage of university students will . . .")

versus individuals (e.g., "how likely is it that a randomly selected class-mate will . . .") (Waytz & Young, 2012; Wildschut, Pinter, Vevea, Insko, & Schopler, 2003). When predicting the behavior of individuals, people give more weight to individual-level influences, such as a person's emotions. By contrast, when predicting group behavior, people give more weight to group-level forces such as social norms and group pressures to conform (Critcher & Dunning, 2013). Thus, people may demonstrate less pronounced empathy gaps when predicting group behavior.

Combating the Empathy Gap

Desire can alter attention and behavior in maladaptive ways, ultimately undermining individuals' goals. Uncovering the factors that lessen the negative impact of desire is therefore an important goal for future research. In contrast to other decision-making domains, having ample cognitive resources does not seem to help, and instead exacerbates the negative effects of affective states on self-regulatory efforts (see Nordgren & Chou, 2013; Van Dillen, Papies, & Hofmann, 2013). One interesting possibility, then, is that the negative impact of a given affective state may be best fought with other affective states. For example, a dieter overwhelmed by cravings for fattening foods might instead try to rally vivid imagery of his or her own weight gain to elicit feelings of disgust or shame that might compete with the cravings. This tactic resonates with the idea of "matching" in the persuasion literature. If attitudes are rooted in affect (versus cognition), persuasion attempts rooted in affect (versus cognition) are more likely to succeed (e.g., Fabrigar & Petty, 1999; Petty & Wegener, 1998). Like persuasion, managing affective states may require other affective states.

In addition to directly undermining self-control efforts, a major problem presented by the empathy gap is the inability of the "cold" self to gain insights from the "hot" self. As a result, individuals overestimate their capacity to control desires, leading them to place themselves in tempting situations that might compromise their goals (Nordgren et al., 2009). Is there a way to "bridge" the empathy gap, merging hot and cold perspectives?

One fruitful approach may be to have people reflect on and take notice of their own struggles while experiencing desires (e.g., by writing down or verbalizing their thoughts while craving during the weight-loss process). This approach aims to bridge the gap between hot and cold perspectives. Given the difficulties involved in reexperiencing affective events, a more promising approach may be to impart the idea that people habitually underestimate the motivational force of impulse. This approach is consistent with Step 1 of Alcoholics Anonymous, during which members admit that they are *powerless over alcohol*. Even if the experience of craving is not actively lived, people may become more wary of exposing themselves to temptation.

Conclusion

Despite the central role that desire plays in our daily lives, people have tremendous difficulty imagining how they (or others) will behave in a state of desire that is different from what they are currently experiencing. We have endeavored to show how these hot–cold empathy gaps present significant challenges for how people perceive, evaluate, and make decisions surrounding desire. We believe that furthering our understanding of empathy gaps will help delineate these challenges, and help steer people toward more desirable decisions and behaviors.

REFERENCES

Ames, D. (2004). Inside the mind-reader's toolkit: Projection and stereotyping in mental state inference. *Journal of Personality and Social Psychology, 87*, 340–353.

Ariely, D., & Loewenstein, G. (2006). The heat of the moment: The effect of sexual arousal on sexual decision making. *Journal of Behavioral Decision Making, 19*, 87–98.

Baer, J. S., Holt, C. S., & Lichtenstein, E. (1986). Self-efficacy and smoking reexamined: Construct validity and clinical utility. *Journal of Consulting and Clinical Psychology, 54*, 846–852.

Banaji, M. R., Bazerman, M. H., & Chugh, D. (2003). How (un)ethical are you? *Harvard Business Review, 81*, 56–65.

Bandura, A. (1977). Self-efficacy: Toward a unifying theory of behavioral change. *Psychological Review, 84*, 191–215.

Baumeister, R. F., & Heatherton, T. F. (1996). Self-regulation failure: An overview. *Psychological Inquiry, 7*, 1–15.

Bechara, A., Damasio, H., Kimball, M. S., & Damasio, A. R. (1997). Deciding advantageously before knowing the advantageous strategy. *Science, 275*, 1293–1295.

Bernabei, R., Gambassi, G., Lapane, K., Landi, F., Gatsonis, C., Dunlop, R., et al. (1998). Management of pain in elderly patients with cancer. *Journal of the American Medical Association, 279*, 1877–1882.

Berridge, K. C., & Winkielman, P. (2003). What is an unconscious emotion: The case for unconscious "liking." *Cognition and Emotion, 17*, 181–211.

Black, D. W. (2007). A review of compulsive buying disorder. *World Psychiatry, 6*, 14–18.

Chochinov, H. M. (1999). Will to live in the terminally ill. *Lancet, 354*, 816–819.

Christensen-Szalanski, J. J. (1984). Discount functions and the measurement of patients' values: Women's decisions during childbirth. *Medical Decision Making, 4*, 47–58.

Crisp, A. H., & Gelder, M. G. (2000). Stigmatisation of people with mental illnesses. *British Journal of Psychiatry, 177*, 4–7.

Critcher, C. R., & Dunning, D. (2013). Predicting persons' goodness versus a person's goodness: Forecasts diverge for populations versus individuals. *Journal of Personality and Social Psychology, 104*, 28–44.

Crocker, J., & Major, B. (1989). Social stigma and self-esteem: The self-protective properties of stigma. *Psychological Review, 96*, 608–630.

Derryberry, D., & Tucker, D. M. (1994). Motivating the focus of attention. In P. M. Niedenthal & K. Shinobu (Eds.), *The heart's eye: Emotional influences in perception and attention* (pp. 167–196). San Diego, CA: Academic Press.

Eibach, R. P., Libby, L. K., & Gilovich, T. D. (2003). When change in the self is mistaken for change in the world. *Journal of Personality and Social Psychology, 84*, 917–931.

Empelen, P., & Kok, G. (2008). Action-specific cognitions of planned and preparatory behaviors of condom use among Dutch adolescents. *Archives of Sexual Behavior, 37*, 626–640.

Epley, N., & Dunning, D. (2000). Feeling "holier than thou": Are self-serving assessments produced by errors in self- or social prediction? *Journal of Personality and Social Psychology, 79*, 861–875.

Epley, N., Keysar, B., Van Boven, L., & Gilovich, T. (2004). Perspective taking as egocentric anchoring and adjustment. *Journal of Personality and Social Psychology, 87*, 312–326.

Fabrigar, L. R., & Petty, R. E. (1999). The role of the affective and cognitive bases of attitudes in susceptibility to affectively and cognitively based persuasion. *Personality and Social Psychology Bulletin, 25*, 363–381.

Fehr, E., & Gächter, S. (2002). Altruistic punishment in humans. *Nature, 415*, 137–140.

Fisher, G., & Rangel, A. (2014). Symmetry in cold-to-hot and hot-to-cold valuation gaps. *Psychological Science, 25*, 120–127.

Foster, G. D. (1995). Reasonable weights: Determinants, definitions, and directions. In D. B. Alison & F. X. Pi-Sunyer (Eds.), *Obesity treatment: Establishing goals, improving outcomes, and reviewing the research agenda* (pp. 35–44). New York: Plenum Press.

Fox, E., Russo, R., & Dutton, K. (2002). Attentional bias for threat: Evidence for delayed disengagement from emotional faces. *Cognition and Emotion, 16*, 355–379.

Gilbert, D. T., Gill, M. J., & Wilson, T. D. (2002). The future is now: Temporal correction in affective forecasting. *Organizational Behavior and Human Decision Processes, 88*, 430–444.

Giordano, L. A., Bickel, W. K., Loewenstein, G., Jacobs, E. A., Marsch, L., & Badger, G. J. (2002). Mild opioid deprivation increases the degree that opioid-dependent outpatients discount delayed heroin and money. *Psychopharmacology, 163*, 174–182.

Grimm, V., & Mengel, F. (2011). Let me sleep on it: Delay reduces rejection rates in ultimatum games. *Economics Letters, 111*, 113–115.

Hassay, D. N., & Smith, M. C. (1996). Compulsive buying: An examination of the consumption motive. *Psychology and Marketing, 13*, 741–752.

Heine, S. J., Lehman, D. R., Markus, H. R., & Kitayama, S. (1999). Is there a universal need for positive self-regard? *Psychological Review, 106*, 766–794.

Hodgkins, M., Albert, D., & Daltroy, L. (1985) Comparing patients' and their physicians' assessments of pain. *Pain, 23*, 273–277.

Hofmann, W., & Van Dillen, L. (2012). Desire: The new hot spot in self-control research. *Current Directions in Psychological Science, 21*, 317–322.

Killen, J. D., & Fortmann, S. P. (1997). Craving is associated with smoking relapse: Findings from three prospective studies. *Experimental and Clinical Psychopharmacology, 5*, 137–142.

Loewenstein, G. (1996). Out of control: Visceral influences on behavior. *Organizational and Human Decision Processes, 65*, 272–292.

Lowenstein, G. (2000). Emotions in economic theory and economic behavior. *American Economic Review, 90*, 426–432.

Loewenstein, G., Nagin, D., & Paternoster, R. (1997). The effect of sexual arousal on predictions of sexual forcefulness. *Journal of Crime and Delinquency, 32*, 443–473.

Loewenstein, G., O'Donaghue, T., & Rabin, M. (2003). Projection bias in predicting future utility. *Quarterly Journal of Economics, 118*, 1209–1248.

Loewenstein, G., & Schkade, D. (1999). Wouldn't it be nice?: Predicting future feelings. In D. Kahneman, E. Diener, & N. Schwarz (Eds.), *Well-being: The foundation of hedonic psychology* (pp. 85–108). New York: Russell Sage Foundation.

Lynch, B. S., & Bonnie, R. J. (1994). Toward a youth-centered prevention policy. In B. S. Lynch & R. J. Bonnie (Eds.), *Growing up tobacco free: Preventing nicotine addiction in children and youths*. Washington, DC: National Academy Press.

Maranto, C. L., & Stenoien, A. F. (2000). Weight discrimination: A multidisciplinary analysis. *Employee Responsibilities and Rights Journal, 12*, 9–24.

Markus, H. R., & Kitayama, S. (1991). Culture and the self: Implications for cognition, emotion, and motivation. *Psychological Review, 98*, 224.

Marquié, L., Raufaste, E., Lauque, D., Mariné, C., Ecoiffier, M., & Sorum, P. (2003). Pain rating by patients and physicians: Evidence of systematic pain miscalibration. *Pain, 102*, 289–296.

Nisbett, R. E., & Kanouse, D. E. (1969). Obesity, food deprivation, and supermarket shopping behavior. *Journal of Personality and Social Psychology, 12*, 289–294.

Nordgren, L. F., & Chou, E. Y. (2011). The push and pull of temptation: The bidirectional influence of temptation on self-control. *Psychological science, 22*, 1386–1390.

Nordgren, L. F., & Chou, E. Y. (2013). A devil on each shoulder: When (and why) greater cognitive capacity impairs self-control? *Social Psychological and Personality Science, 4*, 233–237.

Nordgren, L. F., van der Pligt, J., & van Harreveld, F. (2006). Visceral drives in retrospect: Explanations about the inaccessible past. *Psychological Science, 17*, 635–640.

Nordgren, L. F., van der Pligt, J., & van Harreveld, F. (2007). Evaluating Eve: Visceral states influence the evaluation of impulsive behavior. *Journal of Personality and Social Psychology, 93*, 75–84.

Nordgren, L. F., van der Pligt, J., & van Harreveld, F. (2008). The instability of health cognitions: Visceral states influence self-efficacy and related health beliefs. *Health Psychology, 27*, 722–727.

Nordgren, L. F., van Harreveld, F., & van der Pligt, J. (2009). The restraint bias: How the illusion of self-restraint promotes impulsive behavior. *Psychological Science, 20*, 1523–1528.

O'Brien, E., & Ellsworth, P. (2012). More than skin deep: Visceral states are not projected onto dissimilar others. *Psychological Science, 23*, 391–396.

Pasero, C., & McCaffery, M. (2001). The undertreatment of pain: Are providers accountable for it? *American Journal of Nursing, 101*, 62–65.

Petty, R. E., & Wegener, D. T. (1998). Matching versus mismatching attitude functions: Implications for scrutiny of persuasive messages. *Personality and Social Psychology Bulletin, 24*, 227–240.

Puhl, R. M., & Brownell, K. D. (2006). Confronting and coping with weight stigma: An investigation of overweight and obese adults. *Obesity, 14*, 1802–1815.

Puhl, R. M., & Latner, J. D. (2007). Stigma, obesity, and the health of the nation's children. *Psychological Bulletin, 133*, 557–580.

Read, D., & van Leeuwen, B. (1998). Time and desire: The effects of anticipated and experienced hunger and delay to consumption on the choice between healthy and unhealthy snack food. *Organizational Behavior and Human Decision Processes, 76*, 189–205.

Read, D., & Loewenstein, G. (1999). Enduring pain for money: Decisions based on the perception and memory of pain. *Journal of Behavioral Decision Making, 12*, 1–17.

Robinson, M. D., & Clore, G. L. (2002). Belief and feeling: Evidence for an accessibility model of emotional self-report. *Psychological Bulletin, 128*, 934–960.

Rolls, E. T. (1999). *The brain and emotion.* New York: Oxford University Press.

Ruttan, R. L., McDonnell, M. H. M., & Nordgren, L. F. (2015). Having "been there" doesn't mean I care: When prior experience reduces compassion for emotional distress. *Journal of Personality and Social Psychology, 108*, 610–622.

Sayette, M. A., Loewenstein, G., Griffin, K. M., & Black, J. J. (2008). Exploring the cold-to-hot empathy gap in smokers. *Psychological Science, 19*, 926–932.

Seeburger, F. F. (1993). *Addiction and responsibility. An inquiry into the addictive mind.* New York: Crossroads Press.

Shiffman, S., Engberg, J., Patty, J., Perz, W. G., Gnys, M., Kassel, J., et al. (1997). A day at a time: Predicting smoking lapse from daily urge. *Journal of Abnormal Psychology, 106*, 104–116.

Van Boven, L., & Loewenstein, G. (2003). Social projection of transient drive states. *Personality and Social Psychology Bulletin, 29*, 1159–1168.

Van Boven, L., & Loewenstein, G. (2005). Empathy gaps in emotional perspective taking. In B. Malle & S. Hodges (Eds.), *Other minds* (pp. 284–297). New York: Guilford Press.

Van Boven, L., Loewenstein, G., Dunning, D., & Nordgren, L. F. (2013). Changing places: A dual judgment model of empathy gaps in emotional perspective taking. *Advances in Experimental Social Psychology, 48*, 117–171.

Van Dillen, L. F., Papies, E. K., & Hofmann, W. (2013). Turning a blind eye to temptation: How cognitive load can facilitate self-regulation. *Journal of Personality and Social Psychology, 104*, 427–443.

Waytz, A., & Young, L. (2012). The group-member mind trade-off: Attributing mind to groups versus group members. *Psychological Science, 23*, 77–85.

Winkielman, P., & Berridge, K. C. (2004). Unconscious emotion. *Current Directions in Psychological Science, 13*, 120–123.

Wildschut, T., Pinter, B., Vevea, J. L., Insko, C. A., & Schopler, J. (2003). Beyond the group mind: A quantitative review of the interindividual–intergroup discontinuity effect. *Psychological Bulletin, 129*, 698–722.

Wu, S., & Keysar, B. (2007). The effect of culture on perspective taking. *Psychological Science, 18*, 600–606.

Xiao, E., & Houser, D. (2005). Emotion expression in human punishment behavior. *Proceedings of the National Academy of Sciences of the United States of America, 102*, 7398–7401.

Zajonc, R. B. (2000). Closing the debate over the independence of affect. In J. P. Forgas (Ed.), *Feeling and thinking: The role of affect in social cognition* (pp. 31–58). New York: Cambridge University Press.

CHAPTER 12

Want–Should Conflict

A Synthesis of Past Research

T. Bradford Bitterly[1]
Robert Mislavsky
Hengchen Dai
Katherine L. Milkman

In our daily lives we frequently face a tension between what we want to do (or what we desire) and what we believe we should do. After a long week at work, we may want to share an expensive dinner and a few drinks with friends when we know we should go home early and get a good night's sleep. Similarly, we might be tempted to get caught up on the current season of *Homeland* when we know we should focus on drafting a book chapter we promised to send to collaborators.

For decades, researchers have examined battles like these between highly desirable options that provide immediate gratification (e.g., eating junk food, procrastinating, overspending) and options that provide more long-term benefits (e.g., eating healthy food, meeting deadlines, and saving for retirement; see, e.g., Ainslie, 1975, 1992; Bazerman, Tenbrunsel, & Wade-Benzoni, 1998; Loewenstein, 1996; Schelling, 1984; Sen, 1977; Shefrin & Thaler, 1988; Strotz, 1956; Thaler & Shefrin, 1981). Bazerman et al. (1998) refer to the common struggle between choosing what we desire in the heat of the moment and what would be best for us in the long run as *"want–should* conflict." According to their conceptualization, we each face frequent conflicts between "multiple selves"—our *want* self, who desires immediate gratification, and our *should* self, who argues for our long-term interests.

In this chapter, we review and synthesize past research on *want–should* conflict. We begin with a formal definition of relative *wants* and *shoulds* and summarize prior work on the underlying cognitive processes

---

[1]The first two authors contributed equally to this chapter.

that produce *want–should* conflict. We then describe empirical research on the levers that predictably tip the balance in favor of *want* versus *should* choices. In the final section of this chapter, we discuss a series of interventions that policy makers, organizations, and individuals can use to promote more future-oriented, *should* choices.

What Are *Wants* and *Shoulds* and Why Should We Care?

Before discussing the cognitive processes underlying *want–should* conflict, it is important to clarify what we mean when we refer to *want* and *should* selves and the options that each prefers. As described above, Bazerman et al. (1998) proposed that individuals often evaluate decisions through two different lenses, almost as if they are comprised of two competing selves: a *want* self and a *should* self. The *want* self focuses myopically on the here and now, and thus strongly desires instant gratification. In contrast, the *should* self is more far-sighted, guided primarily by long-term interests.

Milkman, Rogers, and Bazerman (2008, p. 326) define options as relative *wants* and *shoulds* based on the following criteria:

1. The instantaneous utility obtained from the *want* option is greater than the instantaneous utility obtained from the *should* option.
2. The sum of the utility (discounted at a standard exponential rate, $\delta = 1 - \varepsilon$) that will be derived from the *want* option in all future periods is less than the sum of the utility that will be derived from the *should* options in all future periods.

While we follow Milkman et al. (2008) and define *wants* relative to *shoulds* and according to the utility they provide over time, it is worth noting that other definitions of *desire* (or *wanting*, in our language) have focused on characteristics distinct from utility, such as the intense affect and/or feelings evoked by wanting something (Kavanagh, Andrade, & May, 2005; Hofmann, Baumeister, Förster, & Vohs, 2012; see also Andrade, May, Van Dillen, & Kavanagh, Chapter 1, this volume). The utility-based definition we adopt provides a precise characterization of *wants* (and *shoulds*) but admittedly overlooks the important role played by affect in experiencing desire.

Also notable is the fact that the definition we adopt for *wants* and *shoulds* articulates the characteristics of relative *want* and *should* options but does not indicate which type of option is optimal and thus rational (i.e., utility-maximizing). The rational choice is the one that provides greater discounted net utility (calculated by summing the discounted short- and long-term utilities across all future periods). Sometimes the *want* option is optimal and thus rational to select—this is the case when the short-term benefits from the *want* option are significant enough to dominate the long-term benefits from the *should* option. At other times, the long-term benefits of the *should* option exceed the short-term gains from the *want* option, making the *should* option optimal and thus rational to select.

There is some evidence that individuals occasionally underindulge in *want* options—a phenomenon referred to as hyperopia (Kivetz & Keinan, 2006). Indulging in the *wants* that we most desire can cause us to feel wasteful, irresponsible, and immoral (Giner-Sorolla, 2001; Kivetz & Simonson, 2002; Prelec & Herrnstein, 1991), and as a result of a distaste for such feelings, some individuals underconsume *want* options. However, it is far more typical for individuals to feel that they have made the opposite mistake (i.e., overindulging in *wants* at the expense of *shoulds*; Milkman et al., 2008) and to regret this irrational behavior later on. Further, overindulging in *want* options typically has a greater cost than overindulging in *should* options. For example, failures to control one's desires (e.g., choosing pizza over vegetables, watching TV instead of exercising, smoking rather than quitting, buying an unnecessary designer handbag rather than depositing this money in a savings account) can contribute over time to serious individual and societal problems, such as obesity, high cancer rates, and undersaving. In many such cases, then, we can say that observed levels of indulgence in *want* options are suboptimal (and thus not rational), as higher net utility would be obtained by selecting *shoulds* overs *wants*. Because this mistake of overindulging in *wants* is generally more common and costly than the opposite error, when we discuss *want–should* conflict throughout this chapter, we will primarily focus our discussion on how individuals and policy makers can increase the rate at which *should* options are selected.

Cognitive Processes Believed to Produce Want–Should Conflict

In order to better understand the outcomes of the tension that individuals experience when faced with a choice between *want* and *should* options, it is useful to examine the cognitive processes believed to underlie *want–should* conflict. In line with the multiple-selves framework put forth by Bazerman et al. (1998), some economic models have proposed that people are controlled by conflicting selves with competing preferences (Fudenberg & Levine, 2006; Read, 2001; Thaler & Shefrin, 1981). Relatedly, psychologists have proposed a model wherein individuals' decision-making processes are guided by two modes of thought, or "systems," which are referred to as System 1 and System 2 (Stanovich & West, 2000). System 1 is an intuitive, automatic system that relies on emotions and makes quick judgments. System 2 engages in slower and more logical, effortful reasoning (Milkman, Chugh, & Bazerman, 2009). In choosing between *wants* and *shoulds*, the instinctive and emotional processing driven by

System 1 tends to favor affectively rich *want* options, whereas the deliberative and analytical processing of System 2 tends to place more weight on long-term consequences and thus favors *shoulds*. For example, when you are contemplating eating a slice of chocolate cake, System 1 will focus on the fact that it is delicious, but System 2 will focus on the impact it will have on your waistline. According to this theory, factors in a decision maker's environment that weaken or strengthen System 1 versus System 2 will affect whether *wants* or *shoulds* are favored. Specifically, when an individual's System 1 is triggered (e.g., by visceral factors) or System 2 is taxed (e.g., tied up with complex thinking) and unable to weigh in with full force on want–should conflicts, *wants* will be more likely to win out. But, when System 1 is dampened or System 2 is triggered, *shoulds* will be preferred at a higher rate. Recent neurological research using functional magnetic resonance imaging (fMRI) technology has provided some evidence that indeed, consistent with this two-system model, different neurological regions are differentially activated by decisions that involve short-term rewards and long-term rewards (McClure, Laibson, Loewenstein, & Cohen, 2004).

In contrast to models of multiple competing systems, other research has proposed that construal level theory (CLT) can explain *want–should* conflict. According to CLT, events and choices can be represented in two fundamental and distinct ways—abstractly or concretely. The proximity of an event impacts how it is mentally represented. Distant events (e.g., events that are distant in space, time, or likelihood) are evaluated at a high level and are associated with schematic, abstract, and goal-relevant characteristics. In contrast, proximal events (e.g., events that are nearby in space, time, or likelihood) are evaluated at a low level and draw people's attention to concrete, specific, and detail-focused characteristics (Liberman, Sagristano, & Trope, 2002; Trope & Liberman, 2003). For example, a low-level construal of exercising would activate thoughts about the pain, discomfort, and time required to work out, pushing an individual to do what she wants and skip the gym, whereas a high-level construal of exercising would focus thoughts on the overarching benefits of exercise for one's physical and psychological well-being, pushing an individual to do what she should and exercise. Building on this notion, recent research has shown that *should* choices are more appealing when construed at a high level than at a low level (Rogers & Bazerman, 2008; Fujita, Trope, Liberman, & Levin-Sagi, 2006). In other words, this line of research posits that one fundamental factor that produces a tension between *want* and *should* choices and tips the scales when we face such choices is the level at which we construe the world, which is shifted by our circumstances.

Another body of research suggests that limited self-regulatory capacity shapes the outcomes of our internal struggles between *wants* and *shoulds* (Muraven & Baumeister, 2000). According this stream of research, self-control (or the ability to select *should* choices) is conceptualized as resembling a muscle that can be weakened through repeated use. The idea is that after resisting something we desire (e.g., a particularly tempting *want*) or, more generally, after engaging in activities that require the use of our executive function (e.g., overriding impulses), we have less self-control "strength" available for subsequent choices, causing us to give in to our short-term desires more readily (Muraven & Baumeister, 2000). According to this theory, giving in to the desires of our *want* self is attributable to a lack of self-control strength and is more likely after we have been called upon to repeatedly exercise self-control. Overall, the research on depletion suggests that when the *should* self is in a weakened state, it is more likely to lose its bouts with the *want* self.

What Factors Shift Whether We Choose *Wants* or *Shoulds*?

Choosing for Now or Later

Much prior research on *want–should* conflict has examined instability in our preferences for *wants* and *shoulds* when we make choices for now versus later. A stylized finding from this literature is that people prefer *should* options at a higher rate when making decisions for the more distant future but prefer *want* options more often the sooner choices will take effect. For example, deciding to go to the gym tomorrow is easier than deciding to go this minute, and committing to save more for retirement next year is easier than committing to forgo a portion of today's paycheck. This pattern has been demonstrated in decision domains ranging widely from those involving money to those involving food and movie rentals (e.g., Thaler, 1981; Ainslie & Haendel, 1983; King & Logue, 1987; Kirby & Herrnstein, 1995; Kirby, 1997; Read, Loewenstein, & Kalyanaraman, 1999; Milkman, Rogers, & Bazerman, 2009; Milkman, Rogers, & Bazerman, 2010).

Economists have modeled the tendency to prefer *wants* over *shoulds* at a higher rate the sooner a choice will be enacted by assuming that people discount utility more steeply in the short term than over the long run (Ainslie, 1992; Laibson, 1997; Loewenstein & Prelec, 1992; Strotz, 1956). Perhaps the most widely used model of impatience in intertemporal choice is Laibson's (1997) quasi-hyperbolic time discounting model in which all periods beyond the present period are discounted steeply by a constant factor, $\beta < 1$, in addition to the rational, exponential discount factor, $\delta = 1 - \varepsilon$. Because *should* options provide more long-term utility but less short-term utility than *want* options, Laibson's model makes a clear prediction about how time will shape the outcomes of *want–should* conflicts: people will prefer *wants* over *shoulds* at a higher rate when choosing for the present period than when choosing for future periods.

Multiple laboratory and field studies investigating impulsiveness have confirmed that people show extremely high discount rates for delayed rewards (Angeletos, Laibson, Repetto, Tobacman, & Weinberg, 2001; Kirby, 1997; Kirby & Herrnstein, 1996; McClure et al., 2004). In an early study of dynamic inconsistency, the average participant opted to receive $50 immediately (a *want* option) rather than $100 in 6 months (a *should* option) but preferred to receive $100 in 18 months rather than $50 in 12 months (Ainslie & Haendel, 1983). These results contradict the predictions of standard economic theory, which suggests that an individual's preferences between two sure sums of money should depend only on the time delay that separates their receipt (6 months in both cases). These results, however, are consistent with a quasi-hyperbolic time discounting model.

Intertemporal preference reversals involving *wants* and *shoulds* have been shown not only with money but also with various other outcomes. For example, in one experiment, subjects randomly assigned to select a film to watch that day were more likely to select lowbrow films (*want* choices) than subjects randomly assigned to select a film they would watch several days in the future (Read et al., 1999). In a field study of dynamic inconsistency and online DVD rentals, Milkman et al. (2009) demonstrated that when people rent a *should* movie before a *want* movie, they are significantly more likely to return their rentals out of order, suggesting a higher tendency to procrastinate when it comes to watching *should* films than *want* films. They also hold *should* movies longer than *want* movies, which is further evidence of procrastination when it comes to doing what we *should*. Interestingly, more experienced renters exhibit this pattern to a lesser extent than inexperienced renters, suggesting that there is some scope for learning how to avoid dynamic inconsistency. In the domain of online grocery shopping, Milkman et al. (2010) found that the percentage of extreme *should* groceries (e.g., fruits and vegetables) in a customer's basket tends to increase and the percentage of extreme *want* groceries (e.g., ice cream and cookies) tends to decrease the further in advance of delivery a customer places her order. In addition, Milkman et al. (2010) showed that customers spent more when ordering for more immediate delivery than for a later delivery (spending is a typical *want* behavior, whereas saving is a *should* behavior), which provides another example of dynamic inconsistency.

Related field research has demonstrated that firms respond to, capitalize on, and profit from consumers' dynamic inconsistency when it comes to *wants* and *shoulds*. For example, Oster and Scott Morton (2005) found that across approximately 300 American magazines, the ratio of the newsstand price to the subscription price is significantly larger for leisure magazines (*wants*) than for investment magazines (*shoulds*). This suggests that magazine pricing has been optimized to take advantage of people's tendency to plan ahead (e.g., subscribing) when it comes to purchasing *should* options but to make spur-of-the-moment decisions (e.g., buying a magazine at the newsstand) when it comes to purchasing *want* options. Additionally, DellaVigna and Malmendier (2006) examined gym attendance (a *should* behavior) and found evidence that people regularly paid a high fee for unlimited gym memberships when they could have saved money by selecting a flat, pay-per-visit fee schedule instead. These results indicate that gym goers often overestimate their future attendance (a *should*) when signing up for a membership (planning in advance) and opt for the *want* option (in this case, skipping gym visits) when deciding whether or not to exercise on a given day. In other words, "now" they prefer the *want* of skipping the gym, but "later" they anticipate preferring the *should* of exercise, and firms are able to extract excess fees from consumers as a result of this type of dynamic inconsistency.

Cognitive Load

As described above, one theory that has been proposed to explain the choices people make when faced with *want–should* tradeoffs is a two-system model. This theory suggests that the relative strengths of System 1 reactions (characterized by emotions and instincts) and System 2 reactions (characterized by deliberative, controlled thinking) influence the outcomes of *want–should* conflicts. Building on this notion, *want* options are expected to be more likely to win out when the cognitive resources available to make a decision are limited (or when System 2 is overburdened), which would allow System 1 to dominate the decision process. In one study designed to test this prediction, Shiv and Fedorikhin (1999) presented participants with two snack options: a piece of chocolate cake (a *want*) or a cup of fruit salad (a *should*). They found that individuals who were randomly assigned to memorize a seven-digit number (and who thus had reduced cognitive resources) were more likely to choose cake over fruit than those who were assigned to memorize a two-digit number. This finding is consistent with a two-system model of *want–should* conflict and highlights the fact that the availability of cognitive resources is critical to making farsighted and deliberative *should* decisions.

Construal Level

As discussed previously, construal level theory (CLT) suggests that we prefer *shoulds* over *wants* more often when we are thinking abstractly and thus focusing on the global and goal-relevant features of options rather than when we are thinking concretely and thus focusing on the contextualized, surface-level, and goal-irrelevant features of options. For instance, abstract representations of exercising bring to mind its long-term benefits, while concrete representations remind us of its in-the-moment pains and required planning. Past experimental research has shown that the tendency to make *should* choices can indeed be enhanced by inducing abstract, high-level representations of events (e.g., by focusing people on more distal events in time, space, and hypotheticality rather than more proximal events; Trope & Liberman, 2003; Rogers & Bazerman, 2008). For example, Fujita et al. (2006) primed some research participants to think abstractly by asking them to describe *why* they maintain good physical health and primed others to think concretely by asking them to describe *how* they maintain good physical health. They found that when a more abstract, high-level mindset was activated, people exhibited stronger preferences for delayed *should* rewards over immediate *want* outcomes. This research highlights that inducing people to adopt a higher-level construal mindset is one way to increase future-oriented, *should* decision making.

Depletion

The process of reining in our short-term desires and choosing *shoulds* over *wants* requires exercising willpower or self-regulation (Carver & Scheier, 1998; Higgins, 1996). As discussed previously, a growing body of research suggests that exerting willpower comes at a cost, and that cost is a reduction in available self-control resources for use in future choices (Baumeister, Bratslavsky, Muraven, & Tice, 1998). In other words, individuals have limited self-regulatory resources, and exerting self-control to avoid *wants* in one situation can decrease one's subsequent ability to exert self-control. For example, in one study designed to test this theory, Baumeister et al. (1998) showed that participants who resisted eating chocolate chip cookies (an obvious *want* for most people) quit working on unsolvable puzzles earlier (where persistence is a *should* behavior) than did individuals who resisted eating radishes, an activity that for most people requires little self-control. Further, in field research, it has been shown that exposure to demanding work environments—which induce repeated exertion of willpower—exhausts executive resources (Danziger, Levav, & Avnaim-Pesso, 2011) and reduces *should* choices (Dai, Milkman, Hoffmann, & Staats, 2015). In one study, hospital employees sanitized their hands (an important *should* behavior) less and less at recommended times later in their work shifts—an effect that was exacerbated by higher work intensity and alleviated by longer breaks between shifts (Dai et al., 2015). Together, these studies illustrate the paradox that by exercising self-control now, we increase the likelihood that we will give in to our desires to indulge later. Fortunately, although the self-control muscle can be weakened through repeated use, it can also be strengthened through proper exercise. Muraven (2010) found evidence that practicing small acts of self-control greatly increased smokers' chances of successfully quitting the habit.

Incidental Uncertainty

Building on prior ego depletion research, Milkman (2012) proposed and demonstrated that facing uncertainty about the future is depleting and can thus reduce self-control resources and increase our tendency to select *want* options. For example, when people were unsure of whether or not they held a winning lottery ticket, they were less persistent on math problems (where persisting is a *should*) than when they knew the outcome of the lottery. When they were unsure which of two movies they would watch tomorrow, they were more likely to choose to eat an unhealthy *want* snack than when they were informed of which movie they would see. Further, when prompted to simply describe uncertain (versus certain) aspects of their lives, participants were more likely to elect to read a *want* magazine over a *should* magazine. The effect of uncertainty on take-up of *should* options was mediated by depletion. Overall, this work suggests that reducing uncertainty in an individual's environment can reduce impulsive choices and increase the likelihood that he or she will select *should* options.

Joint versus Separate Evaluations

The outcomes of *want–should* conflicts are also influenced by whether we evaluate options one at a time or simultaneously. Although *want* options tend to be preferred at a higher rate than *should* options in isolation, we are more likely to think about the costs and benefits of each option and make farsighted *should* choices when multiple options are evaluated at the same time (Bazerman et al., 1998). For example, when viewed in isolation, a charity that saves baby polar bears may seem more alluring and receive more donations than a charity that funds skin cancer research. However, when these choices are compared side by side, people tend to donate to the charity that helps people, viewing its mission as more important, albeit less emotionally resonant (Kahneman & Ritov, 1994). This research highlights the fact that presenting *want* and *should* options simultaneously rather than sequentially is one way to promote more *should* choices.

Mood Effects

Past research has also demonstrated that emotions can shift the outcomes of *want–should* conflicts. First, positive mood has been shown to facilitate future-oriented, *should* decision making (Labroo & Patrick, 2009; Fedorikhin & Patrick, 2010), and a number of explanations have been proposed for this. One account is that experiencing positive affect signals to decision makers that their current situation is nonthreatening, which reduces discounting of the future and thus makes *shoulds* relatively more attractive (Pyone & Isen, 2011; Labroo & Patrick, 2009). Another reason suggested by past research is that positive affect can counteract ego depletion, restoring the depleted willpower resources necessary for selecting *should* options (Tice, Baumeister, Shmueli, & Muraven, 2007). Further, Fedorikhin and Patrick (2010) argued that resisting temptation may be a technique that individuals in a positive mood employ to maintain their emotional state, since giving in to temptation can induce guilt and other negative emotions. In one study, these authors demonstrated that after randomly assigning participants to watch clips of videos that induced either a happy or neutral mood, those placed in a positive mood were more likely to select a *should* option (grapes) over a relative *want* option (M&Ms). However, they found that the tendency for positive moods to increase *should* choices is attenuated by elevated arousal, because arousal is depleting (Fedorikhin & Patrick, 2010). In addition to exploring the impact of positive moods, past research has also explored the impact of negative affect on *want–should* conflict. Recent studies have demonstrated that negative affect can lead to self-control breakdowns (Leith & Baumeister, 1996), whereby sadness increases decision makers' tendency to focus on immediate gratification and to dramatically discount future outcomes (Lerner, Li, & Weber, 2013). Together, this research shows that people who are relaxed and happy are more likely to make *should* choices, whereas individuals who are emotionally aroused or in a negative mood are more likely to reach for the instant gratification produced by indulging in a *want* option.

Licensing Effects

Interestingly, our choices between *wants* and *shoulds* can be affected not only by our current state but also by decisions we have made in the past as well as those we anticipate making in the future. Specifically, past research has shown that people feel "licensed" to make (or justified in making) *want* choices if they believe they have previously engaged in *should* behaviors or if they anticipate having opportunities to engage in *should* behaviors in the future (see also de Ridder, de Witt Huberts, & Evers, Chapter 10, this volume; Dholakia, Chapter 20, this volume). For example, Khan and Dhar (2006) showed that people who were asked to imagine they would partake in a *should* behavior (e.g., donating part of their tax rebate to charity, volunteering for community service), relative to a control group who did not imagine any such future good behavior, were more likely to select an affectively desirable *want* product (e.g., a pair of designer glasses) over a cognitively favorable *should* product (e.g., a less expensive but more utilitarian pair of glasses).[2] Furthermore, *want*

---

[2]Interestingly, licensing effects only hold when participants voluntarily engage in a *should* behavior—there is no licensing effect when individuals are forced to engage in *shoulds*.

products are more likely to be selected when individuals make what they believe is the first of a series of similar decisions rather than a single, isolated choice, presumably because individuals making repeated decisions believe they will have the opportunity to choose *shoulds* in the future to compensate for current indulgences (Khan & Dhar, 2007). These findings highlight that choosing between *wants* and *shoulds* is often not done in isolation but instead hinges on an individual's past choices and anticipated future decisions.

Closeness to Your Future Self

The outcomes of *want–should* conflicts are affected not only by what we think our future self will choose but also by how close we feel to our future self. *Want–should* conflicts fundamentally involve tradeoffs between options that satisfy the present self's desires (*wants*) and options that benefit the future self (*shoulds*). As a result, when we do not feel psychologically connected to our future self, we should be less interested in taking actions to benefit this self and thus shy away from *should* options. Indeed, an emerging stream of research suggests that people are more impatient the more disconnected they feel from their future self. For example, people prefer smaller-sooner rewards over larger-later rewards at a higher rate when they anticipate experiencing life-changing events (rather than events that are unlikely to change their identity and beliefs), since life-changing events induce a greater disassociation between their image of their present self and their image of their future self (Bartels & Rips, 2010). More generally, when people are told that their identity (e.g., beliefs, values, and goals) will change considerably over time, they are more likely to accept immediate benefits (*wants*) and forsake larger deferred benefits (*shoulds*). On the other hand, farsighted decision making can be facilitated by making people feel closer to their future self. For example, Hershfield et al. (2011) increased study participants' reported willingness to save for retirement by allowing them to virtually interact with age-progressed images of themselves—an experience that helped them relate to and imagine their future self.

Fresh Starts

Recent research suggests that there are naturally arising points in time when people are particularly motivated to pursue their long-term interests, or in other words, to prefer *shoulds*. Temporal landmarks, which include personally relevant life events (e.g., anniversaries, birthdays) and reference points on shared calendars (e.g., holidays, the start of a new week, month, year, or semester), demarcate the passage of time and help us organize our activities, memories, and experiences (Robinson, 1986; Shum, 1998). Recent field research by Dai, Milkman, and Riis (2014) has shown that temporal landmarks magnify people's virtuous intentions and increase their engagement in *should* behaviors. Dai et al. (2014) analyzed (1) daily Google search volume for the term "diet," (2) undergraduate students' gym attendance records, and (3) a wide range of goals (pertaining to education, health, finance, etc.) that Internet users committed to pursuing on a goal-setting website (*www.stickK.com*). Each of these three field studies revealed that people engage in *should* behaviors (i.e., dieting, exercising, and goal pursuit) more frequently following temporal landmarks, including the start of the week, month, year, and academic semester, as well as immediately following a birthday, a federal holiday, or a school break. The authors refer to this phenomenon as "the fresh start effect" (Dai et al., 2014).

In another paper, Dai, Milkman, and Riis (2015) explore what types of temporal landmarks are most motivating and examine the mechanism underlying increased motivation. They find that more meaningful landmarks produce a larger uptick than less meaningful landmarks in the rate at which people intend to and choose to engage in *should* behaviors. For example, people expect that they are more likely to begin pursuing their goals following a more meaningful landmark (e.g., their first move to a new home) than following a less meaningful landmark (e.g., moving to a new home for the ninth time). Also, Dai et al. (2015) find that students are more likely to choose to receive reminders about their goals on a date labeled as the beginning of their school's summer break than the same date labeled "Administrative Day." Furthermore, Dai et al. (2015) propose and show that this strengthened motivation to engage in *should* behaviors following more meaningful temporal landmarks is driven by a greater psychological disassociation from one's past imperfections.

This stream of research on the "fresh start effect" suggests several techniques that can potentially be leveraged to promote *should* choices. For example, managers and policy makers may consider encouraging farsighted decisions following temporal landmarks (e.g., a birthday, a work anniversary), particularly those that are perceived as more psychologically meaningful (e.g., a major birthday, a round-number work anniversary). In addition, framing a given day as a meaningful fresh start may increase the likelihood that people will make more *should* decisions.

Prescriptions

Past research examining what shifts decisions when we face *want–should* tradeoffs (reviewed above) highlights that our choices regarding *wants* and *shoulds* are malleable and depend on the context in which we make a decision. Taking advantage of this malleability, an increasing number of "nudges," or interventions that leverage psychology to guide behavior without restricting choice (Thaler & Sunstein, 2008), have been designed with the goal of promoting farsighted, *should* decisions. As discussed previously, many policy makers are seeking ways to increase engagement in *should* behaviors (e.g., increasing savings, reducing smoking, increasing healthy eating and exercise). Here we review a series of different "nudges" that have been shown to successfully increase the rate at which we choose *shoulds* over *wants*.

Prompt Planning

Prompting plan making—or prompting people to stipulate when, where, and how they will enact their goals—is one of the oldest prescriptions for increasing engagement in *should* behaviors, dating back to research conducted in the 1960s. Specifically, in 1965, Leventhal, Singer, and Jones demonstrated that prompting people to form a plan of action for receiving a tetanus shot significantly increased take-up of tetanus inoculations. Since then, plan making has been shown to improve our likelihood of achieving goals in a diverse array of domains, including exercise, dieting, smoking cessation, academic performance, test preparation, recycling, and voting (for more extensive reviews, see Gollwitzer, 1999; Rogers, Milkman, John, & Norton, in press).

Planning prompts are effective for a number of reasons (Dai et al., 2013; Rogers et al., in press), one of which is that they reduce forgetfulness. When people take the time to create and even write down the when, where, and how of a plan, they mentally associate their target actions with cues relating to the when and where of execution. For example, creating a plan with the form "at noon tomorrow, I will vote" links voting to the cue of "noon tomorrow." When a cue arises (e.g., at noon tomorrow), an individual who has formed a plan is more likely to remember and then perform the predetermined actions. Planning also discourages procrastination by creating explicit commitments to oneself and sometimes also to others. For example, people feel internal pressure to follow through on their plans and seek to avoid breaking explicit commitments to themselves because behaving inconsistently with their past actions, beliefs, and attitudes can create discomfort (Festinger, 1962). Further, some plans (e.g., to get a mammogram) may literally require making an appointment (e.g., with a doctor), which may be difficult to cancel or delay.

Recent large-scale field studies have demonstrated the effectiveness of plan making as a means of increasing take-up of two important *should* behaviors—receiving flu shots and receiving colonoscopies (Milkman, Beshears, Choi, Laibson, & Madrian, 2011, 2013). In one three-armed randomized, controlled trial (Milkman et al., 2011), thousands of employees from a Midwestern utility company were informed by mail of where and when free flu shots would be available at their work site. Employees in the control condition only received this logistical information. Employees in two other conditions were encouraged on their reminder mailing to (privately) form a plan about either (1) the date (the general planning condition) or (2) both the date and time (the specific planning condition) when they intended to receive their shot. Prompting employees to make a specific plan increased flu shot uptake significantly from 33% in the control condition to 37% in the specific planning condition. As expected, the take-up rate in the general plan condition of 35% fell between the other two conditions (and did not differ significantly from either). Notably, employees whose on-site clinic was open only for a single day (as opposed to 3 or 5 days) and who thus had the most to lose from forgetfulness or procrastination benefited the most from the prompt (turnout in this group increased from 30% in the control to 38% in the specific plan group). In a similar study by Milkman et al. (2013), planning prompts were demonstrated to significantly increase take-up of colonoscopies. In this study, those predicted to be the most likely to forget to follow through (e.g., older adults, adults with children, and those who did not comply with previous reminders) benefited most from the planning prompt. These field experiments, together with past research, highlight the value of planning prompts as a scalable, low-cost nudge for increasing engagement in *should* behaviors by combating forgetfulness and procrastination.

Commitment Devices

Many people are sophisticated about preventing their self-control problems from getting in the way of their good (or *should*) intentions (O'Donoghue & Rabin, 1999). As a result, another way to increase engagement in *shoulds* is by providing individuals with access to commitment devices—or a means of voluntarily (1) enforcing restrictions on themselves until they have done what they know they should or (2) imposing penalties for failing to do what they should. Commitment devices have existed in many forms throughout the years. For instance, the piggy bank is a commitment device that encourages us to commit to saving by setting aside a certain portion of earnings for future use. More modern forms of commitment devices include Antabuse, a medication that makes alcoholics physically ill after consuming even a small amount of alcohol, and *stickK.com*, a website that takes users' money if they fail to achieve their goals. A definition of commitment devices provided by Rogers, Milkman, and Volpp (2014, p. 2065) states that they have two basic features: "First, people voluntarily elect to use them. This means people must be self-aware enough about the gap between their current goals and their likely future behaviors that they see the value of taking steps to constrain their future selves. . . . Second, commitment devices associate consequences with people's failures to achieve their goals."

Ultimately, commitment devices are mechanisms that allow people to prevent themselves from giving in to unwise *wants*. Past research has shown that they can been used successfully to reduce procrastination (Ariely & Wertenbroch, 2002), undersaving (Ashraf, Karlan, & Yin, 2006; Beshears, Choi, Laibson, Madrian, & Sakong, 2011), smoking (Giné, Karlan, & Zinman, 2010), failures to achieve work goals (Kaur, Kremer, & Mullainathan, 2010), and succumbing to repeated temptations in a laboratory setting (Houser, Schunk, Winter, & Xiao, 2010). A classic example of a commitment device is the Save More Tomorrow™ program, which asks employees to agree to increase their savings rates whenever they receive a raise and has been shown to dramatically increase savings rates (Thaler & Benartzi, 2004).

Some past studies have further shown that people are sometimes willing to pay for products that make a desirable option less attractive in an effort to commit themselves to making *should* choices. Examples of such "value-destroying" options include restrictive savings accounts that penalize withdrawals before a predetermined date or before a savings goal is reached (Ashraf et al., 2006; Beshears et al., 2011) and gym memberships that cost more if one fails to meet a predefined attendance goal (Royer, Stehr, & Sydnor, 2012). Similarly, some people will voluntarily limit the amount of *want* products available for their future consumption because they expect their future self to overconsume, by buying smaller packages of *wants* despite the presence of volume discounts (Wertenbroch, 1998) or by ordering smaller portions of fast-food meals even when a larger portion costs the same price (Schwartz, Riis, Elbel, & Ariely, 2012). In fighting the urge to procrastinate, some will even elect to self-impose earlier deadlines than those externally designated by supervisors or instructors (Ariely & Wertenbroch, 2002). The fact that many choose to restrict their future choice sets to reduce future *want* decisions supports the notion that people value overcoming desires that conflict with their long-term well-being.

Temptation Bundling

Temptation bundling is a new type of commitment device (introduced in 2014 by Milkman, Minson, and Volpp), which has proven an effective means of increasing engagement in one important *should* behavior—exercise. Temptation bundling seeks to increase *should* behaviors by bundling them with tempting *wants*, a strategy that can simultaneously reduce engagement in *wants* and increase engagement in *shoulds*. For example, a doctoral student may have the goal of spending more time writing a manuscript (a *should* behavior) while recognizing that he has been consuming too many Starbucks white chocolate mochas (a *want* behavior). Using temptation bundling, the student might commit to only consuming white chocolate mochas while working on his manuscript, thus increasing time spent writing and reducing white chocolate mocha consumption. In addition to simultaneously tackling two types of self-control problems, temptation bundling has the potential to harness consumption complementarities: working while drinking mochas may make work more enjoyable and efficient as well as reducing one's guilt (and therefore overall enjoyment) associated with mocha consumption.

Milkman et al. (2014) demonstrated the effectiveness of temptation bundling as a means of increasing exercise (a *should* behavior) in a field experiment. Study participants were randomly assigned to (1) a full-treatment condition in which access to tempting lowbrow audio novels (*wants*) was restricted to the gym, (2) an intermediate treatment condition in which participants were simply encouraged to self-restrict their enjoyment of tempting audio novels to the gym, or (3) a control condition. Initial gym attendance among individuals in the full treatment condition was 51% higher than attendance in the control group (a significant difference), and participants in the intermediate treatment condition showed a marginally significant 29% initial increase in gym attendance, although notably, the boosts in gym attendance in both treatment groups decayed significantly over the course of the 9-week study. Furthermore, at the conclusion of the study, 61% of participants were willing to pay to have their access to an iPod containing tempting audio novels restricted to the gym. In other words, people would pay to have access to a possession they could otherwise use freely restricted so they could only enjoy this desirable *want* while exercising (or engaging in a *should* behavior). These findings suggest that temptation bundling may be an effective means of increasing take-up of *shoulds* and that there may be a market for temptation-bundling devices.

Conclusion

This chapter has synthesized research on the internal conflict we face when presented with *want* and *should* options, with particular attention to how we can best encourage more *should* choices. The effectiveness of many of the strategies we have discussed has important implications for public policy. In the realm of public health, for instance, ailments such as addiction and obesity carry tremendous costs. Specifically, it is estimated that unhealthy behaviors may account for up to 40 percent of premature deaths in the United States (Schroeder, 2007), and such behaviors place a significant strain on the nation's health care systems (Finkelstein, Trogdon, Cohen, & Dietz, 2009). In many cases, outcomes such as obesity and addiction can be traced back to individuals' failures to successfully navigate *want–should* conflicts, with our short-term desires (e.g., watching television, eating junk food, smoking) frequently winning out over what is in our long-term best interest (e.g., exercising, eating healthy food, receiving preventive care, quitting smoking).

The research highlighted throughout this chapter shows that even minor interventions (e.g., planning prompts, making individuals feel closer to their future self) can shift behaviors in societally beneficial directions. Policy makers may be able to utilize these types of interventions to "nudge" individuals toward *should* behaviors without restricting their choices (Thaler & Sunstein, 2008). While still a relatively new idea, the notion that "nudging" citizens toward *should* choices without taxing them or restricting their options in any way has gained popularity with politicians around the world. For example, in 2010, Prime Minister David Cameron of the United Kingdom created a Behavioral Insights Team (also known as the "nudge unit") to apply such techniques to public problems (Bell, 2013). For academics to provide policy makers as well as individuals with the greatest possible insight about how to facilitate *should* decision making, additional research on *want–should* conflict is needed. The better we understand *want–should* conflict, the more successful we will become at designing effective interventions that promote *should* choices and help people avoid the temptation to give in to harmful cravings and desires.

REFERENCES

Ainslie, G. (1975). Specious reward: A behavioral theory of impulsiveness and impulse control. *Psychological Bulletin, 82*(4), 463–509.

Ainslie, G. (1992). *Picoeconomics: The interaction of successive motivational states within the individual.* New York: Cambridge University Press.

Ainslie, G., & Haendel, V. (1983). The motives of the will. In E. Gottheil, K. A. Druley, T. E. Skoloda, & H. M. Waxman (Eds.), *Etiologic aspects of alcohol and drug abuse* (pp. 119–140). Springfield, IL: Charles C Thomas.

Angeletos, G., Laibson, D., Repetto, A., Tobacman, J., & Weinberg, S. (2001). The hyperbolic consumption model: Calibration, simulation, and empirical evaluation. *Journal of Economic Perspectives, 15*(3), 48–68.

Ariely, D., & Wertenbroch, K. (2002). Procrastination, deadlines, and performance: Self-control by precommitment. *Psychological Science, 13*(3), 219–224.

Ashraf, N., Karlan, D., & Yin, W. (2006). Tying Odysseus to the mast: Evidence from a commitment savings product in the Philippines. *Quarterly Journal of Economics, 121*(2), 635–672.

Bazerman, M. H., Tenbrunsel, A. E., & Wade-Benzoni, K. (1998). Negotiating with yourself and losing: Making decisions with competing internal preferences. *Academy of Management Review, 23*(2), 225–241.

Bartels, D. M., & Rips, L. J. (2010). Psychological connectedness and intertemporal choice. *Journal of Experimental Psychology, 139*(1), 49–69.

Baumeister, R. F., Bratslavsky, E., Muraven, M., & Tice, D. M. (1998). Ego depletion: Is the active self a limited resource? *Journal of Personality and Social Psychology, 74*(5), 1252–1265.

Bell, C. (2013, February 11). Inside the Coalition's controversial "nudge unit." *Telegraph.* Retrieved from *www.telegraph.co.uk/news/politics/9853384/Inside-the-Coalitions-controversial-Nudge-Unit.html.*

Beshears, J., Choi, J. J., Laibson, D., Madrian, B., & Sakong, J. (2011). *Self control and liquidity: How to design a commitment contract* (RAND Working Paper No.

WR-895-SSA). Available at *http://scholar.harvard.edu/files/laibson/files/self_control_and_liquidity_how_to_design_a_commitment_contract.pdf.*

Carver, C. S., & Scheier, M. F. (1998). *On the self-regulation of behavior.* New York: Cambridge University Press.

Dai, H., Milkman, K. L., Beshears, J., Choi, J. J., Laibson, D., & Madrian, B. C. (2013). Planning prompts as a means of increasing rates of immunization and preventive screening. *Public Policy and Aging Report, 22*(4), 16–19.

Dai, H., Milkman, K. L., Hofmann, D. A., & Staats, B. R. (2015). The impact of time at work and time off from work on rule compliance: The case of hand hygiene in health care. *Journal of Applied Psychology, 100*(3), 846–862.

Dai, H., Milkman, K. L., & Riis, J. (2014). The fresh start effect: Temporal landmarks motivate aspirational behavior. *Management Science, 60*(10), 2563–2582.

Dai, H., Milkman, K. L., & Riis, J. (2015). *Put your imperfections behind you: Why and how meaningful temporal landmarks motivate aspirational behavior.* Philadelphia: University of Pennsylvania.

Danziger, S., Levav, J., & Avnaim-Pesso, L. (2011). Extraneous factors in judicial decisions. *Proceedings of the National Academy of Sciences, 108*(17), 6889–6892.

DellaVigna, S., & Malmendier, U. (2006). Paying not to go to the gym. *American Economic Review, 96*(3), 694–719.

Fedorikhin, A., & Patrick, V. M. (2010). Positive mood and resistance to temptation: The interfering influence of elevated arousal. *Journal of Consumer Research, 37*(4), 698–711.

Festinger, L. (1962). *A theory of cognitive dissonance.* Stanford, CA: Stanford University Press.

Finkelstein, E. A., Trogdon, J. G., Cohen, J. W., & Dietz, W. (2009). Annual medical spending attributable to obesity: Payer- and service-specific estimates. *Health Affairs, 28*(5), 822–831.

Fudenberg, D., & Levine, D. (2006). A dual self model of impulse control. *American Economic Review, 96*(5), 1449–1476.

Fujita, K., Trope, Y., Liberman, N., & Levin-Sagi, M. (2006). Construal levels and self-control. *Journal of Personality and Social Psychology, 90*(3), 351–367.

Giné, X., Karlan, D., & Zinman, J. (2010). Put your money where your butt is: A commitment contract for smoking cessation. *American Economic Journal: Applied Economics, 2*, 213–235.

Giner-Sorolla, R. (2001). Guilty pleasures and grim necessities: Affective attitudes in dilemmas of self-control. *Journal of Personality and Social Psychology, 80*(2), 206–221.

Gollwitzer, P. M. (1999). Implementation intentions: Strong effects of simple plans. *American Psychologist, 54*(7), 493–503.

Hershfield, H. E., Goldstein, D. G., Sharpe, W. F., Fox, J., Yeykelis, L., Carstensen, L. L., et al. (2011). Increasing saving behavior through age-progressed renderings of the future self. *Journal of Marketing Research, 48*, S23–S37.

Higgins, E. T. (1996). The "self digest": Self-knowledge serving self-regulatory functions. *Journal of Personality and Social Psychology, 71*(6), 1062–1083.

Hofmann, W., Baumeister, R. F., Förster, G., & Vohs, K. D. (2012). Everyday temptations: An experience sampling study of desire, conflict, and self-control. *Journal of Personality and Social Psychology, 102*(6), 1318–1335.

Houser, D., Schunk, D., Winter, J., & Xiao, E. (2010). *Temptation and commitment in the laboratory* (Working Paper No. 488, Institute for Empirical Research in Economics, University of Zurich).

Kahneman, D., & Ritov, I. (1994). Determinants of stated willingness to pay for public goods: A study in the headline method. *Journal of Risk and Uncertainty,* *9*(1), 5–37.

Kavanagh, D. J., Andrade, J., & May, J. (2005). Imaginary relish and exquisite torture: The elaborated intrusion theory of desire. *Psychological Review, 112*(2), 446–467.

Kaur, S., Kremer, M., & Mullainathan, S. (2010). Self-control and the development of work arrangements. *American Economic Review, 100*(2), 624–628.

Khan, U., & Dhar, R. (2006). Licensing effect in consumer choice. *Journal of Marketing Research, 43*(2), 259–266.

Khan, U., & Dhar, R. (2007). Where there is a way, is there a will?: The effect of future choices on current preferences. *Journal of Experimental Psychology, 136*(2), 277–288.

King, G. R., & Logue, A. W. (1987). Choice in a self-control paradigm with human subjects: Effects of changeover delay duration. *Learning and Motivation, 18*(4), 421–438.

Kirby, K. N. (1997). Bidding on the future: Evidence against normative discounting of delayed rewards. *Journal of Experimental Psychology, 126*(1), 54–70.

Kirby, K. N., & Herrnstein, R. J. (1995). Preference reversals due to myopic discounting of delayed rewards. *Psychological Science, 6*(2), 83–89.

Kivetz, R., & Keinan, A. (2006). Repenting hyperopia: An analysis of self-control regrets. *Journal of Consumer Research, 33*(2), 273–282.

Kivetz, R., & Simonson, I. (2002). Earning the right to indulge: Effort as a determinant of customer preferences toward frequency program rewards. *Journal of Marketing Research, 39*(2), 155–170.

Labroo, A. A., & Patrick, V. M. (2009). Psychological distancing: Why happiness helps you see the big picture. *Journal of Consumer Research, 35*(5), 800–809.

Laibson, D. (1997). Golden eggs and hyperbolic discounting. *Quarterly Journal of Economics, 112*(2), 444–477.

Leith, K. P., & Baumeister, R. F. (1996). Why do bad moods increase self-defeating behavior? Emotion, risk tasking, and self-regulation. *Journal of Personality and Social Psychology, 71*(6), 1250–1267.

Lerner, J. S., Li, Y., & Weber, E. U. (2013). The financial costs of sadness. *Psychological Science, 24*(1), 72–79.

Leventhal, H., Singer, R., & Jones, S. (1965). Effects of fear and specificity of recommendation upon attitudes and behavior. *Journal of Personality and Social Psychology, 2*(1), 20–29.

Liberman, N., Sagristano, M., & Trope, Y. (2002). The effect of temporal distance on level of construal. *Journal of Experimental Social Psychology, 38*(6), 523–535.

Loewenstein, G. F., & Prelec, D. (1992). Anomalies in intertemporal choice: Evidence and an interpretation. *Quarterly Journal of Economics, 107*(2), 573–597.

Loewenstein, L. K. (1996). Out of control: Visceral influences on behavior. *Organizational Behavior and Human Decision Processes, 65*(3), 272–292.

McClure, S. M., Laibson, D., Loewenstein, G., & Cohen, J. D. (2004). Separate neural systems value immediate and delayed monetary rewards. *Science, 306*(5695), 503–507.

Milkman, K. L. (2012). Unsure what the future will bring? You may overindulge: Uncertainty increases the appeal of wants over shoulds. *Organizational Behavior and Human Decision Processes, 119*(2), 163–176.

Milkman, K. L., Beshears, J., Choi, J. J., Laibson, D., & Madrian, B. C. (2011). Using implementation intentions prompts to enhance influenza vaccination rates. *Proceedings of the National Academy of Sciences, 108*(26), 10415–10420.

Milkman, K. L., Beshears, J., Choi, J. J., Laibson, D., & Madrian, B. C. (2013). Planning prompts as a means of increasing preventive screening rates. *Preventive Medicine, 56*(1), 92–93.

Milkman, K. L., Chugh, D., & Bazerman, M. H. (2009). How can decision making be improved? *Perspectives on Psychological Science, 4*(4), 379–383.

Milkman, K. L., Minson, J., & Volpp, K. (2014). Holding the Hunger Games hostage at the gym: An evaluation of temptation bundling. *Management Science, 60*(2), 283–299.

Milkman, K. L., Rogers, T., & Bazerman, M. H. (2008). Harnessing our inner angels and demons: What we have learned about want/should conflicts and how that knowledge can help us reduce short-sighted decision making. *Perspectives on Psychological Science, 3*(4), 324–338.

Milkman, K. L., Rogers, T., & Bazerman, M. H. (2009). Highbrow films gather dust: Time-inconsistent preferences and online DVD rentals. *Management Science, 55*(6), 1047–1059.

Milkman, K. L., Rogers, T., & Bazerman, M. H. (2010). I'll have the ice cream soon and the vegetables later: A study of online grocery purchases and order lead time. *Marketing Letters, 21*(1), 17–36.

Muraven, M. (2010). Practicing self-control lowers the risk of smoking lapse. *Psychology of Addictive Behaviors, 24*(3), 446–452.

Muraven, M., & Baumeister, R. F. (2000). Self-regulation and depletion of limited resources: Does self-control resemble a muscle? *Psychological Bulletin, 126*(2), 247–259.

O'Donoghue, T., & Rabin, M. (1999). Doing it now or later. *American Economic Review, 89*(1), 103–124.

Oster, S., & Scott Morton, F. M. (2005). Behavioral biases meet the market: The case of magazine subscription prices. *Advances in Economic Analysis and Policy, 5*(1), 1–32.

Prelec, D., & Herrnstein, R. J. (1991). Preferences or principles: Alternative guidelines for choice. In R. J. Zeckhauser (Ed.), *Strategy and choice* (pp. 319–340). Cambridge, MA: MIT Press.

Pyone, J. S., & Isen, A. M. (2011). Positive affect, intertemporal choice, and levels of thinking: Increasing consumers' willingness to wait. *Journal of Marketing Research, 48*(3), 532–543.

Read, D. (2001). Intrapersonal dilemmas. *Human Relations, 54*(8), 1093–1117.

Read, D., Loewenstein, G., & Kalyanaraman, S. (1999). Mixing virtue with vice: Combining the immediacy effect and the diversification heuristic. *Journal of Behavioral Decision Making, 12*(4), 257–273.

Robinson, J. A. (1986). Temporal reference systems and autobiographical memory. In D. C. Rubin (Ed.), *Autobiographical memory* (pp. 159–188). Cambridge, UK: Cambridge University Press.

Rogers, T., & Bazerman, M. H. (2008). Future lock-in: Future implementation increases selection of "should" choices. *Organizational Behavior and Human Decision Processes, 106*(1), 1–20.

Rogers, T., Milkman, K. L., John, L., & Norton, M. I. (in press). Making the best laid plans better: How plan-making increases follow-through. *Behavioral Science and Policy.*

Rogers, T., Milkman, K. L., & Volpp, K. G. M. (2014). Commitment devices: Using initiatives to change behavior. *Journal of the American Medical Association, 311*(20), 2065–2066.

Royer, H., Stehr, M. F., & Sydnor, J. R. (2012). *Incentives, commitments and habit for-*

mation in exercise: Evidence from a field experiment with workers at a Fortune-500 company (Working Paper No. w18580). Cambridge, MA: National Bureau of Economic Research.

Schelling, T. C. (1984). *Choice and consequence: Perspectives of an errant economist.* Cambridge, MA: Harvard University Press.

Schroeder, S. A. (2007). Shattuck lecture: We can do better—Improving the health of the American people. *New England Journal of Medicine, 357*(12), 1221–1228.

Schwartz, J., Riis, J., Elbel, B., & Ariely, D. (2012). Inviting consumers to downsize fast-food portions significantly reduces calorie consumption. *Health Affairs, 31*(2), 399–407.

Sen, A. K. (1977). Rational fools: A critique of the behavioral foundations of economic theory. *Philosophy and Public Affairs, 6*(4), 317–344.

Shefrin, H. M., & Thaler, R. H. (1988). The behavioral life-cycle hypothesis. *Economic Inquiry, 26*(4), 609–643.

Shiv, B., & Fedorikhin, A. (1999). Heart and mind in conflict: The interplay of affect and cognition in consumer decision making. *Journal of Consumer Research, 26*(3), 278–292.

Shum, M. S. (1998). The role of temporal landmarks in autobiographical memory processes. *Psychological Bulletin, 124*(3), 423–442.

Stanovich, K. E., & West, R. F. (2000). Advancing the rationality debate. *Behavioral and Brain Sciences, 23*(5), 701–717.

Strotz, R. H. (1956). Myopia and inconsistency in dynamic utility maximization. *Review of Economic Studies, 23*(3), 165–180.

Thaler, R. H. (1981). Some empirical evidence on dynamic inconsistency. *Economics Letters, 8*(3), 201–207.

Thaler, R. H., & Benartzi, S. (2004). Save more tomorrow: Using behavioral economics to increase employee saving. *Journal of Political Economy, 112*(S1), S164–S187.

Thaler, R. H., & Shefrin, H. (1981). An economic theory of self control. *Journal of Political Economy, 89*(2), 392–406.

Thaler, R. H., & Sunstein, C. R. (2008). *Nudge: Improving decisions about health, wealth, and happiness.* New Haven, CT: Yale University Press.

Tice, D. M., Baumeister, R. F., Shmueli, D., & Muraven, M. (2007). Restoring the self: Positive affect helps improve self-regulation following ego depletion. *Journal of Experimental Social Psychology, 43*(3), 379–384.

Trope, Y., & Liberman, N. (2003). Temporal construal. *Psychological Review, 110*(3), 403–421.

Wertenbroch, K. (1998). Consumption self-control by rationing purchase quantities of virtue and vice. *Marketing Science, 17*(4), 317–337.

PART IV

Desire, Affect, and Well-Being

CHAPTER 13

You Shall Not Always Get What You Want

The Consequences of Ambivalence toward Desires

Frenk van Harreveld
Hannah U. Nohlen
Iris K. Schneider

> I count him braver who overcomes his desires than him who
> conquers his enemies: For the hardest victory is over self.
> —ARISTOTLE

Ever since Aristotle, scholars have acknowledged desire as an important driving force that guides human behavior. Wants and needs are key to our survival. For example, without the desire for food, drink, and sex we would starve, dehydrate, and fail to reproduce. However, we also need to curtail primary urges such as laziness, hunger, and lust to some extent; otherwise modern society would resemble Sodom and Gomorrah. Despite the fundamental importance of desires, they are often accompanied by conflict (Lewin, 1935): we may regret acting on some impulsive desires if they are in conflict with an overarching goal, creating the core of what we view as temptation (Baumeister, 2002; see also Hofmann, Kotabe, Vohs, & Baumeister, Chapter 3, this volume). In the present chapter we will first show that temptations are inherently ambivalent in nature. Subsequently we will discuss the ambivalent nature of temptations along the lines of recent insights into the consequences of ambivalence for information processing and behavior. Thus we will shed light on the unique and important consequences of the mixed feelings often elicited by desire.

The inherent approach–avoidance conflict vis-à-vis temptations is represented in people's ambivalence toward desires such as unhealthy food, sex, and smoking and toward behaviors that are not immediately pleasurable but are desirable in the long run, such as dieting and engaging in regular exercise. The intrinsic relation between ambivalence and temptation is evident from Emmons (1996), who defines ambivalence as "an approach-avoidance conflict—wanting but at the same time not wanting the same goal object." Ambivalence can also be defined as a psychological state in which "a person holds mixed feelings (positive and negative) toward some psychological object" (Gardner, 1987, p. 241) and as such is fundamentally different from indifference, which is defined by the *absence* of positive and negative feelings toward an object (Thompson, Zanna, & Griffin, 1995). In the current chapter we will investigate the consequences of ambivalence in the context of (unhealthy) temptations and discuss how programs aimed at promoting healthier behavioral choices can be improved by taking the ambivalent structure of temptations into account.

Ambivalence is a topic that has been receiving an increasing amount of research attention in recent years (see van Harreveld, Nohlen, & Schneider, 2015, for an overview). As desires are inherently ambivalent, it is not surprising that ambivalence has also been investigated in the context of attitude objects that relate to temptations, such as chocolate (Sparks, Conner, James, Shepherd, & Povey, 2001), meat (Povey, Wellens, & Conner, 2001), drugs and condoms (Kane, 1990), smoking (Lipkus, Green, Feaganes, & Sedikides, 2001), *not* engaging in physical exercise (Sparks, Harris, & Lockwood, 2004), and dieting (Armitage & Arden, 2007).

When taking a closer look at ambivalence in the context of such unhealthy temptations, it becomes apparent that ambivalence toward unhealthy temptations is often characterized by a conflict between immediate pleasures (feeling good) and a superordinate goal (good health). More specifically, while we may be drawn toward sweets, fast food, cigarettes, alcohol, drugs, and unprotected casual sex because they provide us with immediate gratification, these desires are at odds with superordinate goals of losing weight, living healthily, and avoiding sexually transmitted disease. However, the reverse can also be the case. Ambivalence toward physical exercise and dieting is based on a tradeoff between short-term costs (becoming tired, being hungry) and long-term gains (becoming healthier). In both cases, however, the short-term component is more affective in nature, while the long-term component is more cognitive. Ambivalence toward these unhealthy desires therefore reflects what is known as affective–cognitive ambivalence (Lavine, 1998).

A second feature of ambivalence toward unhealthy temptations is that it is often based on a discrepancy between a more automatically activated attitude (e.g., "Smoking feels good") that has been overridden by a more reflective attitude ("Smoking is bad for me"). According to the Past Attitudes are Still There (PAST) model by Petty, Tormala, Brinol, and Jarvis (2006) this coexistence of automatically activated and more reflective attitudes is what is known as *implicit ambivalence*. People may become aware of such a conflict, for example, when they notice they are automatically reaching for the cookie jar and only then realize they are on a diet and have to restrain themselves. We will return to the consequences of such implicit ambivalence later in this chapter.

Finally, ambivalence toward unhealthy temptations often has a social element to it (Priester & Petty, 2001) in the sense that excessively giving in to temptations tends to be evaluated negatively by others. This is, for example, illustrated by the fact that overweight people are not only denigrated by thin people, but also by employers, potential romantic partners, and even by themselves (Crandall, 1994).

The Experience of Ambivalence

Because temptations are inherently tied to feelings of ambivalence it is important to understand the consequences of ambivalence. In general, *experiencing* ambivalence has repeatedly been associated with feelings of unpleasantness. In terms of what may cause this unpleasantness, it has been argued that ambivalence constitutes a violation of fundamental consistency motives (e.g., Jonas, Diehl, & Brömer, 1997; Maio, Bell, & Esses, 1996; McGregor, Newby-Clark, & Zanna, 1999; Newby-Clark, McGregor, & Zanna, 2002; Nordgren, van Harreveld, & van der Pligt, 2006). People are arguably motivated to be consistent in terms of their attitudes and behaviors (e.g., Festinger, 1964), and having mixed thoughts and/ or feelings about a topic does not fit with this motivation, as they make it impossible to keep one's behavior fully in line with one's attitudes, causing negative feelings. This is, for example, indicated by studies relating ambivalence to negative mood (Hass, Katz, Rizzo, Bailey, & Moore, 1992), negative physiological arousal (van Harreveld, Rutjens, Rotteveel, Nordgren, & van der Pligt, 2009a), negative behavior toward stigmatized persons (Katz, 1981) and even burnout, schizophrenia, and victimization (cf. Coser, 1976; Wexler, 1983).

Regardless of this fundamental need for consistency, many people have ambivalent attitudes about matters such as exercise, donating blood, eating fast food, drinking alcohol, or watching television while not constantly feeling torn and conflicted about these topics. In fact, some studies even have indicated that ambivalence can be positive (Pillaud, Cavazza, & Butera, 2013) and can be *negatively* associated with (negatively experienced) physiological arousal (Maio, Greenland, Bernard, & Esses, 2001). Thus it seems that conflicting thoughts and feelings are a prerequisite for ambivalence-induced negative affect but are not sufficient in themselves. Instead, situational factors also play a role.

One important situational factor is simultaneous accessibility. It has been shown that ambivalence is experienced as particularly unpleasant when the positive and negative components of the ambivalent attitude are simultaneously *accessible* and relevant to the situation, because then the ambivalent attitude holder becomes aware of his or her conflicting thoughts or feelings (Newby-Clark et al., 2002). For instance, many people have both positive and negative evaluations toward alcoholic beverages. They may view alcohol as a key ingredient of tasty drinks and as a social lubricant, but also as a potential cause of nausea and hangovers. Often these opposing evaluations are accessible and relevant at different times. The positive feelings toward alcoholic drinks may be more salient in the evening at the bar, while the negative feelings are more salient the following morning. However, there are also instances during which both evaluations are accessible at the same time, for example, when we are enjoying a few drinks after work until we see a colleague misbehave after having had a few too many. This situation causes the positive and negative components of the ambivalent attitude to become simultaneously accessible, resulting in the experience of ambivalence.

The notion that ambivalence can exist in a relatively dormant state on the one hand and can be subjectively experienced as unpleasant on the other is reflected in the different measures of ambivalence. Here a distinction is made between measures of *potential* and *felt* ambivalence. While measures of potential ambivalence (i.e., Kaplan, 1972) aim to assess the extent to which an individual has positive and negative associations with an attitude object, measures of felt ambivalence (i.e., Jamieson, 1993) measure the extent to which one feels "torn" between both sides of the attitude object.

Further exploring the situational influence on the experience of ambivalence, van Harreveld et al. (2009b), in their model of ambivalence-induced discomfort (MAID), argue that having to make a dichotomous evaluative choice for or against an ambivalent topic is a primary cause of simultaneous accessibility, and thus of discomfort. Of course, very often our ambivalent attitudes can remain noncommittal. Topics such as abortion and euthanasia may be associated with ambivalent thoughts for many people, but it is likely that the opposing evaluations will become irreconcilable only when the circumstances demand an unequivocal stance for or against, for example, in an election or due to personal circumstances such as unwanted pregnancy or a relative falling ill. Indeed, studies found ambivalence caused negative physiological arousal and negative emotions, especially when participants were forced to commit to one side or the other, but did not lead to more negative emotions when participants could stay uncommitted (van Harreveld et al., 2009a).

It is not surprising that one of the negative emotions evoked by ambivalent choices in this latter study was *regret*. Actions are associated with higher levels of regret than inaction (e.g., Gilovich & Medvec, 1994), and for an ambivalent attitude holder, having to make a discrete choice is an action and should thus lead to the anticipation of regret. We will return to the relation between regret and ambivalence later in this chapter.

These findings about the link between ambivalence and discomfort provide insight into the circumstances under which people feel bad about unhealthy temptations. Negative feelings are likely to arise when an unhealthy temptation presents itself, for example, in the form of a delicious apple pie, while at the same time we are aware of our commitment to a diet. This is when we become aware of a conflict between a super-ordinate goal (losing weight) and an immediate desire (eating delicious food). Perhaps somewhat counterintuitively, when a tradeoff between an immediate desire and a superordinate goal has to be made in tempting situations, the unpleasant nature of ambivalence may lead people toward unhealthy choices. The reason for this is that negative affective states lead people to let short-term gains prevail over long-term costs (Schwarz & Pollack, 1977; Wertheim & Schwarz, 1983; see also Lopez, Wagner, & Heatherton, Chapter 7, this volume). Thus, when deciding whether or not to order a piece of apple pie with one's coffee, being aware of one's ambivalent feelings about high-calorie foods can lead to negative affect, and this affective response can, in turn, lead to a decreased ability to resist temptation, as short-term gains (e.g., enjoying apple pie) outweigh long-term costs (gaining weight). Later in this chapter we will further discuss this notion that while people are quite bad at resisting temptation to begin with, they are even worse at controlling themselves when experiencing the negative affect that can be the result of ambivalence.

Coping Strategies

Clearly, people often experience ambivalence with regard to their temptations, and ambivalence may be experienced as unpleasant. There are two basic forms of dealing with the negative feelings associated with ambivalence: *emotion-focused* coping and *problem-focused* coping (cf. van Harreveld et al., 2009b). The former kind of coping is focused on diminishing the negative affective experience of ambivalence without targeting the source of ambivalence itself. The latter form of coping involves resolving ambivalence altogether and is aimed at obtaining an unequivocal— positive *or* negative—stance toward the cause of the ambivalence.

Emotion-focused coping involves efforts to feel better about an ambivalent choice without solving the problem itself (i.e., conflicting evaluations). When an ambivalent choice is imminent, for example whether to go to the gym or to sleep in, a very direct way to do this is postponing the ambivalent decision. A recent study by Nohlen, van Harreveld, van der Pligt, and Rotteveel (2014) has indeed shown that ambivalence leads to the delay of an ambivalent choice. A unique feature of ambivalence in the context of temptations is, of course, that this kind of ambivalence is based on a tradeoff between a desire for immediate gratification versus a long-term goal (see also Bitterly, Mislavsky, Dai, & Milkman, Chapter 12, this volume). Delaying the decision, therefore, often is a decision in itself, either one that reflects self-control (going to the gym) or the lack thereof (staying in bed).

Another form of emotion-focused coping is the attempt to redefine the situation, for example by denying one's responsibility for the decision. In the aforementioned example, one could downplay one's responsibility by exaggerating a slight injury.

Downplaying one's responsibility is likely to play an important role in the context of coping with ambivalence. Earlier we showed that feelings of (anticipated) regret play a role in causing discomfort for ambivalent attitude holders facing a decision. As there has to be a sense of responsibility for one's behavior for regret to occur (e.g., Zeelenberg, van Dijk, & Manstead, 1998), it is plausible that denial of responsibility for the chosen alternative can be effective in reducing the agony of ambivalence. Whether (and when) ambivalent attitude holders indeed employ this particular kind of emotion-focused coping has yet to be examined empirically.

Emotion-focused coping is thus aimed at making the experience of ambivalence less unpleasant. These coping strategies cannot always be employed, however. Some decisions cannot be postponed, and sometimes personal responsibility for one's decision cannot be denied. In these situations, problem-focused coping comes into play.

Problem-focused coping is more directly aimed at the root of the problem: the ambivalent attitude itself. Problem-focused coping with ambivalence-induced discomfort is aimed at eliminating the problem by (temporarily) changing the attitude and reducing ambivalence. For example, when one is ambivalent about whether or not to try an illicit drug one has never used before, a problem-focused approach is to increase confidence about the decision by attempting to swing the balance within the attitude to one evaluative side. This can be achieved by putting more emphasis on either the risky or on the pleasant nature of the drug. Similarities with research on cognitive dissonance can be drawn here (see McGregor et al., 1999), in the context of which it has been argued that bolstering consonant cognitions (Sherman & Gorkin, 1980) or trivializing or denying dissonant cognitions (Simon, Greenberg, & Brehm, 1995) can be effective in reducing feelings of dissonance by changing the attitude.

Whereas dissonance generally concerns situations where one has committed to a choice alternative, ambivalence often occurs in predecisional stages. This makes for an important difference between the two. As a result, ambivalent attitude holders are likely to be more motivated to invest cognitive resources in contemplating their decision than their postdecisional (dissonant) counterparts. Indeed, research has indicated that ambivalence is associated with increased cognitive activity (Monteith, Devine, & Zuwerink, 1993), more systematic processing (Jonas et al., 1997), a larger difference in effectiveness between strong and weak persuasive messages (Maio et al., 1996), greater ventrolateral prefrontal cortex (PFC) activity (Cunningham, Johnson, Gatenby, Gore, & Banaji, 2003), and a relatively more effortful process of integrating attributes when forming an attitude (van Harreveld, van der Pligt, De Vries, Wenneker, & Verhue, 2004; van Harreveld & van der Pligt, 2004). The idea that ambivalent attitude holders process information more extensively to reduce their ambivalence is supported by the aforementioned research by Maio and colleagues (1996) who found that ambivalent attitude holders were not only more receptive to the strong persuasive message, but this message also reduced their ambivalence.

It thus seems that ambivalent attitude holders are (at least sometimes) motivated to scrutinize attitude-relevant information with the aim of reducing ambivalence. This may not always be an effective tool in reaching this aim, however, as the available information may be ambivalent in itself. Scrutinizing such ambivalent information may only further increase ambivalence. Therefore, if the aim is to *reduce* ambivalence, a more selective kind of information processing may be more effective, where the ambivalent attitude holder selectively focuses on either the positive or the negative aspects of the topic at hand.

There are various ways in which selective focus on one side or the other can help one to obtain a less ambivalent attitude. For example, when the decision is imminent whether or not to eat a delicious but very rich piece of pie, one may either emphasize its positive attributes (it may in fact be the most delicious piece of pie one has ever tasted), downplay its negative attributes ("We will just go to the gym afterwards to burn the extra calories"), emphasize its negative attributes (one piece of pie equals an hour of suffering in the gym), or downplay its positive attributes ("It's probably not that good anyway"), a process much like that of the fox in the fable who cannot reach the grapes and decides they are sour). It appears that at least in the context of temptations, people may most effectively reduce their ambivalence by downplaying the immediate, positive attributes of the temptation. Johnson and Rusbult (1989) have, for example, shown that people who are most committed to their relationship particularly devalue potential alternative partners rather than enhance the attractiveness of their existing partner. Interestingly, people committed to their relationship do not devalue other potential partners indiscriminately, but do this especially with the attractive and threatening ones, underlining the likely motivational nature of this effect.

Aiming to tip the balance within one's attitude to one side may be an especially fruitful route in combating the unpleasant nature of ambivalence because such biased processing is cognitively less effortful than unbiased processing. Clark, Wegener, and Fabrigar (2008), for example, found that ambivalent attitude holders tend to focus on pro-attitudinal information and avoid counterattitudinal information. In other words, ambivalent attitude holders process information in accordance with the slight evaluative inclinations they may have.

More recent studies by Sawicki and colleagues (e.g., Sawicki et al., 2013) shed more light on this effect as they show that the effects of ambivalence on information seeking depend on knowledge about the ambivalent topic. Specifically, ambivalence was found to facilitate attitude-consistent exposure *only* when issue knowledge was low, arguably because less familiar information is perceived to be potentially effective in reducing ambivalence. However, when knowledge about the ambivalent topic was relatively high, more univalent attitudes were predictive of attitude-consistent information seeking.

Research has thus related ambivalence to both psychological discomfort and to more biased processing of information. Nordgren and colleagues (2006) tied these two effects together. First, they found that when ambivalent participants were able to attribute their discomfort to an external source (a placebo pill), they did not feel any ambivalence-induced discomfort. When such an external attribution was not possible (because they thought the pill would make them feel relaxed), ambivalence *was* associated with psychological discomfort. Second, the placebo pill manipulation also had an effect on information processing as measured with a thought-listing task. Participants who could not attribute their discomfort to an external source were more biased in their thoughts about the attitude object as compared to those who did have the possibility of attributing their discomfort to the pill. Moreover, the direction of this bias was predicted by the initial attitude. Participants who reported being ambivalent but in their overall attitudes leaned slightly toward one side of the evaluative continuum also tended to report more thoughts in relation to that particular side. This is plausible because it represents the most direct route toward a less ambivalent and more univalent attitude. This selective focus in terms of attitude-related thoughts was also effective in reducing ambivalence, as assessed by comparing the two measures of ambivalence. The results of this study thus indicate that biased systematic processing is a potentially effective tool in reducing the discomfort caused by ambivalence.

While this study indicates that ambivalent attitude holders can go through the effortful process of generating relatively one-sided thoughts (cf. biased systematic processing, Killeya & Johnson, 1998) with the aim of swinging the balance within their attitude to one side or the other, heuristic processing (Chaiken, 1980) can be a cognitively even more efficient way of obtaining a more one-sided attitude. Indeed, ambivalent attitude holders have been shown to process more heuristically than their non-ambivalent counterparts. For example, ambivalent attitude holders are less likely to check the reliability of information about the attitude object before being persuaded (Zemborain & Johar, 2007), and they are more persuaded by consensus information than those who are not ambivalent (Hodson, Maio, & Esses, 2001).

Adaptive Flexibility

Thus far we have shown several ways in which ambivalent attitude holders cope with the unpleasant nature of facing a decision that forces them to "jump off the fence" (van Harreveld et al., 2009a). Strategies range from changing aspects of the situation (by avoiding the decision or by cognitively redefining the situation) to addressing the root of the problem (the attitude itself) and striving toward a more unequivocal and less ambivalent attitude. According to the MAID (van Harreveld et al., 2009b), ambivalent attitude holders are flexible in the sense that they are likely to employ different coping strategies depending on the specific characteristics of the decision.

In the MAID model it is argued that when facing a decision, ambivalent attitude holders go through an effort–accuracy tradeoff that determines the preferred coping strategy. This is in accordance with Payne and colleagues (Payne, Bettman, & Johnson, 1993), who believe that decision makers have to trade off between two goals: minimizing cognitive effort and maximizing accuracy in terms of making the best possible decision. These incompatible goals drive the ambivalent decision maker toward different coping strategies. The goal of minimizing effort on the one hand leads decision makers toward the least demanding coping strategies (i.e., emotion-focused coping strategies). In accordance with a cognitive miser view, it has indeed been argued that delay is the first coping strategy that people are likely to turn to when facing a difficult decision (Luce, 1998; Luce, Bettman, & Payne, 1997). Cognitively redefining one specific decisional situation is also likely to be a strategy requiring less cognitive effort than changing one's preexisting attitude altogether. According to the MAID model, the accuracy motivation drives decision makers toward the problem-focused coping strategies, but these strategies also differ in terms of their required cognitive effort. Whether one goes through a process of carefully weighing the pros and cons of a decision or processes information in a more selective or heuristic way is also likely to be influenced by the relative strength of effort and accuracy motives.

The outcome of the tradeoff between the motive to maximize accuracy on the one hand and the motive to reduce cognitive effort on the other is thought to be determined by the extent to which regret is anticipated about potentially making the wrong decision (van Harreveld et al., 2009b). Take the example where you are asked by friends to join them and go out for drinks on a Friday night. On the one hand, you may be enthusiastic about going out after a week of hard work but anticipate an inconvenient hangover, especially because you have committed to spending the next day with your in-laws. The difficulty of the decision may be exacerbated by the anticipation of regret about making the wrong decision. If you go out for drinks, this may make the subsequent day even more gruesome than it would already be under normal circumstances.

However, if you decide to spend the night on the couch, you run the risk of being confronted by friends telling you stories about an epic night out on town. Anticipating regret about making the wrong decision in a situation like this is likely to promote accuracy motivations and thus a tendency toward more effortful coping strategies. This could be a careful weighing of the pros and cons of each of the two options. When regret about the decision is *not* anticipated, however (i.e., when the decision is less relevant), for example, because you are not likely to hear a lot of details about that Friday night from your friends, less effortful coping strategies are likely to ensue. Biased systematic processing (e.g., "John is coming as well and he is such a buzz killer" or "I will just take an aspirin in the morning and it will be fine") is an example of such a strategy, because this can be a more efficient way to reduce ambivalence than unbiased systematic processing.

Besides the anticipation of regret, the extent to which the cognitive resources required to process useful information are available also plays a role. Sometimes there simply is not enough time to carefully weigh the pros and cons, and the motivation to minimize cognitive effort will then logically prevail. Under these circumstances ambivalent attitude holders will resort to biased systematic processing or the arguably even less effortful heuristic processing.

There is some reason to believe that emotion-focused and problem-focused coping strategies can also be employed simultaneously. For example, Hanze (2001) found that ambivalence leads to both systematic processing as well as avoidance, and Ferrari and Dovidio (2000) have found that procrastinators search more extensively for attitude-relevant information. While this latter finding suggests that procrastination may be strategically employed to generate the time that is required to engage in more effortful coping, more recent studies by Nohlen et al. (2014) indicate that ambivalent attitude holders delay their choice simply because they want to distract themselves from the difficult (and thus presumably unpleasant) decision.

A final point that has to be made with respect to the prevalence of these coping strategies is that because choice situations are an important and straightforward cause of ambivalence-induced discomfort, we have chosen to discuss coping strategies in that context as well. However, the problem-focused coping strategies discussed here are also applicable to attitude holders who experience discomfort because their opposing evaluations have become salient for a different reason, such as in the example we gave earlier about enjoying a few drinks after work until seeing a colleague misbehave after having had a few too many. Recent research has indicated that simply the process of engaging in introspection about one's ambivalent attitude can render ambivalence unpleasant and spawn subsequent coping efforts (van Harreveld, Rutjens, Schneider, Nohlen, & Keskinis, 2014).

Ambivalence and Unhealthy Temptations

At the beginning of this chapter we argued that temptations are issues people are inherently ambivalent about (e.g., drinking, smoking, having unsafe sex, eating fast food). Above we have shown that ambivalent attitudes can be associated with different kinds of coping behavior, and we have aimed to shed light on the motivations that determine which coping strategies are deployed. In the following section we want to make the point that these insights have direct and indirect consequences for the choices people make about the temptations they are ambivalent about. Also, we aim to provide insights for those who design tools that aim to promote restraint in the context of ambivalent temptations.

Behavioral change campaigns addressing many of the aforementioned unhealthy behaviors involve persuasive messages in which, for example, the negative consequences of the focal behavior are emphasized and/or the positive consequences are downplayed. Such messages obviously require the motivation and ability to process the persuasive arguments. At first sight the role of ambivalence may seem quite clear: making people's ambivalent feelings toward (for example) smoking salient will lead to a negative affective response, which, in turn, will motivate them to carefully think about a persuasive message and generally make them more susceptible to efforts aimed at attitude change (e.g., Armitage, Conner, & Norman, 1999). While this may indeed be a viable strategy sometimes, the MAID model aims to predict *under which circumstances* this is the case. When there is plenty of time and cognitive resources, it seems advisable to rely on strength of persuasive arguments. However, in many cases decisions in tempting situations need to be made more quickly, and this leads ambivalent attitude holders toward less effortful processing primarily aimed at making a decision, not so much at making the best possible decision. Under these circumstances persuasive communication using source characteristics (e.g., reliability or attractiveness of a message source), for instance, is likely to be more effective.

The idiosyncrasies of ambivalence toward temptations also present those who aim to promote healthy behavior with a number of problems, and we will discuss three of them. First of all, as noted earlier, ambivalence toward unhealthy desires is often characterized by a conflict between affect ("the cigarette is going to taste great" "going to the gym is going to make me suffer") and cognition ("smoking is bad for my health," "going to the gym is going to help me lose weight"). Research (Lavine, 1998) indicating that affect usually drives behavior in such cases of affective–cognitive ambivalence is in line with the observation that people are terrible at resisting temptations to behave unhealthily, despite having the best intentions.

Similarly, research has suggested that valence components of an attitude become spontaneously activated when encountering an attitude object (e.g., Bargh, Chaiken, Raymond, & Hymes, 1996). Given that the affective reaction toward temptations is generally positive (one of desire, e.g., not going to the gym; eating chocolate cake), the approach response is initiated before later, more reflective processes can intervene and inhibit the approach response. As with the arguments of Petty and colleagues (2006) in their PAST model, insufficient motivation or capacity to consciously think about one's evaluation may lead to execution of the first response without intervention of more reflective processes. Situational factors may thus determine whether initial affective reactions guide behavior or whether later, more reflective processes adjust the behavioral response in line with overarching goals. For example, with respect to smoking cigarettes, the PAST model argues that when an ex-smoker has sufficient motivation and energy, she will be aware of the fact that she has rejected the initially positive response toward smoking cigarettes. However, in situations where the ex-smoker is tired or in a hurry, the initial (and more positive) reaction toward smoking will no longer be adjusted and the likelihood of succumbing to temptation increases.

The notion that ambivalence can be based on a discrepancy between initial responses and more reflective adjustments thus presents a significant challenge for those aiming to promote healthy behavioral decisions. Presenting one's audience with explicit persuasive arguments may be ineffective in influencing the quick evaluations that are predictive of actual spontaneous behavior. For persuasive communication to be effective, it is therefore important that it not only aim for explicit endorsement, but also target the attitude structure that underlies evaluations (i.e., associations).

The third and final potential pitfall posed by ambivalence in the context of promoting resistance to unhealthy temptations is directly related to the potentially unpleasant nature of ambivalence. More specifically, making people aware of their ambivalence and then expecting that the ensuing negative affect will lead them to carefully think about a subsequently presented persuasive message does not take into account the fact that negative affect also tends to lead to a decreased ability to resist temptation, as short-term gains (e.g., enjoying a cigarette) outweigh long-term costs (damaging one's health) (Schwarz & Pollack, 1977; Wertheim & Schwarz, 1983). In using ambivalence as a tool to make recipients more susceptible to persuasive messages, it is therefore important to realize that while ambivalence-induced negative affect may certainly help to draw the recipient's attention toward a persuasive message, the ambivalence-induced negative affect may also lead to a decreased ability to resist temptation. The idea that the experience of ambivalence may make one less resistant toward temptation is supported, for example, by research showing that when people are exposed to chocolate they are more likely to eat it if they previously were given the instruction to abstain from it (Stirling & Yeomans, 2004; Soetens, Braet, Van Vlierberghe, & Roets, 2008).

The reason behind these effects probably lies in the fact that resisting temptations requires self-control. It is a well-established finding that continuously exerting self-control diminishes the success of subsequent efforts at self-control (Muraven & Baumeister, 2000). In other words, when en route from work to home we drive past a number of tempting bakeries and successfully restrain ourselves from buying a delicious but very rich dessert, we may be less able to control our anger once we come home and see that our children took it upon themselves to paint the garage. Interestingly, self-control strength is specific to behaviors that require self-control. Thus, a task that requires thought suppression impairs subsequent self-control, while solving math problems does not have a similar effect (Muraven, Tice, & Baumeister, 1998).

In the current context, it is relevant that stress and the regulation of negative mood also deplete the resources required for self-control. As we have seen earlier, ambivalence choices (for example vis-à-vis temptations) are likely to be associated with negative mood and physiological arousal (e.g., van Harreveld et al., 2009a). Regulating the negative affective nature of ambivalence might thus draw the cognitive resources that are necessary for restraint. Being aware of one's ambivalence for a prolonged period of time can thus lead our self-control to crumble because of a depletion of resources. It has to be noted that recently the notion that self-control draws from a finite source was challenged by the idea that people strive for a balance between behaviors that satisfy "want-to goals" and those that are in the service of "have-to goals" (Inzlicht, Schmeichel, & Macrae, 2014). After successive satisfaction of "have-to goals" that serve the cognitive side of temptations, people may thus be motivated to shift their attention toward the affective side of temptation and be more inclined to fulfill their desires. Future research should indicate whether such striving for balance also plays a role with respect to coping with ambivalence toward temptations.

As a final note in this discussion about the problems that ambivalence toward temptation poses for attempts to promote healthier choices in the context of temptations, we want to discuss a line of research suggesting that the presentation of an unhealthy temptation can also increase the activation of long-term healthy goals. Kroese, Evers, and De Ridder (2009) showed that participants who saw a picture of a chocolate cake subsequently made a healthier snack choice than participants who saw a picture of a flower. Kroese and colleagues argue that this is because being exposed to the temptation activates goal importance. In this case, of course, the picture of the cake was not an actual temptation as participants could not eat the picture.

Related research by Fishbach and Zhang (2008) suggests that the way the temptation is *presented* may influence whether people are likely to give in to it or let the long-term goal prevail. Their research indicates that when healthy and unhealthy foods (e.g., a can of Coke and a bunch of strawberries) are presented together in a unified choice set (in one image), the two goals complement each other and people balance between them. This leads people to make the unhealthy choice now and balance this decision with the intention to make the healthy choice later. However, if the healthy and unhealthy foods are presented separately (in two images), people conclude that the goals are competing against each other. Because of this incompatibility of the goals, people highlight the pursuit of the more important long-term goal and thus are inclined to resist temptation. More research is certainly needed to elucidate when and why these ironic effects of exposure to temptation occur and when it is better to not lead people into temptation.

Conclusions

While desires direct our behavior toward the fulfillment of important needs, we are also expected to control these desires, as not doing so can be both physically and socially unhealthy. This inherent ambivalence toward certain desires is what defines temptations, and we have aimed to shed more light on the consequences of the ambivalent nature of temptations.

We have first shown that ambivalence can be experienced as unpleasant. This is the case when the conflict between associations becomes salient, for example, when a decision has to be made, or even through introspecting about one's ambivalence. Experiencing negative affect as a consequence of ambivalence initiates efforts to reduce discomfort. This can be achieved either through the relatively low-effort emotion-focused coping or through a more effortful process of problem-focused coping. While the former involves changing the context in such a way that the ambivalence is no longer experienced as problematic (e.g., by delaying the decision), the latter directly targets the ambivalent attitude and leads to a more one-sided, unequivocal attitude. Because of the less effortful nature of emotion-focused coping, this is what ambivalent attitude holders first turn to when facing a decision. When emotion-focused coping is not possible, however, problem-focused coping strategies are deployed, including both high-effort and low-effort strategies. Which of these is used depends on the tradeoff between the motivation to make the best possible decision and the motivation to minimize expended cognitive effort. Besides motivation, ability obviously also plays a role. For example, when we are tired after a long day at work and shopping for food, we may be too depleted to invest the cognitive resources required to adequately weigh the pros and cons of the unhealthy but convenient pizza.

While motivation and ability are important factors in determining how we cope with ambivalence, they also have a more direct influence on the decisions we make with regard to temptations. Initial reactions to temptations are positive, and only with sufficient motivation and ability can the initial reaction be overridden by more reflective processes that take future consequences into account. Thus, motivation and ability are crucial in sustaining healthy behavior.

We have discussed these insights into the consequences of ambivalence in the context of aims to promote healthy choices in tempting situations. Awareness about ambivalence is a potentially useful tool in this respect. Making people aware of their ambivalence toward temptations might help draw attention to a persuasive message because this message may help reduce the unpleasant experience of ambivalence. However, there are a number of pitfalls one has to be aware of in this respect. For example, negative affect (which can result from ambivalence) is known to lead people to let short-term goals (e.g., having a few "relaxing" drinks) prevail over long-term goals (protecting one's liver) because emotion regulation is also cognitively effortful. When cognitive efforts that are in line with "have-to goals" are spent continuously, we strive for a balance and are more likely to shift our attention to "want-to goals," thus giving in to unhealthy short-term gratifications (Inzlicht et al., 2014). Being aware of our ambivalence can thus even backfire.

It becomes all the more clear why it is so extremely difficult to promote healthy behavioral decisions in tempting situations. Many temptations present themselves when we are tired, distracted, or perhaps even drunk, circumstances under which we are not very willing or able to think carefully about the pros and cons of the available options. This is when the want-to goals (usually in favor of giving in to the temptation) are a more likely determinant of choice than have-to goals, which are usually in favor of restraint. The fact that cravings (e.g., for cigarettes, sex, alcohol, fatty foods) also play a role in many tempting situations only adds to the strength of short-term motives in these situations.

The frequent lack of motivation and/or resources to think about our attitudes and decisions is a challenge when aiming to promote healthy choices in tempting situations. Given the low-effort nature of delay as a strategy to cope with ambivalence, it may be that persuading tempted decision makers to delay their choice is a relatively fruitful strategy. As argued above, procrastination is employed as a coping strategy simultaneously with strategies that require more elaborate thinking (Hanze, 2001; Ferrari & Dovidio, 2000). Choice delay may, for example, not be merely an avoidant strategy; it may also create the time that is needed to carefully weigh one's options (Nohlen et al., 2014). Persuading tempted decision makers to defer their choice may eventually lead them toward healthier decisions.

Even without the time created through procrastination, there are fortunately cases in which we have time to decide whether to indulge or not, for example, when the choice to indulge is made throughout a certain period of time. Think of a situation where one had decided to go to the gym first thing Saturday morning but upon waking up has chosen to sleep in instead. In certain cases, going to the gym will remain an option throughout the day, and the choice to indulge will therefore have to be reevaluated continuously. In such cases there is time for a more careful assessment of the (tempting) situation, and the conscious attitude based on long-term goals has a greater chance to (eventually) influence our behavior. It thus appears that in promoting healthier choices in the context of temptations, "buying time" may be an important strategy simply because it gives tempted decision makers more time to think and the long-term goals a greater chance to prevail.

In this chapter we have discussed the consequences of ambivalence for human behavior in the context of temptations. We have aimed to make clear that using the ambivalent nature of temptations as a tool to promote restraint is a double-edged sword. On the one hand, the negative affect that may be associated with ambivalence can lead short-term goals (and thus indulgences) to prevail. On the other hand, it also makes ambivalent attitude holders more susceptible to processing persuasive information that promotes restraint. While these insights provide a number of guidelines for those aiming to promote healthy decisions in tempting situations, there is sufficient reason to be ambivalent about our ambivalence toward temptations.

REFERENCES

Armitage, C. J., & Arden, M. A. (2007). Felt and potential ambivalence across the stages of change. *Journal of Health Psychology, 12,* 149–158.

Armitage, C. J., Conner, M., & Norman, P. (1999). Differential effects of mood on information processing: Evidence from the theories of reasoned action and planned behaviour. *European Journal of Social Psychology, 29,* 419–433.

Baumeister, R. F. (2002). Yielding to temptation: Self-control failure, impulsive purchasing, and consumer behaviour. *Journal of Consumer Research, 28,* 670–676.

Bargh, J. A., Chaiken, S., Raymond, P., & Hymes, C. (1996). The automatic evaluation effect: Unconditional automatic attitude activation with a pronunciation task. *Journal of Experimental Social Psychology, 32,* 104–128.

Chaiken, S. (1980). Heuristic versus systematic information processing and the use of source versus message cues in persuasion. *Journal of Personality and Social Psychology, 39,* 752–766.

Clark, J. K., Wegener, D. T., & Fabrigar, L. R. (2008). Attitudinal ambivalence and message-based persuasion: Motivated processing of proattitudinal information and avoidance of counterattitudinal information. *Personality and Social Psychology Bulletin, 34,* 565–577.

Coser, R. L. (1976). Authority and structural ambivalence in the middle-class family. In L. A. Coser & B. Rosenberg (Eds.), *Sociological theory.* New York: Macmillan.

Crandall, C. S. (1994). Prejudice against fat people: Ideology and self-interest. *Journal of Personality and Social Psychology, 66,* 882–894.

Cunningham, W. A., Johnson, M. K., Gatenby, J. C. G., Gore, J. C., & Banaji, M. R. (2003). Neural components of social evaluation. *Journal of Personality and Social Psychology, 85,* 639–649.

Emmons, R. A. (1996). Strivings and feeling: Personal goals and subjective well-being. In P. M. Gollwitzer & J. A. Bargh (Eds.), *The psychology of action: Linking cognition and motivation to behavior* (pp. 313–337). New York: Guilford Press.

Ferrari, J. R., & Dovidio, J. F. (2000). Examining behavioral processes in indecision: Decisional procrastination and decision-making style. *Journal of Research in Personality, 34*, 127–137.

Festinger, L. (1964). *Conflict, decision, and dissonance.* Stanford, CA: Stanford University Press.

Fishbach, A., & Zhang, Y. (2008). Together or apart: When goals and temptations complement versus compete. *Journal of Personality and Social Psychology, 94*, 547–559.

Gardner, P. L. (1987). Measuring ambivalence to science. *Journal of Research in Science Teaching, 24*, 241–247.

Gilovich, T., & Medvec, V. H. (1994). The temporal pattern to the experience of regret. *Journal of Personality and Social Psychology, 67*, 357–365.

Hanze, M. (2001). Ambivalence, conflict, and decision making: Attitudes and feelings in Germany toward NATO's military intervention in the Kosovo war. *European Journal of Social Psychology, 31*, 693–706.

Hass, R. G., Katz, I., Rizzo, N., Bailey, J., & Moore, L. (1992). When racial ambivalence evokes negative affect, using a disguised measure of mood. *Personality and Social Psychology Bulletin, 18*, 786–797.

Hodson, G., Maio, G. R., & Esses, V. M. (2001). The role of attitudinal ambivalence in susceptibility to consensus information. *Basic and Applied Social Psychology, 23*, 197–205.

Inzlicht, M., Schmeichel, B. J., & Macrae, C. N. (2014). Why self-control seems (but may not be) limited. *Trends in Cognitive Sciences, 18*, 127–133.

Jamieson, D. W. (1993, August). *The attitude ambivalence construct: Validity, utility, and measurement.* Paper presented at the annual meeting of the American Psychological Association, Toronto, Ontario, Canada.

Johnson, D. J., & Rusbult, C. E. (1989). Resisting temptation: Devaluation of alternative partners as a means of maintaining commitment in close relationships. *Journal of Personality and Social Psychology, 57*, 967–980.

Jonas, K., Diehl, M., & Brömer, P. (1997). Effects of attitudinal ambivalence on information processing and attitude-intention consistency. *Journal of Experimental Social Psychology, 33*, 190–210.

Kane, S. (1990). AIDS, addiction and condom use: Sources of sexual risk for heterosexual women. *Journal of Sex Research, 27*, 427–444.

Kaplan, K. J. (1972). On the ambivalence–indifference problem in attitude theory and measurement: A suggested modification of the semantic differential technique. *Psychological Bulletin, 77*, 361–372.

Katz, I. (1981). *Stigma: A social psychological analysis.* Hillsdale, NJ: Erlbaum.

Killeya, L. A., & Johnson. B. T. (1998). Experimental induction of biased systematic processing: The directed-thought technique. *Personality and Social Psychology Bulletin, 23*, 17–33.

Kroese, F. M., Evers, C., & de Ridder, D. T. D. (2009). How chocolate keeps you slim: The effect of food temptations on weight watching goal importance, intentions and eating behaviour. *Appetite, 53*, 430–433.

Lavine, H. (1998). On the primacy of affect in the determination of attitudes and behavior: The moderating role of affective–cognitive ambivalence. *Journal of Experimental Social Psychology, 34*, 398–421.

Lewin, K. (1935). Environmental forces in child behavior and development. In K. Lewin (Ed), *A dynamic theory of personality* (pp. 66–113). New York: McGraw-Hill.

Lipkus, I. M., Green, J. D., Feaganes, J. R., & Sedikides, C. (2001). *Journal of Applied Social Psychology, 31,* 113–133.

Luce, M. F. (1998). Choosing to avoid: Coping with negatively emotion-laden consumer decisions. *Journal of Consumer Research, 24,* 409–433.

Luce, M. F., Bettman, J. R., & Payne, J. W. (1997). Choice processing in emotionally difficult decisions. *Journal of Experimental Psychology: Learning, Memory, and Cognition, 23,* 384–405.

Maio, G. R., Bell, D. W., & Esses, V. M. (1996). Ambivalence and persuasion: The processing of messages about immigrant groups. *Journal of Experimental Social Psychology, 32,* 513–536.

Maio, G. R., Greenland, K., Bernard, M., & Esses, V. M. (2001). Effects of intergroup ambivalence on information processing: The role of physiological arousal. *Group Processes and Intergroup Relations, 4,* 355–372.

McGregor, I., Newby-Clark, I. R., & Zanna, M. P. (1999). "Remembering" dissonance: Simultaneous accessibility of inconsistent cognitive elements moderates epistemic discomfort. In E. Harmon-Jones & J. Mills (Eds.), *Cognitive dissonance: Progress on a pivotal theory in social psychology* (pp. 325–352). Washington, DC: American Psychological Association.

Monteith, M. J., Devine, P. G., & Zuwerink, J. R. (1993). Self-directed versus other-directed affect as a consequence of prejudice-related discrepancies. *Journal of Personality and Social Psychology, 64,* 198–210.

Muraven, M., & Baumeister, R. F. (2000). Self-regulation and depletion of limited resources: Does self-control resemble a muscle? *Psychological Bulletin, 126,* 247–259.

Muraven, M., Tice, D. M., & Baumeister, R. F. (1998). Self-control as a limited resource: Regulatory depletion patterns. *Journal of Personality and Social Psychology, 74,* 774–789.

Newby-Clark, I. R., McGregor, I., & Zanna, M. P. (2002). Thinking and caring about cognitive inconsistency: When and for whom does attitudinal ambivalence feel uncomfortable? *Journal of Personality and Social Psychology, 82,* 157–166.

Nohlen, H. U., Van Harreveld, F., van der Pligt, J., & Rotteveel, M. (2014). *A waste of time?: The prevalence and effectiveness of choice delay in ambivalent decision-making.* Manuscript under review.

Nordgren, L. F., Van Harreveld, F., & van der Pligt, J. (2006). Ambivalence, discomfort, and motivated information processing. *Journal of Experimental Social Psychology, 42,* 252–258.

Payne, J. W., Bettman, J. R., & Johnson, E. J. (1993). *The adaptive decision maker.* Cambridge, UK: Cambridge University Press.

Petty, R. E., Tormala, Z. L., Brinol, P., & Jarvis, W. B. G. (2006). Implicit ambivalence from attitude change: An exploration of the PAST model. *Journal of Personality and Social Psychology, 90,* 21–41.

Pillaud, V., Cavazza, N., & Butera, F. (2013). The social value of being ambivalent: Self-presentational concerns in the expression of attitudinal ambivalence. *Personality and Social Psychology Bulletin, 39,* 1139–1151.

Povey, R., Wellens, B., & Conner, M. (2001). Attitudes towards following meat, vegetarian and vegan diets: an examination of the role of ambivalence. *Appetite, 37,* 15–26.

Priester, J. R., & Petty, R. E. (2001). Extending the bases of subjective attitudinal ambivalence: Interpersonal and intrapersonal antecedents of evaluative tension. *Journal of Personality and Social Psychology, 80,* 19–34.

Sawicki, V., Wegener, D. T., Clark, J. K., Fabrigar, L. R., Smith, S. M., & Durso, G. R. O. (2013). Feeling conflicted and seeking information: When ambivalence enhances and diminishes selective exposure to attitude-consistent information. *Personality and Social Psychology Bulletin, 39*, 735–747.

Schwarz, J. C., & Pollack, P. R. (1977). Affect and delay of gratification. *Journal of Research in Personality, 11*, 147–164.

Sherman, S. J., & Gorkin, L. (1980). Attitude bolstering when behavior is inconsistent with central attitudes. *Journal of Experimental Social Psychology, 16*, 388–403.

Simon, L., Greenberg, J., & Brehm, J. (1995). Trivialization: The forgotten mode of dissonance reduction. *Journal of Personality and Social Psychology, 68*, 247–260.

Soetens, B., Braet, C., Van Vlierbergh, L., & Roets, A. (2008). Resisting temptation: Effects of exposure to a forbidden food on eating behaviour. *Appetite, 51*, 202–205.

Sparks, P., Conner, M., James, R., Shepherd, R., & Povey, R. (2001). Ambivalence about health behaviours: An exploration in the domain of food choice. *British Journal of Social Psychology, 6*, 53–68.

Sparks, P., Harris, P. H., & Lockwood, N. (2004). Predictors and predictive effects of ambivalence. *British Journal of Social Psychology, 43*, 371–383.

Stirling, L. J., & Yeomans, M. R. (2004). Effect of exposure to a forbidden food on eating in restrained and unrestrained women. *International Journal of Eating Disorders, 35*, 59–68.

Thompson, M. M., Zanna, M. P., & Griffin, D. W. (1995). Let's not be indifferent about (attitudinal) ambivalence. In R. E. Petty & J. A. Krosnick (Eds.), *Attitude strength: Antecedents and consequences* (pp. 361–386). Hillsdale, NJ: Erlbaum.

van Harreveld, F., Nohlen, H. U., & Schneider, I. K. (2015). The ABC of ambivalence: Affective, behavioral and cognitive consequences of attitudinal conflict. In M. P. Zanna & J. Olson (Eds.), *Advances in experimental social psychology* (vol. 52). New York: Academic Press.

van Harreveld, F., Rutjens, B. T., Rotteveel, M., Nordgren, L. F., & van der Pligt (2009). Ambivalence and decisional conflict as a cause of psychological discomfort: Feeling tense when jumping off the fence. *Journal of Experimental Social Psychology, 45*, 167–173.

van Harreveld, F., Rutjens, B. T., Schneider, I. K., Nohlen, H. U., & Keskinis, K. (2014). In doubt and disorderly: Ambivalence promotes compensatory perceptions of order. *Journal of Experimental Psychology: General, 143*, 1666–1676.

van Harreveld, F., & van der Pligt, J. (2004). Attitudes as stable and transparent constructions. *Journal of Experimental Social Psychology, 40*, 666–674.

van Harreveld, F., van der Pligt, J., & de Liver, Y. N. (2009). The agony of ambivalence and ways to resolve it: Introducing the MAID model. *Personality and Social Psychology Review, 13*, 45–61.

van Harreveld, F., van der Pligt, J., De Vries, N. K., Wenneker, C., & Verhue, D. (2004). Ambivalence and information integration in attitudinal judgment. *British Journal of Social Psychology, 43*, 431–447.

Wertheim, E. H., & Schwarz, J. C. (1983). Depression, guilt, and self-management of pleasant and unpleasant events. *Journal of Personality and Social Psychology, 45*, 884–889.

Wexler, P. (1983). *Critical social psychology.* London: Routledge & Kegan Paul.

Zeelenberg, M., van Dijk, W. W., & Manstead, A. S. R. (1998). Reconsidering the relation between regret and responsibility. *Organizational Behavior and Human Decision Processes, 74*, 254–272.

Zemborain, M. R., & Johar, G. V. (2007). Attitudinal ambivalence and openness to persuasion: A framework for interpersonal influence. *Journal of Consumer Research, 33*, 506–514.

CHAPTER 14

Desires and Happiness

Aristotelian, Puritan, and Buddhist Approaches

Shigehiro Oishi
Erin Westgate
Jane Tucker
Asuka Komiya

What Is Desire? What Is Happiness?

In this volume, desire is defined as wants that are linked to motivation, pleasure, and reward. In conventional terms, then, desire includes low-level physical cravings (e.g., water, food, sex), acquired cravings (e.g., alcohol, cigarettes, the *New York Times*), and, in a broader sense, even ideals that do not necessarily involve craving or withdrawal (e.g., a big house, promotion). In this chapter, we discuss the role of desire in happiness, centering on two questions: "Are desires a blessing or a curse?" and "Does the satisfaction of desires lead to happiness?" First, we provide our definition of happiness. We then summarize the existing literature on (1) the possession of desire and happiness, and (2) the satisfaction of desire and happiness. Next, we review various theoretical accounts of desires and happiness, after which we present two approaches to the dilemma of desires: a Puritan approach and a Buddhist approach. Finally, we provide our own framework that classifies desire according to two types (cravings versus ideals) and two targets of desire (self versus others) to integrate our diverse and sometimes confusing findings.

According to Aristotle, happiness (Greek *eudaimonia*) is not a fleeting feeling but consists of a series of activities in accordance with one's virtues, ultimately culminating in a fulfilling life (Thomson, 1953). Far from an idle state, the Aristotelian conception of happiness requires the full utilization of one's mental and physical faculties. For this reason,

Aristotle often equates the happy life with the contemplative life, yet contemplation is not enough. In addition to leading a fulfilling life, Aristotelian happiness requires favorable objective conditions such as a minimum level of wealth, good looks, physical health, and good relationships. He states, "We are now in a position to define the happy man as 'one who is active in accordance with complete virtue, and who is adequately furnished with external goods, and that not for some unspecified period but throughout a complete life'" (Thomson, 1953, p. 84). In short, Aristotelian happiness captures the virtuous and philosophical life of the privileged. He also emphasizes that virtuous actions give rise to the feeling of pleasure or pain in the *right* manner and at the *right* time (Nussbaum, 1986, 2001). A virtuous life is not just a merry life, but a deeply satisfying one.

Whereas a virtuous life evokes ideals of moral loftiness and integrity, some of which may elude reliable self-report, a satisfying life is more amenable to self-disclosure. Wayne Sumner (1996), a philosopher, conceptualizes authentic happiness as a subjective sense of life satisfaction. A shift from the Aristotelian virtue-centric concept of happiness to Sumner's subjective sense of satisfaction makes it easier for psychologists to investigate happiness. In the present chapter, therefore, we use Sumner's definition of happiness as "a subjective sense of life satisfaction" rather than the Aristotelian definition of a virtuous life.

To be sure, no one can make a fully informed judgment about his or her overall life. Our life satisfaction judgments, like any other complex judgments, may be distorted or biased in certain ways (Schwarz & Strack, 1999). However, despite some inevitable distortion from objective reality, people's self-reported levels of life satisfaction tend to be reliably corroborated by their spouse, family members, and friends (Schneider & Schimmack, 2009). Thus, in a typical survey context, people are able to form an informed judgment about their life satisfaction and seem to report their life satisfaction honestly, and a well-validated life satisfaction scale such as the Satisfaction with Life Scale (SWLS; Diener, Emmons, Larsen, & Griffin, 1985) may therefore capture reliable variance in people's long-term happiness. In this chapter, we use the term *happiness* to refer to a relatively stable sense of life satisfaction, or a sense that life is going well. When we use it to refer to a fleeting momentary mood of pleasantness and cheerfulness, we denote it as a happy mood.

The Role of Desires in Happiness

Is Having Desires a Blessing or a Curse?

When it comes to happiness, desires can be something of a double-edged sword. A life devoid of desire might strike many as bleak, and, indeed, apathy and amotivation are widely considered symptoms of depression (Beck, 1967, pp. 263–264; see also Treadway, Chapter 15, this volume). In fact, desires can certainly have a positive impact on our happiness (see also Kringelbach & Berridge, Chapter 6, this volume); the desire to achieve personal goals positively influences our lives, and commitment to and attainment of personal goals enhances satisfaction with life (Brunstein, 1993). People who are pursuing their most important goals are happier, both in terms of life satisfaction (Brunstein, 1993) and positive affect (Emmons, 1986) than those who are not. Indeed, many researchers have found that it is not enough to look at people's objective life circumstances in determining their happiness; instead, it is the concordance between objective circumstances and our desires or aspirations that predicts how happy we are (Diener & Fujita, 1995; Plagnol & Easterlin, 2008; Stutzer, 2004).

At the same time, however, research cautions that the *desire* to attain personal goals is not, by itself, enough. In order for personal goals to contribute to happiness, one must actually *attain* them. Discrepancies between what you desire and what you have actually achieved can lead to hopelessness, unhappiness, and dissatisfaction. In a longitudinal study, Nickerson, Schwarz, Diener, and Kahneman (2003) found that desiring financial success was negatively associated with overall happiness, job satisfaction, and satisfaction with friends. However, this was true only for people with lower incomes. That is, wealthy people who desired (and had achieved) financial success experienced few negative consequences with regard to their friendships, happiness, or job satisfaction, but poorer people who desired (but had not achieved) financial success were likely to be unhappy and less satisfied with their jobs and friendships. However, even for wealthy people, the desire for financial success was not wholly benign; despite being financially well off, wealthy people who desired financial success expressed less satisfaction with their family lives.

Several studies by Solberg, Diener, Wirtz, Lucas, and Oishi help to further illustrate the dangers of desires that seem to lie tantalizingly out of reach. In one such study (2002), participants were asked to imagine that they were middle class and that people wealthier than them possessed items that were either more or less desirable than their own—items which, by virtue of their lesser wealth, the participants presumably could not afford. They were then asked how satisfied they were with their imagined middle-class income. In a second similar study, participants were asked to imagine their current desires as well as their actual anticipated future annual income. After being informed that they either would or would not be able to afford what they desired in the future, they were then asked how satisfied they were with their anticipated future income. In both cases, participants who perceived more discrepancy between their desires and their actual states felt less satisfied with their income than those who did not. That is, people were less satisfied with their own income when they were told that wealthier people owned more desirable items as well as when they were told that they could not achieve their desires with their anticipated future income, all highlighting the fact that while desire may sometimes positively influence our lives, this is less likely to be the case for desires that we expect to go unfulfilled.

Research on materialism, or the tendency to place value on material acquisitions, has also suggested that desire can impair happiness, and that the desire for material goods can be a symptom of unhappiness. A meta-analysis concluded that on the whole, materialists are less happy than nonmaterialists (see Burroughs & Rindfleisch, 2002; Kasser, 2002, for review). Norris and Larsen (2011) hypothesized that since materialists want more than what they have and focus on the discrepancy between the two, they should feel less life satisfaction than nonmaterialists. Supporting this hypothesis, they found that materialists were indeed less happy than nonmaterialists, a discrepancy explained by the extent to which materialists wanted more than they had.

What about education? By opening the door to greater opportunity, might education serve as a buffer against some of the pitfalls of desire, such as the unhappiness that comes from desiring what one cannot realistically obtain? Unfortunately, the answer appears to be "no." In fact, more educated people are even more likely to desire what they do not have and less likely to be happy. Campbell, Converse, and Rodgers (1976) found that college graduates live in nicer houses in nicer neighborhoods, yet they are no more satisfied with their housing or neighborhood than high school graduates. By opening the door to more options and opportunities, education may actually foster ambition and desires for things that may or may not ultimately be attainable (see also Michalos, 1985).

Always wanting "the best" might also be particularly pernicious. People who actively seek the best possible outcomes may be successful in terms of occupational status and income, but they tend to be less happy (Schwartz et al., 2002; Iyengar, Wells, & Schwartz, 2006; see, however, Diab, Gillespie, & Highhouse, 2008, for the null findings). Barry Schwartz and his colleagues conducted a series of studies, showing that "maximizers," who want to make the best choice possible and thus closely examine every available option, feel less happy and experience less life satisfaction than "satisficers," who are satisfied with the first choice that is "good enough" to meet their basic requirements (Schwartz et al., 2002). Maximizers may expect greater success and thus compare their current situation (no matter how good) to potentially better outcomes. They often do this by comparing themselves to other successful people, which can only confirm their own relative perceived "shortcomings." Accordingly, dissatisfaction quickly arises despite the fact that maximizers actually fare quite well by objective standards. For example, Iyengar et al. (2006) reported that maximizers are more likely to be admitted to top-15 universities in the United States and obtain higher-salary jobs following graduation than their satisficer counterparts (indeed, every one-unit increase in the composite maximizing score was associated with a $2,630 increase in annual salary!). However, despite being objectively more successful, maximizers were actually *less* happy than satisficers, because maximizers tended to focus on what they could not obtain, opening themselves up to strong feelings of regret. In the end, the satisficers, who were not as successful as the maximizers in terms of occupational status or income, were the happier of the two.

Related to satisficing, when goals are too difficult or simply impossible to attain, disengagement from goals appears to be conducive for happiness. For instance, Miller and Wrosch (2007) found that adolescents high in ability to disengage from difficult or impossible goals showed healthy levels of C-reactive protein, whereas those low in goal disengagement showed an increase in C-reactive protein over time. Thus, although the pursuit of personally important goals is associated with happiness in general (e.g., Emmons, 1986), mindless pursuit of impossible goals is not.

Finally, recent studies found that wanting to be happy itself might be detrimental to happiness (see Gruber, Mauss, & Tamir, 2011, for review). For instance, wanting to be happy was associated with loneliness and social disconnection. Of course, the causal direction could lead from loneliness to wanting to be happy rather than the other way around. Nevertheless, wanting to be happy might not be a productive desire for happiness.

Does the Satisfaction of Desires Lead to Happiness?

Desires by themselves may be a mixed blessing, but what about satisfying one's desires? Surely getting what you want must make people happy. To answer this question, Oishi, Schimmack, and Diener (2001) asked undergraduates to keep a daily diary, which they used to examine the relationship between participants' daily experiences of physical pleasures (e.g., food and sex) and happiness on that day. They found that people generally felt happier on days when they fulfilled their physical desires, compared to days when they did not (the average within-person $r = .43$, $p < .01$). In addition, average physical pleasure over the 23 days was positively associated with life satisfaction ($r = .28$, $p < .01$). Thus, overall, the satisfaction of physical pleasures was moderately associated with daily satisfaction and long-term life satisfaction. Interestingly, not everyone experienced this boost in happiness. Sensation seekers, who look for novel, exciting experiences, obtained more happiness from physical pleasure than non–sensation seekers. Overall, though, these findings suggest that at least some kinds of pleasure can lead to happiness, depending on what people seek and desire.

In a similar study, Tay and Diener (2011) analyzed nationally representative data from 123 nations and found that the satisfaction of basic needs (e.g., food, shelter) was moderately and positively associated with life evaluation (the appraisal of where one's current life stands on a ladder scale from 0 to 10, $r = .31$). Satisfaction of basic needs was much more strongly associated with positive life evaluation than satisfaction of the need for safety/security, social support/love, mastery, or autonomy (r's ≤ .18). In contrast, satisfaction of the need for social support/love ($r = .29$), respect ($r = .36$), mastery ($r = .29$), and autonomy ($r = .26$) was more strongly associated with positive feelings than the satisfaction of basic needs ($r = .12$). In general, the satisfaction of various desires is positively associated with life satisfaction and positive affect, although the magnitude of the association varies depending on the indicator of happiness used, as well as the types of desires.

What about with regard to more high-level desires, such as the desire for financial success, or the attention of a loved one? Of course, satisfying a desire generally indicates that the current situation has improved, and it is natural to expect that such satisfaction should bring happiness. As noted earlier, achieving personal goals does in fact lead to happiness (Brunstein, 1993; Emmons, 1986), particularly if they are the right kinds of goals. For instance, Sheldon and Kasser (1998) showed that the satisfaction of goals consistent with a person's intrinsic psychological needs (e.g., self-acceptance, intimacy, or community involvement) leads to greater happiness than achieving more extrinsic goals, such as financial success, physical attractiveness, or popularity. To the extent that a desire involves the satisfaction of intrinsic psychological needs, fulfilling it may afford similar benefits to happiness (see, however, Oishi & Diener, 2001; Oishi, Diener, Lucas, & Suh, 1999, for cultural differences in the type of goal attainment). Likewise, as discussed earlier, many studies have shown that people are happier when the gap between their current circumstances and aspirations is small, suggesting that satisfying one's aspirations may be generally associated with well-being (Plagnol & Easterlin, 2008; Stutzer, 2004).

Even if the satisfaction of some desires or aspirations leads to happiness, however, it would be premature to conclude that desires are, on the whole, a good thing to have. Might we be better off if we did not have any desires that required satisfaction in the first place? Even fulfilled desires can breed their own problems, which may acquire a life of their own and endure even after the initial desire is achieved. Richard Easterlin, a very prominent economist and researcher on happiness, noted this fact as early as the 1970s in what has come to be called the "Easterlin paradox." Easterlin (1974) argued that material wealth was strongly related to happiness at the individual level, but not nearly so much at the national level. He looked at happiness data from the United States during a period of rapid economic growth—from 1946 to 1970—and found that levels of happiness remained essentially unchanged throughout the period, despite the rapid increase in personal income. Easterlin attributed this stability in happiness to the influence of social comparison processes:

people judge their levels of financial well-being not against some objective criterion but against that of others. Thus, economic development did not necessarily lead to greater happiness because as incomes rose, the standard of consumption rose with them. As the economy grows, people's desires grow, too: they want a newer car, a larger house, more expensive jewelry, leaping from one desire to the next as each is "fulfilled" in turn. Even worse, because such success is relative to the success of others, it invites people to embark on an infinite consumption race, leading everyone to nearly inevitable dissatisfaction and unhappiness (Frank, 1997).

That increases in income are accompanied by a nearly inevitable increase in material aspirations has been documented extensively by economists since Easterlin first pointed out this paradox. Thus, although income may temporarily lead to increased happiness, the desires and aspirations that accompany it largely negate many of its positive effects and quickly erode any chance of lasting happiness (Clark, Frijters, & Shields, 2008; Stutzer, 2004).

Likewise, because the standards for success are relative rather than objective, people easily adapt once their desires are achieved and revert to their baseline level of happiness (e.g., Brickman & Campbell, 1971; Kahneman, 1999). For many individuals, happiness boosted by winning a lottery (Gardner & Oswald, 2007), moving to a new house (Nakazato, Schimmack, & Oishi, 2011), or marrying the love of your life (Lucas, Clark, Georgellis, & Diener, 2003) does not seem to last. Eventually people become dissatisfied with their present situation, even if that situation or outcome was previously highly desired. As people adapt to this "new normal," they interpret this dissatisfaction as a sign that something is missing. In their quest to reexperience the temporary boost in happiness that they experienced initially before adaptation set in, they set their sights even higher. Such disappointment might be exacerbated by the fact that they likely expected happiness much more intense and lasting than what they actually experienced (Wilson & Gilbert, 2008). In this revolving cycle of desires, the standard for success rises higher and higher and people want more and more.

In addition to unstable and relativistic standards of happiness, another impediment standing in the way of happiness is that people often experience conflicting goals and desires. Hofmann, Kotabe, and Luhmann (2013) found that people felt no happier upon satisfying their desires if the desire they achieved conflicted with other goals. In their study, participants reported their current desires and emotional experiences for 1 week using their cell phones. When their desires (e.g., eating chocolate) did not conflict with other personal goals (which was the norm), satisfying that desire did increase happy moods (see also Oishi et al., 2001). However, if those desires did conflict with other goals (e.g., going on a diet), then satisfying the desire did not intensify happy moods. In such cases, satisfying those desires did result in some positive feelings, but the accompanying feelings of guilt and loss of pride undermined the positive effects of satisfying the desire, resulting in no net gain in happiness.

Existing Theoretical Accounts

In sum, desire can be a blessing and a curse. Furthermore, while the satisfaction of some desires appears to lead to happiness, the satisfaction of many other desires does not. In this section, we will summarize existing theoretical accounts that might help explain these divergent findings.

Hierarchy of Desires

Like Aristotle, Plato also argued that happiness is distinct from pleasures (Waterfield, 1993). While pleasure may be enjoyable, he argued that it can never bring lasting happiness, because pleasure (especially sensual pleasure) is the relief experienced by the removal of pain rather than a distinct good in its own right. When we drink because we are thirsty or sleep because we are tired, it feels good because the water alleviates our thirst and the sleep alleviates our tiredness. Yet neither water nor sleep can be expected to bring us true happiness. Likewise, satisfying our desires may resemble the removal of pain, in that its chief reward consists of relief from wanting. Happiness can come only from pursuing what is good for its own sake, not merely from escaping the bad. Both Plato and Aristotle maintained that the pleasure of the mind differs from worldly pleasure. The pleasure of the mind is pure and more conducive to happiness because it is arises not from relief at the removal of pain but out of the goodness of the pursuit of virtuous pleasure. According to Aristotle and Plato, then, desire is a blessing if it is the desire for knowledge, logic, art, and so forth. In contrast, desire is a curse if it is the desire for food, sex, and other low-level needs, or for acquired needs, such as alcohol and gambling, which are characterized by uncontrollable cravings and strong withdrawal symptoms.

This classical division of pleasure into two classes, one consisting of "high-level" desires amenable to lasting happiness and the second consisting of "low-level" needs unlikely to contribute to real happiness, has parallels in contemporary psychological science. Hofmann et al. (2013) classify desires into two classes: temptation versus nontemptation. They define nontemptation desires as "low conflict desires" (p. 2) that people do not attempt to resist (see also Hofmann, Kotabe, Vohs, & Baumeister, Chapter 3, this volume). Temptation desire thus typically includes low-level physical needs such as sex and acquired desires such as sweets, whereas nontemptation desire includes the desire to work and experience leisure (although for nondieting individuals, sweets are not "high conflict" desires and are therefore considered nontemptation desires). Hofmann et al. (2013) found that temptation desire, when satisfied, gives rise to mixed emotions, whereas nontemptation desire, when satisfied, does not. Thus, temptation desire is a curse because even when we satisfy it, we experience undesirable emotions as well as pleasure, whereas nontemptation desire may be more of a blessing because its satisfaction produces only positive feelings. Overall, then, Hofmann et al.'s temptation account provides a clean psychological explanation for why the satisfaction of some desires is conducive to happiness while that of other desires is not.

Spiral of Desires: Why Is the Satisfaction of Desire Not Enough?

One of the reasons why the satisfaction of temptation desires is problematic is that giving in to them often makes it difficult for individuals to pursue other important goals in life (Hofmann et al., 2013). Continually satisfying your desire for sweets can lead to poor health; continually satisfying your desire for alcohol or drugs can lead to even worse outcomes. However, nontemptation desire is not entirely free of problems either. Fame and financial success may both be nontemptation desires, but seeking fame and fortune rarely leads to happiness in the end. However, whereas the fulfillment of temptation desires (e.g., eating sweets) often puts one at odds with other conflicting goals (e.g., losing weight), that is not the primary problem with nontemptation desires. The main issue with nontemptation desires isn't that they lead to conflicts with other goals, but rather that the act of satisfying a nontemptation desire only strengthens and magnifies it. The rich want to become richer; the famous yearn to become ever more famous. As our achievements grow, so do our aspirations. Aspirations and new desires stem from a variety of sources: they evolve from past experience (e.g., past gains in income spur increased aspirations and less happiness), are provoked by social comparison (e.g., observing the material goods of wealthier peers), and accompany positive expectations about the future (e.g., by aspiring to what one expects to gain; McBride, 2001; McBride, 2010; Stutzer, 2004). When there is a discrepancy between one's evolving aspirations and one's actual situation, it can lead to diminished happiness, even when the person's original desire was achieved. As discussed earlier, Easterlin (1974) has documented this effect with growing national income. Even though wealthier countries tend to be happier, people within those countries do not become happier as their income increases, due in part to social comparison and in part to growing desire. This issue of growing desire is conceptually akin to Brickman and Campbell's (1971) hedonic treadmill; just as an old desire is satisfied, a new desire emerges.

Building on the hedonic treadmill theory, Sheldon and Lyubomirsky (2012) suggest that bottom-up and top-down processes combine to prevent desire from leading to lasting changes in happiness. Bottom-up processes (such as adaptation and habituation) lead us to feel fewer and fewer positive emotions from our satisfied desires. For example, the owner of a new car experiences diminishing enjoyment of the car once he or she has become accustomed to it and the car is no longer "new and shiny." At the same time, through top-down processes, the satisfaction of one desire simply breeds new desires and aspirations to replace it, instigating a cycle of desire that can never quite be fulfilled. The owner of the new Toyota soon sets his or her sights on a new Lexus instead. Positive events (e.g., losing weight, becoming popular) lead to even greater aspirations (e.g., losing even more weight, making even more friends), which highlights the discrepancy between what one has and what one wants, which then leads to even more negative feelings.

Kasser (2002) describes this process neatly with the example of Netscape founder Jim Clark. At first, Clark thought that he would be really happy if he made $10 million. But when he made $10 million, he wasn't happy. Instead he wanted to make $100 million. When he actually made $100 million, he still wasn't happy. Instead he wanted to make $1 billion. When he actually made $1 billion, he presumably said, "Once I have more money than Larry Ellison [Oracle], I'll be satisfied" (Kasser, 2002, p. 43). We all doubt if Clark will ever be happy if and when he overtakes Larry Ellison. But it is clear that new desires can grow in tandem with the satisfaction of old desires, a process that is exacerbated by social comparison in a never-ending feedback loop.

In addition to social comparison and the hedonic treadmill, another reason why the satisfaction of a desire does not lead to greater happiness may be our lack of self-knowledge. As shown by Wilson, Gilbert, and their colleagues (see Wilson & Gilbert, 2008, for review), research on affective forecasting suggests that we are not always very good at predicting how we will feel about events and achievements in the future. We overestimate how long we will feel good after a positive event, and we overestimate the length and negativity of unpleasant events. In short, we expect the good things to be better and the bad things to be worse than they really are. Unsurprisingly, this may be true of desires as well. We desire things that we hope will bring us happiness, not realizing that this happiness may be neither as intense nor as enduring as we expect and hope for. A variety of research suggests that we often want things that we think will make us happy, even though ultimately they do not bring us lasting happiness, such as winning the lottery (Gardner & Oswald, 2007), buying a new house (Nakazato et al., 2011), and getting married (Lucas et al., 2003). It is important to examine whether the satisfaction of desires fails to bring us happiness because we want the "wrong" things, or because we simply habituate. Indeed, it is difficult for desires to bring us happiness if we desire something we don't really want, need, or like. If the self-knowledge hypothesis is correct, better self-knowledge might increase the chance that the satisfaction of desires will lead to greater happiness. Yet it is not clear how one might go about achieving this goal.

According to self-determination theory (e.g., Ryan & Deci, 2000), processes like habituation and evolving aspirations are not the main reason that achieving our desires fails to bring us greater happiness. Instead, its proponents argue that the type of desire is crucial, offering a taxonomy that provides an alternative to the temptation/nontemptation distinction discussed above. According to Ryan and Deci, the satisfaction of desires leads to happiness when the desires are based on intrinsic motivations, but not on extrinsic motivations (Sheldon & Lyubomirsky, 2012). Even in the pursuit of material wealth (which is typically classified as an extrinsic goal), achieving such financial goals is positively associated with satisfaction of life when that desire is motivated more broadly by the intrinsic pursuit of success (i.e., when intrinsic interest in success, which enables people to distinguish themselves from others, is the primary motivation; Garðarsdóttir, Dittmar, & Aspinall, 2009).

From the self-determination perspective, intrinsically motivated goals, which come from the self and have their origin in people's own lives and intimate relationships rather than being externally imposed, are regarded as basic psychological needs, in the same way that food and water are basic physical needs. When goals and desires represent intrinsic and basic psychological needs, satisfying them may well lead to happiness. From the self-determination perspective, then, it is not necessarily knowing what is desirable for the self and pursuing it that brings greater happiness, but pursuing so-called intrinsic goals.

Two Approaches to the Dilemma of Desire

In the previous section, we summarized existing theoretical accounts explaining why the satisfaction of desire does not always lead to happiness, ranging from hedonic adaptation to social comparison to self-determination theory. As seen above, desires in general, and sensuous ones in particular, pose hurdles for the path to happiness. In this section, we present two approaches to handling the dilemma of desire (for a summary, see Figure 14.1). One is a Puritan (Protestant work ethic) approach, or trying to satisfy one's desires via self-discipline. Instead of removing or reducing the main desires (goals) themselves, this approach tries to satisfy one's higher-level desires or attain one's main goals through hard work and the exertion of self-control to resist temptation (lower-level desires). It is the equivalent of trying to save $20,000 by working more while exercising self-discipline to spend less. An alternative approach is offered by Buddhism. Rather than seeking to attain one's higher-level desires, this approach instead advocates trying to remove, reduce, and accommodate the desires themselves. Instead of working more (as the

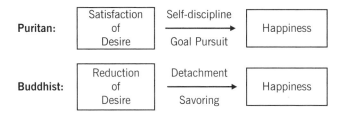

FIGURE 14.1. Two approaches to desire and happiness.

Protestant work ethic would advocate) or spending less (the Puritan virtue of self-control), the Buddhist approach might question the desire to save $20,000 in the first place ("Why need more?"). Thus, this approach might lead you to modify the goal (i.e., to save $10,000 instead) or give up on the goal entirely.

The Puritan Approach

Hofmann, Luhmann, Fisher, Vohs, and Baumeister (2014) examined the Puritan approach to desire, namely, self-control. Puritan concepts of self-control involve not only discipline in working hard to achieve one's high-level desires (e.g., hard work, focus, perseverance), but also discipline in abstaining from indulgence in low-level desires that may impede or interfere with those goals. And, in fact, Hofmann et al. (2014) found that trait self-control (the ability to resist temptations) was positively associated with long-term happiness because it helps participants stay on target with their goals. Interestingly, however, they also found that individuals high in self-control felt happier than others moment to moment as well. So it was not the case that these individuals were laboriously and painfully exerting self-control to resist temptation and achieve their goals; rather they seemed to do this with pleasure. This might be partly because individuals high in self-control also tend not to have many temptation desires that conflict with their larger goals in life, or it might simply be that when self-control comes easily, it can be invoked to overcome such temptations relatively painlessly. In a similar vein, Quoidbach and Dunn (2013) found that college students randomly assigned to give up chocolate for 1 week later savored and enjoyed chocolate more. This is somewhat surprising because people might presumably feel guilty while eating chocolate, especially since eating chocolate may conflict with many college students' fitness and weight-loss goals. However, it is likely that the successful resistance to temptation for 1 week gave them moral license to indulge in chocolate without guilt later. In other words, self-control may lead to moderation in consumption and simultaneously greater enjoyment of the occasional consumption of a highly desired object. These findings suggest that Puritan self-control might actually increase the intensity of pleasure when the desire is eventually satisfied. Temptation desires generally pose a challenge to everyone. However, individuals low in self-control tend to have a particularly difficult time navigating temptations. Thus, temptation desires are especially bad for individuals without good self-control.

The Puritan approach to desire teaches that high-level desire is not itself a problem. High-level desire may be a motivation to engage in hard work or perseverance (e.g., working hard to achieve a high-level desire). It is low-level desire that must be resisted by exercising self-control in the face of temptation. By advocating that one aggressively pursue the "right" desires and resolutely resist the "wrong" ones, the Puritan approach promises that happiness is largely a matter of self-discipline. However, despite being the focus of most empirical psychological work, the Puritan approach is not the only approach to desire and temptation.

The Buddhist Approach

The other approach to handling the temptation problem can be found in both traditional Buddhist philosophy as well as ancient Greek Stoicism, which both hold that, far from fostering happiness, desires are a primary cause of unhappiness. The path to happiness, according to Buddhism, lies not in the satisfaction of desires, but in freedom from desire itself. Likewise, the ancient Greek and Roman Stoic philosophers warned against wanting things beyond one's grasp, suggesting that people should instead desire that which they already have (Irvine, 2008).

Although both Buddhism and Stoicism posit that desire breeds unhappiness, their practical approaches differ. Desire, the Stoics suggested, is a fact of life, which can even potentially be used to our benefit if understood and handled wisely. Because it is the absence of something that makes us desire it, the Stoics reasoned that we should routinely imagine the loss of the things that we have and hold dear so that we might desire them instead (see Koo, Algoe, Wilson, & Gilbert, 2008, for empirical evidence). By making us want what we've already got, Stoicism turns desire into a tool that works for rather than against us. Far from holding that people should never have any aspirations or ambition, the Stoics simply cautioned that people should concern themselves only with things within their control, as concerning oneself with anything else is a waste of time. According to one modern interpretation, this means that rather than desiring to win a tennis match (something not wholly within your control), you should make it your goal simply to practice hard and play to the best of your abilities (something presumably within your control). That way, it is wholly within your power to meet your goal and to avoid the disappointment of an aspiration thwarted, the outcome of the match notwithstanding.

Buddhism, on the other hand, takes a different approach. Unhappiness, Buddhism teaches, is not only a result of desire, but an inherent aspect of it. If desire is the longing for something you do not have, then wanting what you do not or cannot have is in itself a form of suffering that can only end when desire ceases. However, desire does not cease simply because it has been satisfied. The problem is that, in truth, it cannot ever be fully satisfied. Because all things in the world are temporary in the end, they can never truly satisfy desire; ultimately any sense of success is (necessarily) an illusory and a temporary one. The person who eats today will be hungry again tomorrow. Buddhism teaches that the failure to understand this is what gives rise to desire in the first place, and that one path to reducing desire lies in understanding that all things are temporary. Ultimately, however, Buddhist philosophy advocates that only the cessation of desire can bring lasting happiness and an end to suffering. Wanting what you don't have, Buddhism teaches, can never be a good thing, no matter how much self-control or discipline you exercise.

If we use the analogy of Puritan versus Buddhist/Stoic approaches, self-determination theory is a variant of the Puritan approach, or seeking *primary control* by trying to obtain what you want. The Buddhist, or Stoic, approach to happiness, on the other hand, might be seen as advocating what some researchers have identified as *secondary control* (Morling & Evered, 2006)—not getting what we want (primary control), but wanting what we've already got. Norris and Larsen (2011) found that the satisfaction of desires leads to happiness when people are satisfied with and attending to the things they actually have and nothing more. Similarly, nonmaterialists tend to be happier than materialists because nonmaterialists are more easily satisfied with what they already have. Brown, Kasser, Ryan, Alex Linley, and Orzech (2009) showed that mindfulness, a state of receptive attention to present events and experience, narrowed the perceived discrepancy between desires and people's actual states and also enhanced happiness. Several mindfulness intervention studies also found that participants randomly assigned to the mindfulness intervention show reduced craving for alcohol (e.g., Garland, Gaylord, Boettiger, & Howard, 2010) or smoking (e.g., Brewer et al., 2011). Together, these findings suggest that curbing desires by finding satisfaction with one's current state (accommodating desire to one's current situation), rather than trying to satisfy ever-growing desires, may be one of the keys to avoiding the trap of desire.

Research on satisficing suggests several other strategies that may help people pursue greater happiness without invoking greater desire as well. Schwartz et al.'s (2002) work on choice shows that although people think they want more choices, they are actually happier with their decisions when their choices are limited. Voluntarily choosing to limit one's options (such as by looking at only one or two televisions when shopping) or evaluating one object at a time (single evaluation) instead of evaluating multiple objects simultaneously (joint evaluation) may enhance satisfaction with one's eventual choice and reduce the temptation to engage in upward comparisons (Hsee, Hastie, & Chen, 2008). In short, ignorance may (sometimes) be bliss—you can't want what you don't know exists, so you're better off not knowing! Iyengar et al.'s (2006) work on satisficers suggests that some people naturally tend to pursue this strategy by pursuing available options only until a suitable choice is found, rather than looking for the perfect option. And as we've seen, this strategy seems to work—satisficers are, on the whole, happier than people who don't satisfice.

Kurtz (2008) suggests another strategy for enhancing happiness without feeding desire. The art of savoring, she explains, is the art of wanting what you have, rather than trying to have what you want. Focusing on day-to-day pleasures and savoring the moment may increase appreciation and desire for what one already possesses, thus leading to greater happiness without the desire for more. In this vein, Sheldon and Lyubomirsky (2012) suggest that continued appreciation of the positive changes in one's life can prevent adaptation to them, and advocate variety as a further prophylactic against habituation. Tatzel (2003) makes a similar point in proposing that even material goods may make us happier if we focus on the experiential aspect of owning such goods, including focusing on the aesthetics, functionality, and pleasure afforded by them (see also Van Boven & Gilovich, 2003).

Taking a slightly different tack, Dunn, Aknin, and Norton (2008) suggest that the path to personal happiness lies in focusing not on ourselves and our own situation but on others, and on making them happy instead. In a study comparing personal purchases with purchases for others, these researchers found that people experienced longer-lasting and more positive boosts to their happiness after spending money on a friend as compared to spending money on themselves. Such purchases may be less likely to provoke desires for more and may be more resistant to the effects of habituation and adaptation. Perhaps instead of attending to our own desires, we should attempt to fulfill the desires of others if we hope to achieve happiness.

Finale: A Synthesis

Although we use Sumner's (1996) definition of happiness as authentic life satisfaction, we use Aristotelian concepts of pleasure in our attempt to understand desire and happiness. Aristotle did not view all kinds of pleasures equally, declaring that "intellectual pleasures are superior to sensuous ones" (Thomson, 1953, p. 324), which he regards as transient. We likewise distinguish between two types of desires: (1) low-level physical

TABLE 14.1. The Type and the Target of Desire: Does the Satisfaction of Desire Lead to Happiness?

Desire	Self	Other
Craving	No	Sometimes
Ideal	Sometimes	Yes

or acquired craving ("I've got to have it") and (2) noncraving, or ideals ("I would ideally like to have it"). This classification is similar to Hofmann et al.'s (2013) classification of temptation versus nontemptation desires. In addition, we distinguish between two targets of our desires: (1) ourselves, and (2) others. Most desires concern the self ("I want *X*"), whereas some concern others ("I want *Y* to be/behave *Z*"). Table 14.1 summarizes our conceptualization.

Desire: Cravings versus Ideals

As seen above, the satisfaction of low-level physical or acquired desires does not generally lead to an increase in happiness. The satisfaction of these desires (or cravings) simply restores the individual back to baseline, or the equilibrium point. They are the psychological equivalent of eating because you are hungry, or sleeping because you are tired. In Aristotelian terms, they are pleasant because they offer relief from pain, not because they are good in their own right. As we have seen, cravings may also be particularly susceptible to conflict with other goals, so that even those pleasant feelings of relief are mixed with negative feelings in other regards. However, it should be noted that deprivation with respect to these low-level cravings is not healthy either (Hofmann et al., 2013; Oishi et al., 2001).

In contrast to low-level desires, which rarely lead to enduring happiness, we propose that the satisfaction of higher-level ideals *can* sometime lead to an increase in happiness over time, as the satisfaction of such ideals often entails a positive change in life circumstances (e.g., more freedom, Inglehart, Foa, Peterson, & Welzel, 2008; see also Diener, Lucas, & Scollon, 2006, for long-term changes in baseline happiness). Such desires are also less likely to conflict with other desires, and achieving them may be a wholly positive experience rather than a mixed emotional experience. Yet even ideals may still be problematic for happiness. Ideals are not immune to hedonic treadmill, adaptation, and habituation effects, and ideals, once achieved, have a tendency to spawn new ones. So while ideals may not always lead to happiness, they at least have the potential to contribute to it in a way that cravings do not.

Origins of Desire: Self versus Others

Although most research on desire and happiness has been concerned with the desire of the individual him- or herself (i.e., "I want X"), the key to delaying hedonic adaptation might lie in positive feedback from others (e.g., hearing "thank you" from a friend, or a returned favor). Because of the positive feedback, in the form of expressions of gratitude and reciprocal actions, that often accompanies acts done for others (Algoe, 2012), acting to fulfill others' desires might give rise to a more significant and lasting change in happiness than acting solely on one's own behalf. Illustrating this feedback loop, Muise, Impett, Kogan, and Desmarais (2013) recently found that couples high in partner-oriented sexual desires (high scores on items such as "How far would you be willing to go to meet your partner's sexual needs?" and "How high a priority for you is meeting the sexual needs of your partner?") maintain their own sexual desire for a longer period of time, a strong predictor of sexual and relationship satisfaction among long-term couples (Muise, Impett, & Desmarais, 2013). These findings suggest, then, that rather than being a sacrifice, satisfying your partner's desire can simultaneously increase your own happiness as well, as your partner's satisfaction tends to have a positive impact on your own happiness but without the negative drawbacks that usually accompany desires. Of course, however, the type of desire is important as well. If a partner's desire took the form of a craving for cocaine, helping to satisfy his desire might not increase your own happiness, even if he thanked you and gave or did something in return. In the case of sexual behaviors, though, the satisfaction of a partner's desire *can* satisfy one's own desire. In a sense, this is a situation where two individuals desire the same thing, and each of them helps the other to achieve the goal. The satisfaction of a partner's desire can produce happiness, especially when it also satisfies one's own desire. Then, the satisfaction of a *shared* desire might be the most potent path to happiness.

So, in the end, are desires a blessing or a curse? As with many things, the answer is "it depends." In clarifying the link between desires and happiness, it is important to distinguish between desires-as-cravings and desires-for-ideals, as the underlying mechanisms between the two are very different. Cravings, or low-level physical or acquired desires, are likely to be a curse, because they invite people to step aboard a nonstop hedonic treadmill, in which any boost in happiness is both temporary and fleeting. On the other hand, ideals (although not without their own pitfalls) are more likely to have the potential to be a blessing, leading to positive changes in an individual's life, especially if we satisfy the desires of others rather than our own. However, even ideals may not always lead to happiness. In addition to distinguishing between cravings and ideals, it is equally important to investigate the interpersonal nature of some desires. Somewhat counterintuitively, the satisfaction of another's ideals (instead of one's own) might be most conducive to achieving long-term happiness. Especially if the desires are shared, satisfying them can create a positive feedback loop: the happiness of both people is even further enhanced by knowing that the other person is likewise happy. Future research might apply these insights and important distinctions in further illuminating why it is that some desires leads to happiness whereas others does not.

Finally, as stated above, most empirical approaches to desire have adopted a viewpoint that could be considered decidedly Puritan in nature. This approach accepts desire as a given, and focuses on how people achieve the "right" desires through discipline and hard work while resisting the "wrong" desires by exercising self-control. The Buddhist approach offers an alternative: rather than regulating how we respond to a desire, it advocates regulating the desire itself. Although some desires may simply be out of our control, it would be ideal to investigate the effectiveness of a Buddhist or Stoic approach in the future: namely, how to increase happiness by reducing one's desires, or by working to shift them to conform to one's present circumstances.

Desire is and will remain a significant part of people's lives. It shapes our day-to-day actions, from trivial tasks such as deciding what to eat or which shoes we want, to larger decisions with far-ranging implications, such as the craving for drugs and alcohol or the thirst for knowledge. It, without a doubt, has a large impact on our happiness and unfortunately, as we have discovered, that impact is often a negative one. The question of how to live happily with our desires is an ancient one that has concerned philosophers and religions around the world, from the ancient Greek Stoics and Aristotle to Buddhism and our own more recent Puritan tradition. Learning to live with, channel, and perhaps even regulate or reduce desires may be a challenge, but it is one that is potentially fruitful for people's overall well-being and happiness in life. The research discussed here can help us understand how to live a happy life with (or even perhaps one day even without) desires.

REFERENCES

Algoe, S. B. (2012). Find, remind, and bind: The functions of gratitude in everyday relationships. *Social and Personality Psychology Compass, 6*, 455–469.

Beck, A. (1967). *Depression: Causes and treatments*. Philadelphia: University of Pennsylvania Press.

Brewer, J. A., Mallik, S., Babuscio, T. A., Nich, C., Johnson, H. E., et al. (2011). Mindfulness training for smoking cessation: Results from a randomized controlled trial. *Drug and Alcohol Dependence, 119*, 72–80.

Brickman, P., & Campbell, D. T. (1971). Hedonic relativism and planning the good society. In M. H. Appley (Ed.), *Adaptation level theory: A symposium* (pp. 287–305). New York: Academic Press.

Brown, K. W., Kasser, T., Ryan, R. M., Alex Linley, P., & Orzech, K. (2009). When what one has is enough: Mindfulness, financial desire discrepancy, and subjective well-being. *Journal of Research in Personality, 43,* 727–736.

Brunstein, J. (1993). Personal goals and subjective well-being: A longitudinal study. *Journal of Personality and Social Psychology, 65,* 1061–1070.

Burroughs, J. E., & Rindfleisch, A. (2002). Materialism and well-being: A conflicting values perspective. *Journal of Consumer Research, 29,* 348–370.

Campbell, A., Converse, P. E., & Rodgers, W. L. (1976). *The quality of American life: Perceptions, evaluations, and satisfactions.* New York: Russell Sage Foundation.

Clark, A., Frijters, P., & Shields, M. (2008). Relative income, happiness, and utility: An explanation for the Easterlin paradox and other puzzles. *Journal of Economic Literature, 46,* 95–144.

Diab, D. L., Gillespie, M. A., & Highhouse, S. (2008). Are maximizers really unhappy?: The measurement of maximizing tendency. *Judgment and Decision Making, 3,* 364–370.

Diener, E., Emmons, R. A., Larsen, R. L., & Griffin, S. (1985). The Satisfaction with Life Scale. *Journal of Personality Assessment, 49,* 71–75.

Diener, E., & Fujita, F. (1995). Resources, personal strivings, and subjective well-being: A nomothetic and idiographic approach. *Journal of Personality and Social Psychology, 68,* 926–935.

Diener, E., Lucas, R. E., & Scollon, C. N. (2006). Beyond the hedonic treadmill: Revising the adaptation theory of well-being. *American Psychologist, 61,* 305–314.

Dunn, E. W., Aknin, L. B., & Norton, M. I. (2008). Spending money on others promotes happiness. *Science, 319,* 1687–1688.

Easterlin, R. A. (1974). Does economic growth improve the human lot?: Some empirical evidence. In P. A. David & W. R. Melvin (Eds.), *Nations and households in economic growth* (pp. 89–125). New York: Academic Press.

Emmons, R. A. (1986). Personal strivings: An approach to personality and subjective well-being. *Journal of Personality and Social Psychology, 51,* 1058–1068.

Frank, R. H. (1997). The frame of reference as a public good. *Economic Journal, 107,* 1832–1847.

Garðarsdóttir, R. B., Dittmar, H., & Aspinall, C. (2009). It's not the money, it's the quest for a happier self: The role of happiness and success motives in the link between financial goals and subjective well-being. *Journal of Social and Clinical Psychology, 28,* 1100–1127.

Gardner, J., & Oswald, A. (2007). Money and mental wellbeing: A longitudinal study of medium-sized lottery wins. *Journal of Health Economics, 26,* 49–60.

Garland, E. L., Gaylord, S. A., Boettiger, C. A., & Howard, M. O. (2010). Mindfulness training modifies cognitive, affective, and physiological mechanisms implicated in alcohol dependence: Results of a randomized controlled pilot trial. *Journal of Psychoactive Drugs, 42,* 177–199.

Gruber, J., Mauss, I. B., & Tamir, M. (2011). A dark side of happiness?: How, when, and why happiness is not always good. *Perspectives on Psychological Science, 6*(3), 222–233.

Hsee, C. K., Hastie, R., & Chen, J. (2008). Hedonomics: Bridging decision research with happiness research. *Perspectives on Psychological Science, 3,* 224–243.

Hofmann, W., Kotabe, H., & Luhmann, M. (2013). The spoiled pleasure of giving in to temptation. *Motivation and Emotion, 37,* 733–742.

Hofmann, W., Luhmann, M., Fisher, R. R., Vohs, K. D., & Baumeister, R. F. (2014). Yes, but are they happy?: Effects of trait self-control on affective well-being and life satisfaction. *Journal of Personality, 82*(4), 265–277.

Inglehart, R., Foa, R., Peterson, C., & Welzel, C. (2008). Development, freedom, and rising happiness: A global perspective (1981–2007). *Perspectives on Psychological Science, 3*, 264–285.

Irvine, W. (2008). *A guide to the good life: The ancient art of Stoic joy.* New York: Oxford University Press.

Iyengar, S. S., Wells, R. E., & Schwartz, B. (2006). Doing better but feeling worse: Looking for the "best" job undermines satisfaction. *Psychological Science, 17*, 143–150.

Kahneman, D. (1999). Objective happiness. In D. Kahneman, E. Diener, & N. Schwarz (Eds.), *Well-being: Foundations of hedonic psychology* (pp. 3–25). New York: Russell Sage Foundation.

Kasser, T. (2002). *The high price of materialism.* Cambridge, MA: MIT Press.

Koo, M., Algoe, S. B., Wilson, T. D., & Gilbert, D. T. (2008). It's a wonderful life: Mentally subtracting positive events improves people's affective states, contrary to their affective forecasts. *Journal of Personality and Social Psychology, 95*, 1217–1224.

Kurtz, J. L. (2008). Looking to the future to appreciate the present: The benefits of perceived temporal scarcity. *Psychological Science, 19*, 1238–1241.

Lucas, R. E., Clark, A. E., Georgellis, & Diener, E. (2003). Reexamining adaptation and the set point model of happiness. *Journal of Personality and Social Psychology, 84*, 527–539.

McBride, M. (2001). Relative-income effects on subjective well-being in the cross-section. *Journal of Economic Behavior and Organization, 45*, 251–278.

McBride, M. (2010). Money, happiness, and aspirations: An experimental study. *Journal of Economic Behavior and Organization, 74*, 262–276

Michalos, A. C. (1985). Multiple discrepancies theory (MDT). *Social Indicators Research, 16*, 347–413.

Miller, G. E., Wrosch, C. (2007). You've gotta know when to fold'em: Goal disengagement and systemic inflammation in adolescence. *Psychological Science, 18*, 773–777.

Morling, B., & Evered, S. (2006). Secondary control reviewed and defined. *Psychological Bulletin, 132*, 269–296.

Muise, A., Impett, E. A., & Desmarais, S. (2013). Getting it on versus getting it over with: Sexual motivation, desire, and satisfaction in intimate bonds. *Personality and Social Psychology Bulletin, 39*, 1320–1332.

Muise, A., Impett, E. A., Kogan, A., & Desmarais, S. (2013). Keeping the spark alive: Being motivated to meet a partner's sexual needs sustains sexual desire in long-term romantic relationships. *Social Psychological and Personality Science, 4*, 267–273.

Nakazato, N., Schimmack, U., & Oishi, S. (2011). Effect of changes in living condition on well- being: A prospective top-down bottom-up model. *Social Indicators Research, 100*, 115–135.

Nickerson, C., Schwarz, N., Diener, E., & Kahneman, D. (2003). Zeroing in on the dark side of the American dream: A closer look at the negative consequences of the goal for financial success. *Psychological Science, 14*, 531–536.

Norris, J. I., & Larsen, J. T. (2011). Wanting more than you have and its consequences for well-being. *Journal of Happiness Studies, 12*, 877–885.

Nussbaum, M. C. (1986). *The fragility of goodness: Luck and ethics in Greek tragedy and philosophy.* Cambridge, UK: Cambridge University Press.

Nussbaum, M. C. (2001). *Upheavals of thought: The intelligence of emotions.* Cambridge, UK: Cambridge University Press.

Oishi, S., & Diener, E. (2001). Goals, culture, and subjective well-being. *Personality and Social Psychology Bulletin, 27,* 1674–1682.

Oishi, S., Diener, E., Lucas, R. E., & Suh, E. M. (1999). Cross-cultural variations in predictors of life satisfaction: Perspectives from needs and values. *Personality and Social Psychology Bulletin, 25,* 980–990.

Oishi, S., Schimmack, U., & Diener, E. (2001). Pleasures and subjective well-being. *European Journal of Personality, 15,* 153–167.

Plagnol, A. C., & Easterlin, R. A. (2008). Aspirations, attainments, and satisfaction: Life cycle differences between American women and men. *Journal of Happiness Studies, 9,* 601–619.

Quoidbach, J., & Dunn, E. W. (2013). Give it up: A strategy for combating hedonic adaptation. *Social Psychological and Personality Science, 4*(5), 563–568.

Ryan, R. M., & Deci, E. L. (2000). Self-determination theory and the facilitation of intrinsic motivation, social development, and well-being. *American Psychologist, 55,* 68–78.

Schneider, L., & Schimmack, U. (2009). Self-informant agreement in well-being ratings: A meta-analysis. *Social Indicators Research, 94,* 363–376.

Schwarz, N., & Strack, F. (1999). Reports of subjective well-being: Judgmental processes and their methodological implications. In D. Kahneman, E. Diener, & N. Schwarz (Eds.), *Well-being: The foundations of hedonic psychology* (pp. 61–84). New York: Russell Sage Foundation.

Schwartz, B., Ward, A., Monterosso, J., Lyubomirsky, S., White, K., & Lehman, D. R. (2002). Maximizing versus satisficing: Happiness is a matter of choice. *Journal of Personality and Social Psychology, 83,* 1178–1197.

Sheldon, K. M., & Kasser, T. (1998). Pursuing personal goals: Skills enable progress, but not all progress is beneficial. *Personality and Social Psychology Bulletin, 24,* 1319–1331.

Sheldon, K. M., & Lyubomirsky, S. (2012). The challenge of staying happier: Testing the hedonic adaptation prevention model. *Personality and Social Psychology Bulletin, 38,* 670–680.

Solberg, E. C., Diener, E., Wirtz, D., Lucas, R. E., & Oishi, S. (2002). Wanting, having, and satisfaction: Examining the role of desire discrepancies in satisfaction with income. *Journal of Personality and Social Psychology, 83,* 725–734.

Stutzer, A. (2004). The role of income aspirations in individual happiness. *Journal of Economic Behavior and Organization, 54,* 89–109.

Sumner, L. W. (1996). *Welfare, happiness, and ethics.* Oxford, UK: Oxford University Press.

Tatzel, M. (2003). The art of buying: Coming to terms with money and materialism. *Journal of Happiness Studies, 4*(4), 405–435

Tay, L., & Diener, E. (2011). Needs and subjective well-being around the world. *Journal of Personality and Social Psychology, 101,* 354–365.

Thomson, J. A. K. (1953). *The ethics of Aristotle: The Nicomachean ethics.* London: Penguin Books.

Van Boven, L., & Gilovich, T. (2003). To do or to have?: That is the question. *Journal of Personality and Social Psychology, 85,* 1193–1202.

Waterfield, R. (1993). *Plato: Republic.* New York: Oxford University Press.

Wilson, T. D., & Gilbert, D. T. (2008). Explaining away: A model of affective adaptation. *Perspectives on Psychological Science, 3,* 370–386.

CHAPTER 15

Liking Little, Wanting Less
On (Lacking) Desire in Psychopathology

Michael T. Treadway

Anhedonia: What's in a Name?

The term *anhedonia* was originally coined as an antonym to *analgesia*, and was intended to describe severe bouts of melancholia. In contemporary practice, it is often used to describe any significant reduction of positive emotionality in daily life. Patient descriptions of anhedonia often involve reports of decreased interest, pleasure, motivation, or connection associated with everyday activities such as socializing, eating, and working. All of these domains have traditionally been subsumed under the anhedonia construct. The goal of this chapter, however, is to emphasize some of the important subdomains of anhedonia that relate to the distinct cognitive and biological process of reinforcement and pleasure.

For most of its century-old history in the psychiatric literature, the anhedonia construct remained relatively obscure. Only in recent decades has anhedonia become a central feature in the current nosology of multiple psychiatric conditions, most notably in major depressive disorder (MDD) and schizophrenia. This growing conceptual relevance has been reflected by a sharp rise in empirical research devoted to the understanding and treatment of anhedonia as distinct from common comorbid symptoms. Mounting interest in this particular symptom likely results from the confluence of several distinct currents, which include influential theoretical frameworks regarding the diagnostic importance of anhedonia in MDD and schizophrenia (Klein, 1974; Meehl, 1975), the observation of comparatively poorer treatment outcomes for anhedonic symptoms (Shelton & Tomarken, 2001), and a surge in preclinical discoveries regarding the molecular and systems-level mechanisms underlying reward processing generally (for reviews see Berridge & Kringelbach, 2008; Rushworth,

Noonan, Boorman, Walton, & Behrens, 2011; Salamone, Correa, Farrar, & Mingote, 2007). This last trend is of particular importance, as the field of psychiatry often relies on translational neuroscience approaches in its quest to elucidate the etiopathophysiology of mental disorders (Insel et al., 2010). Thus, the availability of a rich basic science literature is crucial.

Despite this heightened focus, many fundamental questions remain regarding the nature of anhedonic symptoms, their etiology, phenomenology, biological underpinnings, and specificity to psychiatric illness. Indeed, several recent theoretical reviews have called for a critical reexamination of the anhedonia construct (D. M. Barch & Dowd, 2010; Foussias & Remington, 2008; Strauss & Gold, 2012; M. T. Treadway & Zald, 2011). Much of this critique has hinged on the question of what alterations in reward processing are included in a definition of anhedonia. Does anhedonia describe a singular problem in experiencing pleasure, or does it include deficiencies in a number of reward-related domains? The answer to this question has substantial implications for the theoretical conceptualization of anhedonia and related constructs, for the assessment of psychopathology involving these symptoms, for understanding the neural substrates of psychiatric symptoms, and for the treatment or reward processing abnormalities.

The need for clarity on this issue is highlighted by the diagnostic criteria for major depressive episode as enshrined in DSM-IV and DSM-5. One can meet the A2 criteria for a depressive episode either by a loss of pleasure or a loss of interest. If pleasure and interest are reflections of a singular process, then this collapsing of terms should cause little problem. However, if pleasure and interest reflect different processes, they may have dramatically different pathophysiological substrates. That is to say, circuit-level mechanisms underlying interest, such as reward prediction, anticipation, and motivation, which relate to potential future rewards, may be distinct from those involved in the experience of pleasure, enjoyment, or satisfaction that occurs following reward receipt (Barch & Dowd, 2010; Treadway & Zald, 2011; see also Kringelbach & Berridge, Chapter 6, this volume).

Unfortunately, most clinical measures of psychopathology and dimensional assessments of anhedonia fail to discriminate between these various domains of reward processing. While such measures have had a useful place in the context of clinical assessment and care, they may mask important behavioral and biological distinctions that are critical for understanding pathophysiology.

Anhedonia and the Many Components of Reward Processing

It has long been recognized that reward processing behavior involves multiple subprocesses, such as anticipation, motivation, prediction, subjective pleasure, and satiety. It has only been more recently, however, that investigators have been able to clearly show that these subcomponents are neurobiologically dissociable; manipulations of specific neurochemicals can alter a single dimension of reward-related behavior without affecting others. For example, it is possible to ablate goal-directed behavior without any apparent change in hedonic responsiveness to received rewards. This particular distinction is frequently referred to as a difference between "wanting" (defined as the desire to obtain a reinforcer) and "liking" (defined as the subjective experience of pleasure that may arise upon consumption of the reinforcer) (Berridge, 2007; Berridge & Robinson, 1998; see also Kringelbach & Berridge, Chapter 6, this volume). For the purposes of this chapter, the term *desire* will be used to denote anticipatory responses to reward (e.g., effort to obtain a reward), and *pleasure* or *hedonic impact* will be used to describe subjective experiences of positive feeling states resulting from reward attainment.

A key implication of this work is that a reduction in reward-seeking behavior may result from impairments in one or many subcomponent processes, which in turn implies that they may have shared or unshared neurobiological origins across different individuals. Despite this new understanding of the biological divisions involved in reward and reinforcement in the preclinical literature, current clinical methods have largely continued to construe anhedonic symptoms along a unitary dimension with a focus on reduced hedonic capacity. Consistent with this orientation, until recently, most clinical and laboratory measures of anhedonia have either focused exclusively on subject pleasure and/or positive feeling states, or treated different subdomains of desire and pleasure as being equivalent.

To date, the assessment of anhedonic symptom severity in most clinical research and practice settings continues to rely almost exclusively on self-report instruments. Moreover, these self-report measures tend to emphasize only reports of hedonic response to positive stimuli, with little or no attention to diminished drive or motivation. This emphasis on the experience of pleasure can be seen in the Chapman Anhedonia Scale (Chapman, Chapman, & Raulin, 1976), the Scale of Negative Symptoms (SANS; Andreasen, 1982), the Fawcett–Clark Pleasure Scale (FCPS; (Fawcett, Clark, Scheftner, & Hedeker, 1983), and the Snaith–Hamilton Pleasure Scale (SHAPS; Snaith et al., 1995). Importantly, none of these scales have made an explicit attempt to dissociate the pleasure and motivational aspects of anhedonia.

As the importance of desire has been increasingly acknowledged in anhedonia research (Treadway & Zald, 2013) a number of scales have recently been developed that attempt to distinguish desire from hedonic components of anhedonia. These include the Temporal Experience of Pleasure Scale (TEPS; Gard, Gard, Kring, & John, 2006), which seeks to measure both anticipatory and consummatory aspects of pleasure; the

Grit questionnaire (Duckworth, Peterson, Matthews, & Kelly, 2007), a trait-like measure of sustained motivation in pursuit of long-term goals; the approach motivation scale (Elliot & Thrash, 2010); the appetitive motivation scale (AMS; Cooper, Smillie, & Jackson, 2008); and the Specific Loss of Interest or Pleasure Scale (SLIPS; Winer, Veilleux, & Ginger, 2014).

A limitation of these measures, however, is that they often do not discriminate between different types of emotion reporting. Recent empirical and theoretical advances have shown that different types of verbal reports access distinct types of self-knowledge: the "experiencing self" that is able to report on the qualities of a positive experience in that moment, the "retrospective self" that attempts to remember past experiences, and the "believing" self, which attempts to average past experiences into a trait-like summation (Robinson & Clore, 2002). While these three types of verbal report would be theoretically expected to correlate quite highly, empirical research has increasingly revealed that they are often only moderately correlated in practice (Conner & Barrett, 2012; Edmondson et al., 2013; Kagan, 2007; Kahneman & Deaton, 2012; Schwartz, Neale, Marco, Shiffman, & Stone, 1999). This is also true in clinical populations experiencing anhedonia, where there is a noted discrepancy between in-the-moment responses to affective stimuli and trait measures of enjoyment (Strauss & Gold, 2012).

One way to address this problem is the use of laboratory-based measures that focus exclusively on "in-the-moment" affective experiences. Interestingly, these measures often yield contradictory results with retrospective or trait assessments. While some studies find that individuals with depression generally rate positively valenced stimuli as being less enjoyable, less arousing, or less able to affect their mood as compared to controls (for a meta-analytic review, see Bylsma, Morris, & Rottenberg, 2008), a large number of studies have reported no group differences in these ratings (Allen, Trinder, & Brennan, 1999; Dichter, Tomarken, Shelton, & Sutton, 2004; Forbes & Dahl, 2005; Gehricke & Shapiro, 2000; Kaviani et al., 2004; Keedwell, Andrew, Williams, Brammer, & Phillips, 2005a, 2005b; Mitterschiffthaler et al., 2003; Renneberg, Heyn, Gebhard, & Bachmann, 2005; Surguladze et al., 2005; Tremeau et al., 2005; Tsai, Pole, Levenson, & Munoz, 2003). Moreover, four separate studies using the sweet taste test found that depressed patients and matched controls exhibited no differences in the reported hedonic impact of sucrose (Amsterdam, Settle, Doty, Abelman, & Winokur, 1987; Berlin, Givry-Steiner, Lecrubier, & Puech, 1998; Dichter, Smoski, Kampov-Polevoy, Gallop, & Garbutt, 2009; Kazes et al., 1994). In schizophrenia, the evidence for deficits of "in-the-moment" experience is even weaker, with many reports suggesting absolutely no difference between schizophrenia patients and healthy controls when rating responses to positively valenced stimuli. Gold and colleagues have demonstrated a striking distinction between self-reported anhedonia using the Chapman Anhedonia Scale and affective reports of pleasure emotions in response to positively valenced laboratory stimuli; while schizophrenia patients rated themselves as significantly more anhedonic according to the Chapman Scales, their affective ratings were identical to those of controls (J. M. Gold, Waltz, Prentice, Morris, & Heerey, 2008; Kring & Moran, 2008). Overall, these studies cast doubt on the extent to which blunted hedonic capacity is truly impaired in disorders commonly associated with anhedonic symptoms.

Although the interpretability of these studies is aided by a focus on "in-the-moment" experience, they are still susceptible to other potential biases associated with verbal report. Alternative approaches to the assessment of anhedonia have emphasized behavioral measures. One well-replicated finding has been that individuals with depression fail to develop a response bias toward rewarded stimuli (Henriques, Glowacki, & Davidson, 1994; Pizzagalli, Iosifescu, Hallett, Ratner, & Fava, 2008; Pizzagalli, Jahn, & O'Shea, 2005). These paradigms use discrimination tasks in which subjects must categorize a briefly presented stimulus as belonging to category A or B. A payoff matrix is used so that subjects are more rewarded for correctly guessing category A, as opposed to category B, with no punishment associated with incorrect guesses. Healthy control subjects typically develop a response bias toward the more rewarding option, whereas patients with MDD do not (Pizzagalli et al., 2008, 2005). Importantly, this finding has been specifically linked with anhedonic symptom severity and treatment of anhedonic symptoms (Pizzagalli et al., 2008; Vrieze et al., 2013). Anhedonia—but not overall depression—has also been associated with blunted learning using instrumental conditioning tasks (Chase et al., 2010). Not all studies support clear learning impairments in reinforcement learning, however, as several reward-based Pavlovian and instrumental conditioning studies have found comparable learning rates across depressed and nondepressed subjects (Kumar et al., 2008; Whitmer, Frank, & Gotlib, 2012).

Further laboratory studies have also sought to assess desire more directly by assessing an individual's willingness to expend effort in order to obtain various rewards. To isolate this construct behaviorally, a number of groups have recently employed various effort-based decision-making tasks in which subjects must expend physical or mental effort in order to earn varying levels of rewards. One such task developed by our group is the Effort-Expenditure for Rewards Task (EEfRT, pronounced "effort"; Treadway, Buckholtz, Schwartzman, Lambert, & Zald, 2009). During this task, participants perform a series of trials in which they are asked to choose between completing a "high effort" and "low effort" task in exchange for monetary compensation. Using the EEfRT and a similar effort-based paradigm, two studies have found evidence for impairment in motivation for rewards in MDD (Clery-Melin et al., 2011; Treadway, Bossaller, Shelton, & Zald, 2012a). A similar pattern was observed in schizophrenia patients (Barch, Treadway, & Schoen, 2014; Gold et al., 2012). Critically, in each study differences in effort expenditure between anhedonic patients and controls were found to result from the fact that controls modulated their effort output as a function of how much reward was at stake, while patients did not. This suggests that, rather than a pure effort-mobilization deficit, anhedonic symptoms may be more directly linked to ineffective allocation of effort in pursuit of rewards.

Taken together, the reviewed behavioral evidence suggests that although deficits in the experience of pleasure figure prominently in clinical diagnoses, the lack of consistent group differences in laboratory tests involving subjective responses to positive stimuli raises potential doubts as to whether a narrowly defined conceptualization of anhedonia as a specific deficit in the capacity to feel pleasure is accurate or useful in characterizing the most common reward processing abnormalities in depression and schizophrenia. In contrast, these behavioral studies have supported the claim that altered motivational states are common features of these disorders. Indeed, these reinforcement learning and motivational deficits may be key drivers of deficient reward-related behavior in these conditions, possibly to an even greater extent than an altered hedonic capacity.

Mapping Subdomains
of Reward Abnormalities to Distinct Neural Circuits

As described in the introduction, circuit-level mapping of anhedonic pathophysiology will likely require disaggregating anhedonic symptoms into their constituent elements of desire, hedonic response, and so forth. A number of behavioral studies have already begun to provide support for this approach, as anhedonic populations can exhibit either normal or abnormal symptom profiles depending on whether motivation or hedonic response is assessed. This distinction has important ramifications for the study of neurobiological mechanisms, as preclinical research has already demonstrated clear distinctions in neural systems responsible for motivation and pleasure.

Animal models have long suggested that the mesolimbic dopamine system may be selectively involved in reward motivation, but not hedonic response. The mesolimbic dopamine system encompasses a specific subpopulation of dopamine neurons that innervate the ventral striatum (VS), a key region involved in the processing of reward-relevant information (Haber & Knutson, 2010; see also Lopez, Wagner, & Heatherton, Chapter 7, this volume). Evidence for the necessity of intact mesolimbic dopamine function as an underpinning of motivated behavior has been demonstrated through the use of effort-based decision-making tasks. In these models, animals must choose whether to consume freely available but less desirable food rewards (low effort), or to exert physical effort in exchange for more palatable food rewards (high effort). Healthy rats exhibit a strong preference for the high-effort option, while attenuation or blockade of dopamine—especially in the ventral striatum—results in a behavioral shift toward low-effort options (Cousins & Salamone, 1994; Salamone et al., 2007). Critically, dopamine blockade does not reduce overall consumption, highlighting a selective role in willingness to work rather than appetitive drive. Moreover, potentiation of dopamine produces the opposite effects, resulting in an increased willingness to work for preferred rewards (Bardgett, Depenbrock, Downs, Points, & Green, 2009). In contrast to these dramatic effects of dopamine manipulations on effort production, attenuation or even complete absence of dopamine appears to have no consequences for hedonic responsiveness (for a review, see Berridge & Kringelbach, 2008).

In humans, effort-based decision-making tasks have also been used to explore the role of mesolimbic dopamine circuitry in normal and abnormal reward motivation. Mirroring the effects of dopamine potentiation in rats, one study found that administration of the dopamine agonist *d*-amphetamine produced a dose-dependent increase in the willingness to work for rewards (Wardle, Treadway, Mayo, Zald, & de Wit, 2011). Interestingly, these effects were strongest during trials for which probability of reward receipt was low, suggesting that dopamine may be involved in helping animals overcome probabilistic discounting as well as effort-related response costs. Similar effects of dopamine enhancement using the dopamine precursor L-DOPA have been observed on measures of vigorous effortful responding (Beierholm et al., 2013) as well reward anticipation and an optimism bias (Sharot, Guitart-Masip, Korn, Chowdhury, & Dolan, 2012; Sharot, Shiner, Brown, Fan, & Dolan, 2009), two constructs that are closely related to motivation.

To further elucidate the role of dopamine function as a predictor of individual differences, a follow-up study used positron emission tomography (PET) imaging to test associations between amphetamine-induced dopamine release (a probe of dopamine system reactivity) and willingness to exert physical effort for rewards (Treadway et al., 2012b). Here we found that the magnitude of dopamine release in the striatum positively predicted the proportion of high-effort choices subjects made during low-probability trials. Localization to this region is consistent with preclinical findings (Cousins & Salamone, 1994; Salamone et al., 2007) as well as human functional neuroimaging studies (Croxson, Walton, O'Reilly, Behrens, & Rushworth, 2009; Kurniawan et al., 2010; Schmidt, Lebreton, Clery-Melin, Daunizeau, & Pessiglione, 2012). Intriguingly, our study also found a negative relationship between percentage of high-effort choices and dopamine release in the insula. While insula dopamine function has not traditionally been a focus for rodent models of effort-based decision making, recent work suggests that insular dopamine receptor mRNA expression is predictive of effort-related behaviors (Simon et al., 2013). Moreover, other human imaging studies have observed insula activation when participants chose not to expend effort (Prevost, Pessiglione, Metereau, Clery-Melin, & Dreher, 2010). Although further investigation is necessary, these data suggest that the insula and striatum may play somewhat antagonistic roles in determining whether an individual is willing to overcome effort costs.

Similar convergence between clinical and preclinical studies has been observed in reinforcement learning studies. Using a rodent version of a signal-detection task developed by Pizzagalli and colleagues, researchers found that a pharmacological blockade of dopamine release abolished the development of a reward response bias, a pattern that mirrors behavioral effects in depressed patients (Der-Avakian, D'Souza, Pizzagalli, & Markou, 2013). In humans, dopamine PET imaging revealed that reinforcement learning during this task was associated with dopamine release in medial prefrontal reward areas (Vrieze et al., 2011). The role of dopamine in reinforcement learning has also received substantial validation from computational modeling approaches, which have been found to successfully predict the effects of pharmacological and optogenetic manipulations in both animals and humans (Frank, 2005; Maia & Frank, 2011; Montague, Dolan, Friston, & Dayan, 2012).

Finally, it is worth noting that abnormalities in corticostriatal circuitry have increasingly been reported in anhedonic patient populations. Blunted striatal engagement in response to reward-predicting cues has been frequently reported in individuals with schizophrenia (Juckel et al., 2006) as well as unaffected first-degree relatives (Winton-Brown, Fusar-Poli, Ungless, & Howes, 2014; Wolf et al., 2014). Similarly, a number of human fMRI studies have found reduced prediction-error signaling in the VS in MDD (Kumar et al., 2008; Pizzagalli et al., 2009; Steele, Meyer, & Ebmeier, 2004). In addition to these psychiatric conditions, individuals experiencing significant reductions in energy and desire as a consequence of a medical treatment, such as interferon-alpha therapy, also show reduced neural responses to reward anticipation, as well as decreased dopamine synthesis capacity (Capuron et al., 2012). These findings further implicate the role of corticostriatal systems in the pathophysiology of anhedonia.

Summary and Conclusions

In this chapter, I have reviewed some of the conceptual and methodological challenges to studying anhedonia and its biological bases. Anhedonic symptoms have distinct components related to motivation, learning, and subjective responses to stimuli and life events, each of which maps onto a distinct aspect of circuitry. It is therefore likely that anhedonic symptoms have distinct subtypes. Other subtypes are likely to exist, and further refinement of the anhedonic construct—and its pathophysiology—through the use of multiple measurements will be required to better understand, prevent, and treat this symptom. Going forward, mapping distinct facets of anhedonia to specific circuits will be critical in the development of biological markers that can reliably aid in diagnosis and treatment prediction. As the DSM-based nosology has been found to lack a clear biological basis (Kapur, Phillips, & Insel, 2012), the use of circuit-level measures will become increasingly important (Akil et al., 2010). Ultimately, this approach will help contribute to a biologically based nosology of psychiatric symptoms.

REFERENCES

Akil, H., Brenner, S., Kandel, E., Kendler, K. S., King, M. C., Scolnick, E., et al. (2010). The future of psychiatric research: Genomes and neural circuits. *Science, 327*(5973), 1580–1581.

Allen, N. B., Trinder, J., & Brennan, C. (1999). Affective startle modulation in clinical depression: Preliminary findings. *Biological Psychiatry, 46*(4), 542–550.

Amsterdam, J. D., Settle, R. G., Doty, R. L., Abelman, E., & Winokur, A. (1987). Taste and smell perception in depression. *Biological Psychiatry, 22*(12), 1481–1485.

Andreasen, N. C. (1982). Negative symptoms in schizophrenia: Definition and reliability. *Archives of General Psychiatry, 39*(7), 784–788.

Barch, D., Treadway, M. T., & Schoen, N. (2014). Effort, anhedonia and function in schizophrenia: Reduced effort allocation predicts amotivation and functional impairment. *Journal of Abnormal Psychology, 123,* 387.

Barch, D. M., & Dowd, E. C. (2010). Goal representations and motivational drive in schizophrenia: The role of prefrontal-striatal interactions. *Schizophrenia Bulletin, 36*(5), 919–934.

Bardgett, M. E., Depenbrock, M., Downs, N., Points, M., & Green, L. (2009). Dopamine modulates effort-based decision making in rats. *Behavioral Neuroscience, 123*(2), 242–251.

Beierholm, U., Guitart-Masip, M., Economides, M., Chowdhury, R., Duzel, E., Dolan, R., et al. (2013). Dopamine modulates reward-related vigor. *Neuropsychopharmacology, 38,* 1495–1503.

Berlin, I., Givry-Steiner, L., Lecrubier, Y., & Puech, A. J. (1998). Measures of anhedonia and hedonic responses to sucrose in depressive and scizophrenic patients in comparison with healthy subjects. *European Psychiatry, 13,* 303–309.

Berridge, K. C. (2007). The debate over dopamine's role in reward: The case for incentive salience. *Psychopharmacology, 191*(3), 391–431.

Berridge, K. C., & Kringelbach, M. L. (2008). Affective neuroscience of pleasure: Reward in humans and animals. *Psychopharmacology, 199*(3), 457–480.

Berridge, K. C., & Robinson, T. E. (1998). What is the role of dopamine in reward: Hedonic impact, reward learning, or incentive salience? *Brain Research Reviews, 28*(3), 309–369.

Bylsma, L. M., Morris, B. H., & Rottenberg, J. (2008). A meta-analysis of emotional reactivity in major depressive disorder. *Clinical Psychology Review, 28*(4), 676–691.

Capuron, L., Pagnoni, G., Drake, D. F., Woolwine, B. J., Spivey, J. R., Crowe, R. J., et al. (2012). Dopaminergic mechanisms of reduced basal ganglia responses to hedonic reward during interferon alfa administration. *Archives of General Psychiatry, 69*(10), 1044–1053.

Chapman, L. J., Chapman, J. P., & Raulin, M. L. (1976). Scales for physical and social anhedonia. *Journal of Abnormal Psychology, 85*(4), 374–382.

Chase, H., Frank, M., Michael, A., Bullmore, E., Sahakian, B., & Robbins, T. (2010). Approach and avoidance learning in patients with major depression and healthy controls: Relation to anhedonia. *Psychological Medicine, 40*(3), 433.

Clery-Melin, M. L., Schmidt, L., Lafargue, G., Baup, N., Fossati, P., & Pessiglione, M. (2011). Why don't you try harder? An investigation of effort production in major depression. *PLoS ONE, 6*(8), e23178.

Conner, T. S., & Barrett, L. F. (2012). Trends in ambulatory self-report: The role of momentary experience in psychosomatic medicine. *Psychosomatic Medicine, 74*(4), 327–337.

Cooper, A. J., Smillie, L. D., & Jackson, C. J. (2008). A trait conceptualization of reward-reactivity. *Journal of Individual Differences, 29*(3), 168–180.

Cousins, M. S., & Salamone, J. D. (1994). Nucleus accumbens dopamine depletions in rats affect relative response allocation in a novel cost/benefit procedure. *Pharmacology, Biochemistry and Behavior, 49*(1), 85–91.

Croxson, P. L., Walton, M. E., O'Reilly, J. X., Behrens, T. E., & Rushworth, M. F. (2009). Effort-based cost-benefit valuation and the human brain. *Journal of Neuroscience, 29*(14), 4531–4541.

Der-Avakian, A., D'Souza, M. S., Pizzagalli, D. A., & Markou, A. (2013). Assessment of reward responsiveness in the response bias probabilistic reward task in rats: implications for cross-species translational research. *Translational Psychiatry, 3*, e297.

Dichter, G. S., Smoski, M. J., Kampov-Polevoy, A. B., Gallop, R., & Garbutt, J. C. (2009). Unipolar depression does not moderate responses to the Sweet Taste Test. *Biological Psychiatry, 66*, 886–897.

Dichter, G. S., Tomarken, A. J., Shelton, R. C., & Sutton, S. K. (2004). Early- and late-onset startle modulation in unipolar depression. *Psychophysiology, 41*(3), 433–440.

Duckworth, A. L., Peterson, C., Matthews, M. D., & Kelly, D. R. (2007). Grit: Perseverance and passion for long-term goals. *Journal of Personality and Social Psychology, 92*(6), 1087–1101.

Edmondson, D., Shaffer, J. A., Chaplin, W. F., Burg, M. M., Stone, A. A., & Schwartz, J. E. (2013). Trait anxiety and trait anger measured by ecological momentary assessment and their correspondence with traditional trait questionnaires. *Journal of Research in Personality, 47*(6), 843–852.

Elliot, A. J., & Thrash, T. M. (2010). Approach and avoidance temperament as basic dimensions of personality. *Journal of Personality, 78*(3), 865–906.

Fawcett, J., Clark, D. C., Scheftner, W. A., & Hedeker, D. (1983). Differences between anhedonic and normally hedonic depressive states. *American Journal of Psychiatry, 140*(8), 1027–1030.

Forbes, E. E., & Dahl, R. E. (2005). Neural systems of positive affect: Relevance to understanding child and adolescent depression? *Development and Psychopathology, 17*(3), 827–850.

Foussias, G., & Remington, G. (2008). Negative symptoms in schizophrenia: Avolition and Occam's razor. *Schizophrenia Bulletin, 36*(2), 359–369.

Frank, M. J. (2005). Dynamic dopamine modulation in the basal ganglia: A neurocomputational account of cognitive deficits in medicated and nonmedicated Parkinsonism. *Journal of Cognitive Neuroscience, 17*(1), 51–72.

Gard, D. E., Gard, M. G., Kring, A. M., & John, O. P. (2006). Anticipatory and consummatory components of the experience of pleasure: A scale development study. *Journal of Reserch in Personality, 40*, 1086–1102.

Gehricke, J., & Shapiro, D. (2000). Reduced facial expression and social context in major depression: Discrepancies between facial muscle activity and self-reported emotion. *Psychiatry Research, 95*(2), 157–167.

Gold, J. M., Strauss, G. P., Waltz, J. A., Robinson, B. M., Brown, J. K., & Frank, M. J. (2012). Negative symptoms of schizophrenia are associated with abnormal effort-cost computations. *Biological Psychiatry, 74*(2), 130–136.

Gold, J. M., Waltz, J. A., Prentice, K. J., Morris, S. E., & Heerey, E. A. (2008). Reward processing in schizophrenia: A deficit in the representation of value. *Schizophrenia Bulletin, 34*(5), 835–847.

Haber, S. N., & Knutson, B. (2010). The reward circuit: Linking primate anatomy and human imaging. *Neuropsychopharmacology, 35*(1), 4–26.

Henriques, J. B., Glowacki, J. M., & Davidson, R. J. (1994). Reward fails to alter response bias in depression. *Journal of Abnormal Psychology, 103*(3), 460–466.

Insel, T., Cuthbert, B., Garvey, M., Heinssen, R., Pine, D. S., Quinn, K., et al. (2010). Research domain criteria (RDoC): Toward a new classification framework for research on mental disorders. *American Journal of Psychiatry, 167*(7), 748–751.

Juckel, G., Schlagenhauf, F., Koslowski, M., Wustenberg, T., Villringer, A., Knutson, B., et al. (2006). Dysfunction of ventral striatal reward prediction in schizophrenia. *NeuroImage, 29*(2), 409–416.

Kagan, J. (2007). A trio of concerns. *Perspectives on Psychological Science, 2*(4), 361–376.

Kahneman, D., & Deaton, A. (2012). High income improves evaluation of life but not emotional well-being. *Proceedings of the National Academy of Sciences, 107*(38), 16489–16493.

Kapur, S., Phillips, A. G., & Insel, T. R. (2012). Why has it taken so long for biological psychiatry to develop clinical tests and what to do about it? *Molecular Psychiatry, 17*(12), 1174–1179.

Kaviani, H., Gray, J. A., Checkley, S. A., Raven, P. W., Wilson, G. D., & Kumari, V. (2004). Affective modulation of the startle response in depression: Influence of the severity of depression, anhedonia, and anxiety. *Journal of Affective Disorders, 83*(1), 21–31.

Kazes, M., Danion, J. M., Grange, D., Pradignac, A., Simon, C., Burrus-Mehl, F., et al. (1994). Eating behaviour and depression before and after antidepressant treatment: A prospective, naturalistic study. *Journal of Affective Disorders, 30*(3), 193–207.

Keedwell, P. A., Andrew, C., Williams, S. C., Brammer, M. J., & Phillips, M. L. (2005a). A double dissociation of ventromedial prefrontal cortical responses to sad and happy stimuli in depressed and healthy individuals. *Biological Psychiatry, 58*(6), 495–503.

Keedwell, P. A., Andrew, C., Williams, S. C., Brammer, M. J., & Phillips, M. L. (2005b). The neural correlates of anhedonia in major depressive disorder. *Biological Psychiatry, 58*(11), 843–853.

Klein, D. F. (1974). Endogenomorphic depression: A conceptual and terminological revision. *Archives of General Psychiatry, 31*(4), 447–454.

Kring, A. M., & Moran, E. K. (2008). Emotional response deficits in schizophrenia: Insights from affective science. *Schizophrenia Bulletin, 34*(5), 819–834.

Kumar, P., Waiter, G., Ahearn, T., Milders, M., Reid, I., & Steele, J. D. (2008). Abnormal temporal difference reward-learning signals in major depression. *Brain, 131*(8), 2084–2093.

Kurniawan, I. T., Seymour, B., Talmi, D., Yoshida, W., Chater, N., & Dolan, R. J. (2010). Choosing to make an effort: The role of striatum in signaling physical effort of a chosen action. *Journal of Neurophysiology, 104*(1), 313–321.

Maia, T. V., & Frank, M. J. (2011). From reinforcement learning models to psychiatric and neurological disorders. *Nature Neuroscience, 14*(2), 154–162.

Meehl, P. E. (1975). Hedonic capacity: Some conjectures. *Bulletin of the Menninger Clinic, 39*(4), 295–307.

Mitterschiffthaler, M. T., Kumari, V., Malhi, G. S., Brown, R. G., Giampietro, V. P., Brammer, M. J., et al. (2003). Neural response to pleasant stimuli in anhedonia: An fMRI study. *NeuroReport, 14*(2), 177–182.

Montague, P. R., Dolan, R. J., Friston, K. J., & Dayan, P. (2012). Computational psychiatry. *Trends in Cognitive Sciences, 16*(1), 72–80.

Pizzagalli, D. A., Holmes, A. J., Dillon, D. G., Goetz, E. L., Birk, J. L., Bogdan, R., et al. (2009). Reduced caudate and nucleus accumbens response to rewards in unmedicated individuals with major depressive disorder. *American Journal of Psychiatry, 166*(6), 702–710.

Pizzagalli, D. A., Iosifescu, D., Hallett, L. A., Ratner, K. G., & Fava, M. (2008). Reduced hedonic capacity in major depressive disorder: Evidence from a probabilistic reward task. *Journal of Psychiatric Research, 43*(1), 76–87.

Pizzagalli, D. A., Jahn, A. L., & O'Shea, J. P. (2005). Toward an objective characterization of an anhedonic phenotype: A signal-detection approach. *Biological Psychiatry, 57*(4), 319–327.

Prevost, C., Pessiglione, M., Metereau, E., Clery-Melin, M. L., & Dreher, J. C. (2010). Separate valuation subsystems for delay and effort decision costs. *Journal of Neuroscience, 30*(42), 14080–14090.

Renneberg, B., Heyn, K., Gebhard, R., & Bachmann, S. (2005). Facial expression of emotions in borderline personality disorder and depression. *Journal of Behavior Therapy and Experimental Psychiatry, 36*(3), 183–196.

Robinson, M. D., & Clore, G. L. (2002). Belief and feeling: Evidence for an accessibility model of emotional self-report. *Psychological Bulletin, 128*(6), 934.

Rushworth, M. F., Noonan, M. P., Boorman, E. D., Walton, M. E., & Behrens, T. E. (2011). Frontal cortex and reward-guided learning and decision-making. *Neuron, 70*(6), 1054–1069.

Salamone, J. D., Correa, M., Farrar, A., & Mingote, S. M. (2007). Effort-related functions of nucleus accumbens dopamine and associated forebrain circuits. *Psychopharmacology, 191*(3), 461–482.

Schmidt, L., Lebreton, M., Clery-Melin, M. L., Daunizeau, J., & Pessiglione, M. (2012). Neural mechanisms underlying motivation of mental versus physical effort. *PLoS Biology, 10*(2), e1001266.

Schwartz, J. E., Neale, J., Marco, C., Shiffman, S. S., & Stone, A. A. (1999). Does trait coping exist?: A momentary assessment approach to the evaluation of traits. *Journal of Personality and Social Psychology, 77*(2), 360.

Sharot, T., Guitart-Masip, M., Korn, C. W., Chowdhury, R., & Dolan, R. J. (2012).

How dopamine enhances an optimism bias in humans. *Current Biology, 22*(16),1477–1481.

Sharot, T., Shiner, T., Brown, A. C., Fan, J., & Dolan, R. J. (2009). Dopamine enhances expectation of pleasure in humans. *Current Biology, 19*(24), 2077–2080.

Shelton, R. C., & Tomarken, A. J. (2001). Can recovery from depression be achieved? *Psychiatric Services, 52*(11), 1469–1478.

Simon, N. W., Beas, B. S., Montgomery, K. S., Haberman, R. P., Bizon, J. L., & Setlow, B. (2013). Prefrontal cortical–striatal dopamine receptor mRNA expression predicts distinct forms of impulsivity. *European Journal of Neuroscience, 37*(11), 1779–1788.

Snaith, R. P., Hamilton, M., Morley, S., Humayan, A., Hargreaves, D., & Trigwell, P. (1995). A scale for the assessment of hedonic tone: The Snaith–Hamilton Pleasure Scale. *British Journal of Psychiatry, 167*(1), 99–103.

Steele, J. D., Meyer, M., & Ebmeier, K. P. (2004). Neural predictive error signal correlates with depressive illness severity in a game paradigm. *NeuroImage, 23*(1), 269–280.

Strauss, G. P., & Gold, J. M. (2012). A new perspective on anhedonia in schizophrenia. *American Journal of Psychiatry, 169*, 364–373.

Surguladze, S., Brammer, M. J., Keedwell, P., Giampietro, V., Young, A. W., Travis, M. J., et al. (2005). A differential pattern of neural response toward sad versus happy facial expressions in major depressive disorder. *Biological Psychiatry, 57*(3), 201–209.

Treadway, M. T., Bossaller, N. A., Shelton, R. C., & Zald, D. H. (2012a). Effort-based decision-making in major depressive disorder: A translational model of motivational anhedonia. *Journal of Abnormal Psychology, 121*(3), 553–558.

Treadway, M. T., Buckholtz, J. W., Cowan, R. L., Woodward, N. D., Li, R., Ansari, M. S., et al. (2012b). Dopaminergic mechanisms of individual differences in human effort-based decision-making. *Journal of Neuroscience, 32*(18), 6170–6176.

Treadway, M. T., Buckholtz, J. W., Schwartzman, A. N., Lambert, W. E., & Zald, D. H. (2009). Worth the "EEfRT"? The effort expenditure for rewards task as an objective measure of motivation and anhedonia. *PLoS ONE, 4*(8), e6598.

Treadway, M. T., & Zald, D. H. (2011). Reconsidering anhedonia in depression: Lessons from translational neuroscience. *Neuroscience and Biobehavioral Reviews, 35*(3), 537–555.

Treadway, M. T., & Zald, D. H. (2013). Parsing anhedonia: Translational models of reward-processing deficits in psychopathology. *Current Directions in Psychological Science, 22*(3), 244–249.

Tremeau, F., Malaspina, D., Duval, F., Correa, H., Hager-Budny, M., Coin-Bariou, L., et al. (2005). Facial expressiveness in patients with schizophrenia compared to depressed patients and nonpatient comparison subjects. *American Journal of Psychiatry, 162*(1), 92–101.

Tsai, J. L., Pole, N., Levenson, R. W., & Munoz, R. F. (2003). The effects of depression on the emotional responses of Spanish-speaking Latinas. *Cultural Diversity and Ethnic Minority Psychology, 9*(1), 49–63.

Vrieze, E., Ceccarini, J., Pizzagalli, D. A., Bormans, G., Vandenbulcke, M., Demyttenaere, K., et al. (2011). Measuring extrastriatal dopamine release during a reward learning task. *Human Brain Mapping.*

Vrieze, E., Pizzagalli, D. A., Demyttenaere, K., Hompes, T., Sienaert, P., de Boer, P., et al. (2013). Reduced reward learning predicts outcome in major depressive disorder. *Biological Psychiatry.*

Wardle, M. C., Treadway, M. T., Mayo, L. M., Zald, D. H., & de Wit, H. (2011). Amping up effort: Effects of d-amphetamine on human effort-based decision-making. *Journal of Neuroscience, 31*(46), 16597–16602.

Whitmer, A. J., Frank, M. J., & Gotlib, I. H. (2012). Sensitivity to reward and punishment in major depressive disorder: Effects of rumination and of single versus multiple experiences. *Cognition and Emotion, 26*(8), 1475–1485.

Winer, E. S., Veilleux, J. C., & Ginger, E. J. (2014). Development and validation of the Specific Loss of Interest and Pleasure Scale (SLIPS). *Journal of Affective Disorders, 152*, 193–201.

Winton-Brown, T. T., Fusar-Poli, P., Ungless, M. A., & Howes, O. D. (2014). Dopaminergic basis of salience dysregulation in psychosis. *Trends in Neurosciences, 37*(2), 85–94.

Wolf, D. H., Satterthwaite, T. D., Kantrowitz, J. J., Katchmar, N., Vandekar, L., Elliott, M. A., et al. (2014). Amotivation in schizophrenia: Integrated assessment with behavioral, clinical, and imaging measures. *Schizophrenia Bulletin,40*(6),1328–1337.

PART V

Applied Content Domains

CHAPTER 16

Desire for Food and the Power of Mind

Anne Roefs
Katrijn Houben
Jessica Werthmann

In the Western world, overweight and obesity rates are high and continue to rise. Globally, 35% of adults are overweight, and 11% are obese (World Health Organization, 2013). Obesity is related to many detrimental health consequences and a reduced quality of life (Jia & Lubetkin, 2005, 2010; Kolotkin, Meter, & Williams, 2001). Examples include cardiovascular diseases, diabetes, and psychological problems such as depression (e.g., Blaine, 2008; Luppino et al., 2010). Ultimately, the cause of obesity is an energy imbalance, that is, more calories are consumed than are expended (Westerterp, 2010). This energy imbalance seems mainly due to the overconsumption of high-caloric palatable foods (Swinburn, Jolley, Kremer, Salbe, & Ravussin, 2006; Swinburn et al., 2009; Westerterp, 2010). A more interesting question is *why* so many people have an unfavorable energy balance, which has led them to be overweight, or even obese. Why do so many people overconsume high-caloric palatable foods when it is common knowledge that these foods are detrimental for your health and waistline?

An obvious possibility seems to be that people's control of homeostasis is disturbed (Gale, Castracane, & Mantzoros, 2004). However, at the very least, this homeostatic explanation is not sufficient, and nonhomeostatic factors have been shown to play an important role (Shin, Zheng, & Berthoud, 2009). That is, people consume foods because of the expected experience of reward. Homeostatic and nonhomeostatic factors may interact, as foods may, for example, become more attractive when one is hungry (e.g., Siep et al., 2009; Uher, Treasure, Heining, Brammer, & Campbell, 2006). So an important contribution to the obesity epidemic likely is so-called hedonic hunger (Lowe & Butryn, 2007). That is, "some individuals experience frequent thoughts, feelings and urges about food in the absence of any short- or long-term energy deficit" (Lowe & Butryn, p. 432).

Desire for food is thought to be reflected in the brain as food-cue-elicited activity in brain regions involved in reward processing (Berthoud, Lenard, & Shin, 2011; Kringelbach, 2009; van der Laan, de Ridder, Viergever, & Smeets, 2011; see also Lopez, Wagner, & Heatherton, Chapter 7, this volume). These brain regions are listed as follows in Frankort et al. (2012): "the amygdala, hippocampus, ventral pallidum, nucleus accumbens and striatum, the ventral tegmental area and substantia nigra, as well as the anterior cingulate, orbitofrontal, insular, posterior fusiform, dorsolateral prefrontal and medial prefrontal cortices" (p. 627).

With regard to the experience of desire, a highly relevant finding is that activity elicited by visual food stimuli in the insular cortex, the left operculum, and the right putamen was modulated positively by the subjective feeling of appetite in lean healthy participants (Porubská, Veit, Preissl, Fritsche, & Birbaumer, 2006). Moreover, in a study in which participants were put on a monotonous diet and asked during scanning to imagine sensory properties of a favorite food, craving-specific brain activity was found in the hippocampus, insula, and caudate (Pelchat, Johnson, Chan, Valdez, & Ragland, 2004).

With our Western environment being full of food temptations (e.g., Wadden, Brownell, & Foster, 2002), the experience of desire for food is always lurking. So it has become a challenge to attain or retain a healthy weight. However, the food-replete environment is not a problem for everyone, as an approximately equally large number of people have a healthy weight. Therefore, a reasonable hypothesis is that high-caloric foods in the environment may be more attractive for certain people, making it harder for them to resist these foods, thereby possibly leading to overconsumption and ultimately to overweight or obesity.

From a cognitive perspective, this increased attractiveness is thought to be reflected in *biased* cognitive processing of food stimuli in people with overeating problems, such as overweight and obese people and high-restrained eaters. In other words, their desire for food may influence their cognitive processing of food stimuli, making it harder to resist these desires. Moreover, a biased cognitive processing of food stimuli may also maintain and/or further increase food desires. More specifically, their attention may be drawn preferentially to (high-caloric) food cues (e.g., Werthmann et al., 2011), they may have more positive associations with (high-caloric) foods (e.g., Roefs et al., 2011), and (high-caloric) food cues may trigger more activity in the reward centers of their brains (e.g., Frankort et al., 2012). These cognitive processes all may contribute to the degree of experienced craving, desire, and thereby to food consumption (see also Hofmann, Kotabe, Vohs, & Baumeister, Chapter 3, this volume).

Further adding to the potential power of high-caloric food cues in the environment is the hypothesized *automaticity* of the increased cognitive hedonic reactivity to these food cues, while simultaneously assuming that cognitive resources are needed to activate the longer-term goal of a healthy weight (e.g., Hofmann, Friese, & Strack, 2009). As argued recently (Hofmann & Van Dillen, 2012), these initial automatic responses can lead to habitual or impulsive eating behavior, but they may also enter into working memory and can become a conscious desire, which may grow increasingly stronger (see also Kavanagh, Andrade, & May, 2005; Andrade, May, Van Dillen, & Kavanagh, Chapter 1, this volume). If this desire escalates, conscious pursuit of the desire may follow, resulting in the consumption of the desired foods.

Taken together, the idea is that attention, associations, and food-reward processing in the brain are all *automatically* biased toward a *hedonic* response to food in susceptible people. This implies that people with overeating problems will show evidence of all three types of biased cognitive processing. But what is the current status of empirical evidence for this idea? Attention bias for food, implicit measures of associations with food, and brain reward activity in response to food cues will be considered successively in this chapter. The chapter focuses on research done with people with overeating problems, that is, overweight people and restrained eaters. Restrained eaters have a chronic intention of losing weight but are frequently unsuccessful, and then indulge in the high-caloric foods they attempt to avoid (Herman & Polivy, 1980, 2004). The frequent alternations between restraint and disinhibited eating may increase the attractiveness of the high-caloric foods that they actually consider as forbidden (e.g., Gendall & Joyce, 2001).

Biased Attention Toward Foods

A large number of studies have addressed biased attention toward food in various groups of people with eating problems: obesity and overweight, eating disorders, and restrained eating (for meta-analyses, see Brooks, Prince, Stahl, Campbell, & Treasure, 2011; Dobson & Dozois, 2004). The hypothesized increased attractiveness of high-caloric foods to overweight people and high-restrained eaters is thought to be reflected in biased attention toward high-caloric foods.

How Is Attention Bias Measured?

Attention bias for food is frequently assessed using either a food variant of the emotional Stroop task (Williams, Mathews, & MacLeod, 1996) or with the visual probe paradigm (MacLeod, Mathews, & Tata, 1986) measuring response latencies and/or eye movements. In the food Stroop task, participants name the color of (different types of) food words and neutral words. If participants are slower on the food word trials, it is concluded that the food words produce more interference, and this interference is often taken as evidence for an attention bias *toward* food. However, the interpretation of the emotional Stroop effect is not straightforward, as attentional *avoidance* of the stimulus altogether would also cause a slow-down in response latency (e.g., Field & Cox, 2008). Generally, the exact cognitive mechanism underlying the emotional Stroop effect is unclear (see Williams et al., 1996), which complicates the interpretation of interference scores.

The visual probe paradigm (e.g., MacLeod et al., 1986) is an improvement in that sense, as it can be clearly determined whether the participant shows relative attentional approach or avoidance as compared to a contrast category of stimuli. Typically, in this paradigm a pair of cues (e.g., one food and one neutral picture) is presented on screen, and after a certain interstimulus interval (ISI) (e.g., 1,000 msec), a dot replaces one of these pictures. The participant has to decide as quickly as possible in what location (typically left vs. right side of the screen) the dot appeared. If participants are on average faster on trials in which the dot replaces the food picture as compared to the neutral pictures, it is concluded that they have an attention bias toward food. A reverse effect is taken as evidence for attentional avoidance of food. If eye movements are measured, conclusions are reached in a similar way. It is tested whether a first eye movement more often goes to either the food or the control picture, and the gaze duration on both pictures is determined and compared.

Attention Bias for High-Caloric Foods in Obesity and Restrained Eating

There is indeed some evidence for the idea that obese people preferentially attend to (high-caloric) foods as compared to healthy-weight people. Using a visual probe task with eye tracking, Castellanos and colleagues (2009) found that sated obese participants, as compared to sated healthy-weight participants, preferentially attended to food as compared to neutral items, as apparent both in initial orientation and gaze duration. No group differences were observed in the hungry state. Another study using the dot-probe task reported similar results: on a response-latency-based measure, obese people, but not healthy-weight controls, showed a bias toward food pictures, with the effect being primarily due to high-caloric foods (Kemps, Tiggemann, & Hollitt, 2014).

Partly converging evidence was found using event-related potentials (ERPs; Nijs, Franken, & Muris, 2010). Obese people showed evidence of an increased early attention bias for high-caloric food (reflected in the P200 component), but no difference between obese and healthy-weight participants was seen on a later component (P300; see also Nijs, Franken, & Muris, 2008), or on a behavioral measure (response latency in the food Stroop paradigm). This pattern of results was partly observed in eye-tracking data (Werthmann et al., 2011) as well: Obese people more frequently oriented toward a high-caloric food picture than a neutral picture as compared to healthy-weight people, but their fixation duration on these food stimuli was shorter than that in healthy-weight people, suggesting an approach–avoidance response in obese people. Taken together, the three studies described above all found evidence for a relatively early attention bias toward food specifically in overweight or obese people, but diverged in their findings regarding later components of this attention bias (approach, no difference, or even avoid).

Partly in keeping with the previously discussed studies are the results from Nijs, Muris, Euser, and Franken (2010). They measured multiple indices of attention bias for high-caloric food—eye tracking (initial orientation and gaze duration), response latency in a dot-probe task with 100 and 500 msec presentation of cue pair, and P300. They found a difference between obese and healthy-weight participants only on their response latency data in the visual probe task with 100 msec cue-pair presentation, with obese people showing increased attention bias toward high-caloric foods. This partly fits with the above findings that the only difference between obese and healthy-weight participants was observed in an early component of attention bias. However, it is surprising that no differences were found in Nijs et al.'s (2010) eye-tracking data (cf. Werthmann et al., 2011, in which effects were found in eye-tracking data but not in response latency data).

Finally, on a food Stroop task, clear differences were observed between obese and healthy-weight children. That is, obese children specifically showed greater interference by food words than did healthy-weight children (Braet & Crombez, 2003). Note, however, that it is unclear exactly how to interpret the results from this paradigm (see above). One cannot be certain whether increased interference actually reflects more or less attention toward the word itself.

So far it seems there is some evidence for an increased attention bias toward food in overweight and obese people, albeit most convincingly in relatively early attention processes. However, quite a few studies, using various types of methodology, reported no relationship between body mass index (BMI) and attention bias for food: dot-probe tasks comparing attention to healthy and unhealthy food words (Pothos, Tapper, & Calitri, 2009), attention to food and neutral words with a very brief cue-pair presentation of 50 msec (Loeber et al., 2012), or attention to high-caloric foods and neutral control stimuli in obese versus healthy-weight children (Werthmann, Jansen, Vreugdenhil, Nederkoorn, Schyns, et al., in press); an emotional Stroop task with healthy and unhealthy food words (Phelan et al., 2011; Pothos et al., 2009); and gaze time at high- and low-calorie foods in a free-viewing paradigm (Graham, Hoover, Ceballos, & Komogortsev, 2011). Finally, some studies even reported a reverse association between BMI and attention bias toward high-caloric foods. That is, they found a reduced attention bias for these foods with increasing

BMI. More specifically, Graham et al. (2011) found that their healthy-weight group oriented more frequently toward high-caloric sweet foods than low-caloric foods, while they did not find differences in frequency of initial orientation between food types in their overweight group. In addition, in a visual search paradigm, participants showed increasingly faster detection of food compared to nonfood items with lower BMIs (Nummenmaa, Hietanen, Calvo, & Hyönä, 2011). So, it is evidently too simplistic to conclude that obese people are characterized by an exceptionally strong attention bias toward high-caloric foods.

Another group of people who are hypothesized to be especially vulnerable to the tempting foods in our environment are the restrained eaters. Whether this increased vulnerability to tempting food cues is reflected in biased attention toward food cues has been the topic of many studies, but again, it is hard to draw a general conclusion. In particular, the food Stroop task has been employed frequently. Two meta-analyses (Brooks et al., 2011; Dobson & Dozois, 2004) conclude that there is a small food interference effect specifically in restrained eaters, but one meta-analysis (Johansson, Ghaderi, & Andersson, 2005) concludes that there are no differences between restrained and unrestrained eaters in this regard. Bear in mind the interpretation problems with the emotional Stroop task as well.

Using a visual probe paradigm, most studies found no evidence for a stronger attention bias toward food in restrained than unrestrained eaters (Ahern, Field, Yokum, Bohon, & Stice, 2010; Boon, Vogelzang, & Jansen, 2000; Brignell, Griffiths, Bradley, & Mogg, 2009; Werthmann et al., 2013b), whereas Hepworth, Mogg, Brignell, and Bradley (2010) did. Notably, when using a free-viewing paradigm combined with eye-tracking, a reverse effect was found. More specifically, restraint was associated with a reduced frequency of orientation to high-calorie sweet foods in an overweight group (Graham et al., 2011).

So, taken together, there is no clear evidence for either attentional approach or attentional avoidance of high-caloric foods in either overweight people or restrained eaters. Reaching a general conclusion about these studies is complicated by the great diversity in paradigms, timing parameters, stimulus details, and comparison categories (e.g., high-caloric vs. low-caloric foods or foods vs. neutral items). Though the between-group approach did not prove to be particularly elucidating, what about studies that actually assessed craving for food and consumption of food?

Relationship between Attention Bias and Craving and Consumption

Another highly relevant question is obviously whether an attention bias toward food is actually (causally) related to craving and food intake, as this is frequently assumed in studies assessing attention bias for food. However, it may also be argued that the attention bias toward food is caused by worry or anxiety about food. It is relevant in this respect that attention bias for food has also been frequently studied in patients with anorexia nervosa (AN). Clinically, one could expect both worry/anxiety about food and craving for food in this group of patients.

There have been a number of studies with the food Stroop task in patients with AN, but a meta-analysis (Dobson & Dozois, 2004) concluded that the food interference effect was not consistently observed in these patients. In a study using the visual probe paradigm, an attention bias toward high-caloric foods was observed (Shafran, Lee, Cooper, Palmer, & Fairburn, 2007), and in another study, increased distraction by high-caloric and low-caloric foods was observed in patients with AN (Smeets, Roefs, van Furth, & Jansen, 2008). Note that exactly the reverse—that is, reduced attention for food stimuli in patients with AN—was observed in a recent eye-tracking study (Giel et al., 2011). So, again, research focusing on group differences is not particularly elucidating, and the overall picture is not very consistent. Therefore, research that actually measures craving, or studies in which either craving or attention bias is manipulated, may help us further.

Correlations have been observed between attention bias toward food and momentary craving in an overweight group but not in a healthy-weight group (Werthmann et al., 2011), and between attention bias toward chocolate and chronic chocolate craving (Kemps & Tiggeman, 2009; Smeets, Roefs, & Jansen, 2009; Werthmann, Roefs, Nederkoorn, & Jansen, 2013a). Supporting the association between attentional processing and the control of craving, a recent ERP study (Harris, Hare, & Rangel, 2013) found evidence for early attentional modulation by successful versus unsuccessful self-control, but only when weight loss was made relevant for the participants by monetary incentive. More specifically, in trials in which participants made a food choice indicative of unsuccessful self-control (e.g., chose an unhealthy liked food), the N1 amplitude was more negative (reflecting more attentive processing) than on trials in which participants made a food choice indicative of successful self-control (e.g., chose a healthy but disliked food). So successful self-control in the context of food choice was associated with attention suppression.

In addition, there is also evidence for a causal relationship, that is, evidence that induced craving for chocolate leads to an attention bias for chocolate in chocolate likers (Kemps & Tiggeman, 2009) and high-trait chocolate cravers (Smeets et al., 2009). Relatedly, it was observed that attention bias toward a food decreased from premeasure (before the food was eaten to satiety) to postmeasure (after the food was eaten to satiety) (Di Pellegrino, Magarelli, & Mengarelli, 2011).

Interestingly, there is also evidence for a causal relation in the other direction, with manipulated attention for food affecting craving and/or food intake. More specifically, in two experiments (Kemps, Tiggemann, Orr, & Grear, 2014a) it was shown that participants who were trained to attend to chocolate cues consumed more chocolate in a so-called taste test afterwards as compared to participants who were trained to avoid chocolate cues. Moreover, in one of these experiments (but not the other), the attend-chocolate training was associated with an increase in craving, whereas the avoid-chocolate training was associated with a decrease in craving. Similar results were obtained in a study in which participants were either trained to attend to healthy or to unhealthy foods. It was found that participants who were trained to attend to healthy foods consumed relatively more healthy than unhealthy foods afterwards as compared to the participants who were trained to attend to unhealthy foods (Kakoschke, Kemps, & Tiggeman, 2013). Note that in both Kemps, Tiggemann, Orr, and Grear (2014b) and in Kakoschke et al. (2013), the training procedure also successfully altered the attention bias for the targeted food. This was corroborated in a later study in which it was also found that an attentional training procedure changed the attentional bias, both on the dot-probe task and on a word-stem completion task (Kemps et al., 2014a).

Using a novel attention bias modification procedure based on the anti-saccade task (e.g., Hallett, 1978), converging evidence was obtained (Werthmann, Field, Roefs, Nederkoorn, & Jansen, 2014). Here it was found that participants who were trained to avoid looking at chocolate and who performed highly accurately during the training showed a reduced chocolate intake as compared to a group of participants who were trained to look toward chocolate. No effects of the training on craving were observed, though. In stark contrast to these three studies are results from a study that manipulated attention bias toward cake. Only weak evidence was found for a change in the attention bias itself, and no effects on hunger or food intake were found (Hardman, Rogers, Etchells, Houstoun, & Munafò, 2013).

Taken together, there is a substantial amount of evidence for an association between biased attention for food and craving for food, and even some evidence in support of a causal relationship between these two variables. This conclusion is in line with the results from a meta-analysis on the association between attention bias and craving for addictive substances (Field, Munafò, & Franken, 2009; see also Franken, Chapter 19, this volume). In this meta-analysis, the association between attention bias and craving was small but significant, with some indications for a larger correlation when the measure that was used reflected attentional disengagement. Importantly, the correlation was substantially higher for studies employing a direct measure of attention bias (i.e., eye movement monitoring and ERP measurements) as compared to indirect response-latency-based measures.

Top-Down Influences on Attention Bias

As partially reviewed above, there is quite a large literature on group differences in attention bias toward high-caloric foods, the hypothesis under investigation being that overweight/obese people and chronically restrained eaters show attentional approach toward these foods. The findings have been disappointingly inconsistent. Part of the problem, of course, is the huge diversity in employed paradigms, stimuli, and timing parameters, compromising comparability across studies.

A more general problem is the double-faceted nature of high-caloric foods. In daily life the investigated groups typically fluctuate frequently between a momentary focus on taste versus a focus on health/weight consequences, reflecting this double-faceted nature of high-caloric foods. These fluctuations may be especially pronounced for people with weight problems. The possibility that attention focus (i.e., focus on taste vs. healthiness of food) is an overlooked factor with the potential to explain the divergence of findings in the field has received relatively little attention. It may be the case that such a momentary focus is a stronger determinant of attention bias for food than are more stable differences in weight and restraint status.

One hint that this may be the case is provided by studies that induced craving for food or an addictive substance. The inducement of craving may have led to a strong focus on taste or reward at the cost of health considerations. Indeed, inducing craving for chocolate led to an attention bias toward chocolate in two studies (Kemps & Tiggeman, 2009; Smeets et al., 2009). In a related finding, Werthmann et al. (2013c) discovered an association between self-endorsed eating permission (i.e., whether participants reported that they allowed themselves to consume chocolate in a taste test of the experiment) and a relatively long dwell time on chocolate. Similarly, using eye-tracking methodology as well, it was found that an attention bias for rewarding stimuli was enlarged when participants expected to receive these rewards (Jones et al., 2012). It is relevant here as well that an attentional bias for food was completely eliminated by providing participants with a concurrent high cognitive load, suggesting that some resources are necessary to recognize temptations (Van Dillen, Papies, & Hofmann, 2013).

In addition, from the meta-analysis by Field and colleagues (2009), it became apparent that the correlation between attention bias toward addictive substances and craving for these substances was particularly large when craving was induced in participants as compared to no-craving-induction control conditions. The craving induction possibly had the effect of focusing all the participants on the same aspect of the addictive substance, the positive rewarding aspect. Thus, the participants may have alternated less between focusing on positive versus negative consequences of the addictive substance, leading to a higher correlation between attention bias and craving.

Also supporting the relevance of attention focus is an ERP study (Meule, Kübler, & Blechert, 2013) in which participants were asked to focus either on the immediate or on the long-term consequences of consuming high-caloric and low-caloric foods. The late positive potential (LPP), which is thought to be driven by arousal (Olofsson, Nordin,

Sequeira, & Polich, 2008, as cited in Meule et al., 2013), was sensitive to the immediate versus long-term manipulation. More specifically, the LPP was most positive when participants focused on the long-term consequences of high-caloric food consumption, which the authors interpreted to reflect negative arousal. In a similar vein, the LPP was modulated by a food availability manipulation. That is, restrained eaters, but not unrestrained eaters, showed a less positive LPP for available than for unavailable food cues, which according to the authors might reflect a down-regulation of reactivity to available food stimuli, in order to adhere to their diet later.

A line of research that focuses on the malleability of attention biases in general supports top-down influences as well. Both in an emotional Stroop task and in a dot-probe task, an attention bias toward negative stimuli was observed only when participants were required to focus on the affective stimulus information, but not when they were required to focus on the nonaffective semantic stimulus information (Everaert, Spruyt, & De Houwer, 2013). This suggests that the way stimuli are processed (i.e., top-down influences: focus on affect versus focus on semantics) determines the attention bias. Similarly, in a dot-probe paradigm it was shown that attention was biased toward stimuli reflecting a prioritized goal (Experiment 1) or a goal with a high expectancy of success (Experiment 2) (Vogt, De Houwer, & Crombez, 2011).

Taken together, the double-faceted nature of high-caloric foods, that is, their high-caloric value being a threat to a healthy BMI on the one hand and their high palatability on the other hand, may be part of the explanation for the great diversity of research findings in this field. The attention focus (health versus taste) may fluctuate within participants across and within studies, making it more difficult to observe consistent group differences. Characteristics of the paradigm (e.g., pitting high-caloric foods against low-caloric foods versus pitting high-caloric foods against a neutral category) may inadvertently elicit either an increased focus on health or on palatability, and thereby may affect the observed group differences.

Currently it is unclear whether craving and food-related worry/anxiety are related to attention bias for high-caloric foods in a similar way. That is, are they both related to attention approach, or is craving related to attention approach and food-related worry/anxiety related to attention avoidance? This cannot be inferred from studies focusing on group differences, as it is unclear what attention focus the participants had while performing most studies, and the observed group differences go in multiple directions. In obese as well as restrained eaters both types of attention focus may be equally likely.

Moreover, the study of attention bias may be considered a quantitative approach, in the sense that one can only conclude whether a participant pays *more* or *less* attention to high-caloric foods as compared to neutral nonfood or low-caloric food stimuli. That is, this approach does not inform us to what feature of the food the participant pays attention. Is attention captured by the high-caloric content's negative BMI consequences or by the high palatability? Maybe the attention bias depends on stimulus relevance (Broeren & Lester, 2013), without distinguishing between positive versus negative valence. If the attention bias happened to be driven by craving, then one observes the expected correlations with craving and possibly the expected group differences. If the attention bias happened to be driven by food-related worry/anxiety, then no correlations with craving would be observed, and possibly group differences would go in a different direction.

Implicit Measures of Associations with Food

A related field of research is focused on the positive versus negative associations that are triggered by different types of food. Quite a number of studies have obtained so-called implicit measures of association with food in obese/overweight people and high-restrained eaters. Before briefly explaining the paradigms that are used to obtain these measures, it is important to specify what the term *implicit* means. De Houwer, Teige-Mocigemba, Spruyt, and Moors (2009) defined an *implicit* measure as "a measurement *outcome* that is causally produced by the to-be-measured attribute in the absence of certain goals, awareness, substantial cognitive resources, or substantial time" (p. 350). It is important to keep in mind that implicitness is not an all-or-none feature of a measure (Moors & De Houwer, 2006), and in what sense implicit measures of association can be considered implicit is heavily debated (De Houwer et al., 2009; Roefs, Huijding, Smulders, Jansen, & MacLeod, 2015), and beyond the scope of the current chapter. For now it suffices to say that these implicit measures are generally obtained with the goal of circumventing the problems associated with direct self-reports (i.e., reliance on introspection). Implicit measures (i.e., measurement outcomes) are obtained by indirect measurement procedures such as the Implicit Association Test (IAT; Greenwald, McGhee, & Schwartz, 1998) and the Affective Priming Paradigm (APP; Fazio, Sanbonmatsu, Powell, & Kardes, 1986). *Indirect* means that the participants are not directly asked to report on their associations, but their associations are inferred from their behavior (their pattern of response latencies in the computer task). This pattern of latencies is considered informative regarding associations people have with, for example, high-caloric foods.

Measurement Procedures

In the APP (Fazio et al., 1986), two stimuli are presented in quick succession: a prime followed by a target. In food research the primes are typically different types of foods and the targets general positive and negative stimuli. The prime is briefly presented and can be ignored by the participant. The target is then presented, and the participant is required to evaluate it as quickly as possible. The logic of the paradigm is that affectively congruent prime–target pairs (e.g., strawberry–paradise) should lead to shorter response latencies than affectively incongruent prime–target pairs (e.g., strawberry–disaster). The extent to which this pattern of response latencies is indeed observed reflects the person's evaluation of the prime (e.g., strawberry).

In the IAT (Greenwald et al., 1998), the participant is asked to categorize each presented stimulus as quickly as possible, either according to a target dimension (e.g., high-caloric versus low-caloric foods) or an attribute dimension (e.g., positive versus negative). In the two critical phases of the task these dimensions are combined. That is, targets (i.e., high-caloric and low-caloric foods) and attributes (positive and negative adjectives) are presented in an alternating random order. In a first critical phase, the target category "high-caloric food" and attribute category "positive" share a response key, as well as the target category "low-caloric food" and attribute category "negative." So participants press the same key if a high-caloric food item or a positive attribute is presented, and press the other key if a low-caloric food item or a negative attribute is presented. In a second critical phase these combinations are reversed, such that "high-caloric food" and "negative" now share a response key, as well as the categories "low-caloric food" and "positive." The IAT effect is computed by taking a difference score between these two critical phases, with the logic being that participants perform faster if associated categories share a response key than when nonassociated categories share a response key. So, in the current example, if participants are faster in the first critical phase than in the second critical phase, this is taken as evidence of a preference for high-caloric foods over low-caloric foods.

Group Differences in Food Associations in Obesity and Restrained Eating

According to the hypothesis of increased positive hedonic reactivity, it was expected that overweight people and restrained eaters' implicit measures of associations with food would be positive. That is, that overweight people and restrained eaters would have more positive associations with high-caloric than with low-caloric foods, as compared to healthy-weight people and unrestrained eaters. The empirical evidence mostly goes in exactly the opposite direction though.

On IAT measures, obese (Roefs & Jansen, 2002) as well as restrained eaters (Vartanian, Polivy, & Herman, 2004) had more negative associations with high-caloric foods than with low-caloric foods as compared to healthy-weight people and unrestrained eaters respectively. In addition, using the APP, it was found that all participants, regardless of BMI, preferred low-caloric palatable foods to high-caloric palatable foods (Roefs et al., 2005). In a similar vein, Werrij et al. (2009) found that obese as well as healthy-weight people associated palatable high-caloric foods more with restraint than with disinhibition. Obese children are no exception in this respect, as it was observed that obese and lean children alike had more positive association with healthy than with unhealthy foods (Craeynest, Crombez, Haerens, & De Bourdeaudhuij, 2007).

Top-Down Influences on Implicit Measures of Associations with Food

Importantly, the studies reviewed above all share a methodological characteristic: high-caloric foods are compared to low-caloric foods within the same task, which may elicit an attention focus on the health consequences of high-caloric foods. Houben, Roefs, and Jansen (2010) addressed this possibility using variants of the IAT. In their first experiment high- and low-restrained eaters both showed more negative associations with high-caloric than low-caloric foods, in the absence of positive associations with high-caloric foods, which is in line with earlier work. In their second experiment, they tested positive and negative associations with only high-caloric foods. In this experiment they did find that high-restrained eaters showed more positive associations with high-caloric foods than did low-restrained eaters. The absence of the low-caloric food alternative may have led to an attention focus on palatability.

Roefs et al. (2006) more directly tested the role of attention focus in associations with high-caloric and low-caloric foods using the APP. They found that manipulated attention focus (palatability vs. health) influenced the observed associations with the food stimuli in the expected way. More specifically, when focused on palatability, participants showed more positive associations with high-caloric and palatable food, whereas they showed more positive associations with low-caloric and unpalatable food when they were focused on health. So this implicit measure of associations with food was influenced by a manipulation of attention focus rather than by weight status (obese vs. healthy weight).

Taken together, also for implicit measures of associations with food, it may be too simplistic to just study group differences such as overweight versus healthy-weight people or high- versus low-restrained eaters. Even though these implicit measures are considered to reflect relatively fast processes, these too are likely affected by top-down influences. That is, it matters which aspect of the double-faceted nature of high-caloric foods is in focus: palatability or health/weight consequences. The final part of this chapter is concerned with brain imaging studies that measured neural activation in reward-related areas of the brain in response to visual food stimuli.

Reward Processing in the Brain

The last decade has witnessed a large number of functional magnetic resonance imaging (fMRI) studies addressing activity in reward-related areas of the brain in response to different types of food cues, and comparing obese/overweight and healthy-weight people. Again, the general hypothesis is that obese people would be characterized by stronger hedonic reactivity to (high-caloric) food cues. The dependent measure in these studies is the so-called blood oxygen level–dependent response of the brain (BOLD response), with the logic being that active brain regions require more oxygen, and oxygen-rich blood has different magnetic properties than does oxygen-poor blood.

Food Reward Processing in the Brain in Obesity and Restrained Eating

Indeed, research findings indicated that obese and overweight participants showed a greater BOLD response to visual food stimuli in several reward-related areas of the brain than did healthy-weight participants (e.g., Bruce et al., 2010; Martin et al., 2010; Rothemund et al., 2007; Stoeckel et al., 2008). Only a few fMRI studies have compared high- and low-restrained eaters (Coletta et al., 2009; Schur et al., 2012), and they also found evidence for group differences in brain reward activity, which were modulated by hunger state (Coletta et al., 2009) and the provision of a preload (Schur et al., 2012).

Importantly, though these studies observed differences in several reward-related areas of the brain (e.g., amygdala, insula, striatum, orbitofrontal cortex), the exact areas in which group differences were observed varied considerably over studies. Highly relevant in this respect is a meta-analysis conducted on studies on the neural correlates of processing visual food cues in healthy-weight participants, using a whole-brain approach (van der Laan et al., 2011). The results were remarkable, in the sense that at best 41% concurrence over studies was observed. The three areas that most consistently showed an increased BOLD response to food versus neutral cues included the lateral occipital complex, the left lateral orbitofrontal cortex, and the insula. A similar lack of consistency was apparent in a meta-analysis of fMRI studies including overweight and healthy-weight participants (Brooks, Cedernaes, & Schiöth, 2013; see also Ziauddeen, Farooqi, & Fletcher, 2012).

Top-Down Influences on Reward Processing in the Brain

Of course, several methodological reasons can be offered that may explain the limited concurrence over studies, such as small n, technical differences (i.e., different scanners), design choices (i.e., blocked vs. event-related presentation of stimuli), and so forth. But another important point to consider again is the attention focus of the participants. In many of these studies, participants generally had no other task than to simply pay attention to the presented stimuli, giving no control over what participant actually cognitively do with these food stimuli. As in other types of research, the attention focus of participants likely varies within and across participants, and within and across studies. There is likely a lot of fluctuation between a focus on the palatability of the foods on the one hand and the negative consequences of the high-caloric value on the other hand.

The role of attention focus in this type of study has been addressed recently. Frankort and colleagues (2012) had overweight and healthy-weight participants focus on the palatability of the presented visual food stimuli in half of the runs (biased viewing: focus on palatability), provided no such prime in the other half of runs (unbiased viewing), and compared patterns of BOLD. The overweight sample showed increased activity in reward-related brain areas, but only when the focus was on palatability. Strikingly, the group difference was reversed in the unbiased viewing condition: it was the healthy-weight sample that showed increased activation of the reward system. In addition, Siep and colleagues (2009) showed that food-cue-related activity in the amygdala and medial orbitofrontal cortex critically depended on the explicit evaluation of the palatability of the foods.

In a similar vein, Siep and colleagues (2012) showed that activity in important regions of the mesocorticolimbic circuitry was influenced by the specific instructions provided to participants regarding their processing task for the presented food stimuli. Generally, this activity was enhanced when participants were instructed to up-regulate food palatability thoughts, but diminished when participants were instructed to suppress these thoughts and cravings. In line with these findings, Giuliani and colleagues (Giuliani, Calcott, & Berkman, 2013) showed that cognitive reappraisal with the goal of reducing food desires indeed caused a reduction in self-reported desirability of food. A later study from this lab (Giuliani, Mann, Tomiyama, & Berkman, 2014) found that this type of cognitive reappraisal caused activation in top-down self-regulation brain regions (e.g., dorsolateral prefrontal cortex), which is in line with findings of an earlier study that investigated the effect of cognitive control of food desire on brain activation (Hollmann, Hellrung, Pleger, Schlögl, Kabisch, et al., 2012).

Moreover, a manipulation of mindset (focus on health vs. focus on taste) modulated value- (taste and health ratings) related neural activity (Bhanji & Beer, 2012), and the provision of health cues with the visual presentation of food cues modulated value signals in the ventromedial prefrontal cortex (Hare, Malmaud, & Rangel, 2011). In sum, activity in reward regions of the brain appears differentially impacted not only by physical characteristics (e.g., body weight), but also by cognitive factors like attention focus (e.g., focus on palatability) and processing goals (e.g., up-regulation vs. suppression).

Conclusion: The Power of Mind

Taking all three discussed lines of research into consideration—attention bias toward high-caloric foods, implicit measures of association with high-caloric foods, and food-cue-elicited activity in reward processing related areas of the brain—it seems fair to conclude that top-down processes may play an important role that has not been sufficiently studied yet. High-caloric foods have a double-faceted nature of which many people are aware. They represent, on the one hand, highly palatable foods to indulge in, and on the other hand represent a threat to one's waistline. So, top-down processes may influence the way one conceptualizes a food stimulus, which in turn may determine further cognitive processing and, ultimately, behavior.

Even when obtaining measures that are considered to be relatively automatic (e.g., attention bias and implicit measures of association), no clear, consistent evidence was obtained for increased hedonic reactivity to high-caloric food cues in obese/overweight people or high-restrained eaters. So even at this relatively early stage of cognitive processing, top-down influences may already bias our attention and associations, which conflicts with a strictly serial model of increasingly complex cognitive processing.

So obese/overweight people and restrained eaters are not necessarily always "plagued" by hedonically driven associations and cognitive biases. Instead, top-down processes may determine whether cognitive biases are driven by hedonics or health concerns, even when measures are considered implicit. As a consequence, it is likely too simplistic to just study group differences, that is, to compare, for example, obese/overweight people and healthy weight controls, or high- and low-restrained eaters. The attention focus likely shifts frequently between palatability and health, both within and across people, and within and across studies, making it difficult to observe clear group differences.

Curbing Problematic Food Desires

One approach to reducing food desires is to target the behavioral impulses that are evoked upon encountering palatable food cues. Though obese people are not necessarily always plagued by hedonic reactivity when confronted with high-caloric food cues, as argued above, their attention focus will at least be set on hedonics for a substantial amount of time. So targeting these behavioral impulses could be a viable approach.

However, previous attempts to decrease food desire and overweight by training general inhibition abilities have shown disappointing results. For instance, food intake was higher following impulsivity induction compared to inhibition induction, but this effect was mainly due to increased food intake in the impulsivity condition, while general inhibition training was unsuccessful in reducing food intake (Guerrieri, Nederkoorn, & Jansen, 2012). Recent efforts in inhibitory control training specifically for food show more promising results. Specifically, these lines of research suggest that impulses triggered by palatable food can be reduced by pairing such cues with behavioral stop signals in a go/no-go task. Work from different laboratories has found that consistently withholding responses to palatable food cues is effective in reducing choice for palatable food (Veling, Aarts, & Stroebe, 2013), consumption of palatable food (Houben, 2011; Houben & Jansen, 2011; Veling, Aarts, & Papies, 2011), and body weight (Veling, van Koningsbruggen, Aarts, & Stroebe, 2014) relative to control conditions in which participants are allowed to respond to palatable food cues.

Other cognitive-behavioral approaches include "attention retraining," as discussed earlier in this chapter, and food-cue exposure with response prevention. Food-cue exposure with response prevention is based on principles of Pavlovian conditioning and consists of a prolonged exposure to food cues (e.g., intense smelling of the foods) while actual eating is not allowed, with the goal of breaking the bond between the conditioned stimulus (food cues) and the unconditioned stimulus (actual eating) (Jansen, 1994).

Some studies on attention retraining have indeed provided promising results, in that training attention away from unhealthy foods actually led to a decrease in food consumption afterwards (e.g., Kakoschke et al., 2013; Werthmann et al., 2014), whereas others were not successful (Hardman et al., 2013). For food-cue exposure with response prevention, some small-scale studies with promising results have been published. Cue exposure with response prevention successfully extinguished binges in bulimic patients, with effects sustained at 1-year follow-up (Jansen, Broekmate, & Heymans, 1992), and reduced binges and eating in the absence of hunger in children (Boutelle et al., 2011). Moreover, recently, in a neuroimaging study (Frankort, Roefs, Siep, Roebroeck, Havermans, et al., 2014), it was found that prolonged exposure to chocolate led to extinction on a neural level without a parallel extinction on a self-report level. So the extinction of the neural response in reward-related areas of the brain may precede the self-reported extinction of craving for chocolate.

Taken together, treatments targeted at increasing inhibition or self-control or reducing food desires may be helpful (see also Hofmann, Kotabe, Vohs, & Baumeister, Chapter 3, this volume; Lopez, Wagner, & Heatherton, Chapter 7, this volume). Initial results certainly are promising, but more research is needed to learn what types of training are most effective in reducing food desire and increasing inhibition. It is interesting in this respect that successful post-obese dieters showed reduced cue reactivity, that is, a reduced salivation response to food cues, as compared to currently obese participants (Jansen, Stegerman, Roefs, Nederkoorn, & Havermans, 2010). So successful weight loss seems to go hand in hand with reduced cue reactivity. Moreover, a neuroimaging study showed that successful weight-loss maintainers showed more activity in response to food cues in brain regions associated with inhibition as compared to obese and healthy-weight controls (McCaffery et al., 2009).

Finally, in line with the proposed importance of attentional focus on either hedonics or health, as argued in the current chapter, a treatment focused on changing attentional focus could also be an option worth exploring. One could argue that frequent reminders would be necessary to keep people's attentional focus set on health. One possibility may be the use of e-health, in which treatment delivery is automated via smartphones. This allows frequent and enduring intervention at the times it matters most, that is, in the eating situation.

REFERENCES

Ahern, A. L., Field, M., Yokum, S., Bohon, C., & Stice, E. (2010). Relation of dietary restraint scores to cognitive biases and reward sensitivity. *Appetite, 55*, 61.

Berthoud, H. R., Lenard, N. R., & Shin, A. C. (2011). Food reward, hyperphagia, and obesity. *American Journal of Physiology: Regulatory, Integrative and Comparative Physiology, 300*, R1266–R1277.

Bhanji, J. P., & Beer, J. S. (2012). Taking a different perspective: Mindset influences neural regions that represent value and choice. *Social Cognitive and Affective Neuroscience, 7*, 782–793.

Blaine, B. (2008). Does depression cause obesity?: A meta-analysis of longitudinal studies of depression and weight control. *Journal of Health Psychology, 13*, 1190–1197.

Boon, B., Vogelzang, L., & Jansen, A. (2000). Do restrained eaters show attention toward or away from food, shape and weight stimuli? *European Eating Disorders Review, 8*, 51–58.

Boutelle, K. N., Zucker, N. L., Peterson, C. B., Rydell, S. A., Cafri, G., & Harnack, L. (2011). Two novel treatments to reduce overeating in overweight children: A randomized controlled trial. *Journal of Consulting and Clinical Psychology, 79*, 759–771.

Braet, C., & Crombez, G. (2003). Cognitive interference due to food cues in childhood obesity. *Journal of Clinical Child and Adolescent Psychology, 32*, 32–39.

Brignell, C., Griffiths, T., Bradley, B. P., & Mogg, K. (2009). Attentional and approach biases for pictorial food cues: Influence of external eating. *Appetite, 52*, 299–306.

Broeren, S., & Lester, K. J. (2013). Relevance is in the eye of the beholder: Attentional bias to relevant stimuli in children. *Emotion, 13*, 262–269.

Brooks, S. J., Cedernaes, J., & Schiöth, H. B. (2013). Increased prefrontal and parahippocampal activation with reduced dorsolateral prefrontal and insular cortex activation to food images in obesity: A meta-analysis of fMRI studies. *PLoS ONE, 8*, e60393.

Brooks, S., Prince, A., Stahl, D., Campbell, I. C., & Treasure, J. (2011). A systematic review and meta-analysis of cognitive bias to food stimuli in people with disordered eating behaviour. *Clinical Psychology Review, 31*, 37–51.

Bruce, A. S., Holsen, L. M., Chambers, R. J., Martin, L. E., Brooks, W. M., Zarcone, J. R., et al. (2010). Obese children show hyperactivation to food pictures in brain networks linked to motivation, reward and cognitive control. *International Journal of Obesity, 34*, 1494–1500.

Castellanos, E. H., Charboneau, E., Dietrich, M. S., Park, S., Bradley, B. P., Mogg, K., et al. (2009). Obese adults have visual attention bias for food cue images: evidence for altered reward system function. *International Journal of Obesity, 33*, 1063–1073.

Coletta, M., Platek, S., Mohamed, F. B., van Steenburgh, J. J., Green, D., & Lowe, M. R. (2009). Brain activation in restrained and unrestrained eaters: An fMRI study. *Journal of Abnormal Psychology, 118*, 598–609.

Craeynest, M., Crombez, G., Haerens, L., & De Bourdeaudhuij, I. (2007). Do overweight youngsters like food more than lean peers? Assessing their implicit attitudes with a personalized Implicit Association Task. *Food Quality and Preference, 18*, 1077–1084.

De Houwer, J., Teige-Mocigemba, S., Spruyt, A., & Moors, A. (2009). Implicit measures: A normative analysis and review. *Psychological Bulletin, 135*, 347–368.

Di Pellegrino, G., Magarelli, S., & Mengarelli, F. (2011). Food pleasantness affects visual selective attention. *Quarterly Journal of Experimental Psychology, 64*, 560–571.

Dobson, K. S., & Dozois, D. J. (2004). Attentional biases in eating disorders: A meta-analytic review of Stroop performance. *Clinical Psychology Review, 23*, 1001–1022.

Everaert, T., Spruyt, A., & De Houwer, J. (2013). On the malleability of automatic attentional biases: Effects of feature-specific attention allocation. *Cognition & Emotion, 27*, 385–400.

Fazio, R. H., Sanbonmatsu, D. M., Powell, M. C., & Kardes (1986). On the automatic activation of attitudes. *Journal of Personality and Social Psychology, 50*, 229–238.

Field, M., & Cox, W. M. (2008). Attentional bias in addictive behaviors: A review of its development, causes, and consequences [review]. *Drug and Alcohol Dependence, 97*, 1–20.

Field, M., Munafò, M. R., & Franken, I. H. A. (2009). A meta-analytic investigation of the relationship between attentional bias and subjective craving in substance abuse. *Psychological Bulletin, 135*, 589–607.

Frankort, A., Roefs, A., Siep, N., Roebroeck, A., Havermans, R., & Jansen, A. (2012). Reward activity in satiated overweight women is decreased during unbiased viewing but increased when imagining taste: An event-related fMRI study, *36*, 627–637.

Frankort, A., Roefs, A., Siep, N., Roebroeck, A., Havermans, R., & Jansen, A. (2014). The craving stops before you feel it: Neural correlates of craving during cue exposure with response prevention. *Cerebral Cortex, 24*, 1589–1600.

Gale, S. M., Castracane, V. D., & Mantzoros, C. S. (2004). Energy homeostasis, obesity and eating disorders: Recent advances in endocrinology. *Journal of Nutrition, 134*, 295–298.

Gendall, K. A., & Joyce, P. R. (2001). Characteristics of food cravers who binge eat. In M. M. Hetherington (Ed.), *Food cravings and addiction* (pp. 567–583). London: Leatherhead.

Giel, K. E., Friederich, H. C., Teufel, M., Hautzinger, M., Enck, P., & Zipfel, S. (2011). Attentional processing of food pictures in individuals with anorexia aervosa: An eye-tracking study. *Biological Psychiatry, 69*, 661–667.

Giuliani, N. R., Calcott, R. D., & Berkman, E. T. (2013). Piece of cake. Cognitive reappraisal of food craving. *Appetite, 64*, 56–61.

Giuliani, N. R., Mann, T., Tomiyama, A. J., & Berkman, E. T. (2014). Neural systems underlying the reappraisal of personally craved foods. *Journal of Cognitive Neuroscience, 26*, 1390–1402.

Graham, R., Hoover, A., Ceballos, N. A., & Komogortsev, O. (2011). Body mass index moderates gaze orienting biases and pupil diameter to high and low calorie food images. *Appetite, 56*, 577–586.

Greenwald, A. G., McGhee, D. E., & Schwartz, J. L. K. (1998). Measuring individual differences in implicit cognition: The implicit association test. *Journal of Personality and Social Psychology, 74*, 1464.

Guerrieri R., Nederkoorn C., & Jansen, A. (2012). Disinhibition is easier learned than inhibition: The effects of (dis)inhibition training on food intake. *Appetite, 59*, 96–99.

Hallett, P. E. (1978). Primary and secondary saccades to goals defined by instructions. *Vision Research, 18*, 1279–1296.

Hardman, C. A., Rogers, P. J., Etchells, K. A., Houstoun, K. V. E., & Munafò, M. R. (2013). The effects of food-related attentional bias training on appetite and food intake. *Appetite, 71*, 295–300.

Hare, T. A., Malmaud, J., & Rangel, A. (2011). Focusing attention on the health aspects of foods changes value signals in vmPFC and improves dietary choice. *Journal of Neuroscience, 31*, 11077–11087.

Harris, A., Hare, T., & Rangel, A. (2013). Temporally dissociable mechanisms of self-control: Early attentional filtering versus late value modulation. *Journal of Neuroscience, 33*(48), 18917–18931.

Hepworth, R., Mogg, K., Brignell, C., & Bradley, B. P. (2010). Negative mood increases selective attention to food cues and subjective appetite. *Appetite, 54*, 134–142.

Herman, C. P., & Polivy, J. (1980). Restrained eating. In A. J. Stunkard (Ed.), *Obesity* (pp. 208–225). Philadelphia: Saunders.

Herman, C. P., & Polivy, J. (2004). The self-regulation of eating: Theoretical and practical problems. In R. F. Baumeister & K. D. Vohs (Eds.), *Handbook of self-regulation: Research, theory and applications* (pp. 492–508). New York: Guilford Press.

Hofmann, W., Friese, M., & Strack, F. (2009). Impulses and self-control from a dual-systems perspective. *Perspectives on Psychological Science, 4*, 162–176.

Hofmann, W., & Van Dillen, L. (2012). Desire: The new hot spot in self-control research. *Current Directions in Psychological Science, 21*, 317–322.

Hollmann, M., Hellrung, L., Pleger, B., Schlögl, H., Kabisch, S., Stumvoll, M., et al. (2012). Neural correlates of the volitional regulation of the desire for food. *International Journal of Obesity, 36*, 648–655.

Houben, K. (2011). Overcoming the urge to splurge: The role of inhibitory control in eating behavior. *Journal of Behavior Research and Experimental Psychiatry, 42*, 384–388.

Houben K., & Jansen A. (2011). Training inhibitory control: A recipe for resisting sweet temptations. *Appetite, 56*, 345–349.

Houben, K., Roefs, A., & Jansen, A. (2010). Guilty pleasures. Implicit preferences for high calorie food in restrained eating. *Appetite, 55*, 18–24.

Jansen, A. (1994). The learned nature of binge eating. In C. Legg & D. A. Booth (Eds.), *Appetite: Neural and behavioural bases* (pp. 193–211). Oxford, UK: Oxford University Press.

Jansen, A., Broekmate, J., & Heymans, M. (1992). Cue-exposure vs. self-control in the treatment of binge eating: A pilot study. *Behaviour Research and Therapy, 30*, 235–241.

Jansen, A., Stegerman, S., Roefs, A., Nederkoorn, C., & Havermans, R. (2010). Decreased salivation to food cues in formerly obese successful dieters. *Psychotherapy and Psychosomatics, 79*, 257–258.

Jia, H., & Lubetkin, E. I. (2005). The impact of obesity on health-related quality-of-life in the general adult US population. *Journal of Public Health, 27*(2), 156–164.

Jia, H., & Lubetkin, E. I. (2010). Trends in quality-adjusted life-years lost contributed by smoking and obesity. *American Journal of Preventive Medicine, 38*, 138–44.

Johansson, L., Ghaderi, A., & Andersson, G. (2005). Stroop interference for food- and body-related words: A meta-analysis. *Eating Behaviors, 6*, 271–281.

Jones, A., Hogarth, L., Christiansen, P., Rose, A. K., Martinovic, J., & Field, M. (2012). Reward expectancy promotes generalized increases in attentional bias for rewarding stimuli. *Quarterly Journal of Experimental Psychology, 65*, 2333–2342.

Kakoschke, N., Kemps, E., & Tiggemann, M. (2013). Attentional bias modification encourages healthy eating. *Eating Behaviors*, 1–22.

Kavanagh, D., Andrade, J., & May, J. (2005). The imaginary relish. A cognitive–emotional account of craving. *Psychological Review, 112*, 446–467.

Kemps, E., & Tiggemann, M. (2009). Attentional bias for craving-related (chocolate) food cues. *Experimental and Clinical Psychopharmacology, 17*, 425–433.

Kemps, E., Tiggemann, M., & Hollitt, S. (2014a). Biased attentional processing of food cues and modification in obese individuals. *Health Psychology, 33*, 1391–1401.

Kemps, E., Tiggemann, M., Orr, J., & Grear, J. (2014b). Attentional retraining can reduce chocolate consumption. *Journal of Experimental Psychology: Applied, 20*, 94–102.

Kolotkin, R. L., Meter, K., & Williams, G. R. (2001). Quality of life and obesity. *Obesity Reviews, 2*, 219–229.

Kringelbach, M. L. (2009). The hedonic brain: A functional neuroanatomy of human pleasure. In M. L. Kringelbach & K. C. Berridge (Eds.), *Pleasures of the brain* (pp. 202–221). New York: Oxford University Press.

Loeber, S., Grosshans, M., Korucuoglu, O., Vollmert, C., Vollstädt-Klein, S., Schneider, S., et al. (2012). Impairment of inhibitory control in response to food-associated cues and attentional bias of obese participants and normal-weight controls. *International Journal of Obesity, 36*, 1334–1339.

Lowe, M. R., & Butryn, M. L. (2007). Hedonic hunger: A new dimension of appetite? *Physiology and Behavior, 91*, 432–439.

Luppino, F. S., de Wit, L. M., Bouvy, P. F., Stijnen, T., Cuijpers, P., Penninx, B. W. J. H., et al. (2010). Overweight, obesity, and depression: A systematic review and meta-analysis of longitudinal studies. *Archives of General Psychiatry, 67*, 220–229.

MacLeod, C., Mathews, A., & Tata, P. (1986). Attentional bias in emotional disorders. *Journal of Abnormal Psychology, 95*, 15–20.

Martin, L. E., Holsen, L. M., Chambers, R. J., Bruce, A. S., Brooks, W. M., Zarcone, J. R., et al. (2010). Neural mechanisms associated with food motivation in obese and healthy weight adults. *Obesity, 18*, 254–260.

McCaffery, J. M., Haley, A. P., Sweet, L. H., Phelan, S., Raynor, H. A., Del Parigi, A., et al. (2009). Differential functional magnetic resonance imaging response to food pictures in successful weight-loss maintainers relative to normal-weight and obese controls. *American Journal of Clinical Nutrition, 90*, 928–934.

Meule, A., Kübler, A., & Blechert, J. (2013). Time course of electrocortical food-cue responses during cognitive regulation of craving. *Frontiers in Psychology, 4*, 669.

Moors, A., & De Houwer, J. (2006). Automaticity: A theoretical and conceptual analysis. *Psychological Bulletin, 132*, 297–326.

Nijs, I. M. T., Franken, I. H. A., & Muris, P. (2008). Food cue-elicited brain potentials in obese and healthy-weight individuals. *Eating Behaviors*, 1–9.

Nijs, I. M. T., Franken, I. H. A., & Muris, P. (2010). Food-related Stroop interference in obese and normal-weight individuals: Behavioral and electrophysiological indices. *Eating Behaviors, 11*, 258–265.

Nijs, I. M. T., Muris, P., Euser, A. S., & Franken, I. H. A. (2010). Differences in attention to food and food intake between overweight/obese and normal-weight females under conditions of hunger and satiety. *Appetite, 54*, 243–254.

Nummenmaa, L., Hietanen, J. K., Calvo, M. G., & Hyönä, J. (2011). Food catches the eye but not for everyone: A BMI-contingent attentional bias in rapid detection of nutriments. *PLoS ONE, 6*, e19215.

Pelchat, M. L., Johnson, A., Chan, R., Valdez, J., & Ragland, J. D. (2004). Images of desire: Food-craving activation during fMRI. *NeuroImage, 23*, 1486–1493.

Phelan, S., Hassenstab, J., Mccaffery, J. M., Sweet, L., Raynor, H. A., Cohen, R. A., et al. (2011). Cognitive interference from food cues in weight loss maintainers, normal weight, and obese individuals. *Obesity, 19*, 69–73.

Porubská, K., Veit, R., Preissl, H., Fritsche, A., & Birbaumer, N. (2006). Subjective feeling of appetite modulates brain activity. *NeuroImage, 32*, 1273–1280.

Pothos, E. M., Tapper, K., & Calitri, R. (2009). Cognitive and behavioral correlates of BMI among male and female undergraduate students. *Appetite, 52*, 797–800.

Roefs, A., & Jansen, A. (2002). Implicit and explicit attitudes toward high-fat foods in obesity. *Journal of Abnormal Psychology, 111*, 517–521.

Roefs, A., Huijding, J., Smulders, F. T. Y., Jansen, A., & MacLeod, C. M. (2015). Implicit measures of associations: A case of exaggerated promises? In G. Brown & D. Clarke (Eds.), *Cognitive behavioral assessment, diagnosis and case formulation* (pp. 291–315). New York: Guilford Press.

Roefs, A., Huijding, J., Smulders, F. T. Y, MacLeod, C. M., de Jong, P. J., Wiers, R. W., et al. (2011). Implicit measures of association in psychopathology research. *Psychological Bulletin, 137*, 149–193.

Roefs, A., Quaedackers, L., Werrij, M. Q., Wolters, G., Havermans, R., Nederkoorn, C., et al. (2006). The environment influences whether high-fat foods are associated with palatable or with unhealthy. *Behaviour Research and Therapy, 44*, 715–736.

Roefs, A., Stapert, D., Isabella, L. A. S., Wolters, G., Wojciechowski, F., & Jansen, A. (2005). Early associations with food in anorexia nervosa patients and obese people assessed in the affective priming paradigm. *Eating Behaviors, 6*, 151–163.

Rothemund, Y., Preuschhof, C., Bohner, G., Bauknecht, H. C., Klingebiel, R., Flor,

H., et al. (2007). Differential activation of the dorsal striatum by high-calorie visual food stimuli in obese individuals. *NeuroImage, 37*, 410–421.

Schur, E. A., Kleinhans, N. M., Goldberg, J., Buchwald, D. S., Polivy, J., Del Parigi, A., et al. (2012). Acquired differences in brain responses among monozygotic twins discordant for restrained eating. *Physiology and Behavior, 105*, 560–567.

Shafran, R., Lee, M., Cooper, Z., Palmer, R. L., & Fairburn, C. G. (2007). Attentional bias in eating disorders. *International Journal of Eating Disorders, 40*, 369–380.

Shin, A. C., Zheng, H., & Berthoud, H. R. (2009). An expanded view of energy homeostasis: Neural integration of metabolic, cognitive, and emotional drives to eat. *Physiology and Behavior, 97*, 572–580.

Siep, N., Roefs, A., Roebroeck, A., Havermans, R., Bonte, M. L., & Jansen, A. (2009). Hunger is the best spice: An fMRI study of the effects of attention, hunger and calorie content on food reward processing in the amygdala and orbitofrontal cortex. *Behavioural Brain Research, 198*, 149–158.

Siep, N., Roefs, A., Roebroeck, A., Havermans, R., Bonte, M. L., & Jansen, A. (2012). Fighting food temptations: The modulating effects of short-term cognitive reappraisal, suppression and up-regulation on mesocorticolimbic activity related to appetitive motivation. *NeuroImage, 60*, 213–220.

Smeets, E., Roefs, A., & Jansen, A. (2009). Experimentally induced chocolate craving leads to an attentional bias in increased distraction but not in speeded detection. *Appetite, 53*, 370–375.

Smeets, E., Roefs, A., van Furth, E., & Jansen, A. (2008). Attentional bias for body and food in eating disorders: Increased distraction, speeded detection, or both? *Behaviour Research and Therapy, 46*, 229–238.

Stoeckel, L. E., Weller, R. E., Cook, E. W., III, Twieg, D. B., Knowlton, R. C., & Cox, J. E. (2008). Widespread reward-system activation in obese women in response to pictures of high-calorie foods. *NeuroImage, 41*, 636–647.

Swinburn, B. A., Jolley, D., Kremer, P. J., Salbe, A. D., & Ravussin, E. (2006). Estimating the effects of energy imbalance on changes in body weight in children. *American Journal of Clinical Nutrition, 83*, 859–863.

Swinburn, B. A., Sacks, G., Lo, S. K., Westerterp, K. R., Rush, E., Rosenbaum, M., et al. (2009). Estimating the changes in energy flux that characterize the rise in obesity prevalence. *American Journal of Clinical Nutrition, 89*, 1723–1728.

Uher, R., Treasure, J., Heining, M., Brammer, M. J., & Campbell, I. C. (2006). Cerebral processing of food-related stimuli: Effects of fasting and gender. *Behavioural Brain Research, 169*, 111–119.

van der Laan, L. N., de Ridder, D. T. D., Viergever, M. A., & Smeets, P. A. M. (2011). The first taste is always with the eyes: A meta-analysis on the neural correlates of processing visual food cues. *NeuroImage, 55*, 296–303.

Van Dillen, L. F., Papies, E. K., & Hofmann, W. (2013). Turning a blind eye to temptation: How cognitive load can facilitate self-regulation. *Journal of Personality and Social Psychology, 104*, 427–443.

Vartanian, L. R., Polivy, J., & Herman, C. P. (2004). Implicit cognitions and eating disorders: Their application in research and treatment. *Cognitive and Behavioral Practice, 11*, 160–167.

Veling, H., Aarts, H., & Papies, E. K. (2011). Using stop signals to inhibit chronic dieters' responses toward palatable foods. *Behaviour Research and Therapy, 49*, 771–780.

Veling, H., Aarts, H., & Stroebe, W. (2013). Stop signals decrease choices for palatable foods through decreased food evaluation. *Frontiers in Psychology, 4*, 875.

Veling, H., van Koningsbruggen, G., Aarts, H., & Stroebe, W. (2014). Targeting impulsive processes of eating behavior via the internet: Effects on body weight. *Appetite, 78*, 102–109.

Vogt, J., De Houwer, J., & Crombez, G. (2011). Multiple goal management starts with attention. *Experimental Psychology, 58*, 55–61.

Wadden, T. A., Brownell, K. D., & Foster, G. D. (2002). Obesity: Responding to the global epicemic. *Journal of Consulting and Clinical Psychology, 70*, 510–525.

Werrij, M. Q., Roefs, A., Janssen, I., Stapert, D., Wolters, G., Mulkens, S., et al. (2009). Early associations with palatable foods in overweight and obesity are not disinhibition related but restraint related. *Journal of Behavior Therapy and Experimental Psychiatry, 40*, 136–146.

Werthmann, J., Field, M., Roefs, A., Nederkoorn, C., & Jansen, A. (2014). Attention bias for chocolate increases chocolate consumption: An attention bias modification study. *Journal of Behavior Therapy and Experimental Psychiatry, 45*, 136–143.

Werthmann, J., Roefs, A., Nederkoorn, C., & Jansen, A. (2013a). Desire lies in the eyes: Attention bias for chocolate is related to craving and self-endorsed eating permission. *Appetite, 70*, 81–89.

Werthmann, J., Roefs, A., Nederkoorn, C., Mogg, K., Bradley, B. P., & Jansen, A. (2011). Can(not) take my eyes off it: Attention bias for food in overweight participants. *Health Psychology, 30*, 561–569.

Werthmann, J., Roefs, A., Nederkoorn, C., Mogg, K., Bradley, B. P. & Jansen, A. (2013b). Attention bias for food is independent of restraint in healthy weight individuals: An eye tracking study. *Eating Behaviors, 14*, 397–400.

Werthmann, J., Jansen, A., Vreugdenhil, A. C., Nederkoorn, C., Schyns, G., & Roefs, A. (in press). Food through the Child's Eye: An eye-tracking study on attentional bias for food in healthy-weight children and children with obesity. *Health Psychology*.

Westerterp, K. R. (2010). Physical activity, food intake, and body weight regulation: Insights from doubly labeled water studies. *Nutrition Reviews, 68*, 148–154.

Williams, J. M., Mathews, A., & MacLeod, C. (1996). The emotional Stroop task and psychopathology. *Psychological Bulletin, 120*, 3–24.

World Health Organization. (2013). *Obesity and overweight* (Fact Sheet 311). Retrieved February 7, 2013, from *http://amro.who.int/common/Display.asp?Lang=E&RecID=10203*.

Ziauddeen, H., Farooqi, I. S., & Fletcher, P. C. (2012). Obesity and the brain: How convincing is the addiction model? *Nature Reviews Neuroscience, 13*(4), 279–286.

CHAPTER 17

Sexual Desire
Conceptualization, Correlates, and Causes

Pamela C. Regan

Sexual desire is among the very first sexual responses that people experience in their lives, and it remains one of the most frequent. By the time they reach adolescence and young adulthood, almost all men and women report having felt sexual desire (more than report having experienced intercourse and other sexual responses), and most experience it on a daily or at least weekly basis (see Regan & Atkins, 2006). Moreover, although people can and do express a variety of sexual responses within their romantic relationships, a growing body of scientific research reveals that sexual desire is the aspect of sexuality that plays the most significant role in the attraction process and the initial stages of relationship development, particularly as people fall in love, and that it continues to have important implications for the emotional tenor of established relationships (see Regan, 2004).

This chapter explores the topic of sexual desire. We begin by considering how sexual desire is conceptualized—how it is defined, the ways it is related to (and different from) other human sexual responses, such as sexual arousal and sexual activity, and how it is measured. Next, a framework for understanding the myriad causes and correlates of sexual desire is presented. The remainder of the chapter is devoted to examining several of the personal/individual, relational/interpersonal, and environmental factors that serve to facilitate or inhibit the expression and experience of sexual desire.

Conceptualizing Sexual Desire

Sexual desire (also commonly referred to as *sexual interest, sexual attraction, passion, libido,* or *lust*) is the motivational component of human sexuality, and it is most typically experienced as an interest in sexual activities, a drive to seek out sexual objects or to engage in sexual acts, or a wish, need, or craving for sexual contact (Bancroft, 1988; Kaplan, 1979; Levine, 1984, 2003; Regan & Berscheid, 1999). The experience of sexual desire is presumed to be distinct from other sexual responses, including (1) *sexual arousal* (which has both a *physiological/genital component* consisting of physiological arousal and genital excitement, and a *subjective component* consisting of the perception and awareness of one's physiological/genital arousal), (2) *sexual activity* (which consists of overt sexual behaviors, such as masturbation, kissing, or intercourse), and (3) *sexual affect and cognitions* that are associated with these responses (such as satisfaction, fulfillment, and pleasure).

Because sexual desire, arousal, and activity frequently co-occur, they often are experienced relatively simultaneously (see Basson, 2001; DeLamater, 1991; Kaplan, 1979; see Figure 17.1). For example, a sexual cue of some sort may trigger sexual desire. (This cue might also trigger sexual arousal, which then may lead to desire and/or activity, but for purposes of illustration—and since the focus of this chapter is on desire—we will assume that the cue initially triggers desire. Keep in mind, however, that the sexual response cycle illustrated in Figure 17.1 may initiate with any of the responses depicted.) Perhaps an individual is viewing erotic material or having a sexually themed daydream. Perhaps he or she notices a sexually appealing other person, or receives a sexual invitation or romantic gesture from his or her partner. Any one of these internal or external cues may cause that individual to feel an urge to engage in sexual activities; these desirous feelings may then produce physiological arousal (e.g., increased voluntary muscle tension, increased heart rate, elevated blood

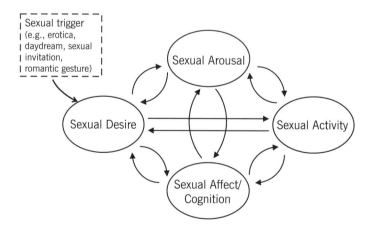

FIGURE 17.1. The interrelationship among sexual responses. Sexual desire, arousal, activity, and related affective/cognitive responses can and do co-occur and thus are often experienced relatively simultaneously.

pressure) and genital excitement (e.g., penile tumescence, vaginal lubrication). The subjective awareness of this physiological and genital arousal may, in turn, increase the desire for sexual contact and may result in sexual activity (e.g., masturbation, intercourse). During and after such activity, the individual may experience various positive (or negative) thoughts and feelings (e.g., pleasure, satisfaction, curiosity, shame, guilt, sadness, beliefs about the appropriateness and quality of the sexual event), which, in turn, may increase or decrease desire, arousal, and/or activity. Assuming that the end result of the sexual interaction is orgasm or sexual satiation, the individual's body will return to its pre-aroused state, and his or her degree of sexual desire also may decrease.

As illustrated in Figure 17.1, the interrelationship among desire, arousal, activity, and associated affective/cognitive responses is quite complex: an initial cue can trigger any one of the various sexual responses, each sexual response can trigger the others (either simultaneously or sequentially), and these responses frequently co-occur. Most researchers nonetheless consider each experience to be a distinct component of sexuality (see Regan & Berscheid, 1999).

Sexual desire varies along at least three dimensions. The first dimension is quantitative and concerns the magnitude of the desire that is experienced. Both the intensity and the frequency with which desire is experienced can vary within any one individual over time. For example, a person may experience sexual desire on numerous occasions over the course of a single day (or week or month) and then feel absolutely no desire at all the following day (or week or month). Similarly, he or she may have a powerful sexual craving at one point in time and a much less intense need at another. In addition, people differ in the chronic amount of desire that they experience, with some individuals possessing a very low level of sexual appetite and others habitually occupying the higher end of the desire spectrum.

The second dimension along which sexual desire varies is qualitative and concerns the specificity of the desired sexual goal and sexual object. An individual may experience an urge to engage in a specific or diffuse sexual activity with a specific or diffuse sexual object. For example, a bored, restless young woman lying awake at night may experience a diffuse desire for some sort of sexual activity with some sort of object. That is, she is interested in engaging in sexual activity, but her general state of interest has not crystallized into the shape of a specific interest in masturbation, intercourse, or other particular activity. The object of her desire is similarly diffuse; she wishes to engage in sexual activity but not necessarily with a specific person. However, if the young woman wants to engage in sexual activity of some nature with her partner, she is experiencing desire for a diffuse goal with a specific object. Similarly, a man watching an erotic scene from a movie featuring his favorite actress may feel the urge to engage in intercourse with that particular individual (a specific goal with a specific object); alternately, he may simply experience an urge to engage in intercourse with an unspecified object (a specific goal with a diffuse object).

The third dimension along which sexual desire varies concerns the originating source of the sexual urge. *Spontaneous sexual desire* refers to a sexual urge that arises from some innate or internally generated cause, whereas *responsive sexual desire* is produced by an external event, cue, or situation (Basson, 2002; but see Meana, 2010, for a critical analysis and alternate view of this distinction). For example, the young woman described in the preceding paragraph is experiencing spontaneous sexual desire. There is no obvious external cue that has triggered her sexual urge; rather, the desire she feels has arisen automatically and spontaneously, as the result of some internal mechanism over which she has little conscious control (see also Hofmann, Kotabe, Vohs, & Baumeister, Chapter 3, this volume). The man described in the preceding paragraph, however, is experiencing responsive sexual desire. His interest has been piqued by an erotic stimulus that has pulled a sexual response from him. Within any one sexual episode, a person may experience both forms of sexual desire, with one augmenting the other (e.g., the young woman in our scenario may call her partner and communicate her desire to him; if he responds in kind, perhaps with a sexually suggestive comment, this external cue may serve to enhance her initial, internally generated desire). In addition, people may experience relatively equal amounts of spontaneous and responsive sexual desire, or they may experience one type more often than the other (see Basson & Brotto, 2009; Goldhammer & McCabe, 2011a; Štulhofer, Carvalheira, & Træen, 2013).

Because desire is a subjective experience rather than an overt physical or behavioral event that can be readily observed, scientists can generally measure it via self-report (see also Sayette & Wilson, Chapter 5, this volume). People might be asked to respond to questions about their feelings in general or for a specific other person (e.g., a dating partner or spouse), and they might be asked to rate their overall level or amount of desire ("How much sexual desire do you experience?"), the frequency of their sexual urges ("How often do you experience sexual desire?"), or the intensity or degree of their sexual attraction to their current partner ("How intensely do you desire _____ sexually?" "How sexually attracted are you to _____?"). Commonly used multi-item self-report measures of sexual desire include the Sexual Desire Inventory–2 (Spector, Carey, & Steinberg, 1996) and the Female Sexual Desire Questionnaire (Goldhammer & McCabe, 2011b).

Exploring Sexual Desire: A Conceptual Framework

As with so many human experiences, sexual desire is a complex phenomenon with multiple causes and correlates. As a result, researchers interested in understanding sexual desire have explored a diversity of factors located at varying levels of analysis. In general, these factors can be divided into three broad classes or categories: personal factors, relational or interpersonal factors, and environmental factors (see Figure 17.2).

Personal factors are variables that are associated with individual partners, who are often referred to as P (Person) and O (Other). These factors include demographic attributes, such as age, gender or biological sex, and race/ethnicity; hormonal or biological processes; affect, mood, or emotional state; self-esteem and body image; physical and mental health variables; sex-related attitudes, preferences, values, and beliefs; various life events (e.g., sexual trauma); sexually appealing characteristics (such as physical attractiveness); and any other personally experienced events or relatively enduring attributes each person brings to the sexual interaction and/or relationship that may affect his or her ability, motivation, and opportunity to experience and express sexual desire. For example, how much sexual desire a person feels is partly a reflection of his or her age (desire decreases with increasing age), physical and mental health (chronic and debilitating physical and mental illnesses are associated with reduced sexual desire), self-esteem and body image issues (people with low self-esteem and poor body image report less sexual interest), partner's sex appeal (some partner attributes stimulate desire more than others), and a host of other individual, P- and O-level factors.

Relational factors are located in neither the desiring individual nor the desired other, but instead emerge from the duo's interactions or result from the combination of their characteristics. Proximity, feelings of mutual attraction and/or passionate love, and the overall health of the partners' relationship, as well as their degree of sexual communication, responsiveness, and similarity (of preferences, attitudes, and level of desire) fall into this category. For example, partners in a healthy relationship characterized by feelings of mutual attraction and love, open sexual communication, and similar sexual preferences are more likely to experience and express desire for each other than are partners in a dysfunctional relationship characterized by anger, hostility, dissatisfaction, and sexual incompatibility.

Environmental factors include variables located in the physical and social environments surrounding the individual and the desired other and in which their sexual interaction/relationship is embedded. Examples of physical environmental factors include access to pornographic or erotic materials as well as to drugs, alcohol, or other substances that might provoke lustful feelings, and economic, occupational, or living conditions that might affect an individual's physical, mental, or sexual health and help or hinder access to sexual partners. For example, some people report heightened feelings of sexual desire after consuming small to moderate amounts of alcohol and various stimulant drugs. Social environmental factors include sociocultural norms or customs, laws, and

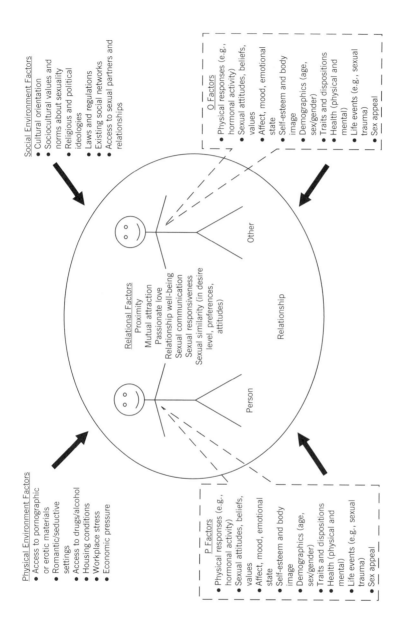

Physical Environment Factors
- Access to pornographic or erotic materials
- Romantic/seductive settings
- Access to drugs/alcohol
- Housing conditions
- Workplace stress
- Economic pressure

Social Environment Factors
- Cultural orientation
- Sociocultural values and norms about sexuality
- Religious and political ideologies
- Laws and regulations
- Existing social networks
- Access to sexual partners and relationships

O Factors
- Physical responses (e.g., hormonal activity)
- Sexual attitudes, beliefs, values
- Affect, mood, emotional state
- Self-esteem and body image
- Demographics (age, sex/gender)
- Traits and dispositions
- Health (physical and mental)
- Life events (e.g., sexual trauma)
- Sex appeal

Relational Factors
Proximity
Mutual attraction
Passionate love
Relationship well-being
Sexual communication
Sexual responsiveness
Sexual similarity (in desire level, preferences, attitudes)

Other

Relationship

Person

P Factors
- Physical responses (e.g., hormonal activity)
- Sexual attitudes, beliefs, values
- Affect, mood, emotional state
- Self-esteem and body image
- Demographics (age, sex/gender)
- Traits and dispositions
- Health (physical and mental)
- Life events (e.g., sexual trauma)
- Sex appeal

FIGURE 17.2. Sexual desire is a complex phenomenon that is affected by many factors. In general, these factors can be grouped into three broad categories or levels of analysis: (1) personal factors associated with the desiring person (P) and the object of his or her desire (O); (2) relational factors that reflect the combination of the two partners' characteristics or emerge from their interaction and/or relationship; and (3) environmental factors located in the physical and sociocultural environments that surround the individuals and in which their sexual interaction/relationship is embedded.

religious doctrine pertaining to sexuality, as well as the existing political climate. Cultural stereotypes (often widely promulgated by the media) about male and female sexuality, the elderly, and the role of passion in romantic relationships (to name a few) may inhibit or facilitate the individual experience of desire. Indeed, the concept of inhibited or low sexual desire is based on a cultural view of "normal" human sexuality that presupposes that both partners in a relationship must experience at least some desire for each other and that decreases in sexual interest signal personal ("I am not normal") and interpersonal ("We no longer love each other," "My partner no longer finds me attractive") dysfunction.

As we will consider throughout the remainder of this chapter, each of these many factors can serve to encourage or restrain the experience of sexual desire.

Personal Factors Associated with Sexual Desire

Most scientists have focused on personal factors in their quest to understand the nature of sexual desire, and a number of individual-level factors do appear to play a role in this particular sexual experience. For example, men and women dealing with serious physical illnesses (e.g., cancer, cardiovascular disease, diabetes, Parkinson's disease, fibromyalgia) typically report decreases in their overall level of sexual interest following the onset of their illness, and their desire levels are usually lower than those reported by healthy adults (Koller et al., 1990; Rico-Villademoros et al., 2012; Schover, Evans, & von Eschenbach, 1987; Schreiner-Engel, Schiavi, Vietorisz, Eichel, & Smith, 1985). Depression and other forms of major mental illness similarly are associated with decreased desire (Bodenmann & Ledermann, 2007; Hintikka et al., 2009; Lourenço, Azevedo, & Gouveia, 2011; for a review, see Regan & Berscheid, 1999). So, too, are various sex-related affective, cognitive, and attitudinal variables, including restrictive sexual attitudes; feelings of fear, anxiety, shame, sadness, or guilt about sexuality; concerns about body image, sexual attractiveness, and sexual performance; and so forth (Brotto, Woo, & Gorzalka, 2012; Carvalho, 2010; Carvalho & Nobre, 2011; Murray & Milhausen, 2012; Sims & Meana, 2010).

Demographic variables also are associated with sexual desire. Chronological age is negatively correlated with desire, with studies consistently revealing a decline in sexual interest with advancing age among both men and women (Birnbaum, Cohen & Wertheimer, 2007; Eplov, Giraldi, Davidsen, Garde, & Kamper-Jørgensen, 2007; Purifoy, Grodsky, & Giambra, 1992; Schiavi, Schreiner-Engel, Mandeli, Schanzer, & Cohen, 1990). In addition, although relatively few researchers have specifically investigated sex differences in desire, the available studies suggest that women experience lower amounts, and less frequent occurrences, of sexual desire than do men (Beck, Bozman, & Qualtrough, 1991; Useche, Villegas, & Alzate, 1990). For example, in one investigation (Regan & Atkins, 2006), women university students reported having felt sexual desire less often than did their male counterparts and, when asked to estimate the actual frequency with which they experienced desire, women's estimated frequency (about 9 times per week) was significantly lower than men's estimated frequency (about 37 times per week).

To some extent, these sex differences may reflect the fact that most research focuses on spontaneous rather than responsive sexual desire. Some theorists argue that the initial triggers of sexual desire differ for men and women, with men's desire primarily arising internally and women's desire primarily arising as a response to external, contextual cues (see Basson, 2002; Laan & Both, 2008). Empirical evidence supports this supposition (Goldhammer & McCabe, 2011a; Regan & Berscheid, 1995, 1996). Thus, questions that ask participants to report on spontaneous sexual desire—that is, on desire that is internally generated and experienced as an autonomous and conscious sexual urge—may do a better job of measuring male sexual desire than female sexual desire. A clearer understanding of the magnitude of sex differences in desire might be provided by research that also includes questions on responsive desire (i.e., desire that is stimulated by external cues, produced by the social or interpersonal context, and/or emerges after sexual arousal or during a sexual interaction).

It is also possible that sex differences in desire may partly be a function of differences in the hormonal milieu that characterizes the bodies of healthy men and women. Research reveals that both endogenous (internally generated) and exogenous (externally administered) sex hormones—in particular, the androgenic hormone *testosterone*—contribute to the timing and intensity of sexual desire. For example, reviews of the medical, clinical, and psychological sexuality literatures (Davis & Braunstein, 2012; Regan, 1999) reveal the following:

• Levels of testosterone are positively correlated with self-reported levels of sexual desire and frequency of sexual thoughts in healthy adult men and women. That is, the higher the level of available (free or active) testosterone in a person's bloodstream, the more sexual desire he or she reports experiencing and the more often he or she indicates having sexual thoughts.

• Treatment with synthetic steroids that suppress the synthesis of testosterone produces diminished sexual desire. This result has been observed in three groups of individuals: (1) male sex offenders who receive antiandrogenic substances (such as cyproterone and medroxyprogesterone acetate) in order to reduce or control their sexual urges; (2) women who are given androgen antagonists to treat various androgen-dependent hair and skin problems (e.g., acne, alopecia, hirsutism, seborrhea); and (3) prostate cancer patients who receive antiandrogenic treatment as part of their medical regimen. In all three groups, such treatment often is associated with a reduction in self-reported sexual desire, fantasies, and urges.

• The administration of testosterone (and other androgens) has been noted to result in an increase in the strength and frequency of sexual desire in three groups of individuals: (1) otherwise healthy men and women complaining of low sexual interest; (2) men with hypogonadism or eugonadism (conditions caused by endocrine system disorders that result in abnormally low levels of testosterone); and (3) women with androgen deficiency syndrome (an androgen deficiency caused by chemotherapy, hysterectomy [removal of the uterus], or oophorectomy [removal of the ovaries]).

These findings not only suggest that some minimum level of testosterone is necessary for the experience of sexual desire in both men and women, but they also may partly explain the reported sex differences in (spontaneous) sexual desire. Specifically, under normal circumstances, a man's bloodstream contains a much higher quantity of testosterone (and other androgens) than a woman's bloodstream, and this greater quantity may allow men to generate and experience spontaneous desire more readily than women.

It is also the case that women are subject to greater variation in hormone levels than men and as a result are particularly prone to fluctuations in desire. The menstrual cycle, pregnancy, and perimenopause are all hormonally mediated life events specific to women, and the hormonal changes that occur during those events are reliably associated with alterations in sexual desire (for reviews, see Regan, 1996, 2013). Consequently, it is difficult to determine the true nature and extent of sex differences in desire without acknowledging the hormonal fluctuations that women's bodies undergo and examining the pattern of men's and women's feelings of desire over time. For example, it is possible that men and women experience roughly the same total amount of (spontaneous and/or responsive) sexual desire on some occasions but vastly different frequencies or intensities of desire on others.

Clearly, many individual-level attributes are associated with sexual desire. In addition, a person's level of sexual interest is likely to be affected by individual-level attributes possessed by the partner or desired other ("Other" in Figure 17.2). In particular, research on "sex appeal" suggests that physical appearance is the partner characteristic most likely to provoke sexual desire in men and women (for a review, see Regan, 2004). For example, in one early investigation of sexual desirability, Regan and Berscheid (1995) asked a group of (heterosexual) university students to list all the characteristics a man or woman could possess that would cause him or her to be sexually desirable. According to their participants, the single most important desire-causing characteristic was a physically attractive appearance (with 90% and 76% of participants specifying this attribute as an essential ingredient in female and male sexual desirability, respectively). A good overall personality and various dispositional attributes (including kindness, self-confidence, and a good sense of humor) also were mentioned as important components of sex appeal.

The results of mate preference studies, in which participants rank order or rate a variety of characteristics in terms of importance or desirability in a potential partner, corroborate these findings. For example, when considering their "ideal partner," high school students in Regan and Joshi's (2003) study rated attributes related to physical appearance (e.g., physical attractiveness, sexy appearance) as most sexually desirable, followed by attributes related to sexual drive (e.g., sexually passionate, sexually responsive, high sex drive) and interpersonal skill and responsiveness (e.g., relaxed in social settings, friendly, easygoing, attentive to others' needs). Research conducted with heterosexual and homosexual adults (e.g., Regan, 1998a; Regan & Berscheid, 1997; Regan, Medina, & Joshi, 2001; Sprecher & Regan, 2002) reveals a similar preference pattern. In one such investigation (Regan, Levin, Sprecher, Christopher, & Cate, 2000), more than 500 university students indicated their preferences for a large variety of characteristics. Interpersonal attributes, including expressiveness and openness, a good sense of humor, and friendliness and sociability, were rated as most sexually appealing. Almost equally important were characteristics related to physical appearance—men and women also desired a partner who possessed high levels of physical attractiveness, athleticism, physical health, and "sexy looks." Third in importance were attributes related to intellect and mental drive, such as intelligence, ambition, and education. The least sexually appealing characteristics concerned similarity (on demographic characteristics, attitudes, interests, and hobbies) and social status (e.g., earning potential, material resources). In sum, a person's sexual interest is most likely to be piqued by someone who possesses an attractive physical appearance, a sexually passionate nature, a kind disposition and good overall personality, and a humorous, relaxed, and responsive interpersonal style. In addition, because individuals who possess high(er) levels of those attributes tend to incite sexual interest in others (who may, in turn, act on their feelings by making sexual and/or romantic overtures), they may have more opportunities to experience and express sexual desire themselves.

Relational Factors Associated with Sexual Desire

Although a person's subjective experience of sexual desire is related to the various individual-level factors considered above (both his or her own and those of the partner), those factors alone do not determine whether or not desire will arise. A host of other factors also come into play, some of which involve the interpersonal or relational context.

One of the most important relational factors associated with feelings of desire is passionate love. Scholars from diverse disciplines have long argued that passionate love is intimately connected with sexual desire (see Berscheid, 1988; Ellis, 1954; Lewis, 1960/1988; Regan, 1998c; Tennov, 1979), and a growing body of empirical research substantiates this theoretical claim. When Ridge and Berscheid (1989) asked a sample of undergraduates whether they thought there was a difference between the experience of "being in love with" and that of "loving" another person, almost all (87%) of them responded affirmatively. Later, when asked to specify the nature of the difference, participants pointed to sexual attraction (which they felt was characteristic of being passionately in love with someone; also see Regan, Kocan, & Whitlock, 1998).

Similar results were provided by a person perception experiment conducted by Regan (1998b, Study 2) a decade later. (Person perception experiments are commonly used in social psychological research and essentially involve manipulating people's perceptions of a relationship and then measuring the impact of that manipulation on their subsequent evaluations and beliefs.) A sample of undergraduates received information about the members of a heterosexual, dating "student couple" who ostensibly reported that they were currently passionately in love with each other, that they loved each other, or that they liked each other. Participants then estimated the likelihood that the members of the couple experienced sexual desire for each other and the amount of desire that they felt for each other. Analyses revealed that men and women perceived partners who were characterized as being passionately in love as more *likely* to experience sexual desire, and as experiencing a greater *amount* of sexual desire, than partners who loved each other or who liked each other. In sum, people strongly believe that this particular relational factor— mutual feelings of passionate love—is associated with sexual attraction.

Moreover, there is evidence that passionate love and sexual desire actually do co-occur in ongoing romantic relationships. For example, during the process of scale validation, Hatfield and Sprecher (1986) administered their Passionate Love Scale (PLS) and a battery of other measures to people involved in romantic (e.g., dating, cohabiting) relationships. Their results revealed that PLS scores for both men and women were significantly positively correlated with several measures of current desire for sexual interaction with the partner (including self-reported desire to be held by the partner, to kiss the partner, and to engage in sex with the partner). A more recent investigation (Regan, 2000) revealed similar results. Here, a sample of men and women in dating relationships were asked to indicate the amount of passionate love and sexual desire they currently felt for their partners. The results indicated that sexual desire and passionate love were positively correlated; that is, the more passionate love participants reported feeling for their dating partners, the more they reported desiring those partners sexually. Passionate love is a potent predictor of sexual attraction.

The overall health of a relationship (which may encompass feelings of passionate love and which often is assessed via measures of relationship satisfaction, adjustment, commitment, or stability) is another interpersonal variable that is significantly linked with sexual desire. For example, Regan (2000) found that the more satisfied men and women were with their current dating relationship, and the less often they actively thought about ending that relationship, the more sexual desire they reported feeling for their partner. Similar results were obtained by Brezsnyak and Whisman (2004), whose survey of married couples revealed that the level of relationship satisfaction husbands and wives experienced was strongly positively correlated with the amount of sexual desire they felt for each other (also see Davies, Katz, & Jackson, 1999). Clinical research using samples of adults (usually women) diagnosed with sexual desire disorders provides additional evidence for the association between overall relationship health and sexual desire (e.g., Dennerstein, Koochaki, Barton, & Graziottin, 2006). In one early investigation, Stuart, Hammond, and Pett (1987) administered a marital adjustment scale to a sample of married women diagnosed with inhibited sexual desire (ISD), married women who reported normal sexual desire, and the spouses of women in both groups. Not only did the women in the ISD group have significantly lower marital adjustment scores than did women in the non-ISD group, but their spouses also reported significantly lower overall adjustment in their marriages than did the spouses of women in the non-ISD group.

Many clinicians believe that dysfunctional dynamics between partners—including poor social support and conflict resolution strategies, interpersonal anger and hostility, maladaptive communication patterns, and power struggles—can have a corrosive effect on sexual desire (Arnett, Prosen, & Toews, 1986; Kaplan, 1979, 1996; Maurice, 2007; McCarthy, Ginsberg, & Fucito, 2006; Trudel, 1991). Indeed, "emotional conflict with partner" was cited as the most common cause of low sexual desire among married men and women in a survey of 400 physicians (Pietropinto, 1986). Moreover, even when the relationship is not overtly hostile, if it is not conducive to open communication and emotional support, sexual desire is likely to be affected. In a longitudinal study of married and cohabiting women, Hällström and Samuelsson (1990) found that those who reported a decrease over time in their level of sexual desire also tended to perceive insufficient emotional support from, and a lack of a confiding relationship with, their partner. It is no surprise that many clinicians now conceptualize desire disorders as a "couple issue" rather than a "personal problem," focus on the dynamics of the couple's relationship during treatment, and apply therapeutic techniques that involve both partners (such as communication skills training and sexual intimacy exercises; Hartmann, Rüffer-Hesse, Krüger, & Philippsohn, 2012; for reviews and additional discussion, see Leiblum, 2010, and Ullery, Millner, & Willingham, 2002).

This is not to imply, of course, that partners in a healthy, well-adjusted relationship will always feel a constant level or an intense degree of sexual desire for one another. In fact, although there is little empirical research that directly examines this issue, many scholars believe that the partners' degree of sexual interest in each other is quite likely to change over the course of marital and other long-term unions (see Regan & Berscheid, 1999). It is even possible for the closeness and intimacy that characterize functional romantic relationships to create a sexual environment that actually dampens desire (for an in-depth discussion, see Ferreira, Narciso, & Novo, 2012). Sims and Meana (2010) asked a sample of married women who had experienced a self-reported loss of sexual interest to identify the factors that had reduced their desire and were preventing its reinstatement. Interestingly, very few women mentioned general relational issues when explaining their reduction in desire—they perceived their marriages as satisfying and healthy and they valued their husbands and viewed them in a positive light. Rather, these women uniformly pointed to sexual dynamics that had developed over time within their marriages, including (1) sexual habituation and over-familiarity (i.e., the loss of novelty, adventure, spontaneity, and excitement that had characterized sexual encounters earlier in the relationship, when sex was riskier and less available and consequently more valuable); (2) "mechanical" or monotonous sexual activity (i.e., orgasm-focused sexual interactions that deemphasized foreplay, creativity, and technique and that had become highly routine and predictable); and (3) sexual advances from the partner that lacked effort, subtlety, tenderness, and ingenuity. As partners grow comfortable and familiar with each other, they may experience a type of sexual stagnation that makes it increasingly difficult for them to feel sexually interested in one another.

Of course, it is also possible for partners, over time, to experience a heightened motivation to meet each other's sexual needs, along with increased openness about sexuality and ease with sexual communication; this sexual dynamic is likely to have a positive impact on sexual desire (see McCarthy & Farr, 2012; Metts, Sprecher, & Regan, 1998; Muise, Impett, Kogan, & Desmarais, 2013). Indeed, at least one study (Birnbaum et al., 2007) has found a strong correlation between sexual intimacy and sexual desire in long-term romantic relationships—women whose sexual interactions with their partners were characterized by high levels of intimacy (e.g., affectionate behavioral exchanges) reported experiencing correspondingly high levels of sexual desire for those partners.

In short, some interpersonal environments are more conducive to the growth and maintenance of sexual desire than others. A relational climate characterized by love, satisfaction, and commitment—and a sexual climate characterized by open, playful, responsive communication and intimate, innovative, partner-oriented interactions—is likely to create and sustain sexual attraction between partners.

Environmental Factors Associated with Sexual Desire

In addition to the relational context, each individual is embedded in an existing physical and social environment that may exert a powerful influence on his or her ability, motivation, and opportunity to experience desire (as well as other sexual responses). For example, people dealing with high levels of stress related to their work or school environment often report lacking sufficient time and energy to feel desire and to act on their sexual urges (see Murray & Milhausen, 2012). Similarly, both men and women report that certain environmental cues, such as pornographic or erotic material and "romantic" or "seductive" settings (e.g., a bedroom staged with dim lights and soft music) can stimulate their sexual interest (McCall & Meston, 2006; Murray & Milhausen, 2012; Regan & Berscheid, 1995).

Many people believe that alcohol, drugs, and various other external agents can function as aphrodisiacs that arouse or enhance sexual desire (see Regan & Berscheid, 1999). The number of putative naturally occurring aphrodisiacs is legion, encompassing a host of herbs (e.g., rosemary), spices (e.g., saffron, cinnamon), plant roots (e.g., ginseng), tree bark extracts (e.g., yohimbine), and almost any fruit or vegetable that bears the slightest resemblance to male or female external genitalia (e.g., asparagus, bananas, celery stalks, figs, peaches, apricots) (see Connell, 1965; Rätsch & Müller-Ebeling, 2013). However, there is virtually no empirical evidence supporting a connection between ingestion of these substances and sexual desire in healthy adults (see, for example, Shamloul, 2010). With respect to nonprescription or so-called recreational drugs, the (albeit limited and often anecdotal) research suggests that (1) small to moderate amounts of alcohol and certain stimulant drugs (cocaine, amphetamine) are related to increased sexual desire (possibly as the result of an expectancy effect rather than any direct influence); (2) small to moderate doses of opiates (opium, morphine, heroin) are related to reduced sexual desire; and (3) higher amounts and chronic use of alcohol and other depressant drugs (e.g., barbiturates), cocaine, and opiates are related to reduced sexual desire (Regan & Berscheid, 1999).

A variety of social forces also are likely to have an impact on sexual desire. People learn the "rules" of sexual attraction—the situations in which, and individuals for whom, it is acceptable to feel desire, how desire should be communicated, and the meanings to attach to desire—from sociocultural norms about male and female sexuality, laws and religious doctrines that govern sexual behavior, media portrayals of sexual encounters and romantic relationships, and the sexual attitudes and behaviors of friends, family, and other social network members (Regan & Berscheid, 1999; Tiefer, 1995). For example, although the cultural messages aimed at both sexes have changed over time, researchers continue to find evidence of what has been called the "sexual double standard" (see Metts et al., 1998; Oliver & Hyde, 1993). Specifically, men are commonly believed to have a stronger sexual drive and need for sexual release than are women (Richgels, 1992; Tolman, 1991). Men also receive more positive reinforcement than do women for expressing their sexual urges, seeking out sexual opportunities, and gaining sexual experience, whereas women generally receive more reinforcement than do men for restraining their sexual needs, establishing limits on sexual intimacy, and confining their sexual activity to committed, love-based relationships (Gagnon & Simon, 1973; Hogben & Byrne, 1998; Reiss, 1967, 1986).

Researchers and clinicians have observed that cultural stereotypes and media portrayals that depict male desire as innate, urgent, and ever present may make it difficult for men to successfully negotiate the reductions in sexual desire (and other aspects of sexuality) that are a natural part of the aging process (see McCarthy & Farr, 2011). These male stereotypes also affect women. In one recent study, women reported participating in unwanted (consensual) intercourse in order to satisfy what they perceived as their male partners' natural or inherent "need" for sex (Hayfield & Clarke, 2012). Similarly, stereotypes and media representations that, for example, depict women as sexually undeveloped relative to men, the elderly as fundamentally asexual, and the physically different (e.g., obese, disabled) as sexually unappealing may conspire to teach individuals from those social groups (and their potential partners) that any sexual desire they experience is "abnormal" or "wrong" and that they are undeserving of having their sexual needs met. This, in turn, may inhibit their opportunities to express, explore, and act on their desires.

To date, scientists have paid less attention to environmental causes and correlates of sexual desire than they have to personal and relational factors. This may reflect the fact that variables at the individual and interpersonal levels of analysis are more clearly visible and readily measured than are variables at the environmental level. Additional investigation into the impact of these factors (particularly social environmental factors) on sexual desire certainly is warranted.

Future Directions

What is sexual desire? How is it similar to and different from other sexual responses? How do researchers and clinicians typically assess or measure sexual desire? What factors are associated with sexual desire? What variables influence its expression and experience? The purpose of this chapter was to provide some answers to these questions by considering current conceptualizations of sexual desire (definition, relation to other human sexual responses, measurement) and by reviewing existing empirical research on the personal/individual, relational/interpersonal, and environmental factors that are associated with this particular experience.

Although there is no small amount of information available about sexual desire, much remains to be learned.

For example, most theorists and researchers interested in sexual desire have focused on exploring its nature and correlates. Less is known about the individual and interpersonal *consequences* of sexual desire. For example, the fact that many men and women believe passionate love and sexual attraction are associated may have important implications for understanding the dynamics of sexual interactions. Consider the following interpersonal scenario. Partner A may express feelings of love, intimacy, and commitment in an attempt to excite Partner B's feelings of sexual desire and increase the likelihood of sexual activity. Moreover, assuming that sexual desire is triggered by declarations of love and commitment, Partner A may view these "romantic" events as adequate justification for the occurrence of sexual activity—regardless of Partner B's expressed consent. Conversely, Partner B, who believes that desire is the appropriate or "normal" response to expressions of intimacy or love from a romantic partner, may be uncertain about how to interpret a nonconsensual sexual encounter that follows any such "romantic" cues.

There is some research that supports these suppositions. Regan (1997) asked men and women to read one of two versions of a scenario involving an interaction between a heterosexual, dating couple. In each scenario, the couple has rented a movie and returned to the man's room in order to view the video; during the movie, "Bob" expresses to "Cathy" his interest in sexual activity. Half of the participants read a scenario in which Bob confesses his feelings of love for Cathy prior to requesting sex; the other half simply read his sexual request. Both scenarios continue with Bob initiating sexual activity, Cathy verbally refusing, and the date ending in sexual intercourse. The results revealed that when Cathy received a verbal declaration of love from Bob, she was viewed as more likely to have experienced sexual desire and to have wanted sexual intercourse—despite her clearly stated unwillingness—than when she received an expression of sexual interest. Additionally, the sexual interaction was perceived as significantly more consensual (i.e., reflecting the mutual desires of the partners) when Bob professed love than when he professed sexual intent. More importantly, however, Cathy's perceived sexual desire level mediated the effect of Bob's sexual request style (romantic vs. sexual) on the perceived likelihood of consensual sex. In other words, the expression of love by Bob significantly increased the likelihood that his subsequent sexual interaction with the unwilling Cathy was labeled "consensual" *because participants assumed that this expression of love caused Cathy to feel sexual desire and to want sex.* The fact that we in this culture have so firmly linked passionate love with sexual desire may influence the labels we place on sexual interactions and possibly contribute to sexual (mis)communication. It is important for future researchers to continue to explore not only the consequences of beliefs about sexual desire, but the ways in which men and women allow their behaviors to be guided by these beliefs and expectations in their actual, ongoing interactions.

And this raises another issue. Because sexual desire is often experienced for a relationship partner and expressed within an existing close relationship, it is related to many other interpersonal phenomena. Unfortunately, there has been relatively little research that considers both the experience and the expression of sexual desire from within a relational context. As noted earlier in this chapter, most empirical research on sexual desire has focused on personal factors (e.g., age, hormones, health) that are associated with the amount and frequency of desire experienced by the individual. Most researchers have not recognized that there may be a significant difference between a person's feelings of sexual desire in general and his or her feelings of sexual desire for a specific relationship partner. In addition, most have not asked their participants about other, interpersonal factors that may influence self-reported desire.

Similarly, we know very little about the role that sexual desire plays within ongoing, interpersonal relationships (in particular, healthy, functioning relationships). For example, among nonclinical (i.e., nondistressed) samples, how does sexual desire for the partner change over time? What is the "typical" progression of sexual desire in long-term romantic relationships? How common is it for couples to experience discrepancies in their levels of desire (i.e., one partner experiences more desire than the other, or one partner experiences desire for a nonreciprocating partner)? What are the consequences of such discrepancies for relationship quality and adjustment? How do couples typically respond to discrepancies or changes in desire? It remains for future (longitudinal) research to investigate whether the waxing and waning of sexual desire within a relationship actually correspond to the ebb and flow of other interpersonally significant events.

In sum, sexual desire is a complex, multiply determined response that is affected by—and that, in turn, has implications for—virtually every aspect of our lives. Understanding sexual desire—what it is, how it differs from other sexual responses, what personal, relational, and environmental factors influence its expression—represents one very important step in learning how to communicate about sexual desire. And learning how to communicate one's feelings of sexual desire (or lack thereof) to a sexual and/or romantic partner is critical to personal well-being and interpersonal satisfaction.

REFERENCES

Arnett, J. L., Prosen, H., & Toews, J. A. (1986). Loss of libido due to stress. *Medical Aspects of Human Sexuality, 20*, 140–148.

Bancroft, J. (1988). Sexual desire and the brain. *Sexual and Marital Therapy, 3*, 11–27.

Basson, R. (2001). Human sex-response cycles. *Journal of Sex and Marital Therapy, 27*, 33–43.

Basson, R. (2002). Women's sexual desire: Disordered or misunderstood? *Journal of Sex and Marital Therapy, 28*, 17–28.

Basson, R., & Brotto, L. A. (2009). Disorders of sexual desire and subjective arousal in women. In R. Balon & R. T. Segraves (Eds.), *Clinical manual of sexual disorders* (pp. 119–159). Arlington, VA: American Psychiatric Publishing.

Beck, J. G., Bozman, A. W., & Qualtrough, T. (1991). The experience of sexual desire: Psychological correlates in a college sample. *Journal of Sex Research, 28*, 443–456.

Berscheid, E. (1988). Some comments on love's anatomy: Or, whatever happened to old-fashioned lust? In R. J. Sternberg & M. L. Barnes (Eds.), *The psychology of love* (pp. 359–374). New Haven, CT: Yale University Press.

Birnbaum, G. E., Cohen, O., & Wertheimer, V. (2007). Is it all about intimacy?: Age, menopausal status, and women's sexuality. *Personal Relationships, 14*, 167–185.

Bodenmann, G., & Ledermann, T. (2007). Depressed mood and sexual functioning. *International Journal of Sexual Health, 19*, 63–73.

Brezsnyak, M., & Whisman, M. A. (2004). Sexual desire and relationship functioning: The effects of marital satisfaction and power. *Journal of Sex and Marital Therapy, 30*, 199–217.

Brotto, L. A., Woo, J. S. T., & Gorzalka, B. B. (2012). Differences in sex guilt and desire in East Asian and Euro-Canadian men. *Journal of Sex Research, 49*, 594–602.

Carvalho, J. (2010). Predictors of women's sexual desire: The role of psychopathology, cognitive-emotional determinants, relationship dimensions, and medical factors. *Journal of Sexual Medicine, 7*, 928–937.

Carvalho, J., & Nobre, P. (2011). Predictors of men's sexual desire: The role of psychological, cognitive-emotional, relational, and medical factors. *Journal of Sex Research, 48*, 254–262.

Connell, C. (1965). *Aphrodisiacs in your garden*. London: Arthur Barker.

Davies, S., Katz, J., & Jackson, J. L. (1999). Sexual desire discrepancies: Effects on sexual and relationship satisfaction in heterosexual dating couples. *Archives of Sexual Behavior, 28*, 553–567.

Davis, S. R., & Braunstein, G. D. (2012). Efficacy and safety of testosterone in the management of hypoactive sexual desire disorder in postmenopausal women. *Journal of Sexual Medicine, 9*, 1134–1148.

DeLamater, J. (1991). Emotions and sexuality. In K. McKinney & S. Sprecher (Eds.), *Sexuality in close relationships* (pp. 49–70). Hillsdale, NJ: Erlbaum.

Dennerstein, L., Koochaki, P., Barton, I., & Graziottin, A. (2006). Hypoactive sexual desire disorder in menopausal women: A survey of Western European women. *Journal of Sexual Medicine, 3*, 212–222.

Ellis, A. (1954). *The American sexual tragedy*. New York: Twayne.

Eplov, L., Giraldi, A., Davidsen, M., Garde, K., & Kamper-Jørgensen, F. (2007). Sexual desire in a nationally representative Danish population. *Journal of Sexual Medicine, 4*, 47–56.

Ferreira, L. C., Narciso, I., & Novo, R. F. (2012). Intimacy, sexual desire and differentiation in couplehood: A theoretical and methodological review. *Journal of Sex and Marital Therapy, 38*, 263–280.

Gagnon, J. H., & Simon, W. (1973). *Sexual conduct: The social sources of human sexuality*. Chicago: Aldine.

Goldhammer, D. L., & McCabe, M. P. (2011a). A qualitative exploration of the meaning and experience of sexual desire among partnered women. *Canadian Journal of Human Sexuality, 20,* 19–29.

Goldhammer, D. L., & McCabe, M. P. (2011b). Development and psychometric properties of the Female Sexual Desire Questionnaire (FSDQ). *Journal of Sexual Medicine, 8,* 2512–2521.

Hällström, T., & Samuelsson, S. (1990). Changes in women's sexual desire in middle life: The longitudinal study of women in Gothenburg. *Archives of Sexual Behavior, 19,* 259–268.

Hartmann, U. H., Rüffer-Hesse, C., Krüger, T. H. C., & Philippsohn, S. (2012). Individual and dyadic barriers to a pharmacotherapeutic treatment of hypoactive sexual desire disorders: Results and implications from a small-scale study with bupropion. *Journal of Sex and Marital Therapy, 38,* 325–348.

Hatfield, E., & Sprecher, S. (1986). Measuring passionate love in intimate relationships. *Journal of Adolescence, 9,* 383–410.

Hayfield, N., & Clarke, V. (2012). "I'd be just as happy with a cup of tea:" Women's accounts of sex and affection in long-term heterosexual relationships. *Women's Studies International Forum, 35,* 67–74.

Hintikka, J., Niskanen, L., Koivumaa-Honkanen, H., Tolmunen, T., Honkalampi, K., Lehto, S. M., et al. (2009). Hypogonadism, decreased sexual desire, and long-term depression in middle-aged men. *Journal of Sexual Medicine, 6,* 2049–2057.

Hogben, M., & Byrne, D. (1998). Using social learning theory to explain individual differences in human sexuality. *Journal of Sex Research, 35,* 58–71.

Kaplan, H. S. (1979). *Disorders of sexual desire and other new concepts and techniques in sex therapy.* New York: Simon & Schuster.

Kaplan, H. S. (1996). Erotic obsession: Relationship to hypoactive sexual desire disorder and paraphilia. *American Journal of Psychiatry, 153,* 30–41.

Koller, W. C., Vetere-Overfield, B., Williamson, A., Busenbark, K., Nash, J., & Parrish, D. (1990). Sexual dysfunction in Parkinson's disease. *Clinical Neuropharmacology, 13,* 461–463.

Laan, E., & Both, S. (2008). What makes women experience desire? *Feminism and Psychology, 18,* 505–514.

Leiblum, S. R. (Ed.). (2010). *Treating sexual desire disorders: A clinical casebook.* New York: Guilford Press.

Levine, S. B. (1984). An essay on the nature of sexual desire. *Journal of Sex and Marital Therapy, 10,* 83–96.

Levine, S. B. (2003). The nature of sexual desire: A clinician's perspective. *Archives of Sexual Behavior, 32,* 279–285.

Lewis, C. S. (1988). *The four loves.* New York: Harcourt Brace. (Original work published 1960)

Lourenço, M., Azevedo, L. P., & Gouveia, J. L. (2011). Depression and sexual desire: An exploratory study in psychiatric patients. *Journal of Sex and Marital Therapy, 37,* 32–44.

Maurice, W. L. (2007). Sexual desire disorders in men. In S. R. Leiblum (Ed.), *Principles and practice of sex therapy* (4th ed., pp. 181–211). New York: Guilford Press.

McCall, K., & Meston, C. (2006). Cues resulting in desire for sexual activity in women. *Journal of Sex and Marital Therapy, 3,* 838–852.

McCarthy, B., & Farr, E. (2011). Male sexual desire and function. *Behavior Therapist, 34,* 133–136.

McCarthy, B., & Farr, E. (2012). Strategies and techniques to maintain sexual desire. *Journal of Contemporary Psychotherapy, 42,* 227–233.

McCarthy, B. W., Ginsberg, R. L., & Fucito, L. M. (2006). Resilient sexual desire in heterosexual couples. *Family Journal, 14,* 59–64.

Meana, M. (2010). Elucidating women's (hetero)sexual desire: Definitional challenges and content expansion. *Journal of Sex Research, 47,* 104–122.

Metts, S., Sprecher, S., & Regan, P. C. (1998). Communication and sexual desire. In P. A. Andersen & L. K. Guerrero (Eds.), *Handbook of communication and emotion: Research, theory, applications, and contexts* (pp. 353–377). Orlando, FL: Academic Press.

Muise, A., Impett, E. A., Kogan, A., & Desmarais, S. (2013). Keeping the spark alive: Being motivated to meet a partner's sexual needs sustains sexual desire in long-term romantic relationships. *Social Psychological and Personality Science, 4,* 267–273.

Murray, S., & Milhausen, R. (2012). Factors impacting women's sexual desire: Examining long-term relationships in emerging adulthood. *Canadian Journal of Human Sexuality, 21,* 101–115.

Oliver, M. B., & Hyde, J. S. (1993). Gender differences in sexuality: A meta-analysis. *Psychological Bulletin, 114,* 29–51.

Pietropinto, A. (1986). Inhibited sexual desire. *Medical Aspects of Human Sexuality, 20,* 46–49.

Purifoy, F. E., Grodsky, A., & Giambra, L. M. (1992). The relationship of sexual daydreaming to sexual activity, sexual drive, and sexual attitudes for women across the life span. *Archives of Sexual Behavior, 21,* 369–385.

Rätsch, C., & Müller-Ebeling, C. (2013). *The encyclopedia of aphrodisiacs: Psychoactive substances for use in sexual practices.* Rochester, VT: Park Street Press.

Reiss, I. L. (1967). *The social context of premarital sexual permissiveness.* New York: Holt, Rinehart, and Winston.

Reiss, I. L. (1986). *Journey into sexuality: An exploratory voyage.* New York: Prentice-Hall.

Regan, P. C. (1996). Rhythms of desire: The association between menstrual cycle phases and female sexual desire. *Canadian Journal of Human Sexuality, 5,* 145–156.

Regan, P. C. (1997). The impact of male sexual request style on perceptions of sexual interactions: The mediational role of beliefs about female sexual desire. *Basic and Applied Social Psychology, 19,* 519–532.

Regan, P. C. (1998a). Minimum mate selection standards as a function of perceived mate value, relationship context, and gender. *Journal of Psychology and Human Sexuality, 10,* 53–73.

Regan, P. C. (1998b). Of lust and love: Beliefs about the role of sexual desire in romantic relationships. *Personal Relationships, 5,* 139–157.

Regan, P. C. (1998c). Romantic love and sexual desire. In V. C. de Munck (Ed.), *Romantic love and sexual behavior: Perspectives from the social sciences* (pp. 91–112). Westport, CT: Praeger.

Regan, P. C. (1999). Hormonal correlates and causes of sexual desire: A review. *Canadian Journal of Human Sexuality, 8,* 1–16.

Regan, P. C. (2000). The role of sexual desire and sexual activity in dating relationships. *Social Behavior and Personality, 28,* 51–60.

Regan, P. C. (2004). Sex and the attraction process: Lessons from science (and Shakespeare) on lust, love, chastity, and fidelity. In J. Harvey, A. Wenzel, & S.

Sprecher (Eds.), *The handbook of sexuality in close relationships* (pp. 115–133). Mahwah, NJ: Erlbaum.

Regan, P. C. (2013). Sexual desire in women. In D. Castañeda (Ed.), *The essential handbook of women's sexuality* (Vol. 1, pp. 3–24). Santa Barbara, CA: Praeger.

Regan, P. C., & Atkins, L. (2006). Sex differences and similarities in frequency and intensity of sexual desire. *Social Behavior and Personality, 34*, 95–102.

Regan, P. C., & Berscheid, E. (1995). Gender differences in beliefs about the causes of male and female sexual desire. *Personal Relationships, 2*, 345–358.

Regan, P. C., & Berscheid, E. (1996). Beliefs about the state, goals, and objects of sexual desire. *Journal of Sex and Marital Therapy, 22*, 110–120.

Regan, P. C., & Berscheid, E. (1997). Gender differences in characteristics desired in a potential sexual and marriage partner. *Journal of Psychology and Human Sexuality, 9*, 25–37.

Regan, P. C., & Berscheid, E. (1999). *Lust: What we know about human sexual desire.* Thousand Oaks, CA: Sage.

Regan, P. C., & Joshi, A. (2003). Ideal partner preferences among adolescents. *Social Behavior and Personality, 31*, 13–20.

Regan, P. C., Kocan, E. R., & Whitlock, T. (1998). Ain't love grand!: A prototype analysis of romantic love. *Journal of Social and Personal Relationships, 15*, 411–420.

Regan, P. C., Levin, L., Sprecher, S., Christopher, F. S., & Cate, R. (2000). Partner preferences: What characteristics do men and women desire in their short-term sexual and long-term romantic partners? *Journal of Psychology and Human Sexuality, 12*, 1–21.

Regan, P. C., Medina, R., & Joshi, A. (2001). Partner preferences among homosexual men and women: What is desirable in a sex partner is not necessarily desirable in a romantic partner. *Social Behavior and Personality, 29*, 625–633.

Richgels, P. B. (1992). Hypoactive sexual desire in heterosexual women: A feminist analysis. *Women and Therapy, 12*, 123–135.

Rico-Villademoros, F., Calandre, E. P., Rodríguez-López, C. M., García-Carrillo, J., Ballesteros, J., Hidalgo-Tallón, J., et al. (2012). Sexual functioning in women and men with fibromyalgia. *Journal of Sexual Medicine, 9*, 542–549.

Ridge, R. D., & Berscheid, E. (1989, May). *On loving and being in love: A necessary distinction.* Midwestern Psychological Association, Chicago, IL.

Schiavi, R. C., Schreiner-Engel, P., Mandeli, J., Schanzer, H., & Cohen, E. (1990). Healthy aging and male sexual function. *American Journal of Psychiatry, 147*, 766–771.

Schover, L. R., Evans, R. B., & von Eschenbach, A. C. (1987). Sexual rehabilitation in a cancer center: Diagnosis and outcome in 384 consultations. *Archives of Sexual Behavior, 16*, 445–461.

Schreiner-Engel, P., Schiavi, R. C., Vietorisz, D., Eichel, J. D. S., & Smith, H. (1985). Diabetes and female sexuality: A comparative study of women in relationships. *Journal of Sex and Marital Therapy, 11*, 165–175.

Shamloul, R. (2010). Natural aphrodisiacs. *Journal of Sexual Medicine, 7*, 39–49.

Sims, K. E., & Meana, M. (2010). Why did passion wane? A qualitative study of married women's attributions for declines in sexual desire. *Journal of Sex and Marital Therapy, 36*, 360–380.

Spector, I. P., Carey, M. P., & Steinberg, L. (1996). The Sexual Desire Inventory: Development, factor structure, and evidence of reliability. *Journal of Sex and Marital Therapy, 22*, 175–190.

Sprecher, S., & Regan, P. C. (2002). Liking some things (in some people) more than others: Partner preferences in romantic relationships and friendships. *Journal of Social and Personal Relationships, 19,* 463–481.

Stuart, F. M., Hammond, D. C., & Pett, M. A. (1987). Inhibited sexual desire in women. *Archives of Sexual Behavior, 16,* 91–106.

Štulhofer, A., Carvalheira, A. A., & Træen, B. (2013). Is responsive sexual desire for partnered sex problematic among men? Insights from a two-country study. *Sexual and Relationship Therapy, 28,* 246–258.

Tennov, D. (1979). *Love and limerence.* New York: Stein & Day.

Tiefer, L. (1995). *Sex is not a natural act and other essays.* Boulder, CO: Westview Press.

Tolman, D. L. (1991). Adolescent girls, women and sexuality: Discerning dilemmas of desire. *Women and Therapy, 11,* 55–69.

Trudel, G. (1991). Review of psychological factors in low sexual desire. *Sexual and Marital Therapy, 6,* 261–272.

Ullery, E. K., Millner, V. S., & Willingham, H. A. (2002). The emergent care and treatment of women with hypoactive sexual desire disorder. *Family Journal: Counseling and Therapy for Couples and Families, 10,* 346–350.

Useche, B., Villegas, M., & Alzate, H. (1990). Sexual behavior of Colombian high school students. *Adolescence, 25,* 291–304.

CHAPTER 18

Aggressive Desires

Thomas F. Denson
Timothy P. Schofield
Emma C. Fabiansson

People experience all sorts of desires, such as wanting to indulge in chocolate, drink fine wines, sleep with beautiful people, and be socially connected. Desires are the conscious experience of wanting to have or do something that brings pleasure—or relief from displeasure (Hofmann & van Dillen, 2012). Moreover, desires differ from general motivations in that the targets of desires are specific people or objects. One universal human desire is wanting to hurt another person when people feel like they or their close others have been unjustly harmed. Such real or perceived harm typically increases anger and approach motivation. Aggression that follows as a consequence of anger provocation is referred to as reactive, affective, or impulsive aggression.[1]

In this chapter, we use the preventive–interventive model of self-control as an organizing framework (Hofmann & Kotabe, 2012) and extend the model to the reactive aggression context. First, we discuss how aggressive desires emerge. We then discuss neurobiological features underlying aggressive desires. Next we discuss how aggressive desires are maintained over time by angry rumination. We then focus on how people may

---

[1]In this chapter, we focus primarily on the desire to engage in reactive aggression. There are no doubt other types of aggressive desires, such as wanting to hurt someone to obtain a secondary goal (e.g., money or notoriety) or wanting to hurt someone for the thrill of it. Understanding these types of desires is important, and scientists are beginning to make progress in that regard (cf. Buckels, Jones, & Paulhus, 2013; Hemphill & Hart, 2002). However, anger provocation has been called "the most important single cause of human aggression" (Anderson & Bushman, p. 37). If left unchecked, reactive aggressive desires can lead to serious acts of violence. Thus, this chapter focuses on the desire to hurt others when angered.

come to view aggressive desires as in conflict with self-regulatory goals (or not). The next section examines individual differences and cultural influences on the desire to aggress. We conclude with a discussion of how people may prevent aggressive desires from emerging and better control aggressive desires that have already entered consciousness.

The Emergence of Aggressive Desires

Evolution has equipped all mammals with the ability to behave aggressively. When people are harmed, they usually feel the desire to retaliate in a tit-for-tat manner (Axelrod, 1984; Eisenberger, Lynch, Aselage, & Rohdieck, 2004). The *preventive–interventive model of self-control* (Hofmann & Kotabe, 2012) is useful for understanding the pathways through which anger provocation can lead to experiencing aggressive desires. The model also suggests that aggressive desires can be controlled or, if left unregulated, may lead to aggressive behavior. A schematic of the preventive–interventive model expanded to fit the reactive aggression context is presented in Figure 18.1.

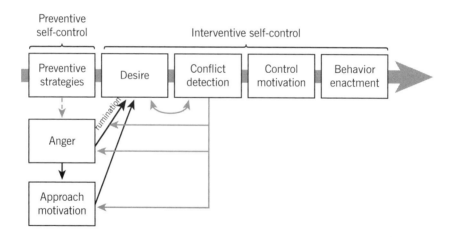

FIGURE 18.1. Expanded schematic of the preventive–interventive model of self-control. The model is specific to instances in which the desire to reactively aggress may be experienced. Preventive strategies inhibit the elicitation of anger, most likely through avoidance of provocation. When one is provoked and anger is experienced, it typically induces an approach motivation. Both anger and approach motivation can elicit the conscious experience of the desire to aggress. Rumination can maintain the desire to aggress over time. Conflict detection can occur at four time points: when anger is experienced, during rumination, when one becomes aware of approach motivational tendencies, and when one consciously experiences the desire to aggress.

The figure depicts the timeline of a potentially aggressive situation partitioned by two forms of self-control. Preventive strategies involve anticipating situations where unwanted desires might emerge and taking proactive steps to ensure that one does not succumb to the problematic desire (see also Hofmann, Kotabe, Vohs, & Baumeister, Chapter 3, this volume). There are very few preventive strategies for preventing aggressive desires, but an example would be avoiding places where one might be provoked (e.g., taking the train to avoid road rage). This specific strategy, called *access restrictions*, is one of the oldest forms of preventive self-control. Thus, preventive strategies preclude the elicitation of aggressive desires, most likely through avoidance of provocation. Unfortunately, it not always feasible to avoid provocative people, nor is it always in one's best interest. However, the important point is the notion that preventive strategies can prevent unconscious impulses from occurring and forming the conscious experience of desire.

At the phenomenological level, anger and the desire to aggress may often be isomorphic. However, we suggest that there is utility in keeping the underlying psychological constructs distinct. We consider anger to be the specific emotion elicited in response to provocation, whereas the desire to aggress is the conscious experience of wanting to hurt someone. In this way, it is possible to examine the distinct influences and neural correlates of each variable. In instances in which provocation produces anger, this anger typically induces a corresponding approach motivation (Carver & Harmon-Jones, 2009; see also Harmon-Jones, Gable, & Harmon-Jones, Chapter 8, this volume). The heightened approach motivation may lead to the awareness of the desire to aggress, particularly if the approach motivation is very strong. However, anger by itself is probably sufficient to elicit an aggressive desire. Indeed, aggressive desires may be experienced in the absence of an immediate motivation to approach the harm doer, as is sometimes the case during a bout of angry rumination (Kelley, Hortensius, & Harmon-Jones, 2013). We suggest that rumination is the fundamental psychological mediator that maintains the desire to aggress over time. We expand upon this notion in a subsequent section of this chapter.

The vast majority of research on self-control has focused on interventive self-control, which is depicted in the next four stages of Figure 18.1. If the preventive strategy is not utilized or fails, aggressive impulses enter working memory and become consciously experienced as the desire to aggress. In the next stage, the desire is either detected as being in conflict with one's goals, social norms, and so forth, or not. Conflict detection can occur at four time points: when anger is experienced, during rumination, when one becomes aware of approach motivational tendencies, and when one consciously experiences the desire to aggress. In today's world there are strong social norms proscribing reactive aggression (cf. Pinker, 2011), suggesting that frequently the aggressive desire will create a self-regulatory conflict. If so, participants may be motivated to inhibit the tendency to aggress. If the desire to behave aggressively is not inhibited and the situation affords the opportunity to aggress, self-control failure occurs.

Neurobiological Mechanisms

A comprehensive understanding of the desire to aggress requires examination of the neural underpinnings of this phenomenon. Neuroimaging research highlights the fact that brain regions implicated in reward may play a critical role in the extent to which aggressive desires influence cognition and behavior. For instance, in one functional magnetic resonance imaging (fMRI) study, participants viewed pictures of people they hated and people for whom they reported neutral feelings (Zeki & Romaya, 2008). Relative to the neutral people, viewing hated people increased activation in the putamen, which is part of the brain's reward circuitry. Similarly, experiencing anger and regulating anger often activates the orbitofrontal cortex (OFC), which is implicated in reward processing (Fabiansson, Denson, Moulds, Grisham, & Schira, 2012; Murphy, Nimmo-Smith, & Lawrence, 2003; Kringelbach, 2005).

In another fMRI study, participants completed a computerized version of the Taylor (1967) aggression paradigm with two fictitious opponents (Krämer, Jansma, Tempelmann, & Münte, 2007). One opponent was scripted to be highly provocative, in that they always selected the loudest blast of noise to be delivered to the actual participant. The other fictitious opponent always selected innocuous blasts. Using a clever design, the authors were able to examine brain activation when participants made the decision to retaliate (or not). In that study, when participants selected the most aggressive levels of retaliation toward the provocative opponent, they showed heightened activation in the dorsal striatum, which is implicated in reward. Similarly, in another neuroimaging study, participants who punished cheaters during an economic exchange game showed heightened activation in the dorsal striatum (de Quervain et al., 2004). Thus, planning and taking revenge toward those who harm us may sometimes feel good.

The preventive–interventive model is compatible with our understanding of the neurobiological consequences and correlates of aggressive desires. In neural terms, self-control involves prefrontal cortical control over impulses from regions implicated in emotion and reward (Heatherton & Wagner, 2011; see also Lopez, Wagner, & Heatherton, Chapter 7, this volume). Braver's (2012) dual mechanisms of control framework distinguishes between proactive and reactive cognitive control (which roughly map onto preventive and interventive self-control, respectively). Proactive cognitive control is characterized by a pattern of anticipatory and/or sustained activation in the lateral prefrontal cortex (PFC). This PFC activation likely reflects the neural representation of actively maintaining goals (e.g., to behave in a socially acceptable manner; Braver, 2012). Reactive cognitive control is characterized by transient activation in the lateral PFC along with activation in a wider network of brain regions such as the anterior cingulate cortex (ACC; Braver, 2012).

The ACC is a particularly important brain region for understanding the emergence and control of aggressive desires. The ACC monitors and detects cognitive conflicts. The ACC shows increased activation when provoked (Denson, Pedersen, Ronquillo, & Nandy, 2009). When provoked, one likely conflict is the desire to retaliate versus the desire to behave nonaggressively in accordance with normative or personal standards or goals. Thus, aggressive desires are likely registered as problematic via activation in the ACC. Through interconnections with the lateral PFC, the ACC contributes to behavior by determining the costs, benefits, and amount of effort needed to exert control in any given situation in which control is required (Gasquoine, 2013; Shenhav, Botvinick, & Cohen, 2013). Although ACC activation may represent a conflict between one's goal of being respected and one's current state of being maltreated, subsequent studies from our laboratory found that increased ACC activation was positively correlated with heightened anger control (Denson, Dobson-Stone, Ronay, von Hippel, & Schira, 2014; Denson, Ronay, von Hippel, & Schira, 2013).

Another defining neurobiological feature of anger provocation is an increase in approach motivation (Carver & Harmon-Jones, 2009). Approach motivation is typically a byproduct of feeling anger and is inextricably linked to aggressive desires. The neural marker of approach motivation is greater relative brain activation in the left lateral PFC than right lateral PFC (Carver & Harmon-Jones, 2009). The approach motivation elicited by aggressive desires in conjunction with increased activation in reward circuitry should facilitate revenge-seeking behavior. However, as is apparent in Figure 18.1, people may experience the competing motivation to override the tendency to aggress. If control is successful, approach motivation may initiate more socially acceptable, assertive behavior or be replaced with avoidance of the source of anger altogether.

In sum, when one is provoked and thinking about revenge, increased reward activation and approach motivation may initiate the conscious experience of desire. The ACC likely plays a critical role in determining whether the desire violates one's self-regulatory goals or standards.

How Is the Desire to Aggress Maintained over Time?

One important aspect of the desire to aggress is that people can experience and revisit the desire over very long periods of time. For instance, in intergroup conflicts, it is not uncommon for the desire to aggress to span multiple generations (cf. Boehm, 1987). We suggest that angry rumination is the principal psychological mechanism that maintains the desire for revenge over time. Angry rumination is perseverative thinking about a personally meaningful anger-inducing event (Denson, 2013). Indeed, the content of rumination often consists of reexperiencing anger provocations as well as planning revenge (Caprara, 1986; Denson, Pedersen, & Miller, 2006; Sukhodolsky, Golub, & Cromwell, 2001).

Angry rumination likely maintains aggressive desires by occupying working memory with aggressive content. In this way, even when angry rumination is intermittent, when actively engaging in rumination, the focus is likely to be on the desire to aggress. No one knows for sure how long angry rumination can maintain aggressive desires, but experimental work shows that angry rumination can heighten aggressive behavior for anywhere from 8 to 24 hours (Bushman & Gibson, 2011; Bushman, Bonacci, Pedersen, Vasquez, & Miller, 2005). One reasonable assumption of this work is that angry rumination maintained aggressive desires over these time periods. As depicted in Figure 18.1, during rumination people may notice that the desire to aggress is becoming problematic. Next, we discuss when aggressive desires may be considered problematic in more detail.

When Are Aggressive Desires Considered Problematic?

Once the desire to aggress has become conscious, the angered individual must decide whether he or she can and should act upon the desire or not. If adequate time and resources are available, this consideration may be reflective in nature. For instance, one may determine whether acting aggressively will advance one's immediate or long-term self-interest. According to Hofmann and Kotabe (2012, p. 709) when "the behavior implied by the desire is at odds with a person's value system and self-regulatory goal standards" people experience a self-control conflict. In the case of aggressive desires, such a conflict occurs when one simultaneously experiences the desire to harm others along with an incompatible desire, such as the desire to be a good member of society. If a conflict is registered (most likely in the ACC), one may view the desire as problematic and subsequently initiate control processes (likely in the PFC). In the instances in which the aggressive desire is deemed problematic, interventive control mechanisms may be initiated. As depicted in Figure 18.1, there are four time points during which aggressive desires may be deemed problematic: when anger is elicited, during rumination, when one becomes aware of approach motivational tendencies (e.g., increasingly getting in the face of someone during an argument), and when one considers the desire to aggress to violate personal or normative standards or goals.

It is worth noting that there may be times when it is not particularly problematic to experience an aggressive desire. These instances may be particularly likely in cases where people experience the desire to aggress to obtain a secondary outcome (e.g., legitimate self-defense, soldiers killing in the line of duty, sadists hurting for a thrill or pleasure, a bully coercing resources from others). In such cases, one would not expect any mechanisms for controlling desire to occur. Indeed, it seems unlikely that a conflict would even be registered in the brain or mind.

There are a number of additional reasons why people may not register aggressive desires as problematic. One reason is suggested by the neuroimaging data showing that in some cases, experiencing the desire to aggress may be rewarding (de Quervain et al., 2004; Krämer et al., 2007; see also Kringelbach & Berridge, Chapter 6, this volume). Depending on the circumstances, some people may actually enjoy thinking about exacting revenge following provocation or when ruminating. Moreover, people may believe that acting out aggressive desires will obviate or attenuate the aggressive desire. These so-called catharsis beliefs are widely held despite scientific evidence showing adverse effects of acting out aggressive catharsis (Bushman, Baumeister, & Phillips, 2001). In these cases, it is unlikely that people would consider acting aggressively to represent a conflict.

Perhaps the most obvious reason that people may not view the desire to aggress to be in conflict with one's self-regulatory goals or standards is caused by the anger itself. For example, people may feel "righteously angry." They may feel like it is their right to get even with their provocateur or teach him or her a lesson. Indeed, in cases of aggressive desires, anger induces a number of cognitive changes that seem to make it unlikely that a conflict will be registered. Next, we review three cognitive processes that may influence the desire to engage in aggression: associative network activation, selective attention, and depth of processing.

Associative Networks

A well-established finding is that priming with aggressive cues (e.g., weapons) increases aggressive behavior when one is provoked (Carlson, Marcus-Newhall, & Miller, 1990). Aggressive cues such as weapons and anger provocation are thought to activate associative networks in which concepts such as anger and aggression are intimately linked (Berkowitz, 1983, 1990). These associative networks for aggression are strengthened for people who are high in trait aggression (Bushman, 1995). For aggressive people, activation of these associative networks can lead to perceiving hostile intent where none exists. For example, participants high in trait aggression perceived stronger associations between aggressive words and ambiguous words that could be interpreted in an aggressive or nonaggressive way (e.g., *alley*). Thus, when provoked, the heightened accessibility of anger and aggression-related constructs is thought to bias downstream judgment and decision-making processes in ways that enhance aggressive desires (cf. Anderson & Bushman, 2002).

Selective Attention and Attentional Scope

Anger can influence what information is attended to and recalled in ways that could bias interpretation of events and enhance the desire to aggress. When angered, people may selectively attend to and process emotion-congruent information. For example, when angered, people are more persuaded by messages framed with anger rather than with sadness (DeSteno, Petty, Rucker, Wegner, & Braverman, 2004). Being angered also increases eye gaze toward reward stimuli over threat stimuli (Ford, Tamir, Gagnon, Taylor, & Brunyé, 2012). This finding is consistent with the approach motivational tendencies induced by anger as well as the neuroscience evidence linking vengeful desires to reward circuitry.

People high in trait levels of anger and aggressiveness show quick responses to hostile stimuli and find such stimuli difficult to ignore (for a review, see Wilkowski & Robinson, 2008). In one clever study that directly monitored eye gaze, Wilkowski, Robinson, Gordon, and Troop-Gordon (2007) presented people high and low in trait anger with scenes that could be interpreted as hostile or not (e.g., kicking a ball through a window). These ambiguous scenes contained hostile cues as well as non-hostile cues. Interestingly, participants high in trait anger seemed puzzled by the nonaggressive cues, likely because they were inconsistent with an automatic judgment of the scene as hostile. Indeed, they spent the majority of the time looking at these innocuous cues, relative to participants low in trait anger.

Another line of research suggests that when people experience desire and the accompanying approach motivation, their attention becomes narrower (Harmon-Jones, Gable, & Price, 2013). Within the context of anger, this attentional narrowing should theoretically facilitate revenge pursuit because abstract peaceful goals or irrelevant goals become less likely to enter consciousness. In this way, anger may induce "tunnel vision" that focuses on retribution and lowers the likelihood of reflective thought, which could lower aggressive desires. Forms of reflective thought that have been shown to reduce the desire for revenge include reappraisal processes, forgiveness, and taking mitigating information into account (Barlett, 2013; Barlett & Anderson, 2011; McCullough, 2008; McCullough, Kurzban, & Tabak, 2013).

Depth of Information Processing

Some evidence suggests that people process information less thoroughly when angered than when not angered. Indeed, angry people are more likely to engage in stereotyping (Bodenhausen, Sheppard, & Kramer, 1994) and to show prejudice, especially toward groups that induce anger (e.g., Arabs) (Dasgupta, DeSteno, Williams, & Hunsinger, 2009; DeSteno, Dasgupta, Bartlett, & Cajdric, 2004), and are less likely to perceive risk (Lerner & Tiedens, 2006). Two psychological dimensions of anger that may determine depth of processing are arousal and certainty. Intense anger is a high arousal emotion that facilitates approach motivation and impulsive action. Interestingly, high arousal may impair memory. For instance, high arousal emotions are more likely to induce false memories than low arousal emotions regardless of the valence of the mood (Corson & Verrier, 2007). Anger also involves appraisals of certainty (Lerner & Keltner, 2001). High certainty emotions such as anger tend to encourage less thorough information processing relative to low certainty emotions (Tiedens & Linton, 2001). Anger, however, does not always lead to shallow information processing. For example, angry people are less swayed by peripheral details and are therefore better able to differentiate between the quality of arguments relative to people in a neutral state (Moons & Mackie, 2007).

To summarize, anger increases the activation in an aggression-related semantic network, which is thought to bias judgment and decision making. Anger also increases processing of anger-relevant stimuli and narrows attention toward goal-relevant pursuits (e.g., exacting revenge). Moreover, anger also largely induces superficial information processing. Together, these three effects on cognition may lower the chances of detecting a self-regulatory conflict as well as bias behavior toward aggression.

Aggressive Desires as a Function of the Person and the Environment

There are no doubt individual differences and contextual determinants of the extent to which people experience intense and frequent desires to hurt others. However, to our knowledge, no research has systematically examined this question. Yet, if we infer the existence of aggressive desire from aggressive behavior, research does implicate certain individual differences. Although it is outside of the scope of this chapter to review all the person and contextual factors implicated in desiring vengeance, and their interactions, we briefly mention a few.

Person Factors

Most serious acts of violence are committed by men. However, when provoked, men and women may not differ in the extent to which they desire revenge. A meta-analysis of the effects of gender on aggression found that when unprovoked, men were more aggressive than women (Bettencourt & Miller, 1996; for consistent effects of gender in the real world, see Archer, 2004). However, provocation greatly reduced this gender difference. Similarly, a meta-analysis of aggression-relevant personality on aggression found that people high in trait aggressiveness were aggressive in laboratory experiments even when not provoked (Bettencourt, Talley, Benjamin, & Valentine, 2006). However, people high in trait anger, narcissism, impulsivity, and angry rumination were only aggressive when provoked. These results suggest that some people may experience "chronic" desires to aggress, whereas many other people only experience the desire to aggress when provoked. Those who are perhaps the most likely to experience the desire to aggress when angered are people high in personality traits associated with "getting even." This includes people likely to ruminate about taking revenge and people who strongly endorse the norm of negative reciprocity (e.g., Caprara, 1986; Denson et al., 2006). People who strongly endorse the norm of negative reciprocity believe that when harmed, they should return the harm in kind (Eisenberger et al., 2004).

Specific genes likely also play a role in the extent to which people are likely to experience aggressive desires. Indeed, twin studies suggest that genes account for approximately half of the variance in aggressiveness (Moffitt, 2005). Recently, molecular geneticists have identified specific genes related to aggression. One of these is the X-linked gene that codes for monoamine oxidase A (MAOA). MAOA is an enzyme that degrades serotonin (as well as norepinephrine and dopamine). Individuals with the low-expression allele (MAOA-L) are at risk for increased aggression and other antisocial behavior relative to individuals with the high-expression allele (MAOA-H), especially when abused as children (Kim-Cohen et al., 2006). Two recent behavioral experiments found that participants with the MAOA-L genotype are more aggressive than participants with the MAOA-H genotype, but only when provoked (McDermott, Tingley, Cowden, Frazzetto, & Johnson, 2009; Kuepper, Grant, Wielpuetz, & Hennig, 2013). There are a number of additional individual biological differences that may predispose people toward experiencing aggressive desires. These include testosterone and cortisol levels, low serotonin, and greater left prefrontal cortical asymmetry.

Cultural Factors

Aggression is a universal phenomenon. All humans are fundamentally equipped with the ability to behave aggressively if need be. However, the cultural environment determines which triggers tend to elicit a desire for vengeance. For instance, in 2005, a Danish newspaper published cartoons of the prophet Muhammad, which sparked outrage in many parts of the Muslim world. Because Islam prohibits depictions of Muhammad, many in the Muslim world viewed this as an insult to their honor. By contrast, many in the West considered the artist to be exercising the right of free speech that is afforded to everyone.

Consistent with this anecdote, research suggests that cultures may differ in the types of triggers that elicit aggressive desires. One cultural dimension that has attracted substantial attention has been so-called "cultures of honor" (Nisbett & Cohen, 1996). Such cultures are characterized by highly aggressive action when one's reputation is impugned. Examples of cultures of honor include areas of the southern and western United States, parts of the Middle East, criminal gangs, and cultures of hypermasculinity. In one often-cited study, Cohen, Nisbett, Bowdle, and Schwarz (1996) found that insulted undergraduate men from the South were more easily angered and showed increases in cortisol and testosterone relative to northern undergraduate men.

Leung and Cohen (2011) recently expanded their cultural typology to include face cultures and dignity cultures in addition to honor cultures. Face cultures are characterized by socially appropriate levels of respect that an individual can obtain from others. Dignity cultures are characterized by a culturally shared belief that, at least in principle, all people are created equal. Using multidimensional scaling, a recent study examined the latent structure of various acts of hostility in Pakistan (honor culture), Japan (face culture), the United States (dignity cultures), and Israel (a hybrid of honor and dignity cultures) (Severance et al., 2013). Results showed that all cultures considered threats to self-worth to be acts of hostility, suggesting that threatening one's self-worth may be a culturally universal trigger that elicits aggressive desires. Interestingly, only the two dignity cultures (the United States and Israel) considered infringements on one's personal resources to be acts of hostility. Presumably, such acts violate the underlying values of autonomy and fairness that are prevalent in dignity cultures. Although these data provide preliminary evidence, much more research is needed on which acts elicit aggressive desires both universally and within different cultures.

What Can People Do about Unwanted Desires to Aggress?

Using the preventive–interventive model of self-control as a guiding framework, this section describes preventive and interventive strategies that may be useful in preventing and regulating aggressive desires.

Preventing the Desire to Aggress: Preventive Strategies

Few forms of proactive/preventive self-control exist in the aggression domain. For instance, avoiding provocative people or alcohol intoxication (i.e., access restrictions), surrounding oneself with peace-loving peers, and limiting consumption of violent media should, in principle, reduce the likelihood of experiencing aggressive desires. However, in many instances these forms of preventive strategies may be impractical to implement for many people. By contrast, there are two social psychological strategies that may prove helpful in preventing aggressive desires: *implementation intentions* and *construal level mindset*. To our knowledge, neither has been tested in the context of aggression, but both should theoretically reduce aggressive desires, anger, and behavior.

Implementation intentions refer to *if–then* plans that people make in response to certain situations (for a review, see Gollwitzer, Gawrilow, & Oettingen, 2010). For example, within the aggression context, implementation intentions may include the following *if-then* contingency: "If people mistreat me, then I will take a deep breath and count to 10." Because implementation intentions become automatized behavioral responses to specific situations or mental states, no conscious desire should be elicited, and hence, there is no need to inhibit the desire to aggress. Although no study has examined the effect of implementation intentions on aggressive desires, affect, or behavior, the effect on other self-regulatory domains and emotions is in the medium-to-large range ($d = 0.65$) (Gollwitzer & Sheeran, 2006).

A second preventive strategy is derived from construal level theory (CLT; Trope & Liberman, 2010). This theory posits that the degree of abstractness versus concreteness with which people think about self-regulatory conflicts can enhance or impair self-control and reactive cognitive control, respectively (Chiou, Wu, & Chang, 2013; Fujita, Trope, Liberman, & Levin-Sagi, 2006; Fujita, Trope, & Liberman, 2010; Schmeichel & Vohs, 2009). Importantly, abstract and concrete mindsets can be primed in one domain and still affect self-control in other domains (Fujita et al., 2006). Thus, it may be possible to induce abstract thinking and hence reduce aggressive desires. No study has examined the effect of abstract mindset on aggressive desires or behavior; however, there is suggestive evidence. Thinking about why an anger-inducing autobiographical event occurred (i.e., an abstract mindset) reduced anger to a greater extent than thinking about the specific details of the event (i.e., a concrete mindset) (Kross, Ayduk, & Mischel, 2005).

Future research may examine the effectiveness of these strategies for reducing aggressive desires. Ideally, research could examine several levels of analysis. For instance, in conjunction with behavior (aggression) and self-report (anger and desire), neuroimaging paradigms could examine activation in the ACC as a neural marker of conflict detection and the initiation of control.

Regulating Aggressive Desires: Interventive Strategies

Despite the best-laid preventive measures, chances are everyone will experience the desire to aggress at some point. However, most people are capable of overriding this desire most of the time. This is a remarkable achievement. In fact, in many parts of the world, on a per capita basis, people are less likely to die by homicide or war than at any other time in human history (Pinker, 2011). Despite this positive trend, unfortunately, the harm invoked by acting out aggressive desires continues to be a pervasive problem for humanity. Fortunately, there are a number of strategies that can be effective in controlling aggressive desires. These include bolstering self-control capacity through training, by consuming glucose, by empathizing with the person who triggered the desire for revenge, by distracting oneself, and by reappraising provocations. We discuss each of these in turn.

Self-Control Training

Recent advances in the science of self-control have repeatedly shown that self-control can be likened to a muscle. This influential "strength model" of self-control has received strong support in over 100 experiments (Inzlicht & Schmeichel, 2012). According to the strength model, self-control capacity can be depleted in the short term, just as exerting a muscle fatigues it. However, the positive implication of this model is that by strengthening self-control through practice, people can improve self-controlled behavior. The idea is that because all acts of self-control rely on a common resource, practicing self-control in one domain will lead to improvements in others. Effective self-control training (SCT) exercises may include any of the following: using one's nondominant hand, practicing better posture, avoiding sweets, recording one's expenditures, and avoiding slang and swearing (Gailliot, Plant, Butz, & Baumeister, 2007; Muraven, 2010; Oaten & Cheng, 2006a, 2006b, 2007; Sultan, Joireman, & Sprott, 2012). All of these SCT manipulations require participants to monitor their ongoing behavior and override habitual responses. Doing so is an act of self-control. Engaging in SCT for 2 to 8 weeks enhances self-controlled behavior in a variety of domains including preventing smoking relapse, saving money, physical persistence, engagement in health-promoting behaviors, increased pain tolerance, and better performance on tests of cognitive functions (Hagger, Wood, Stiff, & Chatzisarantis, 2010).

Importantly, emerging research suggests that just 2 weeks of SCT can increase mastery over aggressive desires. In one experiment, undergraduates participated in a two-session study over 2 weeks (Finkel, DeWall, Slotter, Oaten, & Foshee, 2009). At the first session, participants were depleted of self-control capacity via a mentally demanding task. They subsequently completed a self-report measure of the likelihood that they would want to act aggressively toward their romantic partner if provoked. Participants were then randomly assigned to one of three conditions. In two of the conditions, participants practiced self-control by either using their nondominant hand for everyday tasks (e.g., using a computer mouse) or regulating habitual speech patterns (e.g., saying "yes" instead of "yeah"). In a third control group, participants did not practice self-regulation. At the conclusion of the 2 weeks, participants in both SCT conditions reported a decrease in aggressive desires toward their romantic partner, but as expected, there was no change in the control condition

A recent experiment from our laboratory confirmed the effectiveness of SCT for lowering anger and aggression when provoked (Denson, Capper, Oaten, Friese, & Schofield, 2011). At an initial laboratory session, undergraduates were randomly assigned to the SCT condition or the control condition. In the SCT condition, participants used their nondominant hand for everyday tasks for 2 weeks. The undergraduates in the control condition answered simple math problems during the 2-week interim. In the second laboratory session, participants were insulted (ostensibly by another participant). They reported how angry the provocation made them feel and were given the opportunity to harm the other participant by blasting them with painful noise blasts. Participants who completed 2 weeks of SCT reported significantly lower anger as a result of the provocation than those in the control condition. Moreover, SCT helped aggressive people resist the urge to behave aggressively, quite possibly via reduced desires to aggress. In sum, this study found that boosting self-control capacity can help people better control their desire to aggress.

Glucose Consumption

The strength model of self-control also suggests a second method of improving self-control capacity: consuming glucose (Gailliot & Baumeister, 2007). Glucose improves self-controlled behavior in a variety of domains, although the exact mechanism remains eagerly debated (e.g., Kurzban, 2010; Molden et al., 2012). Recent experimental work suggests that people behave less aggressively after consuming a glucose beverage relative to a placebo (DeWall, Deckman, Gailliot, & Bushman, 2011). Moreover, two experiments from our lab found that consuming glucose helped highly aggressive people behave less aggressively when provoked than consuming a placebo (Denson, von Hippel, Kemp, & Teo, 2010). For people low in trait aggressiveness, glucose had no effect on aggression.

The benefits of adequate glucose availability for lowering aggressive desires may extend to intimate partner violence. One study that followed 107 married couples for 21 days and assessed blood glucose levels and aggressive desires toward their spouse (Bushman, DeWall, Pond, & Hanus, 2014). On days when participants' glucose levels were relatively low, they exhibited stronger desires to aggress as measured by the number of pins stuck in a voodoo doll representing their spouse. Thus, having adequate glucose available in the bloodstream may lower aggressive desires.

Distraction

Perhaps the simplest means of reducing aggressive desires is through distraction, which involves changing the focus of one's thoughts to a neutral or positive topic. Because space in working memory is limited, thinking about something other than revenge takes cognitive "center stage" (Van Dillen & Koole, 2007; see also Andrade, May, Van Dillen, & Kavanagh, Chapter 1, this volume). By loading working memory and attentional capacity, distraction prevents (further) processing of the stimuli and events that elicit aggressive desires. That is, it is not possible to ruminate about revenge when one is distracted. However, to truly reduce the chance that the aggressive desire will recur at a later time, people may need to engage in some type of cognitive processing. Indeed, distraction is useful for reducing anger over the short term, but less so when one must interact with the provocateur at a later time (Fabiansson & Denson, 2012).

Empathy and Mitigating Information

Eisenberg, Eggum, and Di Giunta (2010) reviewed the literature on empathy-related responding, which includes empathy, sympathy, and responding to personal distress. The authors concluded that empathy-related responding can lower aggression. However, much of the intervention research has been conducted in schools with adolescents. Whether or not enhancing empathy can reduce aggressive desires in adults is less clear, but initial results are promising.

In one experiment with undergraduates, before being insulted, participants were informed that the provocateur had been struggling with a diagnosis of multiple sclerosis (Harmon-Jones, Vaughn-Scott, Mohr, Sigelman, & Harmon-Jones, 2004). In the high sympathy condition, participants were asked to imagine how the other person must feel. In the low sympathy condition, participants were asked to remain objective. The results showed that inducing sympathy reduced left prefrontal cortical asymmetry (i.e., an electrophysiological indicator of approach motivation) and hostile attitudes following an insult, but not self-reported anger. Another laboratory experiment found that providing undergraduates with mitigating information immediately after being insulted (e.g., "the reason I graded your essay the way I did was because I broke up with my boyfriend last night") lowered aggression. This effect was mediated by a reduction in the desire for revenge (Barlett & Anderson, 2011). It seems likely that empathy-related responding may have reduced the urge to aggress.

We note that enhancing empathy may be considered a preventive or interventive strategy or both. For instance, it is possible that boosting empathy prevents the occurrence of aggressive desires or helps people regulate aggressive desires when they emerge (or both). Regardless of whether empathy prevents the onset of or helps overcome aggressive desires, the outcomes seem to suggest a strong reduction in aggressive desires. Future research could examine mediating mechanisms.

Conclusion

Whether we like it or not, the desire to aggress is part of being human. Although many nonhuman animals display retaliatory aggression, humans are probably unique in that we consciously experience the motivation to aggress in the form of desire. In this chapter, we reviewed research suggesting how aggressive desires emerge and are maintained over time by angry rumination. We also reviewed evidence from social neuroscience suggesting that changes in reward processing, conflict detection, and approach motivation accompany aggressive desires. We also suggested that, in many circumstances, the cognitive consequences of anger itself may make it unlikely that people will detect a conflict between the desire to aggress and self-regulatory standards or goals. We investigated person and cultural factors that may make some people in some cultures more or less likely to experience the desire to aggress. We concluded with interventions that may prove fruitful in lowering aggressive desire and increasing peace for humanity. Indeed, although all humans have the cognitive architecture for experiencing the desire to hurt others, research shows that we need not be beholden to these desires.

ACKNOWLEDGMENTS

The writing of this chapter and the authors' research were supported by grants from the Australian Research Council's Discovery Projects funding scheme and a Discovery Early Career Researcher Award.

REFERENCES

Anderson, C. A., & Bushman, B. J. (2002). Human aggression. *Annual Review of Psychology, 53*, 27–51.

Archer, J. (2004). Sex differences in aggression in real-world settings: A meta-analytic review. *Review of General Psychology, 8*, 291.

Axelrod, R. (1984). *The evolution of cooperation*. New York: Basic Books.

Barlett, C. P. (2013). Excuses, excuses: A meta-analytic review of how mitigating information can change aggression and an exploration of moderating variables. *Aggressive Behavior, 39*, 472–481.

Barlett, C. P., & Anderson, C. A. (2011). Reappraising the situation and its impact on aggressive behavior. *Personality and Social Psychology Bulletin, 37*, 1564–1573.

Berkowitz, L. (1983). *Aggression: Its causes, consequences, and control.* New York: McGraw-Hill.

Berkowitz, L. (1990). On the formation and regulation of anger and aggression: A cognitive-neoassociationistic analysis. *American Psychologist, 45*, 494–503.

Bettencourt, B. A., & Miller, N. (1996). Gender differences in aggression as a function of provocation: A meta-analysis. *Psychological Bulletin, 119*, 422–447.

Bettencourt, B. A., Talley, A., Benjamin, A. J., & Valentine, J. (2006). Personality and aggressive behavior under provoking and neutral conditions: A meta-analytic review. *Psychological Bulletin, 132*, 751–777.

Bodenhausen, G. V., Sheppard, L. A., & Kramer, G. P. (1994). Negative affect and social judgment: The differential impact of anger and sadness. *European Journal of Social Psychology, 24*, 45–62.

Boehm, C. (1987). *Blood revenge: The enactment and management of revenge in Montenegro and other tribal societies.* Philadelphia: University of Pennsylvania Press.

Braver, T. S. (2012). The variable nature of cognitive control: A dual mechanisms framework. *Trends in Cognitive Sciences, 16*, 106–113.

Buckels, E. E., Jones, D. N., & Paulhus, D. L. (2013). Behavioral confirmation of everyday sadism. *Psychological Science, 24*, 2201–2209.

Bushman, B. J. (1995). The moderating role of trait aggressiveness in the effects of violent media on aggression. *Journal of Personality and Social Psychology, 69*, 950–960.

Bushman, B. J., Baumeister, R. F., & Phillips, C. M. (2001). Do people aggress to improve their mood? Catharsis beliefs, affect regulation opportunity, and aggressive responding. *Journal of Personality and Social Psychology, 81*, 17–32.

Bushman, B. J., Bonacci, A. M., Pedersen, W. C., Vasquez, E. A., & Miller, N. (2005). Chewing on it can chew you up: Effects of rumination on triggered displaced aggression. *Journal of Personality and Social Psychology, 88*, 969–983.

Bushman, B. J., DeWall, C. N., Pond, R. S., & Hanus, M. D. (2014). Low glucose relates to greater aggression in married couples. *Proceedings of the National Academy of Sciences, 11*, 6254–6257.

Bushman, B. J., & Gibson, B. (2011). Violent video games cause an increase in aggression long after the game has been turned off. *Social Psychological and Personality Science, 2*, 29–32.

Caprara, G. V. (1986). Indicators of aggression: The Dissipation-Rumination scale. *Personality and Individual Differences, 7*, 763–769.

Carlson, M., Marcus-Newhall, A., & Miller, N. (1990). Effects of situational aggression cues: A quantitative review. *Journal of Personality and Social Psychology, 58*, 622.

Carver, C. S., & Harmon-Jones, E. (2009). Anger is an approach-related affect: Evidence and implications. *Psychological Bulletin, 135*, 183–204.

Chiou, W. B., Wu, W. H., & Chang, M. H. (2013). Think abstractly, smoke less: A brief construal-level intervention can promote self-control, leading to reduced cigarette consumption among current smokers. *Addiction, 108*, 985–992.

Cohen, D., Nisbett, R. E., Bowdle, B. F., & Schwarz, N. (1996). Insult, aggression, and the southern culture of honor: An "experimental ethnography." *Journal of Personality and Social Psychology, 70*, 945.

Corson, Y., & Verrier, N. (2007). Emotions and false memories valence or arousal? *Psychological Science, 18*, 208–211.

Dasgupta, N., DeSteno, D., Williams, L. A., & Hunsinger, M. (2009). Fanning the flames of prejudice: The influence of specific incidental emotions on implicit prejudice. *Emotion, 9,* 585.

de Quervain, D. J.-F., Fischbacher, U., Treyer, V., Schellhammer, M., Schnyder, U., Buck, A., et al. (2004). The neural basis of altruistic punishment. *Science, 305*(5688), 1254–1258.

Denson, T. F. (2013). The multiple systems model of angry rumination. *Personality and Social Psychology Review, 17,* 103–123.

Denson, T. F., Capper, M. M., Oaten, M., Friese, M., & Schofield, T. P. (2011). Self-control training decreases aggression in response to provocation in aggressive individuals. *Journal of Research in Personality, 45,* 252–256.

Denson, T. F., Dobson-Stone, C., Ronay, R., von Hippel, W., & Schira, M. M. (2014). A functional polymorphism of the MAOA gene is associated with neural responses to induced anger control. *Journal of Cognitive Neuroscience, 26,* 1418–1427.

Denson, T. F., Pedersen, W. C., & Miller, N. (2006). The Displaced Aggression Questionnaire. *Journal of Personality and Social Psychology, 90,* 1032–1051.

Denson, T. F., Pedersen, W. C., Ronquillo, J., & Nandy, A. S. (2009). The angry brain: Neural correlates of anger, angry rumination, and aggressive personality. *Journal of Cognitive Neuroscience, 21,* 734–744.

Denson, T. F., Ronay, R., von Hippel W., & Schira, M. M. (2013). Risk for aggression: Endogenous testosterone and cortisol modulate neural responses to induced anger control. *Social Neuroscience, 8,* 165–177.

Denson, T. F., von Hippel, W., Kemp, R. I., & Teo, L. S. (2010). Glucose consumption decreases impulsive aggression in response to provocation in aggressive individuals. *Journal of Experimental Social Psychology, 46,* 1023–1028.

DeSteno, D., Dasgupta, N., Bartlett, M. Y., & Cajdric, A. (2004). Prejudice from thin air: The effect of emotion on automatic intergroup attitudes. *Psychological Science, 15,* 319–324.

DeSteno, D., Petty, R. E., Rucker, D. D., Wegener, D. T., & Braverman, J. (2004). Discrete emotions and persuasion: The role of emotion-induced expectancies. *Journal of Personality and Social Psychology, 86,* 43.

DeWall, C. N., Deckman, T., Gailliot, M. T., & Bushman, B. J. (2011). Sweetened blood cools hot tempers: Physiological self-control and aggression. *Aggressive Behavior, 37,* 73–80.

Eisenberg, N., Eggum, N. D., & Di Giunta, L. (2010). Empathy-related responding: Associations with prosocial behavior, aggression, and intergroup relations. *Social Issues and Policy Review, 4,* 143–180.

Eisenberger, R., Lynch, P., Aselage, J., & Rohdieck, S. (2004). Who takes the most revenge?: Individual differences in negative reciprocity norm endorsement. *Personality and Social Psychology Bulletin, 30,* 787–799.

Fabiansson, E. C., & Denson, T. F. (2012). The effects of intrapersonal anger and its regulation in economic bargaining. *PLoS One, 7,* e51595.

Fabiansson, E. C., Denson, T. F., Grisham, J. R., Moulds, M. L., & Schira, M. M. (2012). Don't look back in anger: Neural correlates of reappraisal, analytic rumination, and angry rumination during recall of an anger-inducing autobiographical memory. *NeuroImage, 59,* 2974–2981.

Finkel, E. J., DeWall, C. N., Slotter, E., Oaten, M. B., & Foshee, V. A. (2009). Self-regulatory failure and intimate partner violence perpetration. *Journal of Personality and Social Psychology, 97,* 483–499.

Ford, B. Q., Tamir, M., Gagnon, S. A., Taylor, H. A., & Brunyé, T. T. (2012). The angry spotlight: Trait anger and selective visual attention to rewards. *European Journal of Personality, 26*, 90–98.

Fujita, K., Trope, Y., & Liberman, N. (2010). Seeing the big picture: A construal level analysis of self-control. In R. R. Hassin, K. N. Ochsner, & Y. Trope (Eds.), *Self-control in society, mind, and brain* (pp. 408–427). Oxford, UK: Oxford University Press.

Fujita, K., Trope, Y., Liberman, N., & Levin-Sagi, M. (2006). Construal levels and self-control. *Journal of Personality and Social Psychology, 90*, 351–367.

Gailliot, M. T., & Baumeister, R. F. (2007). The physiology of willpower: Linking blood glucose to self-control. *Personality and Social Psychology Review, 11*, 303–327.

Gailliot, M. T., Plant, E. A., Butz, D. A., & Baumeister, R. F. (2007). Increasing self-regulatory strength can reduce the depleting effect of suppressing stereotypes. *Personality and Social Psychology Bulletin, 33*, 281–294.

Gasquoine, P. G. (2013). Localization of function in anterior cingulate cortex: From psychosurgery to functional neuroimaging. *Neuroscience and Biobehavioral Reviews, 37*, 340–348.

Gollwitzer, P. M., Gawrilow, C., & Oettingen, G. (2010). The power of planning: Self-control by effective goal-striving. In R. R. Hassin, K. N. Ochsner, & Y. Trope (Eds.), *Self-control in society, mind, and brain* (pp. 279–296). Oxford, UK: Oxford University Press.

Gollwitzer, P. M., & Sheeran, P. (2006). Implementation intentions and goal achievement: A meta-analysis of effects and processes. *Advances in Experimental Social Psychology, 38*, 69–119.

Hagger, M. S., & Chatzisarantis, N. L. D. (2013). The sweet taste of success: The presence of glucose in the oral cavity moderates the depletion of self-control resources. *Personality and Social Psychology Bulletin, 39*, 28–42.

Hagger, M. S., Wood, C., Stiff, C., & Chatzisarantis, N. L. (2010). Ego depletion and the strength model of self-control: A meta-analysis. *Psychological Bulletin, 136*, 495–525.

Harmon-Jones, E., Gable, P. A., & Price, T. F. (2013). Does negative affect always narrow and positive affect always broaden the mind?: Considering the influence of motivational intensity on cognitive scope. *Current Directions in Psychological Science, 22*, 301–307.

Harmon-Jones, E., Vaughn-Scott, K., Mohr, S., Sigelman, J., & Harmon-Jones, C. (2004). The effect of manipulated sympathy and anger on left and right frontal cortical activity. *Emotion, 4*, 95.

Heatherton, T. F., & Wagner, D. D. (2011). Cognitive neuroscience of self-regulation failure. *Trends in Cognitive Sciences, 15*, 132–139.

Hemphill, J. F., & Hart, S. D. (2002). Motivating the unmotivated: Psychopathy, treatment, and change. In M. McMurran (Ed.), *Motivating offenders to change: A guide to enhancing engagement in therapy* (pp. 193–219). Chichester, UK: Wiley.

Hofmann, W., & Kotabe, H. (2012). A general model of preventive and interventive self-control. *Social and Personality Psychology Compass, 6*, 707–722.

Hofmann, W., & Van Dillen, L. (2012). Desire: The new hot spot in self-control research. *Current Directions in Psychological Science, 21*, 317–322.

Inzlicht, M., & Schmeichel, B. J. (2012). What is ego depletion?: Toward a mechanistic revision of the resource model of self-control. *Psychological Science, 7*, 450–463.

Kelley, N. J., Hortensius, R., & Harmon-Jones, E. (2013). When anger leads to rumination: Induction of relative right frontal cortical activity with transcranial direct current stimulation increases anger-related rumination. *Psychological Science, 24,* 475–481.

Kim-Cohen, J., Caspi, A., Taylor, A., Williams, B., Newcombe, R., Craig, I. W., et al. (2006). MAOA, maltreatment, and gene–environment interaction predicting children's mental health: New evidence and a meta-analysis. *Molecular Psychiatry, 11,* 903–913.

Krämer, U. M., Jansma, H., Tempelmann, C., & Münte, T. F. (2007). Tit-for-tat: The neural basis of reactive aggression. *NeuroImage, 38,* 203–211.

Kringelbach, M. L. (2005). The human orbitofrontal cortex: linking reward to hedonic experience. *Nature Reviews Neuroscience, 6,* 691–702.

Kross, E., Ayduk, O., & Mischel, W. (2005). When asking "why" does not hurt: Distinguishing rumination from reflective processing of negative emotions. *Psychological Science, 16,* 709–715.

Kuepper, Y., Grant, P., Wielpuetz, C., & Hennig, J. (2013). MAOA-uVNTR genotype predicts interindividual differences in experimental aggressiveness as a function of the degree of provocation. *Behavioural Brain Research, 15,* 73–78.

Kurzban, R. (2010). Does the brain consume additional glucose during self-control tasks? *Evolutionary Psychology, 8,* 244–259.

Lerner, J. S., & Keltner, D. (2001). Fear, anger, and risk. *Journal of Personality and Social Psychology, 81,* 146.

Lerner, J. S., & Tiedens, L. Z. (2006). Portrait of the angry decision maker: How appraisal tendencies shape anger's influence on cognition. *Journal of Behavioral Decision Making, 19,* 115–137.

Leung, A. K.-Y., & Cohen, D. (2011). Within- and between-culture variation: Individual differences and the cultural logics of honor, face, and dignity cultures. *Journal of Personality and Social Psychology, 100,* 507.

McCullough, M. E. (2008). *Beyond revenge: The evolution of the forgiveness instinct.* San Francisco: Jossey-Bass.

McCullough, M. E., Kurzban, R., & Tabak, B. A. (2013). Cognitive systems for revenge and forgiveness. *Behavioral and Brain Sciences, 1,* 1–15.

McDermott, R., Tingley, D., Cowden, J., Frazzetto, G., & Johnson, D. D. (2009). Monoamine oxidase A gene (MAOA) predicts behavioral aggression following provocation. *Proceedings of the National Academy of Sciences, 106,* 2118–2123.

Moffitt, T. E. (2005). Genetic and environmental influences on antisocial behaviors: Evidence from behavioral–genetic research. *Advances in Genetics, 55,* 41–104.

Molden, D. C., Hui, C. M., Noreen, E. E., Meier, B. P., Scholer, A. A., D'Agostino, P. R., et al. (2012). The motivational versus metabolic effects of carbohydrates on self-control. *Psychological Science, 23,* 1130–1137.

Moons, W. G., & Mackie, D. M. (2007). Thinking straight while seeing red: The influence of anger on information processing. *Personality and Social Psychology Bulletin, 33,* 706–720.

Muraven, M. (2010). Practicing self-control lowers the risk of smoking lapse. *Psychology of Addictive Behaviors, 24,* 446–452.

Murphy, F. C., Nimmo-Smith, I., & Lawrence, A. D. (2003). Functional neuroanatomy of emotions: A meta-analysis. *Cognitive, Affective, and Behavioral Neuroscience, 3,* 207–233.

Nisbett, R. E., & Cohen, D. (1996). *Culture of honor: The psychology of violence in the South.* New York: Westview Press.

Oaten, M., & Cheng, K. (2006a). Improved self-control: The benefits of a regular program of academic study. *Basic and Applied Social Psychology, 28,* 1–16.

Oaten, M., & Cheng, K. (2006b). Longitudinal gains in self-regulation from regular physical exercise. *British Journal of Health Psychology, 11,* 717–733.

Oaten, M., & Cheng, K. (2007). Improvements in self-control from financial monitoring. *Journal of Economic Psychology, 28,* 487–501.

Pinker, S. (2011). *The better angels of our nature: Why violence has declined.* New York: Viking.

Schmeichel, B. J., & Vohs, K. (2009). Self-affirmation and self-control: Affirming core values counteracts ego depletion. *Journal of Personality and Social Psychology, 96,* 770.

Severance, L., Bui-Wrzosinska, L., Gelfand, M. J., Lyons, S., Nowak, A., Borkowski, W., et al. (2013). The psychological structure of aggression across cultures. *Journal of Organizational Behavior, 34,* 835–865.

Shenhav, A., Botvinick, M. M., & Cohen, J. D. (2013). The expected value of control: An integrative theory of anterior cingulate cortex function. *Neuron, 79,* 217–240.

Sukhodolsky, D. G., Golub, A., & Cromwell, E. N. (2001). Development and validation of the anger rumination scale. *Personality and Individual Differences, 31,* 689–700.

Sultan, A. J., Joireman, J., & Sprott, D. E. (2012). Building consumer self-control: The effect of self-control exercises on impulse buying urges. *Marketing Letters, 23,* 61–72.

Taylor, S. P. (1967). Aggressive behavior and physiological arousal as a function of provocation and the tendency to inhibit aggression. *Journal of Personality, 35,* 297–310.

Tiedens, L. Z., & Linton, S. (2001). Judgment under emotional certainty and uncertainty: The effects of specific emotions on information processing. *Journal of Personality and Social Psychology, 81,* 973.

Trope, Y., & Liberman, N. (2010). Construal-level theory of psychological distance. *Psychological Review, 117,* 440.

Van Dillen, L. F., & Koole, S. L. (2007). Clearing the mind: A working memory model of distraction from negative mood. *Emotion, 7,* 715.

Wilkowski, B. M., & Robinson, M. D. (2008). The cognitive basis of trait anger and reactive aggression: An integrative analysis. *Personality and Social Psychology Review, 12,* 3–21.

Wilkowski, B. M., Robinson, M. D., Gordon, R. D., & Troop-Gordon, W. (2007). Tracking the evil eye: Trait anger and selective attention within ambiguously hostile scenes. *Journal of Research in Personality, 41,* 650–666.

Zeki, S., & Romaya, J. P. (2008). Neural correlates of hate. *PLoS One, 3,* e3556.

CHAPTER 19

The Role of Desire and Craving in Addiction

Ingmar H. A. Franken

Human behavior is largely driven by motivational processes, which can be, in their most basic form, described as two action tendencies: avoidance and approach tendencies (Frijda, 1986; Gray, 1987). Painful or fearful stimuli are usually avoided, and pleasant stimuli are usually approached. The underlying mechanisms of approaching pleasant stimuli are highly relevant for understanding substance use behaviors. Typically, the use of alcohol and drugs results in pleasant feelings. In this way, these substances act as a reward. The perception of stimuli associated with these substances will, by means of Pavlovian conditioning, result in an altered motivational state. More specifically, this perception triggers the approach system. Human appetitive behavior can be explained by the interaction between internal states (e.g., hunger) and incentive stimuli (palatable food) (Toates, 1994). A felt heightened appetitive state can be called desire. Although there are several theories concerning the number of discernable desires, at least two kinds of desires are relevant for substance use (Davis, 1984). There is an emotional (see Goldie, 2002), first-order desire, which, in this case, reflects an appetitive state, for example, the desire to use a substance (mostly an acute state: "I crave a cigarette now"). And there is a volitive, second-order desire, which is synonymous with what we wish (mostly in the long run: "I wish I could stop smoking"). In substance use disorders (SUDs) these two desires are typically (but not necessarily) conflicting: "I have a desire to quit smoking but also a desire to smoke a cigarette right now." The appetitive desire is often felt, although some authors argue that it is not the desire itself that is felt but the feelings toward the imagined object of desire (Goldie, 2002). When desire or craving is mentioned in the remainder of this chapter, I refer to appetitive desire.

Appetite desires (i.e., cravings) play an indisputably important role in the use of psychoactive substances. For many decades the role of craving in addictive behaviors has been acknowledged. More than half a century ago there were already World Health Organization expert meetings on craving for alcohol ("The craving for alcohol," 1955). Although craving has been acknowledged in DSM-5 (American Psychiatric Association, 2013) as one of the criteria for an SUD, its role in SUDs has been debated in recent decades (Kozlowski & Wilkinson, 1987). Today, there seems to be some consensus that craving is relevant in explaining substance use behaviors and clinically relevant for treating SUDs (American Psychiatric Association, 2013; Franken, 2003; Tiffany & Wray, 2011).

Phenomenology

Many review papers have been written on the role of craving in addiction, yet there is little consensus about the exact definition of craving. Most definitions include the notion that craving is an "appetitive desire to take a substance." Desire is an important but often neglected emotion (see, e.g., Ekman, 1992). It reflects both a feeling and an intention regarding behavior (Frijda, 1986) and is accompanied, like other emotions, by bodily sensations. And as with other emotions, an exact and generally accepted definition is difficult to provide (what would be the definition of fear?). A few additional remarks can be made concerning this definition. The word *substance* in the definition above is used to include craving for food, which shares similar characteristics. Further, as indicated by Drummond (2001) and Singleton and Gorelick (1998), it is important to note that although the standard dictionary definition of craving only refers to a *strong* desire, these days most addiction researchers refer to craving as any kind of desire (strong or mild) that can be measured on a continuous scale.

Craving is an important sign of addiction, and is not only present in the "active" phase. Substance craving lasts for several years after the termination of substance use and may even last a lifetime (Hser, Hoffman, Grella, & Anglin, 2001). Stimuli in the environment associated with drug use are still able, by means of Pavlovian conditioning principles (see below), to trigger motivational circuits and elicit a high motivation to use these drugs—so-called cue-elicited craving (Franken, Booij, & Van den Brink, 2005)—which contributes to the continuation of drug use in active drug abusers and relapse in detoxified abusers.

Craving is present among users of all major categories of substances people can get addicted to: alcohol, heroin, cocaine, amphetamines, cannabis, and cigarettes (Carter & Tiffany, 1999). Craving plays an important role in continued substance use and is an important predictor of relapse during a period of abstinence. Many studies find an association between substance use, including relapse and craving (Ferguson & Shiffman, 2009; Tiffany & Wray, 2012), although it should be noted that some do not (Wray, Gass, & Tiffany, 2013).

Biological Factors

Although substance craving is clearly the result of environmental (conditioning) factors and not some kind of innate factor, genetic factors seem to play a role in the experience of craving. To put it another way, some people seem to develop more craving than other people under similar circumstances. Recent evidence from genetic studies shows that genetic variants can partly explain the experience of craving in substance users. In line with biological theories stressing the role of dopamine in craving (see below), there are several studies showing an association between craving and genes that encode dopamine receptors, particularly the dopamine D_4 receptor (e.g., Hutchison, McGeary, Smolen, Bryan, & Swift, 2002; Shao et al., 2006). Carriers of the DRD4 VNTR long type allele experience a stronger craving for alcohol and drugs than persons without this allele. Also relevant to craving are the genes encoding dopamine D_2 receptors (Agrawal et al., 2013; Li et al., 2006). Patients who are carriers of the DRD2 TaqI RFLP A1 allele experience stronger cravings for alcohol (Erblich, Lerman, Self, Diaz, & Bovbjerg, 2004) and heroin (Li et al., 2006) than persons without this allele. It must be noted that these research findings only provide an indication that dopamine receptor genes are involved in craving.

A recent large-scale study found a relation between DRD2 and DRD3 genes and alcohol craving only when using liberal thresholds (Agrawal et al., 2013). There are also some indications that genes encoding the dopamine transporter (DAT) are relevant for craving (Erblich, Lerman, Self, Diaz, & Bovbjerg, 2005; Li et al., 2006). Two studies of smokers showed that the DAT genotype modulates the brain response to craving-eliciting stimuli (Franklin et al., 2009, 2011). Besides dopamine-related genes, the G allele variant of the mu-opioid receptor (OPRM1) also seems to play a role in the experience of alcohol craving (van den Wildenberg et al., 2007). However, caution is needed when interpreting these studies, since a recent genome-wide association study exploring the role of a variety of genes in alcohol craving could not identify signals of genome-wide significance (Agrawal et al., 2013).

One of the most influential recent theories addressing the neural basis of drug craving is Robinson and Berridge's incentive sensitization theory (1993). One of the central aspects of this theory is the notion that in patients with SUD the desire (i.e., "wanting') for a substance does not necessarily run parallel with the hedonic component (i.e., "liking") (see also Kringelbach & Berridge, Chapter 6, this volume). Under normal circumstances these processes are parallel with each other (i.e., you like something you want), but patients with SUD experience strong feelings of wanting without liking the effects of substances anymore. The wanting (craving), whether or not consciously experienced, has taken over the behavior. Importantly, the systems of liking and wanting are hypothesized to have different neurobiological substrates. The liking system is based on the opioid system, which projects on the GABAergic neurons in the nucleus accumbens (Robinson & Berridge, 1993). The neurobiological substrate of the wanting system is the mesolimbic dopamine system. Craving is hypothesized to be associated with the release of dopamine in the nucleus accumbens. Although evidence for this notion is found in animal studies, studies in humans are largely lacking because it is difficult to measure dopamine release in humans. Studies using PET/SPECT scans provide some indication that craving is associated with enhanced dopamine release (Wong et al., 2006; Zijlstra, Booij, van den Brink, & Franken, 2008).

An alternative biological mechanism, which is not mutually exclusive with the account presented above, is the notion that low availability of striatal dopamine D_2 receptors is a vulnerability factor in the development of addictive behaviors (Nader et al., 2006). PET, SPECT, and postmortem studies performed in substance users show that striatal dopaminergic D_2 receptors are reduced (Kish et al., 2001; Volkow et al., 1993, 1997). Long-lasting reduction of DA receptors results in anhedonic feelings that may induce chronic craving (Heinz et al., 2005; Heinz, Schmidt, & Reischies, 1994). An explanation of these apparently contradictory findings—the fact that both enhanced dopamine release and reduced dopamine receptors are associated with craving—is provided by Pilla, Perachon, Sautel, Garrido, Mann, et al. (1999) and Childress and O'Brien (2000). They suggest that craving may be the result of two separate pathways. First, craving might be the result of higher tonic craving levels associated with reduced D_2 receptor densities in the striatum and orbitofrontal cortex (OFC), which results in a chronic anhedonic state. In this case, alcohol or drugs are used to stimulate the dopamine activity in an attempt to alleviate this chronic anhedonic state. Second, phasic increases in *cue-elicited* craving may result from enhanced dopaminergic activity in the reward system (e.g., nucleus accumbens).

Concerning the neuroanatomical substrates of craving, functional imaging studies in humans have repeatedly found that certain brain structures are associated with the subjective experience of craving. This neural network appears similar for all drugs of abuse (Lingford-Hughes et al., 2003). A recent meta-analysis showed that craving was positively correlated with brain activation in the visual cortex, anterior cingulate cortex (ACC), somatosensory cortex, fusiform gyrus, orbitofrontal cortex, ventral striatum (VS), motor cortex, and insula (Yalachkov, Kaiser, & Naumer, 2012). Interestingly, a recent study by Naqvi, Rudrauf, Damasio, and

Bechara (2007) shows a prominent role for the insula. This study demonstrated that smokers with a damaged insula, a region that integrates interoceptive (i.e., bodily) states into conscious feelings, are very likely to no longer experience conscious urges to smoke after quitting. Since other studies also find an association between self-reported craving and insula activation (Luijten et al., 2011) it seems an important to explore the clinical relevance of this finding (Naqvi, Gaznick, Tranel, & Bechara, 2014).

A prominent role for the nucleus accumbens has been reported in animal studies (Ikemoto & Panksepp, 1999). This central area of the dopaminergic reward system seems to be involved in both craving and other motivational aspects of drug use (Robbins & Everitt, 1996; Robinson & Berridge, 1993; Kringelbach & Berridge, Chapter 6, this volume; Lopez, Wagner, & Heatherton, Chapter 7, this volume). However, animal studies do not provide information on whether the nucleus accumbens is involved in experienced/felt craving or appetitive approach behaviors in general.

Psychological Factors

In terms of operant conditioning, craving can be regarded as the result of positive (motivation to feel good; Robinson & Berridge, 1993) and negative (motivation to escape from a negative state; Baker, Piper, McCarthy, Majeskie, & Fiore, 2004) reinforcement. Substance use can be explained by operant conditioning as the result of a drug's pleasant effect (e.g., the rush, euphoria). Typically, drug users want to experience these pleasant effects again (Thorndike's law of effect). In addition, a negative state—for example, stress (Sinha, 2013) or anhedonia (Hatzigiakoumis, Martinotti, Di Giannantonio, & Janiri, 2011)—can be relieved by drug use. Some authors even argue that based on these forms of operant conditioning, two kinds of cravings can be discerned: reward craving and relief craving (Verheul, Van den Brink, & Geerlings, 1999). However, this theoretical distinction is difficult to observe in daily life for patients with SUD (Ooteman, Koeter, Verheul, Schippers, & Van Den Brink, 2006). In addition, it can be questioned whether positive and negative reinforcement result in different subjective experiences of craving; the cause of craving might be the only difference. Although operant conditioning can explain substance use, it can't explain all aspects of craving adequately. For example, why does craving become stronger during the development of an addiction? In addition, sometimes craving is present even when it's not clear that the drug is having a pleasant effect, for example in cigarette smoking and in heroin/cocaine addicts who don't report pleasant effects of drug use anymore after prolonged use but do experience strong cravings. Further, both addicted and nonaddicted persons experience pleasurable effects from using drugs. Lastly, the experience of "sudden" cravings after a long period of abstinence can't be explained by operant conditioning alone.

Pavlovian or classical conditioning might better explain craving in these circumstances. Classical conditioning models explain craving as a conditioned response to a (conditioned) substance-related stimulus (e.g., seeing someone smoking a cigarette) (Childress, McLellan, & O'Brien, 1988; Niaura et al., 1988). This classically conditioned response consists of both a physiological (increased heart rate, sweating, etc.) and a subjective response. In classical conditioning models, craving is regarded as a subjective conditioned response of this type (Tiffany, 1995). Almost all contemporary theories of craving, both biological and psychological, incorporate the idea that the desire for substances is (at least partly) based on classical conditioning. Despite the omnipresence of classical conditioning when it comes to describing the mechanisms of craving and relapse, the therapeutic use of classical conditioning principles (i.e., extinction by cue exposure therapy) in patients with SUD have been rather disappointing so far (Conklin & Tiffany, 2002; Marissen, Franken, Blanken, van den Brink, & Hendriks, 2007).

Cognitive models of craving can be broadly classified into two categories: association models (including expectancy models) and information-processing models. In association models, craving is explained by the expectations of the drug user. Craving is the result of a positive outcome expectancy (e.g., "I will feel great if I take cocaine"), the value which is attributed to this outcome ("feeling great is important") and the experienced possibilities for alternatives ("I can only feel great by using cocaine") (Marlatt, 1985). Recent studies have shown that these drug-related associations can also be present at an implicit level even when there is a negative association on an explicit level (Wiers et al., 2002). In information-processing models (e.g., Franken, 2003) craving is explained partly as the result (and sometimes consequence) of attentional bias (see Figure 19.1). It is known that substance users have a higher level of attention for drug-related stimuli. Attentional bias can be defined as the automatic tendency of patients with SUD to focus their attention predominantly on drugs or drug-related stimuli. This attentional bias is theoretically associated with craving. A heightened motivational state for alcohol or drugs makes the signaling of relevant stimuli easier (i.e., craving results in attentional bias), but vice versa, attentional bias can also result in craving (see also Roefs, Houben, & Werthmann, Chapter 16, this volume). If drug-related cues are signaled more easily, the patient with SUD will be confronted with more stimuli (and probably longer in duration), resulting in more craving. Further, because attention is capacity-limited, persons with high attentional bias will have less attention for other relevant information, such as how to cope with craving (e.g., in treatment). This will also facilitate craving (Franken, 2003). A meta-analysis shows that attentional bias and craving are indeed related phenomena, although the relationship is

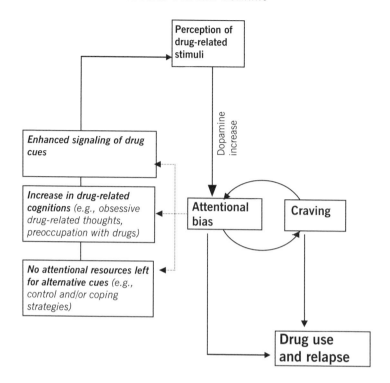

FIGURE 19.1. Attentional bias model. From Franken (2003). Copyright 2003 by Elsevier. Reprinted by permission.

generally modest (Field, Munafo, & Franken, 2009). More direct measures of attention, such as eye tracking, show stronger associations between attentional bias and craving.

Measurement of Craving

One of the major discussions in the scientific literature is about how craving can be measured (Rosenberg, 2009). In general, a distinction can be made between more direct measures, such as self-reported craving, and more distant proxy measures of craving, such as physiological measures. Both have their own advantages and disadvantages and will be discussed in more detail below. Some authors also regard cognitive measures, such as attentional bias and other implicit measures, as proxy measures of craving. However, since these measures primarily measure craving-related cognitive constructs, they will not be discussed here. For a more detailed discussion of craving measurement, see Sayette and Wilson (Chapter 5, this volume).

Self-Report Measures

Since craving is a subjective motivational state, the most obvious choice for measuring it is self-report. Like most emotions and other psychological constructs, craving is not a dichotomous phenomenon but can preferably be measured on a continuous scale. All current craving assessments based on self-report measures do indeed use continuous or interval scales (Rosenberg, 2009). These scales vary from single-item Likert scales (Drobes, Meier, & Tiffany, 1994), to single-item visual analogue scales (Tiffany & Hakenewerth, 1991), to multi-item craving questionnaires (Tiffany & Drobes, 1991), to questionnaires in which craving is a subscale (Anton, Moak, & Latham, 1996). Several authors (Schuster, Greenwald, Johanson, & Heishman, 1995; Tiffany, 1990) stress the fact that multi-item questionnaires are preferred because single-item measures do not capture the broad construct of craving. Another important aspect of the measurement of craving is the time dimension. Craving can be measured both as a more general trait that is more or less continuously present (e.g., craving within the last week/month) or that is the result of a temporary state highly dependent on cue reactivity (e.g., at this moment). There are several questionnaires that capture both components (see, e.g., Nijs, Franken, & Muris, 2007), but most questionnaires capture only one component. For measuring craving during cue reactivity, state measures such as the Desires for Alcohol Questionnaire/Desires for Drug Questionnaire (DAQ/DDQ; Franken, Hendriks, & Van den Brink, 2002; Love, James, & Willner, 1998; Tiffany & Drobes, 1991) are preferred, since they measure craving "now." Arguably, for treatment evaluation purposes, craving "trait" measures (e.g., the OCDS and the OCDUS), are more suitable than craving state measures (e.g., DAQ and DDQ; Anton et al., 1996; Franken et al., 2002).

A relatively new method for investigating craving in a nonlab situation is the ecological momentary assessment (EMA) (see also Hofmann, Kotabe, Vohs, & Baumeister, Chapter 3, this volume; Lopez, Wagner, & Heatherton, Chapter 7, this volume). In EMA studies craving is assessed in the daily life of patients with SUD, typically at several moments during the day (Shiffman et al., 1997). This way craving can be related to activities, cognitions, or feelings in daily life, improving the ecological validity of the measurements (Marhe, Waters, van de Wetering, & Franken, 2013c). Arguably, EMA studies that measure craving might be better predictors of relapse than the typical laboratory studies (see also Sayette & Wilson, Chapter 5, this volume).

Physiological Measures

Although self-report scales provide essential information about subjective emotional or motivational states, they have their limitations, particularly when internal states reflect some kind of taboo. For most people desires are not something that need to be shared with other people (e.g., sexual desires or food cravings). This is particularly true for desires in relation to alcohol and (illicit) drugs, which are influenced by social desirability (Marissen, Franken, Hendriks, & van den Brink, 2005). Therefore, objective measures of motivational state regarding substances can complement the subjective reports. Several physiological measures have been proposed and studied: autonomic measures (Carter & Tiffany, 1999), EEG measures (Littel, Euser, Munafo, & Franken, 2012), and fMRI measures (Hommer, 1999). Although each of these measurements has its own advantages and disadvantages, the general consensus is that their objective results can provide useful information about desires that is not captured by self-report (Marhe, Luijten, & Franken, 2014).

Clinical Implications

There are dozens of studies showing that craving is a predictor of relapse after or during substance use treatment (e.g., Ferguson & Shiffman, 2009; Hartz, Frederick-Osborne, & Galloway, 2001; Soyka, Helten, & Schmidt, 2010; Wray et al., 2013). These studies make it clear that cravings are a potential treatment focus. At the moment there are several treatments that target the reduction of craving. The first is cognitive-behavioral therapy (CBT). An important element of CBT is relapse prevention (Beck, Wright, Newman, & Liese, 1993; Marlatt, 1985), in which craving is typically seen as one of the antecedents of relapse (Barry & Petry, 2009; Larimer, Palmer, & Marlatt, 1999). A typical CBT approach is to teach patients in advance to recognize craving. After that patients are taught how to cope with craving and how to avoid conditioned cues. Another important element of relapse prevention is teaching patients to anticipate and accept the craving reaction as a "normal" conditioned response to a stimulus (Larimer et al., 1999). Relapse prevention in general is an effective method for treating SUDs, particularly alcohol use problems (Irvin, Bowers, Dunn, & Wang, 1999). A second effective approach is a pharmacological approach. In the past decade two pharmacological agents have received considerable attention in clinical trials: acamprosate and naltrexone. Acamprosate is the most prescribed medication for alcohol dependence in the United States. Although the exact mechanism is unknown, it probably attenuates the hyperglutamatergic state that is present during abstinence, possibly by influencing plasma calcium levels (Spanagel et al., 2014). Naltrexone is a nonspecific opioid antagonist and is effective in reducing relapse rates in patients with alcohol use disorder. Both acamprosate and naltrexone have been found to be effective in reducing craving, particularly in alcohol-dependent patients (Maisel, Blodgett, Wilbourne, Humphreys, & Finney, 2013).

More recently, other agents such as baclofen and topiramate have been considered as treatments for reducing alcohol and drug craving. However, so far clinical trials of these drugs have yielded mixed findings, and further research is needed in this area. For smokers varenicline (Tonstad et al., 2006) is an effective agent for treating nicotine addiction. Varenicline is a nicotine receptor partial agonist and reduces both craving and the pleasurable effects of smoking. There are some more experimental options for reducing craving that use direct or indirect neuromodulation. Modulation using surgical techniques (i.e., deep brain stimulation of reward-related brain areas) could have positive effects by normalizing craving levels in alcohol-dependent patients (Kuhn et al., 2011). Nonsurgical stimulation of brain regions in patients with SUD is generally done by transcranial magnetic stimulation (TMS) or transcranial direct current stimulation (tDCS). TMS stimulates or disrupts the neural activity in specific cortical regions and consequently induce changes in the cortical excitability of these areas (Feil & Zangen, 2010); tDCS modulates cortical excitability by altering the neuronal resting membrane potential. These new neuromodulation techniques might be effective in reducing craving in patients with SUD (Feil & Zangen, 2010; Li et al., 2013). Lastly, neurofeedback using EEG or fMRI methodology also seems to be effective in reducing craving (Dehghani-Arani, Rostami, & Nadali, 2013; Li et al., 2013), although more studies are needed in this area.

Conclusions

Although the exact role of craving in addiction behaviors is still unclear, recent studies show that the desire for alcohol and drugs (i.e., craving) is an important aspect of SUDs and related phenomena such as relapse. This is also reflected in the recent addition of craving as one of the criteria for an SUD in DSM-5 (American Psychiatric Association, 2013). Although this inclusion is important, there are many issues that still remain to be addressed in future studies. For example, the striking heterogeneity of the group of persons diagnosed with SUD is hampering further advances in this field. Only 2 out of 11 criteria have to be met for a diagnosis of SUD, resulting in 2,036 different subtypes. Nevertheless, in current treatment practice there is only one diagnosis and a "one-treatment-fits-all" approach (Ozomaro, Wahlestedt, & Nemeroff, 2013). Therefore, specific interventions for subtypes of patients, for example, those with high craving levels, might be another way to improve substance use treatment outcomes.

Another exiting area is the measurement of craving in the natural daily life environment of patients using EMA techniques (Sayette & Wilson, Chapter 5, this volume). Instead of measuring craving in sterile laboratory situations, electronic devices such as PDAs or smartphones can be employed to enhance the ecological validity of craving research (Epstein et al., 2009; Preston et al., 2009; Shiffman, 2009; Waters, Marhe, & Franken, 2012). This is important, since it is known that craving is highly dependent on situational and environmental factors. EMA techniques can also be used in treatment settings by providing "online" relapse prevention techniques (Waters et al., 2012).

Also of particular interest is the relation between craving and neurocognitive markers (e.g., neural indices of attentional bias or inhibitory control) of SUDs that are partly related to craving but also explain additional variance in treatment outcome (Marhe, Luijten, van de Wetering, Smits, & Franken, 2013a; Marhe, van de Wetering, & Franken, 2013b; Marhe et al., 2013c). The interaction between these neurocognitive measures and craving might reveal novel information about the mechanisms of craving, as well as new starting points for craving interventions (e.g., by neuromodulation).

Finally, the development of the Research Domain Criteria (RDoC) initiative by the National Institute of Mental Health has potential repercussions for craving research. The RDoC is an alternative classification system for mental disorders based on neurobiological dimensions and observable behavior (Cuthbert & Insel, 2013), and it has different levels. Craving, measured on the level of self-report (and labeled "approach motivation"), could fit perfectly as a dimension of this system relevant to addictive behaviors. In order to move toward the RDoC approach, it seems important to get some consensus on standardizing ways of measuring craving.

As new knowledge is gained almost every day about the neurobiology of craving and the relation between craving and neurocognitive phenomena, the time when we can apply this knowledge in clinical practice is coming closer (Franken & van de Wetering, 2015).

REFERENCES

Agrawal, A., Wetherill, L., Bucholz, K. K., Kramer, J., Kuperman, S., Lynskey, M. T., et al. (2013). Genetic influences on craving for alcohol. *Addictive Behavior, 38*(2), 1501–1508.

American Psychiatric Association. (2013). *Diagnostic and statistical manual of mental disorders* (5th ed.). Arlington, VA: Author.

Anton, R. F., Moak, D. H., & Latham, P. K. (1996). The obsessive compulsive drinking scale: A new method of assessing outcome in alcoholism treatment studies. *Archives of General Psychiatry, 53*(3), 225–231.

Baker, T. B., Piper, M. E., McCarthy, D. E., Majeskie, M. R., & Fiore, M. C. (2004). Addiction motivation reformulated: An affective processing model of negative reinforcement. *Psychological Review, 111*(1), 33–51.

Barry, D., & Petry, N. M. (2009). Cognitive behavioral treatments for substance use disorders. In P. M. Miller (Ed.), *Evidence-based addiction tyreatment* (pp. 157–174). San Diego, CA: Academic Press.

Beck, A. T., Wright, F. D., Newman, C. F., & Liese, B. S. (1993). *Cognitive therapy of substance abuse.* New York: Guilford Press.

Carter, B. L., & Tiffany, S. T. (1999). Meta-analysis of cue reactivity in addiction research. *Addiction, 94*(3), 327–340.

Childress, A. R., McLellan, A. T., & O'Brien, C. P. (1988). Classically conditioned responses in opioid and cocaine dependence: A role in relapse? *NIDA Research Monograph, 84,* 25–43.

Childress, A. R., & O'Brien, C. P. (2000). Dopamine receptor partial agonists could address the duality of cocaine craving. *Trends in Pharmacological Sciences, 21*(1), 6–9.

Conklin, C. A., & Tiffany, S. T. (2002). Applying extinction research and theory to cue-exposure addiction treatments. *Addiction, 97*(2), 155–167.

The craving for alcohol: A symposium by members of the WHO expert committee on mental health and on alcohol. (1955). *Quarterly Journal of Studies in Alcohol, 16*(1), 34–66.

Cuthbert, B. N., & Insel, T. R. (2013). Toward the future of psychiatric diagnosis: The seven pillars of RDoC. *BMC Medicine, 11,* 126.

Davis, W. A. (1984). The two senses of desire. *Philosophical Studies, 45,* 181–195.

Dehghani-Arani, F., Rostami, R., & Nadali, H. (2013). Neurofeedback training for opiate addiction: Improvement of mental health and craving. *Applied Psychophysiology Biofeedback, 38*(2), 133–141.

Drobes, D. J., Meier, E. A., & Tiffany, S. T. (1994). Assessment of the effects of urges and negative affect on smokers' coping skills. *Behaviour Research and Therapy, 32*(1), 165–174.

Drummond, D. C. (2001). Theories of drug craving, ancient and modern. *Addiction, 96,* 33–46.

Ekman, P. (1992). An argument for basic emotions. *Cognition and Emotion, 6,* 169–200.

Epstein, D. H., Willner-Reid, J., Vahabzadeh, M., Mezghanni, M., Lin, J. L., & Preston, K. L. (2009). Real-time electronic diary reports of cue exposure and mood in the hours before cocaine and heroin craving and use. *Archives of General Psychiatry, 66*(1), 88–94.

Erblich, J., Lerman, C., Self, D. W., Diaz, G. A., & Bovbjerg, D. H. (2004). Stress-induced cigarette craving: Effects of the DRD2 TaqI RFLP and SLC6A3 VNTR polymorphisms. *Pharmacogenomics Journal, 4*(2), 102–109.

Erblich, J., Lerman, C., Self, D. W., Diaz, G. A., & Bovbjerg, D. H. (2005). Effects of dopamine D2 receptor (DRD2) and transporter (SLC6A3) polymorphisms on smoking cue-induced cigarette craving among African-American smokers. *Molecular Psychiatry, 10*(4), 407–414.

Feil, J., & Zangen, A. (2010). Brain stimulation in the study and treatment of addiction. *Neuroscience and Biobehavioral Reviews, 34*(4), 559–574.

Ferguson, S. G., & Shiffman, S. (2009). The relevance and treatment of cue-induced cravings in tobacco dependence. *Journal of Substance Abuse Treatment, 36*(3), 235–243.

Field, M., Munafo, M. R., & Franken, I. H. A. (2009). A meta-analytic investigation of the relationship between attentional bias and subjective craving in substance abuse. *Psychological Bulletin, 135*(4), 589–607.

Franken, I. H. A. (2003). Drug craving and addiction: Integrating psychological and neuropsychopharmacological approaches. *Progress in Neuro-Psychopharmacology and Biological Psychiatry, 27*(4), 563–579.

Franken, I. H. A., Booij, J., & Van den Brink, W. (2005). The role of dopamine in human addiction: From reward to motivated attention. *European Journal of Pharmacology, 526*, 199–206.

Franken, I. H. A., Hendriks, V. M., & Van den Brink, W. (2002). Initial validation of two opiate craving questionnaires: The Obsessive Compulsive Drug Use Scale (OCDUS) and the Desires for Drug Questionnaire (DDQ). *Addictive Behaviors, 27*(5), 675–685.

Franklin, T. R., Lohoff, F. W., Wang, Z., Sciortino, N., Harper, D., Li, Y., et al. (2009). DAT genotype modulates brain and behavioral responses elicited by cigarette cues. *Neuropsychopharmacology, 34*(3), 717–728.

Franken, I. H. A., & van de Wetering, B. J. (2015). Bridging the gap between the neurocognitive lab and the addiction clinic. *Addictive Behaviors, 44*, 108–114.

Franklin, T. R., Wang, Z., Li, Y., Suh, J. J., Goldman, M., Lohoff, F. W., et al. (2011). Dopamine transporter genotype modulation of neural responses to smoking cues: Confirmation in a new cohort. *Addiction Biology, 16*(2), 308–322.

Frijda, N. H. (1986). *The emotions.* Cambridge, UK: Cambridge University Press.

Goldie, P. (2002). *The emotions: A philosophical exploration.* Oxford, UK: Oxford University Press.

Gray, J. A. (1987). *The psychology of fear and stress.* Cambridge, UK: Cambridge University Press.

Hartz, D. T., Frederick-Osborne, L., & Galloway, G. P. (2001). Craving predicts use during treatment for methamphetamine dependence: A prospective, repeated-measures, within-subject analysis. *Drug and Alcohol Dependence, 63*, 269–276.

Hatzigiakoumis, D. S., Martinotti, G., Di Giannantonio, M., & Janiri, L. (2011). Anhedonia and substance dependence: Clinical correlates and treatment options. *Frontiers in Psychiatry, 2*, 10.

Heinz, A., Reimold, M., Wrase, J., Hermann, D., Croissant, B., Mundle, G., et al. (2005). Correlation of stable elevations in striatal (micro)-opioid receptor availability in detoxified alcoholic patients with alcohol craving: A Positron Emission Tomography study using carbon 11-labeled carfentanil. *Archives of General Psychiatry, 62*(1), 57–64.

Heinz, A., Schmidt, L. G., & Reischies, F. M. (1994). Anhedonia in schizophrenic, depressed, or alcohol-dependent patients: Neurobiological correlates. *Pharmacopsychiatry, 27*(Suppl. 1), 7–10.

Hommer, D. W. (1999). Functional imaging of craving. *Alcohol Research and Health, 23*(3), 187–196.

Hser, Y. I., Hoffman, V., Grella, C. E., & Anglin, M. D. (2001). A 33-year follow-up of narcotics addicts. *Archives of General Psychiatry, 58*, 503–508.

Hutchison, K. E., McGeary, J., Smolen, A., Bryan, A., & Swift, R. M. (2002). The DRD4 VNTR polymorphism moderates craving after alcohol consumption. *Health Psychology, 21*(2), 139–146.

Ikemoto, S., & Panksepp, J. (1999). The role of nucleus accumbens dopamine in motivated behavior: A unifying interpretation with special reference to reward-seeking. *Brain Research Reviews, 31*(1), 6–41.

Irvin, J. E., Bowers, C. A., Dunn, M. E., & Wang, M. C. (1999). Efficacy of relapse prevention: a meta-analytic review. *Journal of Consulting and Clinical Psychology, 67*(4), 563–570.

Kish, S. J., Kalasinsky, K. S., Derkach, P., Schmunk, G. A., Guttman, M., Ang, L., et al. (2001). Striatal dopaminergic and serotonergic markers in human heroin users. *Neuropsychopharmacology, 24*(5), 561–567.

Kozlowski, L. T., & Wilkinson, D. A. (1987). Use and misuse of the concept of craving by alcohol, tobacco, and drug researchers. *British Journal of Addiction, 82*(1), 31–36.

Kuhn, J., Grundler, T. O., Bauer, R., Huff, W., Fischer, A. G., Lenartz, D., et al. (2011). Successful deep brain stimulation of the nucleus accumbens in severe alcohol dependence is associated with changed performance monitoring. *Addiction Biology, 16*(4), 620–623.

Larimer, M. E., Palmer, R. S., & Marlatt, G. A. (1999). Relapse prevention. An overview of Marlatt's cognitive-behavioral model. *Alcohol Research and Health, 23*(2), 151–160.

Li, X., Hartwell, K. J., Borckardt, J., Prisciandaro, J. J., Saladin, M. E., Morgan, P. S., et al. (2013). Volitional reduction of anterior cingulate cortex activity produces decreased cue craving in smoking cessation: A preliminary real-time fMRI study. *Addiction Biology, 18*(4), 739–748.

Li, Y., Shao, C., Zhang, D., Zhao, M., Lin, L., Yan, P., et al. (2006). The effect of dopamine D_2, D_5 receptor and transporter (SLC6A3) polymorphisms on the cue-elicited heroin craving in Chinese. *American Journal of Medical Genetics Part B: Neuropsychiatric Genetics, 141*(3), 269–273.

Lingford-Hughes, A. R., Davies, S. J., McIver, S., Williams, T. M., Daglish, M. R., & Nutt, D. J. (2003). *Addiction British Medical Bulletin, 65*, 209–222.

Littel, M., Euser, A. S., Munafo, M. R., & Franken, I. H. A. (2012). Electrophysiological indices of biased cognitive processing of substance-related cues: A meta-analysis. *Neuroscience and Biobehavioral Reviews, 36*(8), 1803–1816.

Love, A., James, D., & Willner, P. (1998). A comparison of two alcohol craving questionnaires. *Addiction, 93*(7), 1091–1102.

Luijten, M., Veltman, D. J., van den Brink, W., Hester, R., Field, M., Smits, M., et al. (2011). Neurobiological substrate of smoking-related attentional bias. *NeuroImage, 54*(3), 2374–2381.

Maisel, N. C., Blodgett, J. C., Wilbourne, P. L., Humphreys, K., & Finney, J. W. (2013). Meta-analysis of naltrexone and acamprosate for treating alcohol use disorders: when are these medications most helpful? *Addiction, 108*(2), 275–293.

Marhe, R., Luijten, M., & Franken, I. H. A. (2014). The clinical relevance of neurocognitive measures in addiction. *Frontiers in Psychiatry, 4*.

Marhe, R., Luijten, M., van de Wetering, B. J., Smits, M., & Franken, I. H. A. (2013). Individual differences in anterior cingulate activation associated with attentional bias predict cocaine use after treatment. *Neuropsychopharmacology, 38*(6), 1085–1093.

Marhe, R., van de Wetering, B. J. M., & Franken, I. H. A. (2013). Error-related brain activity predicts cocaine use after treatment at 3-month follow-up. *Biological Psychiatry, 73*(8), 782–788.

Marhe, R., Waters, A. J., van de Wetering, B. J. M., & Franken, I. H. A. (2013). Implicit and explicit drug-related cognitions during detoxification treatment are associated with drug relapse: An ecological momentary assessment study. *Journal of Consulting and Clinical Psychology, 81*(1), 1–12.

Marissen, M., Franken, I. H. A., Hendriks, V. M., & van den Brink, W. (2005). The relation between social desirability and different measures of heroin craving. *Journal of Addictive Diseases, 24*(4), 91–103.

Marissen, M. A. E., Franken, I. H. A., Blanken, P., van den Brink, W., & Hendriks, V. M. (2007). Cue exposure therapy for the treatment of opiate addiction: Results of a randomized controlled clinical trial. *Psychotherapy and Psychosomatics, 76*(2), 97–105.

Marlatt, G. A. (1985). Relapse prevention: Theoretical rationale and overview of the model. In G. A. Marlatt & J. R. Gordon (Eds.), *Relapse prevention: Maintenance strategies in the treatment of addictive behaviors* (pp. 3–70). New York: Guilford Press.

Nader, M. A., Morgan, D., Gage, H. D., Nader, S. H., Calhoun, T. L., Buchheimer, N., et al. (2006). PET imaging of dopamine D2 receptors during chronic cocaine self-administration in monkeys. *Journal of Neuroscience, 9*(8), 1050–1056.

Naqvi, N. H., Gaznick, N., Tranel, D., & Bechara, A. (2014). The insula: A critical neural substrate for craving and drug seeking under conflict and risk. *Annals of the New York Academy of Sciences, 1316*, 53–70.

Naqvi, N. H., Rudrauf, D., Damasio, H., & Bechara, A. (2007). Damage to the insula disrupts addiction to cigarette smoking. *Science, 315*(5811), 531–534.

Niaura, R. S., Rohsenow, D. J., Binkhoff, J. A., Monti, P. M., Pedraza, M., & Abrams, D. B. (1988). Relevance of cue reactivity to understanding of alcohol and smoking relapse. *Journal of Abnormal Psychology, 97*, 133–152.

Nijs, I. M. T., Franken, I. H. A., & Muris, P. (2007). The modified Trait and State Food-Cravings Questionnaires: Development and validation of a general index of food craving. *Appetite, 49*, 38–46.

Ooteman, W., Koeter, M., Verheul, R., Schippers, G., & Van Den Brink, W. I. M. (2006). Development and validation of the Amsterdam Motives for Drinking Scale (AMDS): An attempt to distinguish relief and reward drinkers. *Alcohol and Alcoholism, 41*(3), 284–292.

Pilla, M., Perachon, S., Sautel, F., Garrido, F., Mann, A., Wermuth, C. G., et al. (1999). Selective inhibition of cocaine-seeking behaviour by a partial dopamine D-3 receptor agonist. *Nature, 400*(6742), 371–375.

Preston, K. L., Vahabzadeh, M., Schmittner, J., Lin, J. L., Gorelick, D. A., & Epstein, D. H. (2009). Cocaine craving and use during daily life. *Psychopharmacology, 207*(2), 291–301.

Robbins, T. W., & Everitt, B. J. (1996). Neurobehavioural mechanisms of reward and motivation. *Current Opinion in Neurobiology, 6*(2), 228–236.

Robinson, T. E., & Berridge, K. C. (1993). The neural basis of drug craving: An incentive-sensitization theory of addiction. *Brain Research Reviews, 18*(3), 247–291.

Rosenberg, H. (2009). Clinical and laboratory assessment of the subjective experience of drug craving. *Clinical Psychology Review, 29*(6), 519–534.

Schuster, C. R., Greenwald, M. K., Johanson, C.-E., & Heishman, S. J. (1995). Measurement of drug craving during naloxone-precipitated withdrawal in methadone-maintained volunteers. *Experimental and Clinical Psychopharmacology, 3*(4), 424–431.

Shao, C., Li, Y., Jiang, K., Zhang, D., Xu, Y., Lin, L., et al. (2006). Dopamine D_4 receptor polymorphism modulates cue-elicited heroin craving in Chinese. *Psychopharmacology, 186*(2), 185–190.

Shiffman, S. (2009). Ecological momentary assessment (EMA) in studies of substance use. *Psychological Assessment, 21*(4), 486–497.

Shiffman, S., Engberg, J. B., Paty, J. A., Perz, W. G., Gnys, M., Kassel, J. D., et al. (1997). A day at a time: Predicting smoking lapse from daily urge. *Journal of Abnormal Psychology, 106*(1), 104–116.

Singleton, E. G., & Gorelick, D. A. (1998). Mechanisms of alcohol craving and their clinical implications. In M. Galanter (Ed.), *Recent developments in alcoholism* (Vol. 14, pp. 177–195). New York: Plenum Press.

Sinha, R. (2013). The clinical neurobiology of drug craving. *Current Opinion in Neurobiology.*

Soyka, M., Helten, C., & Schmidt, P. (2010). OCDS craving scores predict 24-month outcome in alcoholic outpatients. *American Journal on Addictions, 19*(3), 264–269.

Spanagel, R., Vengeliene, V., Jandeleit, B., Fischer, W.-N., Grindstaff, K., Zhang, X., et al. (2014). Acamprosate produces its anti-relapse effects via calcium. *Neuropsychopharmacology, 39*(4), 783–791.

Tiffany, S. T. (1990). A cognitive model of drug urges and drug-use behavior: Role of automatic and nonautomatic processes. *Psychological Review, 97*(2), 147–168.

Tiffany, S. T. (1995). Potential functions of classical conditioning in drug addiction. In C. D. Drummond, S. T. Tiffany, S. Glautier, & B. Remington (Eds.), *Addictive behavior: Cue exposure theory and practice* (pp. 47–71). Chichester, UK: Wiley.

Tiffany, S. T., & Drobes, D. J. (1991). The development and initial validation of a questionnaire on smoking urges. *British Journal of Addiction, 86*(11), 1467–1476.

Tiffany, S. T., & Hakenewerth, D. M. (1991). The production of smoking urges through an imagery manipulation: Psychophysiological and verbal manifestations. *Addictive Behaviors, 16*(6), 389–400.

Tiffany, S. T., & Wray, J. M. (2011). The clinical significance of drug craving. *Annals of the New York Academy of Sciences.*

Tiffany, S. T., & Wray, J. M. (2012). The clinical significance of drug craving. *Annals of the New York Academy of Sciences, 1248,* 1–17.

Toates, F. (1994). Comparing motivational systems: An incentive motivation perspective. In C. R. Legg & D. A. Booth (Eds.), *Appetite: Neural and behavioural bases* (pp. 305–327). Oxford, UK: Oxford University Press.

Tonstad, S., Tonnesen, P., Hajek, P., Williams, K. E., Billing, C. B., Reeves, K. R., et al. (2006). Effect of maintenance therapy with varenicline on smoking cessation: A randomized controlled trial. *Journal of the American Medical Association, 296*(1), 64–71.

van den Wildenberg, E., Wiers, R. W., Dessers, J., Janssen, R. G. J. H., Lambrichs, E. H., Smeets, H. J. M., et al. (2007). A functional polymorphism of the μ-opioid receptor gene (OPRM1) influences cue-induced craving for alcohol in male heavy drinkers. *Alcoholism: Clinical and Experimental Research, 31*(1), 1–10.

Verheul, R., Van den Brink, W., & Geerlings, P. (1999). A three-pathway psychobiological model of craving for alcohol. *Alcohol and Alcoholism, 34*(2), 197–222.

Volkow, N. D., Fowler, J. S., Wang, G. J., Hitzemann, R., Logan, J., Schlyer, D. J., et al. (1993). Decreased dopamine D_2 receptor availability is associated with reduced frontal metabolism in cocaine abusers. *Synapse, 14*(2), 169–177.

Volkow, N. D., Wang, G. J., Fowler, J. S., Logan, J., Gatley, S. J., Hitzemann, R., et al. (1997). Decreased striatal dopaminergic responsiveness in detoxified cocaine-dependent subjects. *Nature, 386*(6627), 830–833.

Waters, A. J., Marhe, R., & Franken, I. H. A. (2012). Attentional bias to drug cues is elevated before and during temptations to use heroin and cocaine. *Psychopharmacology, 219*(3), 909–921.

Wiers, R. W., Stacy, A. W., Ames, S. L., Noll, J. A., Sayette, M. A., Zack, M., et al. (2002). Implicit and explicit alcohol-related cognitions. *Alcoholism: Clinical and Experimental Research, 26*(1), 129–137.

Wong, D. F., Kuwabara, H., Schretlen, D. J., Bonson, K. R., Zhou, Y., Nandi, A., et al. (2006). Increased occupancy of dopamine receptors in human striatum during cue-elicited cocaine craving. *Neuropsychopharmacology, 31*(12), 2716–2727.

Wray, J. M., Gass, J. C., & Tiffany, S. T. (2013). A systematic review of the relationships between craving and smoking cessation. *Nicotine and Tobacco Research, 15*(7), 1167–1182.

Yalachkov, Y., Kaiser, J., & Naumer, M. J. (2012). Functional neuroimaging studies in addiction: Multisensory drug stimuli and neural cue reactivity. *Neuroscience and Biobehavioral Reviews, 36*(2), 825–835.

Zijlstra, F., Booij, J., van den Brink, W., & Franken, I. H. A. (2008). Striatal dopamine D_2 receptor binding and dopamine release during cue-elicited craving in recently abstinent opiate-dependent males. *European Neuropsychopharmacology, 18*, 262–270.

CHAPTER 20

Three Senses of Desire in Consumer Research

Utpal M. Dholakia

Desires to acquire, possess, use, experience, share, and display objects of consumption lie at the heart of consumer behavior. Consumer researchers have conceived of desire variously as "want," "wish," "urge," "craving," "approach motivation," "appetite," and "buying impulse" (e.g., Belk, Ger, & Askegaard, 2003; Dholakia, Gopinath, & Bagozzi, 2005; Hoch & Loewenstein, 1991; Redden & Haws, 2013; Rook & Fisher, 1995). Ontologically, consumer desire possesses the following characteristics: it is conscious and constitutes direct experience rather than a metacognition (Kavanagh, Andrade, & May, 2005; see also Andrade, May, Van Dillen, & Kavanagh, Chapter 1, this volume); it has a "first-person ontology" in the sense that it is meaningful only from the viewpoint of the person experiencing it (Searle, 1999); it has intense, positive affective qualities (Belk et al., 2003; Hirschman & Holbrook, 1982); it is directed toward a particular consumption object, experience, or imagined future state (Hofmann & Van Dillen, 2012); it is motivating and supports a particular goal, choice, or course of action; and it is dynamic with a time-varying intensity.

Despite these shared properties, desire has been conceived of and empirically examined in at least three distinct ways by consumer researchers. In its first sense, desire provides the *motivational impetus* for engaging in decision making and for pursuing enactment of effortful goals. It integrates a series of emotional, cognitive, self-perception, and social appraisals of the consumer and is distinct from, and leads to, formation of the intention. Desire in this sense resides at two levels in the consumer's action hierarchy: at the abstract level in the goal to be pursued as *goal desire*, and in the specific means to reach the goal as *implementation desire*.

Second, in its most popular form, consumer researchers view desire as the *countervailing force that opposes self-control*. In this second sense, the consumer desires to have objects or to perform actions that provide

pleasure in the short term but can produce significant negative consequences in the long run. Upon experiencing desire, processes of self-
regulation kick in, and these processes have been the focus of extensive
attention during the 2000s. Finally, desire is conceived of in consumer
research as *a sudden, spontaneous buying impulse.* In its third sense, desire is
synonymous with an urge or craving to buy, and is produced immediately
upon exposure to the temptation. Over time, unchecked buying impulses
are associated with serious and socially significant syndromes such as
compulsive buying, materialism, and hoarding.

The purpose of this chapter is to provide a critical review of selected
consumer research on desire. A succinct summary of what we know
about these three senses of consumer desire is presented with respect to
its antecedents, constituents, and consequences, and emergent research
questions and opportunities to further enhance our understanding of
consumer desire are pointed out. Each sense of consumer desire is now
considered in more detail.

Sense 1: Consumer Desire as the Motivational Impetus for Decision Making and Effortful Decision Enactment

In research spanning more than two decades and covering a variety
of contexts, the model of goal-directed behavior (MGB) developed by
Bagozzi and colleagues (Bagozzi, 1992, 2006; Dholakia, Bagozzi, & Klein
Pearo, 2004; Perugini & Bagozzi, 2004; Xie, Bagozzi, & Østli, 2013) has
been used extensively to study the role of desire in making and enacting decisions. The MGB describes effortful, nonroutine decisions that are
enacted intentionally by consumers. Rooted in social psychological perspectives on goals (Bagozzi & Dholakia, 1999; Gollwitzer, 1999), the MGB
distinguishes between higher-order goals (e.g., "to maintain a healthy
body weight") and the concrete means to achieve them (e.g., "to run 3
miles every day"). Whereas goals and means refer to specific end-state(s)
chosen after deliberate decision making, desires in the MGB capture the
motivational intensity with which goals and plans are pursued by consumers. Figure 20.1 provides the key constructs in the MGB.

Desire in the MGB

In the MGB, desire is construed as "a state of mind whereby an agent has
a personal motivation to perform an action or to achieve a goal" (Perugini & Bagozzi, 2004, p. 71). Desire provides the motivational impetus
for decision making, serving to integrate a series of emotional, cognitive,
self-perception, and social appraisals, mustering motivation, and leading
to intention formation. It is a necessary antecedent of the consumer's
intentions to pursue a goal and to act. Such a conceptualization of desire

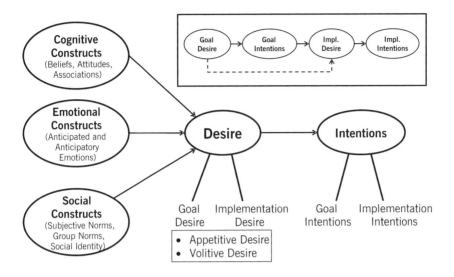

FIGURE 20.1. Graphic representation of key constructs in the MBG.

is grounded in philosophical perspectives, specifically in the distinction between volitive and appetitive desires and in the connection condition for intentions (Davis, 1984), which helps in understanding how desires motivate intentional behavior.

With *volitive desires*, consumers take reasons for acting into account to form self-commitments to act. Philosophers have argued that desires are related to intentions in the sense that once the person is aware of and accepts his or her desire to act, this will motivate him or her to form an intention to act (called the "connection condition" for intentions, Davis, 1984, p. 53). Where volitive desires arouse, *appetitive desires* catalyze reasons for acting to release or free up latent, hidden desires related to biological needs such as food, sex, or safety. Both desires transform reasons for acting into self-regulated motives to act which, in turn, are the proximal causes of intentions. In distinguishing the two, Davis (1984) likens volitive desires to wants and wishes (having a desire), and appetitive desires to yearnings and cravings (desiring something). For a particular consumption object, the consumer's desire may contain either the volitive or appetitive aspect, or both. Consumer culture theory (CCT) researchers have provided rich insights into the experience and expression of both these desires (see Belk et al., 2003, for a review).

Goal and Implementation Desire

In line with extensive research on goal setting and goal striving (Bagozzi & Dholakia, 1999; Gollwitzer, 1999), the MGB distinguishes between *goal desire* and *implementation desire*, which operate at different levels in the consumer's action hierarchy and are antecedents to the *goal* and *implementation intention*, respectively. In a temporal sense, the goal desire precedes the implementation desire, and the effect of the former on the latter is fully mediated through the goal intentions construct. Intentions differ from desires in at least three important aspects: (1) they take feasibility of enactment, including the decision maker's self-efficacy, into account, (2) they are connected more closely to specific physical and mental actions than to desires, and (3) their temporal framing is generally of a shorter duration than that of corresponding desires (see Perugini & Bagozzi, 2004, for further details).

The MGB also makes the distinction between *goal desirability*, the valenced value of outcomes embedded in a particular goal, and *goal desire*, the consumer's motivational state (Trope & Liberman, 2010; Perugini & Bagozzi, 2004). Although it is widely construed in consumer research as an attribute and a descriptor of consumption objects (e.g., how desirable a product or an experience is; Hirschman & Holbrook, 1982), Bagozzi has argued that the notion of desirability is limited and not determinative of action without a consideration of desire, especially for goal-directed, effortful decisions. Specifically, for a consumer to act in relation to a desirable end-state requires that he or she desire to achieve that end-state. For instance, a consumer committed to the voluntary simplicity movement may view a gas-guzzling luxury car as desirable but may not desire to acquire it. On the other hand, a dieter may view oatmeal as bland and undesirable, yet may desire to purchase it because of its nutritional aspects. Goal desire thus represents a necessary condition for decision making to advance beyond the evaluation stage.

Implementation desire transforms the consumer's reasons and motives for choosing a goal and the goal intention into an implementation intention. It reflects how strongly the decision maker wants to enact specific goal-directed behavior(s). While goal desires are directed toward end-states in the MGB, final goals, and the decision maker's intrinsic needs, implementation desires are targeted at means to the chosen ends, energizing the intentions to perform instrumental acts or goal-directed behaviors (see Figure 20.1).

How does the consumer arrive at this motivational state of mind? The MGB describes the cognitive, emotional, and social antecedents of desire. Given space constraints, the emotional and social antecedents of desire in the MGB are considered here, and the reader is referred to Bagozzi (2006) for an extensive discussion of its cognitive antecedents.

Emotional Antecedents of Desire in the MGB

Research involving the MGB makes the distinction between two types of future-oriented emotions that affect the consumer's desire: anticipated emotions and anticipatory emotions.

Anticipated Emotions

When consumers pursuing effortful goals consider and imagine alternative scenarios of achieving and failing to achieve the goal, one aspect of this prefactual appraisal (a type of counterfactual thinking) involves imagining emotions that they will experience (Bagozzi, Baumgartner, & Pieters, 1998). Specifically, imagining goal success leads to positive emotions such as joy, pride, and happiness (e.g., "I will feel happy if I reach my weight loss goal"), and imagined goal failure results in negative emotions like anger, shame, and frustration (e.g., "I will feel ashamed if I am still smoking 3 months from now"). MGB studies have consistently shown that imagined emotional appraisals (i.e., "How I will feel") contribute significantly to the affective and motivational intensity of the experienced desire, providing the basis for deciding to act so as to approach positive or pleasurable anticipated outcomes and corresponding emotional states and to avoid negative or hurtful ones.

Anticipatory Emotions

Whereas anticipated emotions refer to prospective appraisals of imagined future emotional states that are motivating, anticipatory emotions are "currently experienced, phenomenologically real affective responses to possible future events that have positive or negative implications for the self" (Baumgartner, Pieters, & Bagozzi, 2008, p. 686). Unlike anticipated emotions, which can cover a wide range of emotional responses (it is not uncommon for an empirical study to assess 20 or more anticipated emotions), anticipatory emotions are narrower in scope, being limited to hope due to the prospects of a positive future event and fear at the prospect of a negative future event. Although research on anticipatory emotions is in its infancy, one interesting aspect is that their intensity hinges on the event's uncertainty: more uncertainty produces more intense anticipatory emotions. There are also indications that anticipatory emotions play a greater role in influencing and sustaining implementation than goal desire; however, much remains to be known about their nature and functioning, and how they influence desire and other outcomes.

Social Antecedents of Desire in the MGB

The MGB explicitly acknowledges desire's social nature (Belk et al., 2003; Dholakia et al., 2004) by theorizing that its experience, although in the "first person," is influenced materially by others. At least three types of social influences have been studied as antecedents of desire in the MGB by research to date. *Subjective norms* reflect the influence from expectations of significant others (depending on context, these people could be family, friends, coworkers, peers, experts, or members of the community). Because their basis lies in the consumer's need for others' approval, subjective norms characterize compliance processes of social influence and measure the normative pressure experienced by consumers during decision making, such as meeting the spoken, implicit, or inferred expectations of significant others.

Group norms, the second form of social influence on consumer desires, are derived from internalization processes whereby the consumer embraces the goals, values, beliefs, and conventions of the relevant social group. Group norms are particularly relevant in the current social-media-rich environment where marketers create and facilitate so many structured and managed groups for consumers to join and belong to (see Tamir & Ward, Chapter 21, this volume). According to the MGB, internalization occurs when the consumer's values, proclivities, and objectives are consistent with the group to begin with, or converge through a socialization process where over time the person learns about the group's norms and comes to adopt them. Interestingly, group norms emerge even when the group is entirely virtual, far-flung, and sans physical contact (Dholakia et al., 2004).

Third, goal desire is influenced through identification processes, where consumers conceives of themselves in terms of significant features of a particular self-inclusive social category that may or may not be group based (e.g., Harley Davidson rider, *Star Trek* "trekkie"), but which renders the self stereotypically interchangeable with other category members, and stereotypically distinct from outsiders. Identification processes engage aspects of both normative and informational social influence, along with referent power (especially relevant in marketing activities using experts and celebrities), and is characterized by the consumer's *social identity*. This construct is assessed in MGB studies with three dimensions: the consumer's self-awareness of group membership, affective commitment toward the group, and the evaluative significance of group membership for the consumer defined in terms of group-based self-esteem.

Summary

Relative to the remaining two senses of consumer desire, research on goals- and means-oriented desire has provided valuable insights into its emotional and social antecedents when compared to the remaining two senses. Notably, most empirical work involving the MGB to date has relied on surveys and employed structural equation models; there is considerable opportunity to add to knowledge in this research area with an experimental approach to study the processes and moderators involved in the formation, maintenance, and dissipation of goal and implementation desires for effortful goal choices and their enactment.

Sense 2: Consumer Desire as a Countervailing Force to Self-Control

Paralleling social psychology, consumer research on self-control has exploded within the past decade with dozens of articles published annually in the field's major journals. Desire is commonly conceptualized as the countervailing force to self-control in this research. In domains such as food consumption and financial decision making, consumer researchers study decisions and behaviors that have opposing, two-pronged outcomes usually occurring at different times: they yield pleasure in the short term (such as eating a tasty food or spending money to buy a glitzy product) but prove detrimental in some significant way over the longer term (by affecting health adversely or hurting the person's finances, respectively). For such dual-outcome behaviors, the consumer's preferences are seen as "time inconsistent," and because they shift over time, the decision's outcome is the winner of a battle between the opposing motivational forces of desire and willpower (Hoch & Loewenstein, 1991; Hofmann, Friese, & Strack, 2009). The experience and self-regulation of desire is an essential aspect of such decisions.

Virtue and Vice Products

When desire and self-control are countervailing motivational forces, the research is usually about decisions involving "virtue" and "vice" products (e.g., Khan & Dhar, 2007; Wertenbroch, 1998). Such products produce short-term pleasure *and* long-term pain (vice products), or vice versa (virtue products). Consumer behaviors such as eating a chocolate cake, buying cigarettes, or leasing an overly pricey car are all instances of decisions involving vices, while saving money for retirement, skipping a meal, and getting a tooth cavity filled are all virtuous decisions (e.g., Dholakia, Gopinath, Bagozzi, & Nataraajan, 2006; Mukhopadhyay & Johar, 2009).

However, for many consumption objects, consumers' decisions may not entail a motivational tussle, as both short- and long-term outcomes are largely positive. For instance, eating an apple is generally a pleasurable experience in the short term and healthy in the long term for most people. Likewise, a professional football player may consume a steak dinner with much enjoyment after a long day's physical activity without experiencing the conflict that usually badgers a dieter. With respect to desire, such decisions are relatively straightforward in the sense that the consumer's choice to act or not act is dictated simply by the desire's intensity. However, competing options may intrude, each eliciting its own incompatible volitive and appetitive desires, and social, cultural and environmental factors may be considerations. Surprisingly little research has taken up the question of the role played by desires in such decisions even though they likely constitute a majority of decisions that consumers face on a daily basis.

The Strength Model of Self-Control

In studying decisions involving self-regulation, the dominant theoretical perspective is the *strength model of self-control* (Baumeister, 2002;

Baumeister, Vohs, & Tice, 2007). The model posits that engaging in an act of self-regulation depletes this resource; while one is in this ego-depleted state, further attempts at self-control in any domain result in impaired performance. Thus, consumers show deterioration when engaging in consecutive acts of self-control. Dozens of studies, many in consumer settings, have empirically tested and supported the strength model. In most of them, the research focus has been on the self-control side of the motivational struggle between desire and self-control (Baumeister, 2002; Hofmann & Van Dillen, 2012).

However, an increasing body of recent research shows that desire plays a significant, distinct, and nuanced role in the self-regulation process and in determining the outcome. These findings have expanded the strength model of self-control by explicitly considering the role of desire in repeated self-regulation with significant implications for consumer decisions.

Self-Control Increases Subsequent Desire

One such expansion is the *process model of ego depletion* (Inzlicht & Schmeichel, 2012), which posits that in addition to depleting self-control, acts of self-regulation also independently increase an individual's approach motivation in subsequent tasks. Supporting this conjecture, in one study, Schmeichel, Harmon-Jones, and Harmon-Jones (2010) found that when participants had exercised self-control in an initial act by inhibiting their common writing tendencies, they were likely to engage in more low-stakes betting behavior in a subsequent task. In another study, an initial act of self-control facilitated the perception of a reward-relevant symbol, such as a dollar sig,n but did not have any effect on perception of a reward-irrelevant symbol, such as a percent sign.

There is evidence that part of the reason for the increase in desire is that the initial exertion of self-control dulls the consumer's monitoring system responsible for initiating self-regulatory processes. A second reason is that the initial self-control produces a greater sensitivity to rewards so that consumers pay more attention to rewarding stimuli. For consumers, the implications of this finding are significant, and suggest that the effects of making multiple choices and engaging in self-regulatory actions, say during a shopping trip, or an online shopping spree, may be even more tilted toward engaging in vice behaviors than hitherto thought. Not only is self-control depleted, but desire is fueled by prior acts of self-control. More research is needed to study both the magnitude and the moderators of this phenomenon in field settings.

Although desire and self-control are often seen as independent motivational forces that operate against each other, some research indicates that this may not be the case. One distinct way in which the experience of desire is affected is by the consumer's situational self-regulatory tendencies. In particular, those with a temporarily activated *promotion focus*, marked by an ideal-aspirational set of standards, an orientation toward positive outcomes, and a bias toward errors of commission (i.e., making mistakes) in decision making, experience more intense desire when making decisions about tempting products than those who have a temporary *prevention focus* (ought-duty standards, orientation to repel negative outcomes, bias toward errors of omission). In one study, Dholakia and colleagues (2006) found that an initial regulatory focus manipulation resulted in greater intensity of desire for a slice of cheesecake among those whose promotion focus was activated compared to those with prevention focus. Interestingly, even after experiencing more intense desire, promotion focus consumers were able to resist it more successfully than prevention focus consumers because they used more effective approach resistance strategies; in contrast, prevention focus consumers tended to fixate on the tempting stimuli when resisting, and these avoidance strategies did not work as well.

Desire Decreases Subsequent Desire

Self-control is a limited resource, but what about desire? Dholakia and colleagues (2005) provided evidence that much like self-control, the experience of desire consumes desire so that less of it is available for subsequent decisions. In a study of sequential shopping decisions, the authors provided evidence for a "sequential mitigation effect" whereby decision makers experienced less desire for a particular product when they had participated in a prior, desire-laden decision compared to when they did not do so. In one study, for instance, participants' desire for and likelihood of picking up a gourmet sandwich was substantially lower if they had been given an opportunity to impulsively choose a sweater beforehand (even if they did not choose it). These findings are particularly relevant in understanding consumer choices that are made sequentially without implicating self-control.

Within the same decision-making domain, too, there is evidence that many consumers experience lowered desire with repeated consumption (see Redden, Chapter 4, this volume). In studying food consumption, Redden and Haws (2013) demonstrated occurrence of "healthy satiation" such that after eating unhealthy but tasty foods like M&Ms and Skittles, consumers higher in trait self-control (TSC) experienced decreased desire to consume more of these candies. However, consumers who were low in self-control did not experience a corresponding drop in desire. These differences occurred because the former group paid more attention to the amount being consumed. These findings indicate that change in desire intensity during meals may be one reason why so many consumers overeat and suffer adverse effects like ill health and obesity.

The Role of Justification in Enactment of Desires

A key tenet of the strength model of self-control is that acting on one's desires represents a self-regulation failure. Recent research has challenged this view by arguing that consumers actively use justifications based on earlier actions or circumstances to endorse acting on their desire (see de Ridder, de Witt Huberts, & Evers, Chapter 10, this volume, for a review of this research). Specifically, when the consumer engages in or recalls an initial act of restraint, it provides a justification for then acting on one's desires and for subsequent indulgence, referred to as "self-licensing" (de Witt Huberts, Evers, & de Ridder, 2012). In one study, participants were more likely to choose a chocolate cake over a fruit salad after being made to recall an instance in the past when they had restrained themselves from buying an attractive product (Mukhopadhyay & Johar, 2009). In another study, after completing a long and unpleasant task, participants consumed more unhealthy snacks presumably because they felt justified in rewarding themselves (de Witt Huberts et al., 2012). Part of the reason for this subsequent indulgence following control may be a boost in consumers' self-esteem arising from successful restraint (de Witt Huberts et al., 2014).

Desire Resistance Strategies

In addition to studying how desires are enacted, consumer researchers have extensively examined how they are resisted. Resistance strategies may be defined as volitional mechanisms used by consumers to effortfully counter and quell desires for temptations. These strategies involve self-regulation of mental states and processes through different mechanisms. Self-control research has identified several such mechanisms that are helpful in educating consumers and policy makers. One common resistance strategy is to formulate explicit rules or "precommitments" beforehand (Ariely & Wertenbroch, 2002), which are then used as guidelines to resist the desire when it is experienced. For instance, a saving or a dieting program may be regulated effectively by having a well-defined and carefully thought out budget or calorie quota, respectively. Explicit rules are particularly useful for frequently or regularly occurring appetitive consumption desires. Although we know that rules work, research cataloging types of rules and conditions under which they work more or less effectively in the domains of food consumption and financial decision making is still needed.

A second resistance strategy, *selective attention* (Kühl, 1987) refers to the consumer's inclination to attend only to information supporting the volitionally supported course of self-control. Such "closed-mindedness" encourages a focus away from the desire-producing temptation. Applying this strategy has a checkered history going back to Mischel and Mischel's

(1983) seminal finding that children learn to maintain an experimentally induced intention against a more desirable choice by avoiding visual contact with the source of distraction (see also Hoch & Loewenstein, 1991). An alternative approach that many consumers use instead is to shift attention to other cognitively demanding tasks (Kemps, Tiggemann, & Grigg, 2008). Related resistance strategies include *encoding* and *exposure control*, which facilitate the operation of self-control by encoding selective environmental features that are related to fighting the desire, and manipulating the environment to reduce the arousing effects of the desire-producing stimuli (also called as "distancing"), respectively (Fujita, Trope, Liberman, & Levin-Sagi, 2006).

Parsimonious information processing is a strategy about how and when the consumer *stops* processing information during the self-regulation process. To resist a desire successfully often requires minimizing the process of cognitive evaluation, especially when continuing it would favor the desire, or when new information supporting the desire becomes available constantly, such as during consumption episodes that are filled with experiential elements (e.g., a vacation to a tourist destination or a shopping trip through a mall).

Further, the consumer may control his or her emotions to resist the desire by inhibiting negative emotional states and avoiding intrusion of emotional task-related thoughts that could undermine the protective function of volition (Salovey & Mayer, 1990). Emotion control also helps generate positive emotions that may be conducive to successful resistance. M*otivation control*, in contrast, refers to self-regulatory actions that bring attention and effort to bear on the task of resisting the desire. These include such methods as substitution (Hoch & Loewenstein, 1991), where one may give oneself a small immediate reward for successfully resisting a larger and potentially more harmful desire (e.g., buying a smartphone case in lieu of a new smartphone). Motivation control is especially useful for resisting pernicious desires such as breaking a dieting plan or splurging on a big-ticket, unaffordable item.

What happens when the desire proves irresistible and is enacted despite these resistance efforts? Now the consumer has to cope with the failed self-regulation attempt and detach from this failure to resist the desire by inhibiting activation of the resistance elements and preventing excessive ruminations about the desire (e.g., "If only I had restrained myself instead of scarfing down that bowl of chips!").

Summary

The notion that desire and self-control are opposing motivational forces that combat each other like two wolves, "each strong enough to devour the other" and "locked in constant war" (Kenyon, 2012), is currently the most popular way of thinking about desire in consumer research. Over the past decade, this perspective has helped us understand a great deal about how consumers make decisions in domains where self-control is relevant for many people, such as eating and spending money, how they regulate behavior, and the consequences of succeeding and failing to do so.

Sense 3: Consumer Desire as a Sudden, Spontaneous Buying Impulse

Unlike the first two senses of consumer desire, which are marked by a gradual, unfolding process in which cognitive, emotional, social, and motivational forces play roles and determine the effects of desire, a *buying impulse* is marked by a sudden, spontaneous, and strong burst of acquisitive desire directed toward a specific object of consumption. A buying impulse has the following properties: (1) it is experienced immediately when the consumer is exposed to the desirable object; (2) it is intense and short-lived, manifesting as a burst of motivation and impelling the consumer to buy within a very short time period, usually a few moments (e.g., Mukhopadhyay & Johar, 2009); (3) it may produce a state of psychological disequilibrium marked by emotional conflict (referred to as "hedonic complexity" by some researchers, e.g., Kacen & Lee, 2002; Rook, 1987); (4) it discourages inaction or the status quo; and (5) it may occur even in the absence of a deficit state such as physiological deprivation or withdrawal.

Marketing practitioners have long understood the importance of buying impulses in consumer decision making (see Verplanken & Sato, 2011, for a recent review). Over the past half century, retailers have devoted considerable attention to designing and presenting products that will produce the buying impulse in consumers at the point of sale. Store, website, and now mobile site layouts, product aesthetics and packaging, attractive in-store displays, and unexpected spot promotions all try to encourage impulsive purchases. In fact, early consumer research viewed the shopper's buying impulse as a behavioral response triggered by stimuli in the shopping environment (Kollatt & Willett, 1967) and sought to understand the effectiveness of different in-store merchandizing and media stimuli in generating impulses (e.g., Kotler, 1974).

After this early, externally oriented perspective, the eighties and the nineties saw a shift toward understanding the impulsive shopper's psychological state. In one of the first studies using this lens, Rook and Fisher (1995) regarded impulse buying as a trait-driven tendency of consumers that is subject to their internal psychological reactions and emotional experiences rather than the qualities of the desirable object or surrounding stimuli. This shift in perspective opened the doors to the application of motivational and cognitive models to understand how consumers experience buying impulses and the role they play in consumer decisions.

The Buying Impulse Formation and Enactment Model

The integrated buying impulse formation and enactment model[1] (BIFEM; see Dholakia, 2000) is a useful framework for reviewing consumer research on the buying impulse. The BIFEM theorizes that impulsive decisions are preceded by distinct psychological processes (see also Hofmann et al., 2009, and Kavanagh et al., 2005), explains the factors that lead to formation of the buying impulse and its subsequent dissipation or enactment, describing the roles of cognitive and volitional psychological mechanisms. The BIFEM, which is graphically depicted in Figure 20.2, begins with four antecedents of the buying impulse.

Trait Impulsivity

The first antecedent is the consumer's *trait impulsivity*, defined as the tendency to respond quickly and without reflection, and is characterized by rapid reaction times, absence of foresight, and a tendency to act without a careful plan (Rook & Fisher, 1995). Studies have shown that the consumer's buying impulsivity is associated with other traits such

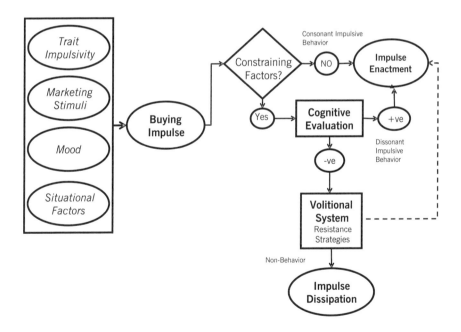

FIGURE 20.2. Graphic representation of key concepts in the BIFEM.

---

[1]The model presented here is an updated version of the model first developed and presented in Dholakia (2000).

as acquisitiveness, variety seeking, sensation seeking, risk aversion, and absorption (a tendency to become immersed in self-involving experiences; Braddock et al., 2011; Weun, Jones, & Beatty, 1998; Youn & Faber, 2000). Those who are impulsive are likely to experience buying impulses more often and with greater intensity. As one example, Stilley, Inman, and Wakefield (2010) found that when consumers shopped through most aisles of a grocery store, only those with high impulsivity were likely to overspend relative to their budget.

Marketing Stimuli

Sensory exposure to the product is a common route to experiencing the buying impulse for many consumers. Product characteristics such as aesthetic appeal, sensory attributes (taste, texture, etc.), and scarcity (e.g., limited quantity or availability) play important roles in stimulating the buying impulse. Moreover, the role of *physical proximity* in impulse experience has been documented in delay-of-gratification research (Mischel & Mischel, 1983) and by marketing practitioners (Schwartz, 2011). Physical proximity may activate positive memories and serve to kindle desire or increase accessibility to the conflicting goals involved (Mukhopadhyay, Sengupta, & Ramanathan, 2008). *Temporal proximity* is another key contributor in impulse formation by producing low-level, concrete construals (Hoch & Loewenstein, 1991; Trope & Liberman, 2010). When seen in concrete, "here-and-now" terms, the product's immediacy may activate an appetitive desire in consumers, triggering the buying impulse. Consistent with this view, low-level, concrete construals have been shown to result in increased preferences for immediate outcomes (vs. delayed ones) and yield more positive assessments of tempting stimuli (Fujita et al., 2006). In the BIFEM, these characteristics are labeled *marketing stimuli* to acknowledge that marketers can significantly influence the presentation of such stimuli (Kotler, 1974).

Mood

Both positive and negative mood states can influence experience of the buying impulse. Positive moods are associated with arousal and encourage open-mindedness, both of which may encourage formation of the buying impulse. Rook and Gardner (1993) found that consumers' positive moods were more conducive to impulsive buying than negative moods, as did Beatty and Ferrell (1998). However, research on mood repair suggests that consumers in negative-valenced moods may also be susceptible to buying urges. Consistent with this idea, research on people with alcohol or cocaine dependence indicates that negative mood increases cravings (see Kavanagh et al., 2005, for a review). More research is needed to better understand the processes by which mood influences experience of the buying impulse.

Situational Factors

Situational factors contextualize the buying decision and increase or decrease the consumer's propensity to experience the buying impulse. One situational factor is the *environmental cues* in which the decision is embedded, aspects of which may favor impulse formation (Kavanagh et al., 2005). For instance, a person who has just received a paycheck may be more susceptible to the impulse's experience. Engaging in unrelated activities may also play a role. Recent research has shown that simply purchasing a lottery ticket or even contemplating its purchase produces concrete thoughts about how any potential winnings will be spent, and the accompanying rush of pleasurable thoughts encourages the buying impulse (Kim, 2013).

Preshopping factors, such as how concretely the consumer has defined the shopping goal, whether a store is chosen for its low prices, and whether the shopper means to go to one particular store (vs. multiple stores) during a shopping trip are all positive contributors to the buying impulse (Bell, Corsten, & Knox, 2011). Finally, *cultural factors* also influence the buying impulse. By emphasizing control and moderation of one's emotions, collectivistic cultures may dampen the buying impulse as these consumers focus more on negative aspects of outcomes and not as much on positive consequences relative to individualistic cultures (Kacen & Lee, 2002).

The Buying Impulse

In the BIFEM, the *buying impulse* is defined as *an irresistible urge to buy*, and its experience is marked by a certain intensity. The buying impulse can be construed as an affectively charged, cognitive event in which the consumption object is in focal attention; it cannot be blocked from being experienced when its antecedents are present with sufficient strength, and multiple eliciting factors will increase probability and strength of its occurrence. The influence of the antecedents (as main effects and as interactions) in producing the buying impulse may vary by consumer or even across occasions for the same person.

Constraining Factors

When the consumer experiences the buying impulse, mental responses are automatically triggered to assess possible *constraints to its enactment* (Vallacher, 1983). Constraints on the impulse's enactment generally fall into one of three categories.

First, the consumer may realize that there are *current impediments* to enactment. For instance, there may not be sufficient time or money, or the consumer may recognize that enactment violates precommitments or longer-term standards (Baumeister, 2002; Hofmann et al., 2009). To allow some leeway, many consumers provide an "in-store slack" in their mental budgets, earmarked specifically for unplanned impulse purchases (Stilley et al., 2010). Second, consumers may consider harmful consequences of impulse enactment. For instance, an overweight person may visualize his or her future appearance. Finally, negative *anticipatory emotions*, particularly fear, may also work against acting on the impulse (Bagozzi et al.,1998).

Many research findings in the extant literature are consistent with the view of *constraining factors* in the BIFEM. First, constraining factors are similar to the construct of an "interrupt" that is experienced by consumers and alerts them to the need for cognitive deliberation (Hoch & Loewenstein, 1991). Many of Rook's (1987) study participants evaluated a particular buying impulse negatively, explicitly recognizing that they were breaking budgetary or dietary rules. Constraining factors are also similar to "attenuating countervailing forces" proposed by psychiatrists studying aggressive impulsive behaviors (Plutchik & van Praag, 1995). This line of research suggests that when one experiences an aggressive impulse, internal factors may serve to attenuate its effect and prevent violent behavior. Examples of such factors include appeasement by others or recalling a previous injury that one has suffered.

Consonant and Dissonant Buying Impulses

If no constraining factors are identified at this point, the buying impulse will be seen as *consonant*, that is, *harmonious with the consumer's goals, resources, standards,* and *situation.* The consumer then responds reflexively and enacts the impulse buying without any further deliberation or hesitation. Self-regulation is not needed here. For example, a stick-thin marathon runner may simply pick up a chocolate cookie and bite into it without a second thought. The strength and interactions of the antecedents determine experience and enactment of the buying impulse, and cognitive evaluation of the impulsive action or its consequences is minimal. The consumer acts and moves on.

However, if constraining factors are identified, the consumer experiences internal conflict and ambivalence. In this case, the buying impulse may be termed "dissonant." According to the BIFEM, its experience results in a more thought-based evaluation of the consequences of enactment, and a shift from a hedonic, impulse-dominated mode to a more evaluative one. The consumer now weighs the pros and cons of enacting the impulse. This evaluative process, which occurs quickly, in real time, guides behavior. If the assessment is positive, the consumer may view the constraining factor(s) as not significant enough and enact the impulse.

Resisting Dissonant Impulses

When the consumer experiences a dissonant buying impulse and evaluates the behavior negatively, an *outcome expectancy* (i.e., the subjective likelihood of successfully resisting the impulse, given continued effort) is derived. This expectancy is directly influenced by impulse strength and valence of negative cognitive evaluation, which determine the motivation available for resistance. If expectancy for successful resistance is sufficiently favorable, the volitional system continues to guide the individual toward resistance until the window of opportunity for impulse enactment closes. Resisting dissonant buying impulses involves engaging processes of self-regulation and using one or more of a combination of desire resistance strategies, discussed earlier in the chapter. On the other hand, if the expectancy is sufficiently unfavorable, resistance to the buying impulse dwindles, and the consumer succumbs to his or her dissonant impulse. Afterwards, conflict may be experienced along with negative emotions such as guilt or regret.

As the volitional resistance processes operate, the strength of the buying impulse eventually dwindles as the antecedent factors responsible for it recede from the consumer's attention. In this case, the buying impulse dissipates without being enacted. The BIFEM represents a parsimonious, yet psychologically rich account of the process through which consumption impulses are formed and get enacted or resisted by consumers.

Compulsive Buying Behavior

For some consumers, the buying impulse is frequently experienced as intense desire to acquire, possess, and hoard objects, and may be a symptom of a cluster of psychological disorders that include substance abuse, impulse control, compulsive gambling, buying, and hoarding behaviors. Consumer researchers have studied compulsive buying, which is exemplified by "chronic, repetitive purchasing . . . [which] becomes a primary response to negative events or feelings [and which] . . . becomes very difficult to stop and ultimately results in harmful consequences" (Faber & O'Guinn, 1992, p. 459) and is marked by a tendency to buy repetitively without adequate impulse control over these behaviors (Ridgway, Kukar-Kinney, & Monroe, 2008, p. 622). Compulsive buying exhibits aspects of both obsessive–compulsive and impulse-control disorders and is of significant scale and scope, with a recent large-scale study reporting that 5.8% of all U.S. consumers are compulsive buyers (Koran, Faber, Aboujaoude, Large, & Serpe, 2006).

Among compulsive shoppers, both physiological and social psychological influences play roles in the experience of the buying impulse and subsequent buying response. Researchers have found a high rate of depression among compulsive buyers, and incidence of disappointment with oneself after shopping episodes, leading to the conclusion that for many, the act of buying represents an attempt at self-medication to relieve negative affective states such as sadness, depression, and anxiety (Hassay & Smith, 1996; see Black, 2007, for a review). Culturally, compulsive buying is found to be more prevalent in developed countries, suggesting that disposable income, access to a variety of consumer goods, and leisure time are supporting factors (Black, 2007). Psychologically, compulsive buying is directed toward protecting one's self-concept in a publicly visible fashion, such that the act of acquiring the product itself (rather than visibly consuming it) becomes the carrier of symbolic meaning for the consumer. Such a psychology is supported by the heavy emphasis marketers place these days on "experiential marketing" whereby the purchase process for the product is metamorphosed into an enjoyable and immersive experience for the consumer. It is also in line with consumer researchers' long-held interest in hedonic consumption (Hirschman & Holbrook, 1982) and the shift from functional aspects of satisfaction delivery to its "fun, emotions, sensory stimulation, fantasy, and amusement elements" (Bloch, Ridgway, & Nelson, 1991, p. 445). It is quite possible that many of the marketing programs meant to provide pleasure to consumers have the unintended consequence of stimulating compulsive desires to buy.

Compulsive buying is pernicious because its consequences for consumers are manifold, serious, and long-lived. Financial harm, often extreme indebtedness and repeated bankruptcy, legal problems, depression, anxiety, and feelings of guilt are mostly personal outcomes, but the person also pays a social price through serious damage to relationships with significant others, family members, and friends, difficulty in maintaining a career, and so on (Lejoyeux & Weinstein, 2010). Although there has been a steady stream of impactful research on compulsive buying by consumer researchers such as Ronald Faber, Thomas O'Guinn, and others, much remains to be known about the role of marketing practices in affecting compulsive buying and factors that moderate these behaviors. There are other correlates of impulsive consumer desires, such as materialism and hoarding, that parallel some of the discussion provided here on compulsive shopping. Extended discussions of these phenomena are beyond the scope of this chapter (see Ahuvia & Wong, 2002, for a discussion of materialism, and Steketee & Frost, 2003, for a discussion on hoarding).

Future Research Questions

As the preceding discussion makes clear, research on consumer desires has advanced significantly over the past decade. We know a lot about the cognitive, emotional, and social mechanisms by which desire influences the choice and enactment of effortful goals; we have made great headway in understanding the motivational tussle between desire and self-regulation, and research on the buying impulse as well as its longer-term consequences, such as buying compulsions, is thriving. In this concluding section of the chapter, two other promising areas for future research concerning consumer desires are considered.

Sexual Desire and Consumer Decision Making

As observed throughout this chapter, researchers have studied consumer desire extensively in domains such as food consumption and personal finances. However, one domain that has received scant attention to date is that of sexual desire, despite the fact that sex plays a significant role in both marketing practice and the lived experience of consumers (Belk et al., 2003; Hirschman & Holbrook, 1982).

Not surprisingly, the few studies that have been reported by consumer researchers unambiguously reveal effects of sexual stimuli on consumer decision making. For instance, Van Den Bergh, Dewitte, and Warlop (2008) showed that exposure to photographs of lingerie-clad female models resulted in increased impatience (i.e., greater discounting of delayed financial rewards) among heterosexual males, leading the authors to conclude that "an induced sexual appetite instigates a greater urgency to consume anything rewarding" (p. 94). Ariely and Loewenstein (2006) reported that sexually aroused male undergraduates found a range of sexual activities to be more appealing, were more willing to engage in morally questionable practices, and to practice unsafe sex compared to those who were not sexually aroused.

Despite these tantalizing hints, many unanswered questions remain about how sexual desire affects other types of consumer desires, the methods of its regulation, and its effects on consumption decisions and actions, particularly those involving food and money. For instance, does quelling sexual desire result in depletion of self-regulatory resources, or does it strengthen one's resolve and encourage virtuous consumption decisions and behaviors? Are there comorbidities in how consumers react to sexual, eating, and spending desires? These gaps in our understanding of sexual desire are particularly telling given the sexualization of marketing symbols and messages in virtually every industry and the vast scale and scope of sexually motivated consumption (Belk et al., 2003).

Just as striking, pornography on the Internet has continued to propagate over the past decade, with estimates indicating that Internet pornography now accounts for close to 70% of the total Internet pay-to-view content and constitutes an industry that earns over $20 billion annually in revenue (although such estimates are likely gross underestimates because major companies in this industry are privately owned and many others operate illegally), and it is responsible for 13% of all Internet searches (see Covenant Eyes, 2013, for detailed pornography statistics).

Despite its significance both as a consumer activity and as a social issue, we know every little about the psychological processes, including sexual desires, involved in consuming pornographic materials or their effects on consumers' subsequent choices and actions.

What can explain the relative lack of research on sexual desire and consumption? One reason could be that this topic is simply an uncomfortable one to grapple with for many consumer researchers given the prevailing religious, political, cultural, and societal mores about sexual desires. For instance, asking subjects to self-stimulate themselves as an experimental manipulation (Ariely & Loewenstein, 2006) is likely to make many researchers (and institutional review boards) queasy. Another reason could be that conventional methods of studying questions about desires, such as standard experimental manipulations and surveys, may not be suitable for studying questions about sexual desire, given its unique aspects and the social desirability and reticence that surround it for most consumers. Despite these challenges, it is clear that the study of sexual desire remains a vast, unexplored frontier with opportunities for pioneering consumer researchers.

Effects of Changing Technological and Cultural Environments on Consumer Desires

One of the truisms about consumer behavior is that it occurs within constantly shifting social, political, technological, and cultural contexts. With significant changes in the context, the types and nature of desire-producing stimuli also change significantly, as do consumer responses to them, yielding promising research opportunities with practical consequences.

As one example, there has been a persistent trend away from ownership of consumer goods and services to renting access, even in categories such as cars and car rides (Lyft, Uber, Zipcar), designer dresses and handbags (Rent the Runway, Le Tote), and even textbooks (Chegg). Suddenly, possession becomes irrelevant for many, and consumption turns into a transactional process. We are only just beginning to study the effects of these changes on consumer desires and decision making. For instance, recent CCT research shows that consumers' ownership desires differ from their access desires (Chen, 2009). Whereas ownership desires are linked with self-identification, oriented toward a longer-term and intimate relationship with the object, and emphasize possession and control, access desires lack self-identification, are associated with a distant circumstantial relationship, and emphasize surprise and imagination.

As a second example, smartphones have emerged as a brand-new product category over the past decade, not only changing consumers' communication and information search behaviors drastically, but also being associated with significant levels of addictive behaviors among a wide swathe of consumers (Kwon et al., 2013). In the span of a few short years, addictive behaviors that were limited to a small fraction of consumers are rampant among most consumers. We currently know little about which aspects of smartphone technology and use are most responsible for this uncontrolled desire in users, nor do we know the roles played by interactivity, connectedness, and constant updating of new information (e.g., in news apps) at ever-increasing rates on consumer desires and self-regulatory strategies in these contexts. Even more important, we have yet to learn the effects of these desires in other functional domains. As these examples make clear, many exciting opportunities to study consumer desires continue to emerge.

Conclusion

The discussion throughout this chapter has supported one somewhat puzzling yet irrefutable conclusion: research on the three senses of consumer desire has proceeded, by and large, along parallel paths with few intersections or overlaps. A significant part of this segregation has to do with the unique perspectives with which consumer desire is conceptualized and measured in the three senses. For instance, its conception as a longer-term motivational state supporting the pursuit of deliberately chosen effortful goals is starkly different from its occurrence as a strong, momentary impulse to buy something. However, at least some of this separation can be attributed to the relatively siloed and paradigmatic methods by which research on these three senses has progressed. Under the MGB and its correlates, for instance, virtually all studies use surveys and analyze the gathered data using structural equation modeling approaches. Likewise, most research on consumer desire as an adversary to self-control employs standard experimental methods, usually in a lab setting.

So, do we need to pick one particular perspective on consumer desire and call it the winner? Absolutely not! As the discussion herein makes amply clear, each perspective has valuable, unique, and additive insights to offer, not only regarding how consumers make and follow through on their decisions, but also how they are able to avoid or fall prey to overtures of marketers. In the future, what would be productive is to loosen the extant methodological reins within each sense. This will allow future researchers to use ideas from one line of consumer desire research to advance knowledge in other lines explicitly. Thus, research under the MGB would benefit greatly by utilizing experimental manipulations to study hitherto unexplored avenues such as interactions and nonlinear relationships between constructs, whereas research on the tussle between desire and self-control would move forward significantly through designing and executing field studies that allow the study of the longer-term (i.e., over weeks or months) evolution and dynamics of desire and self-control experience that cannot be studied in the lab.

ACKNOWLEDGMENTS

I would like to thank Nivriti Chowdhry, Jihye Jung, and Kelly Haws for comments on previous versions of this chapter.

REFERENCES

Ahuvia, A. C., & Wong, N. Y. (2002). Personality and values based materialism: Their relationship and origins. *Journal of Consumer Psychology, 12*(4), 389–402.

Ariely, D., & Loewenstein, G. (2006). The heat of the moment: The effect of sexual arousal on sexual decision making. *Journal of Behavioral Decision Making, 19*(2), 87–98.

Ariely, D., & Wertenbroch, K. (2002). Procrastination, deadlines, and performance: Self-control by precommitment. *Psychological Science, 13*(3), 219–224.

Bagozzi, R. P. (1992). The self-regulation of attitudes, intentions, and behavior. *Social Psychology Quarterly, 55*(2), 178–204.

Bagozzi, R. P. (2006). Automaticity, purposiveness, and self-regulation. In N. K. Malhotra (Ed.), *Review of marketing research* (Vol. 2, pp. 3–42). Armonk, NY: Sharpe.

Bagozzi, R. P., Baumgartner, H., & Pieters, R. (1998). Goal-directed emotions. *Cognition and Emotion, 12*(1), 1–26.

Bagozzi, R. P., & Dholakia, U. M. (1999). Goal setting and goal striving in consumer behavior. *Journal of Marketing, 63*(4), 19–32.

Baumeister, R. F. (2002). Yielding to temptation: Self-control failure, impulsive purchasing, and consumer behavior. *Journal of Consumer Research, 28*(4), 670–676.

Baumeister, R. F., Vohs, K. D., & Tice, D. M. (2007). The strength model of self-control. *Current Directions in Psychological Science, 16*(6), 351–355.

Baumgartner, H., Pieters, R., & Bagozzi, R. P. (2008). Future-oriented emotions: Conceptualization and behavioral effects. *European Journal of Social Psychology, 38*(4), 685–696.

Beatty, S. E., & Ferrell, E. M. (1998). Impulse buying: Modeling its precursors. *Journal of Retailing, 74*(2), 169–191.

Belk, R. W., Ger, G., & Askegaard, S. (2003). The fire of desire: A multisited inquiry into consumer passion. *Journal of Consumer Research, 30*(3), 326–351.

Bell, D. R., Corsten, D., & Knox, G. (2011). From point of purchase to path to purchase: How preshopping factors drive unplanned buying. *Journal of Marketing, 75*(1), 31–45.

Black, D. W. (2007). A review of compulsive buying disorder. *World Psychiatry, 6*(1), 14–18.

Bloch, P. H., Ridgway, N. M., & Nelson, J. E. (1991). Leisure and the shopping mall. *Advances in Consumer Research, 18,* 445–452.

Braddock, K. H., Dillard, J. P., Voigt, D. C., Stephenson, M. T., Sopory, P., & Anderson, J. W. (2011). Impulsivity partially mediates the relationship between BIS/BAS and risky health behaviors. *Journal of Personality, 79*(4), 793–810.

Chen, Y. (2009). Possession and access: Consumer desires and value perceptions regarding contemporary art collection and exhibit visits. *Journal of Consumer Research, 35*(6), 925–940.

Covenant Eyes. (2013). Pornography statistics. Available at *www.covenanteyes.com.*

Davis, W. A. (1984). The two senses of desire. *Philosophical Studies, 45*(2), 181–195.

de Witt Huberts, J. C., Evers, C., & de Ridder, D. T. (2012). License to sin: Self-licensing as a mechanism underlying hedonic consumption. *European Journal of Social Psychology, 42*(4), 490–496.

Dholakia, U. M. (2000). Temptation and resistance: An integrated model of consumption impulse formation and enactment. *Psychology and Marketing, 17*(11), 955–982.

Dholakia, U. M., Bagozzi, R. P., & Klein Pearo, L. (2004). A social influence model of consumer participation in network- and small-group-based virtual communities. *International Journal of Research in Marketing, 21*(3), 241–263.

Dholakia, U. M., Gopinath, M., & Bagozzi, R. P. (2005). The role of desires in sequential impulsive choices. *Organizational Behavior and Human Decision Processes, 98*(2), 179–194.

Dholakia, U. M., Gopinath, M., Bagozzi, R. P., & Nataraajan, R. (2006). The role of regulatory focus in the experience and self-control of desire for temptations. *Journal of Consumer Psychology, 16*(2), 163–175.

Faber, R. J., & O'Guinn, T. C. (1992). A clinical screener for compulsive buying. *Journal of Consumer Research, 19*(2), 459–469.

Fujita, K., Trope, Y., Liberman, N., & Levin-Sagi, M. (2006). Construal levels and self control. *Journal of Personality and Social Psychology, 90*(3), 351–367.

Gollwitzer, P. M. (1999). Implementation intentions: Strong effects of simple plans. *American Psychologist, 54*(7), 493–503.

Hassay, D. N., & Smith, M. C. (1996). Compulsive buying: An examination of the consumption motive. *Psychology and Marketing, 13*(8), 741–752.

Hirschman, E. C., & Holbrook, M. B. (1982). Hedonic consumption: Emerging concepts, methods and propositions. *Journal of Marketing, 46*(3), 92–101.

Hoch, S. J., & Loewenstein, G. F. (1991). Time-inconsistent preferences and consumer self-control. *Journal of Consumer Research, 17*(4), 492–507.

Hofmann, W., Friese, M., & Strack, F. (2009). Impulse and self-control from a dual-systems perspective. *Perspectives on Psychological Science, 4*(2), 162–176.

Hofmann, W., & Van Dillen, L. (2012). Desire: The new hot spot in self-control research. *Current Directions in Psychological Science, 21*(5), 317–322.

Inzlicht, M., & Schmeichel, B. J. (2012). What is ego depletion?: Toward a mechanistic revision of the resource model of self-control. *Perspectives on Psychological Science, 7*(5), 450–463.

Kacen, J. J., & Lee, J. A. (2002). The influence of culture on consumer impulsive buying behavior. *Journal of Consumer Psychology, 12*(2), 163–176.

Kavanagh, D. J., Andrade, J., & May, J. (2005). Imaginary relish and exquisite torture: The elaborated intrusion theory of desire. *Psychological Review, 112*(2), 446–467.

Kemps, E., Tiggemann, M., & Grigg, M. (2008). Food cravings consume limited cognitive resources. *Journal of Experimental Psychology: Applied, 14*(3), 247–254.

Kenyon, S. (2012). *Time untime.* New York: St. Martin's Press.

Khan, U., & Dhar, R. (2007). Where there is a way, is there a will?: The effect of future choices on self-control. *Journal of Experimental Psychology: General, 136*(2), 277–288.

Kim, H. (2013). Situational materialism: How entering lotteries may undermine self-control. *Journal of Consumer Research, 40*(4), 759–772.

Kollat, D. T., & Willett, R. P. (1967). Customer impulse purchasing behavior. *Journal of Marketing Research, 4*(1), 21–31.

Koran, L., Faber, R., Aboujaoude, E., Large, M., & Serpe, R. (2006). Estimated prevalence of compulsive buying behavior in the United States. *American Journal of Psychiatry, 163*(10), 1806–1812.

Kotler, P. (1974). Atmospherics as a marketing tool. *Journal of Retailing, 49*(4), 49–64.

Kühl, J. (1987). Action control: The maintenance of motivational states. In F. Halisch & J. Kühl (Eds.), *Motivation, intention, and volition* (pp. 279–291). Berlin: Springer.

Kwon, M., Lee, J. Y., Won, W. Y., Park, J. W., Min, J. A., Hahn, C., et al. (2013). Development and validation of a smartphone addiction scale (SAS). *PLoS One, 8*(2), e56936.

Lejoyeux, M., & Weinstein, A. (2010). Compulsive buying. *American Journal of Drug and Alcohol Abuse, 36*, 248–253.

Mischel, H. N., & Mischel, W. (1983). The development of children's knowledge of self-control strategies. *Child Development*, 603–619.

Mukhopadhyay, A., & Johar, G. V. (2009). Indulgence as self-reward for prior shopping restraint: A justification-based mechanism. *Journal of Consumer Psychology, 19*(3), 334–345.

Mukhopadhyay, A., Sengupta, J., & Ramanathan, S. (2008). Recalling past temptations: An information-processing perspective on the dynamics of self-control. *Journal of Consumer Research, 35*(4), 586–599.

Perugini, M., & Bagozzi, R. P. (2004). The distinction between desires and intentions. *European Journal of Social Psychology, 34*(1), 69–84.

Plutchik, R., & Van Praag, H. M. (1995). The nature of impulsivity: Definitions, ontology, genetics, and relations to aggression. In E. Hollander & D. J. Stein (Eds.), *Impulsivity and aggression*. Oxford, UK: Wiley.

Redden, J., & Haws, K. (2013). Healthy satiation: The role of decreasing desire in effective self-control. *Journal of Consumer Research, 39*(5), 1100–1114.

Ridgway, N. M., Kukar-Kinney, M., & Monroe, K. B. (2008). An expanded conceptualization and a new measure of compulsive buying. *Journal of Consumer Research, 35*(4), 622–639.

Rook, D. W. (1987) The buying impulse. *Journal of Consumer Research, 14*(2), 87–113.

Rook, D. W., & Fisher, R. J. (1995). Normative influences on impulsive buying behavior. *Journal of Consumer Research, 22*(3), 305–313.

Rook, D. W., & Gardner, M. P. (1993). In the mood: Impulse buying's affective antecedents. In J. Arnold-Costa & R. W. Belk (Eds.), *Research in consumer behavior* (Vol. 6, pp. 1–28). Greenwich, CT: JAI Press.

Salovey, P., & Mayer, J. D. (1990). Emotional intelligence. *Imagination, Cognition, and Personality, 9*, 185–211.

Schmeichel, B. J., Harmon-Jones, C., & Harmon-Jones, E. (2010). Exercising self-control increases approach motivation. *Journal of Personality and Social Psychology, 99*(1), 162–173.

Schwartz, G. (2011). *The impulse economy: Understanding mobile shoppers and what makes them buy.* New York: Altria Books.

Searle, J. R. (1999). *Mind, language and society: Philosophy in the real world.* New York: Basic Books.

Steketee, G., & Frost, R. (2003). Compulsive hoarding: Current status of the research. *Clinical Psychology Review, 23*(7), 905–927.

Stilley, K. M., Inman, J. J., & Wakefield, K. L. (2010). Planning to make unplanned purchases?: The role of in-store slack in budget deviation. *Journal of Consumer Research, 37*(2), 264–278.

Trope, Y., & Liberman, N. (2010). Construal-level theory of psychological distance. *Psychological Review, 117*(2), 440–463.

Vallacher, R. R. (1983). Thinking is believing. *Contemporary Psychology, 28*(2), 104–106.

Van den Bergh, B., Dewitte, S., & Warlop, L. (2008). Bikinis instigate generalized impatience in intertemporal choice. *Journal of Consumer Research, 35*(1), 85–97.

Verplanken, B., & Sato, A. (2011). The psychology of impulse buying: An integrative self-regulation approach. *Journal of Consumer Policy, 34*, 197–210.

Wertenbroch, K. (1998). Consumption self-control by rationing purchase quantities of virtue and vice. *Marketing Science, 17*(4), 317–337.

Weun, S., Jones, M. A., & Beatty, S. E. (1998). The development and validation of the impulse buying tendency scale. *Psychological Reports, 82*, 1123–1133.

Xie, C., Bagozzi, R. P., & Østli, J. (2013). Cognitive, emotional, and sociocultural processes in consumption. *Psychology and Marketing, 30*(1), 12–25.

Youn, S., & Faber, R. J. (2000). Impulse buying: Its relation to personality traits and cues. In S. J. Hoch & R. J. Meyer (Eds.), *Advances in consumer research* (Vol. 27, pp. 179–185). Provo, UT: Association for Consumer Research.

CHAPTER 21

Old Desires, New Media

Diana I. Tamir
Adrian F. Ward

We are social animals. We live, work, and play side by side with other people, constantly communicating, interacting, and connecting. And we take advantage of every opportunity to surround ourselves with yet more social stimuli—the televisions in our homes, computers in our offices, and smartphones in our pockets all serve as portals to social worlds. In fact, the digital social stimuli provided by "new media" seem to dominate our social lives; the average adult American spends over 5 hours of "leisure time" a day watching television, over an hour online, and an additional hour accessing the web via smartphone (Nielsen, 2014). These numbers, particularly those related to Internet use, are growing every year (Rainie, Fox, & Duggan, 2014). Digital supplements to our physical social worlds may even be evolving into replacements for face-to-face social connection. Research shows that time spent online is negatively correlated with going to parties, attending cultural events, and socializing with other people in a variety of offline domains (Wallsten, 2013). As social animals in a digital world, we seem to obsessively log on, tune in, and exchange face-to-face interaction for social content delivered through a screen.

Our insatiable desire to connect with new media may be a product of social minds gone astray. Our social minds, from our most basic to our most advanced neurocognitive processes, encourage us to seek out social connection and enable us to succeed in achieving our social goals. New media offer simple solutions to complex social needs. With the change of a channel, we can connect with our "neighbor" Mr. Rogers or our "friends" on *Friends*; with the tap of a button, we can relive social events through Facebook photos or communicate with relationship partners on the other side of the earth. At times, these solutions may be real. At other times, however, our social minds may motivate behaviors that provide only the *illusion* of adaptive functioning. They may provide immediate cues of social acceptance, without ever actually increasing social connectedness. New media may allow us to swap family dinner for TV dinners and *Family Matters* reruns, or attend social events by simply viewing the Facebook photos—and may motivate us to continue doing so.

In this chapter, we provide an overview of how our pervasive connection to new media is encouraged by our social minds, and what these digitized social interactions might mean for real-world social outcomes. We explore the bases of our need for social connection, the brain's reward system that motivates us to seek out social stimuli, and the mentalizing system that allows us to succeed in our social endeavors. We then turn to an analysis of how these components of our social minds contribute to our desire to find and create social connection through our screens. Finally, we offer some perspective on what this all might mean—whether our social minds are ruining or enhancing our relationships, both online and off.

Building Blocks of a Social Mind

Our motivation to connect with others is not new; Twitter didn't create our desire to share personal experiences, Facebook didn't create our desire to maintain relationships, and Reddit didn't create our desire to find communities consistent with our interests. Rather, our widespread use of new media as a conduit for social connection may stem from a fundamental need to belong—a core need to feel connected with others as a result of both frequent social interaction and strong interpersonal relationships (Baumeister & Leary, 1995).

The adaptive significance of social connection may seem to pale in comparison to basic biological needs such as food and sex. However, interpersonal connections can provide massive adaptive benefits by increasing the likelihood of meeting more basic biological needs. Groups increase proximity, improving the odds of both reproductive success (access to potential mates) and physical survival (safety in numbers); groups allow for cooperation, enabling more efficient food acquisition via cooperative agriculture and hunting; groups give rise to communication, through which people can bypass costly trial-and-error forms of learning in favor of socially provided secondary knowledge about potential dangers and rewards. Groups increase the potential to not just survive, but also to thrive (Holt-Lunstad, Smith, & Layton, 2010); achieving sufficiently strong social bonds enhances psychological well-being and protects individuals from feelings of loneliness and depression (Helliwell & Putnam, 2004).

The evolutionarily adaptive and psychologically positive implications of connection depend on a social structure that encourages repeated positive interactions. Communities are defined by connection, a concept distinct from mere social contact. In connected communities, each individual can reasonably infer that other members of the group can be relied on as hunting companions or mates, they can develop shared experiences, they can pay prosocial behavior back (or forward), and so on. These and other benefits associated with consistent positive interactions in early humans may have led to the emergence of the highly social nature of humans today (Dunbar & Shultz, 2007; Nowak & Sigmund, 2005; Tomasello, 1999) and established social connection as one of our most fundamental motives.

Our ability to satisfy this fundamental need to belong is supported by two systems: our most basic neurocognitive structures and some of our most uniquely human cognitive abilities. Our reward system labels social cues as positive stimuli and encourages behaviors consistent with pursuing social acceptance. Our ability to mentalize—or think about the minds of others—enables us to navigate social interactions in ways likely to maximize connection. Importantly, each of these generally adaptive systems may sometimes get off track—they may motivate us to engage in behaviors that *feel* social, but in fact do nothing to increase our social connectedness.

Social Motivation, and Social Motives Led Astray

Over the last few decades, the emergence of cognitive neuroscience has enabled the identification and exploration of the neural cytoarchitecture and computations involved in motivation and reward processing. One group of structures in particular—the dopaminergic reward system—has been implicated in both identifying rewards and motivating reward-consistent behavior (see also Kringelbach & Berridge, Chapter 6, this volume; Lopez, Wagner, & Heatherton, Chapter 7, this volume). This system plays a fundamental role in motivating goal-directed behavior. It connects instrumental behaviors and cues of reward with experienced outcomes, increasing the likelihood of performing behaviors that result in rewarding outcomes and decreasing the likelihood of performing behaviors likely to result in aversive outcomes. The neural regions (e.g., ventral tegmental area [VTA], ventral striatum [VS]) and neurotransmitters (e.g., dopamine) that compose this system have been implicated in motivating goal-directed behavior related to everything from basic physical needs such as food acquisition (Berridge, 1996) to more complex—but no less adaptive—needs such as social cooperation (Rilling et al., 2002).

Our motivation to connect with others, much like the motivation to pursue basic physiological needs such as food or sex, is associated with activity in the brain's reward system. Social interactions and social stimuli (e.g., faces) recruit these reward-related neural substrates (Aharon et al., 2001; Meshi, Morawetz, & Heekeren, 2013; Mobbs, Greicius, Abdel-Azim,

Menon, & Reiss, 2003; Mobbs et al., 2009; Tricomi, Rangel, Camerer, & O'Doherty, 2010). These regions are also implicated in the formation of intimate attachments: the early stages of romantic love are typified by dopaminergic activity in the VTA (Aron et al., 2005), and analogous dopaminergic systems are implicated in the coupling behavior of a wide range of species that form long-lasting relationships, including (but not limited to) monogamous prairie voles (Gingrich, Liu, Cascio, Wang, & Insel, 2000). Importantly, activity in reward-related neural systems during interpersonal interactions is not just signaling the possibility of sex (a primary reinforce), it is also associated with engaging in cooperative interactions more generally (Rilling et al., 2002). Taken together, this evidence suggests that the reward system motivates a broad range of social behaviors, from the pursuit of acceptance in initial social encounters to the selection of a long-term mate.

The reward system both *labels* and *predicts* rewards. When a particular positive stimulus is encountered for the first time, reward activity serves to call our attention to the presence of this stimulus ("something good is happening"); over repeated experiences, this activity shifts forward in time to call our attention to the *possibility* of encountering this stimulus ("something good is about to happen"). For example, a comedian telling a joke may experience a surge in dopaminergic activity not when the joke "lands" and the audience bursts into laughter, but when the joke is told—when the possibility of laughter is first created. However, unfulfilled expectations of reward result in depressed dopaminergic activity, encouraging the correction of misguided anticipations of reward. If a comedian's joke is met with silence rather than laughter, the silence in the audience—and corresponding depression of dopaminergic activity—will ensure that the joke is never told again.

However, the threshold for positive feedback—for getting the sense that a goal-directed behavior has "landed"—may not always coincide with the actual achievement of a desired outcome. Not all goals are as cut and dried as food acquisition, where one can be reasonably sure that one has or has not eaten a piece of chocolate cake; neither are all social goals as straightforward as moving an audience to laughter. More ambiguous goals, such as those involved in day-to-day social interactions, may rely on "proxy" cues to signal successful goal pursuit. For example, it can often be difficult to know how liked or accepted one is by one's peers, but it's much easier to know whether or not a remark has elicited a smile. In this way, the reward system response may not actually provide any direct insight into the desired outcome (e.g., social acceptance), only the existence of an easily identifiable proxy cue (e.g., a smiling face, or a virtual "like"). These signals commonly co-occur with the desired outcomes, but importantly, they are not perfect indicators. An acquaintance's smile could be no more than a social nicety and a "like" on Facebook may represent only an illusory cue of social acceptance.

The brain's reward system can also be stimulated by cues even further dissociated from actual goal achievement. Research on imagination indicates that positive fantasies about future outcomes allow individuals to simulate goal achievement, and these simulations allow them to experience positive feedback based on imagined—rather than actual—success (see also Andrade, May, Van Dillen, & Kavanagh, Chapter 1, this volume). As a result, positive fantasies undermine motivation and reduce the likelihood of meeting goals related to everything from weight management to relationship acquisition to professional advancement (Oettingen & Mayer, 2002). The reward system motivates us to engage with the social world, but because this system is sensitive to proxy cues of social connection—smiles, "likes," or even imagined acceptance—it may often reinforce behaviors that elicit these cues, even when the cues no longer predict meaningful social connection.

Mentalizing, and Mentalizing Led Astray

Our brain's reward system supports our basic motivations to pursue social connection. Our capacity for *actually* connecting with others depends upon our ability to mentalize, or to think about others' internal thoughts and feelings (Waytz, Zaki, & Mitchell, 2012). This mentalizing system supports a sophisticated and perhaps even uniquely human set of cognitive processes and neural structures (Buckner & Krienen, 2013; Dunbar & Shultz, 2007). Thinking about others' mental states allows us to infer their intentions, make sense of their behaviors, and respond in ways that build trust and demonstrate understanding.

Our capacity for mentalizing is not just an ability, but an overwhelming tendency; the minds of others pervade our own thoughts. When we encounter other people, we automatically think about their mental states, make inferences about their beliefs, and intuit their intentions (Malle, 2005; Malle & Hodges, 2005). These inferences and intuitions grease the wheels of interaction, communication, and connection. Our social orientation is active even in the absence of others. When our minds are not directed toward pursuing specific goals or completing externally imposed tasks, they often turn toward the social world—ruminating about the mental states of relationship partners, replaying and analyzing past social encounters, and imagining future interactions from the banal to the fantastical (Buckner & Carroll, 2007; Mars et al., 2012; Schilbach, Eickhoff, Rotarska-Jagiela, Fink, & Vogeley, 2008a, 2008b). Our dedication of vast amounts of temporal and cognitive resources to mentalizing about others is yet another indication of the extent to which the social world permeates our mental lives.

This remarkable ability to infer others' thoughts, beliefs, and intentions could be devoted to staying one step ahead of those around us, always engaging in some sort of high-stakes rock-paper-scissors. More often than not, however, we use our social minds to form and maintain social connections. While affiliation seems to stand at odds with competition, the bedrock of evolutionary theory, a long history of psychological research suggests that the motivation to maximize social connection is often more powerful than competitive motives. Competitors will unite around a common cause with minimal resistance; mere social contact can trump long-standing prejudices and tensions (Sherif, Harvey, White, Hood, & Sherif, 1961; Wilder & Thompson, 1980). Indeed, the mere presence of subtle social cues prompts people to forgo selfish behaviors for more prosocial ones (Bohnet & Frey, 1999; Ward et al., 2014). Prosociality may even be a more intuitive strategy than selfishness. Recent research has demonstrated that people make more prosocial decisions when forced to make these decisions quickly (Rand, Greene, & Nowak, 2012; Rand et al., 2014; Zaki & Mitchell, 2013)—evidence that cooperation and generosity in our daily lives may represent our default response, rather than a result of effortful control over selfish impulses. Although the dynamics of interpersonal behavior are complex, one motivation seems to stand the strongest and shine the brightest: the motivation to connect with those around us.

Like the brain's reward system, our proclivity for mentalizing may sometimes lead us away from, rather than toward, social connection. The tendency to think in social terms may cause us to see social stimuli (or minds) even where they do not exist. We see faces in the clouds, anthropomorphize invisible deities, accuse malfunctioning computers of intentional sabotage, and treat our pets as confidants, children, and best friends (Epley, Waytz, & Cacioppo, 2007). In the extreme, this ability to imagine alternate realities, combined with our tendency to devote our daydreams to social interactions, allows us to not just imagine social stimuli, but to interact with these stimuli—to communicate with invisible deities, marry animals (Matthews, 1994), and create fantastical relationships with celebrities, characterized by intimacy, acceptance, and belonging (Greenwood & Long, 2010). People are most apt to create their own social worlds at the times when they need actual social connection the most, suggesting that this ability functions to serve our need for social connection and stave off feelings of loneliness (Epley, Akalis, Waytz, & Cacioppo, 2008; Waytz et al., 2010).

Motivation, Mentalizing, and Media

Our brains seem built for social connection. Our reward system encourages us to seek out social interactions and our ability to mentalize enables us to successfully connect with others. These two mechanisms for motivating and maximizing social connection often work in tandem to help us achieve evolutionarily adaptive goals. However, they may also lead us astray: the motivation to pursue social connection may be satisfied by illusory proxy cues of connection—cues that we unwittingly overendow with social significance.

Many of our interactions with new media may present cases of this type, in which these mechanisms for maximizing social connection are redirected not toward actual social connection but merely toward the cues typically associated with connection. The motivation we have for engaging with new media may be remarkably similar to the motivation we have for forming and developing face-to-face relationships. This is because media—even in its most rudimentary forms—presents a perfect environment for social-seeking minds. Humans have the unique ability to drastically reshape their environment, just as much as they are shaped by it (Kareiva, Watts, McDonald, & Boucher, 2007; Pani, 2000), and our desires are now shaping the environment. Our desire for calorie-rich food is exemplified by the proliferation of fast-food joints and an obesity epidemic, and our desire for social connection may be best exemplified by the rapid rise of media. New media put our social minds into overdrive by providing near constant social cues and opening up myriad new avenues of human interaction without the same constraints imposed by offline realities. Here we discuss these two ways in which media capitalize upon our mentalizing and motivational systems, in turn.

Social Connection through a TV Screen

Research on *parasocial interaction*—the illusory "give and take" between media users and media personalities—suggests that people often form interpersonal attachments with media persona (Horton & Wohl, 1956). Even though the viewer may be separated from politicians, performers, and the characters they play by a pane of glass, a thousand miles, or a dozen years, attachments with these people mimic the experience of relationships one might have with a close friend. These attachments can feel significant and intimate, leaving the viewer with a sense that he or she knows and understands a media personality as only a true friend could; in fact, research indicates that people think about media personalities and face-to-face interaction partners in very similar ways (Reeves & Greenberg, 1977; Reeves & Lometti, 1979; Reeves & Nass, 1996). Consistent with the idea that social connection grows from repeated interactions, parasocial relationships seem to form automatically as the viewer spends more time engaging with media; the more hours viewers spend watching television, the more likely they are to develop parasocial relationships, and the more significant these relationships become (Greenwood, 2008). Although these relationships may seem impoverished from the outside, the individuals seeking social connection don't always differentiate between the social and the parasocial.

The similarities between physical and digital social connection suggest that some individuals might use media as a source of social connection in place of face-to-face interaction. Indeed, individuals who feel especially in need of social connection often turn to parasocial relationships to fill this need (Russell, Cutrona, Rose, & Yurko, 1984). That is, individuals who are lonely, introverted, or have low self-esteem experience an increased desire for companionship, and this desire often leads them to seek connection through a TV screen (Finn & Gorr, 1988; Jonason, Webster, & Lindsey, 2008; Rubin, Perse, & Powell, 1985; Tsao, 1996; Weaver, 2003). The resulting strong parasocial attachments to television characters allow these individuals to compensate for their lack of actual social connections by forming imaginary connections with relationship partners they can call up any time, "on demand" (Derrick, Gabriel, & Hugenberg, 2009; Knowles, 2007). Importantly, people would not be able to find social comfort in TV were it not for our ability to mentalize. Research on anthropomorphization suggests that the feeling of loneliness makes people more likely to see social cues and minds even where there are none (Epley et al., 2008; Waytz et al., 2010). When applied to TV characters, this process allows individuals who feel particularly in need of social connection to more readily endow television characters with the social and mental properties with which they so desperately need to interact. These individuals often find the companionship they are seeking. Parasocial relationships decrease loneliness and feelings of exclusion, at least in the short term. Thinking about a favorite television character provides a buffer against feelings of exclusion, much like the buffer provided by thinking about a "real life" friend. Indeed, people who feel lonely or excluded often choose to think about television characters rather than other social figures in their lives as a way regaining a subjective sense of connection (Gardner, Pickett, & Knowles, 2005). Though parasocial relationships may be easy to criticize from the outside, they seem to serve an important function for those seeking connection: the sense of companionship offered by these relationships may protect the formerly disconnected from future feelings of loneliness and isolation (Horton & Wohl, 1956). Even in the absence of loneliness or exclusion, thinking about a favorite TV character causes people to feel a greater sense of global belonging (Derrick et al., 2009).

Television does not simply rely on viewers' tendency to see the world in social terms or fabricate social connection based on subtle cues. Rather than waiting for viewers to create immersive relationships with fabricated minds, broadcasting practices have evolved to intentionally engender this sense of social connection, seducing the viewer into a relationship that remains, at its core, unidirectional. From the earliest days of broadcast journalism, media personalities were instructed to create feelings of friendliness and intimacy (Scannell, 1996), and the hallmarks of their methods—for example, patterns of verbal communication and body language, just the right amount of eye contact, and an informal style—have been shown to increase the intensity of parasocial connections (Hartmann & Goldhoorn, 2011). As the format grew, television personalities became more explicit in their intention to connect with audiences, with Mr. Rogers famously asking every viewer to be his friend, his companion, his "neighbor." More recently, the advent of "reality television" has transformed media personalities from idealized figures to "people like us"; this sense of "hyperauthenticity" (Rose & Wood, 2005) further amplifies the intimacy people feel with the characters on their screens (Rubin et al., 1985).

The evolution of television programming serves as an example of people crafting a world tailor-made to fulfill their social desires. Television media can route our desire for social connection—usually achieved though relationships with our families, friends, or acquaintances—into experiences of connection through a screen. Indeed, these parasocial relationships offer many of the same intrapsychic benefits as real relationships. But interactions offered by television are necessarily limited. Television viewers and media personas remain separated from each other by glass, distance, and time. Even the best attempts at creating a sense of intimacy or reality cannot offer "true" interactions. The efforts of broadcasters and imaginations of viewers notwithstanding, viewers may feel like they are connected to their favorite media personalities—but they might not always feel like these personalities are connected to them.

Social Connection through a Computer Screen

The evolution of media over the past hundred or so years reveals an attempt, whether conscious or not, to create a world consistent with our social desires; formal newsreels gave way to informal broadcasts, informal broadcasts evolved into talk shows with sets inviting viewers to insert themselves into the conversation (e.g., *The Tonight Show*), invitations to public conversation paved the way for invitations into private living rooms (e.g., *Mr. Rogers' Neighborhood*), and these simulations of intimacy ultimately gave way to real (or "real") intimacy (e.g., *The Real World*). The Internet takes this evolution to the extreme and, in doing so, expertly capitalizes on people's desire for social connection. The Internet builds upon the strengths of television to feed our desire for social cues, while also addressing some of the inherent limitations in earlier media's capacity for offering seemingly meaningful interaction.

Although the Internet was originally conceived of as an "information management system" (Leiner et al., 2012), it has quickly transformed into a tool for social connection. The Internet in its current form is capable of satisfying our desire for social connection by providing more extensive, more immersive, and more interactive opportunities to engage with others around the world. And people are taking advantage of this tool in ever-growing numbers. From 2005 to 2014, the number of American adults using the Internet rose at a steady clip, climbing from 66% to 87%, and nearly reaching full saturation (Rainie et al., 2014). In this same time span, adults' use of online social networking sites has risen from just 8% to 67%—an increase of 738% (Brenner, 2013). As a result of this widespread and rapid adoption of digital tools for social connection, social networking has become the number one activity on the web (Tancer, 2008). More and more people are spending more and more time online—and they're dedicating the majority of this time to the pursuit of social connection.

One way in which the Internet has built upon earlier forms of media is by providing users opportunities to "know" others in ways that would not otherwise be possible. Through sites such as Facebook and Twitter, performers, personalities, and political figures can now send their thoughts *directly* to their audiences, unhindered by temporal delays or carefully managed scripts. Social media break down the walls between individuals and media personalities, creating the illusion of direct, unmediated social interaction and communication (Lee & Jang, 2013). Even when the Internet is used for this type of unidirectional communication (much like television), people perceive this communication as being more interactive—as if it were part of an ongoing, real-time, intimate conversation (Pempek, Yermolayeva, & Calvert, 2009). And people value simply receiving information from others in a social context (Tamir & Mitchell, 2014), suggesting that the perceived interactive intimacy afforded by social media may act as a rewarding cue of social connection.

Not only does the Internet allow for more intimate connections with famous media personalities, it also vastly expands the number of nonfamous individuals we can "know" and interact with. In the days of television, parasocial relationships with famous personalities were one of the few options people had for fulfilling the desire for social connection outside the bounds of face-to-face interactions. Creating a connection with nonfamous individuals was not a viable option simply because our ability to connect with others outside of our neighborhoods and television screens was limited. However, the advent of the Internet has created a fundamental change in the scale of our connective abilities. We can now connect with *anyone*, from long-lost relatives to anonymous message board users. In this regard, the Internet trumps not only television, but real life as well, by providing users unparalleled access to others' lives.

As outlined above, the Internet allows for a dramatic increase in the intimacy and access that allow one to "know" others compared to older forms of media. However, fulfilling the need to belong entails much more than just observing others' lives. In order to experience a sense of belonging, people need meaningful social interactions, and the Internet affords users just that: the opportunity to not just observe, but share—to broadcast their own lives and draw others into their personal experiences. By opening up a passageway from the lives of individuals to the outside social world, the Internet marks a fundamental advance over previous forms of media.

In everyday life, people often try to attain the adaptive outcomes associated with social connection by sharing information about themselves with others. Talking about oneself engenders affinity between conversation partners and increases the likelihood of forming strong social bonds (Cozby, 1972, 1973). Much as the level of intimacy conveyed by talk-show hosts determines the intensity of our parasocial relationships, the level of intimacy conveyed through our own speech has a large impact on the intensity and quality of our interpersonal connections. Disclosing personal information may be the most intimate of all forms of communication. Further, when we share information with others, we increase the likelihood of others sharing information with us in the future, a positive feedback loop enabling greater and greater cohesion (Bowles & Gintis, 2002). The immense importance of self-disclosure to our social lives is borne out in analyses of human conversational patterns, where researchers find that approximately 30–40% of our conversations are devoted to talking about our own personal experiences (Dunbar, Marriott, & Duncan, 1997; Dunbar & Shultz, 2007; Emler, 1990, 1994; Landis & Burtt, 1924).

As with other means to adaptive ends, sharing information with others is associated with activity in the reward system (Tamir & Mitchell, 2012; Tamir, Zaki, & Mitchell, 2014). In these studies, not only did sharing information result in activity in the brain's reward system, participants were also willing to give up significant sums of money for opportunities to disclose information with others. Sharing information specifically about the *self*—or engaging in self-disclosure—trumps all other forms of communication in terms of both subjective reward and the level of activity in the reward system (Tamir & Mitchell, 2012; Yamaguchi et al., 2007). This research supports the idea that people are highly motivated to self-disclose.

The Internet has hijacked this extreme desire to self-disclose. Social media platforms such as Facebook, YouTube, and Twitter are built entirely upon user-generated content. People's unusually high drive to provide content has contributed to the remarkable success of these social sharing sites (ranked the number two, three, and nine most visited websites in the world, respectively). However, the Internet does not simply provide a venue for fulfilling our desire to disclose; rather, it exploits these desires by continuously evolving into an environment unconstrained by factors that limit this self-disclosure in offline social interactions. First, whereas face-to-face interactions often necessitate small audiences, the audience for social media is virtually limitless. When sharing information we can choose to tell a few close friends . . . or we can tell hundreds of Facebook friends and Twitter followers in just a fraction of the time. We are no longer constrained by proximity, and larger audiences mean greater opportunities for far-reaching self-disclosure. Second, Internet users don't have to abide by social norms that define face-to-face interactions. For example, in everyday conversation, disclosers must listen to information shared by others in between sharing information about themselves. The Internet releases individuals from this "norm of reciprocity." No longer are individuals limited by social norms such as waiting your turn, or self-disclosing in only limited doses. Instead, people can share unlimited quantities of information, gluttonously feeding their desire to self-disclose without restraint. And while the interactions enabled by new media may still be somewhat impoverished when compared to face-to-face experiences, this has not stymied self-disclosure on the Internet in the least. Instead, this new online social environment built around our self-disclosure desires has allowed this behavior to flourish: self-disclosure is so pervasive online that researchers estimate over 80% of activity on social media sites consists simply of announcing one's own immediate experiences (Naaman, Boase, & Lai, 2010). The Internet allows us to share information with the world to an extent previously unimaginable.

We have a deeply rooted desire to maximize social connection. As we have shaped the Internet, we have created a system uniquely tailored to fulfill our desires. Our habitual use of this system suggests that we have been successful. With its ever-growing and ever-evolving suite of social networking websites, communities, and applications, the Internet appears to provide access to endless venues for our social connection desires.

But are we *really* connecting? Do our mediated social interactions truly fulfill the *need* to belong, a need previously fulfilled only through face-to-face social interactions? Or do they merely fulfill our *desires*, providing an internal sense that we have taken meaningful strides toward achieving our social goals without actually providing any long-term, substantive benefit? Our dopaminergic reward system motivates adaptive behavior by moving rewards forward in time; we experience reward not necessarily when long-term adaptive outcomes are achieved, but when we receive cues suggesting that our actions in the here-and-now are consistent with these more distal outcomes. This focus on short-term cues over long-term outcomes allows for flexible and environment-sensitive behavior, often increasing the chance that we will achieve the desired long-term outcomes; however, this short-term focus also creates the possibility that our behavior may be motivated by short-term cues even when these cues become divorced from long-term adaptive functioning. In the context of face-to-face interactions, self-disclosure often increases our chances of reaping the adaptive rewards offered by increased social connection and group belonging (Cozby, 1973); for much of human existence—indeed, until the last 25 years—the short-term rewards associated with self-disclosure signaled that we were en route to achieving more long-term adaptive goals. However, when we channel our motivation to self-disclose through new media, we may often swap face-to-face conversations for a series of Tweets, or catching up over coffee for a session of Facebook "stalking." In this new world, is the connection between self-disclosure and social connection real, or does it exist only in the mind of the Tweeter, blogger, or chronically oversharing Facebook user?

Consequences of Mediated Connection

The Internet may encourage us to seek out illusory cues related to goal completion without actually moving us any closer to achieving these goals—most notably, the long-term adaptive goal of maximizing social cohesion; we may mistake "likes" and "retweets" for actual social connection. On the other hand, the Internet may allow us to truly expand our social worlds; our online behaviors may still serve as means to an adaptive end—and the ends we can achieve may be greater than we could have ever imagined just twenty-five years ago. As is often the case, the true effects of the Internet on the connection between "social" behavior and long-term social outcomes likely lies somewhere between these two extremes, and may be different for different people in different situations.

Enhancing Social Connection

The types of interactions enabled by social media can both improve pre-existing offline relationships and allow for the formation and maintenance of relationships that may not have been possible without these new forms of communication. Much like the telephone or the postal service, the Internet expands the circle of individuals with whom one can realistically stay in contact. By reducing temporal, spatial, and social barriers to communication, social networking sites allow us to expand our relationship circles beyond close friends and family to include more distant friends and acquaintances (Steijn & Schouten, 2013), and can transform the task of maintaining long-distance relationships from the arduous to the effortless, replacing obligation with enjoyment (Wellman, Haase, Witte, & Hampton, 2001). This ability to reduce social and geographical distance may explain the association between using social network sites (e.g., Facebook) and improvements in both offline friendships and general social capital (Ellison, Steinfield, & Lampe, 2007; Steinfield, Ellison, & Lampe, 2008). Online social interactions can *augment* our offline relationships, increasing the quantity and improving the quality of our social interactions; in these instances, the Internet seems to have overwhelmingly positive effects for both our social lives and our well-being more generally (Ahn & Shin, 2013; Valkenburg, Peter, & Schouten, 2006). Time spent online does reduce time spent face to face (Wallsten, 2013), but this tradeoff may still result in net positive social outcomes (Bargh & McKenna, 2004).

Creating Social Connection

Online social media may be particularly helpful in creating social oppor-tunities for individuals who lack sufficiently fulfilling face-to-face rela-tionships. For example, research suggests that social anxiety leads to defi-cits in both companionship and intimacy (Vernberg, Abwender, Ewell, & Beery, 1992), but the Internet seems to offer a solution for socially anx-ious individuals by providing a safe environment in which to practice social interactions and form interpersonal connections—connections that may never have been established if not for the anxiety-ameliorating environment offered by computer-mediated communication (Hughes, Rowe, Batey, & Lee, 2012). In these cases, social media may not simply *enhance* preexisting relationships, but potentially lead to the *creation* of new ones. Online platforms that allow for anonymous interaction pro-vide the least social pressure, but even non-anonymous interactions may reduce anxiety by allowing individuals the time and space to carefully craft messages. As a result, individuals who are shy, socially anxious, or generally avoidant of face-to-face interactions often turn to the Internet as a functional avenue for self-disclosure and social interaction (Orr et al., 2009; Papacharissi & Rubin, 2000; Sheldon, 2008; Valkenburg & Peter, 2007).

Similarly, individuals who are lonely, upset, or otherwise unsatisfied with their face-to-face relationships often turn to online social networks in an attempt to gain social support (Park, Kee, & Valenzuela, 2009). Though most Facebook users generally report feeling less lonely than non-users (Ryan & Xenos, 2011), the Internet may offer lonely users a source of social interaction left unfulfilled by face-to-face interactions. For some, it may provide their first chance to display themselves as they truly are—or as who they wish to be; for others, it may provide the promise of social support, interpersonal understanding, or simply an escape from unsat-isfying day-to-day and face-to-face interactions. For these individuals in particular need of social connection, the Internet may serve as an acces-sible alternative to face-to-face interactions—and may provide some of the benefits missing from their offline relationships, such as increases in self-esteem and perceived social support (Shaw & Gant, 2002).

Replacing Social Connection

For some, the Internet may appear to be a social paradise, one in which myriad barriers to social connection—the confines of time and space, the limitations created by social anxiety, the biases imposed by surface-level characteristics such as age, gender, or ethnicity, and so on—fall by the way-side. In this light, it is unsurprising that some may use computer-mediated interactions as replacements for face-to-face relationships. Unfortunately, however, evidence suggests that relying on online relationships for social connection—that is, using these interactions not to supplement or augment face-to-face interactions, but to *replace* them altogether—generally fails to result in the positive outcomes associated with more intimate face-to-face relationships (Papacharissi & Rubin, 2000).

Use of social media may have positive effects in the short term (Shaw & Gant, 2002), but getting one "like" on Facebook may not offer the same *sustained* meaning as a real compliment in real life (Forest & Wood, 2012). These opportunities for social connection offered by social media do not seem to fully satisfy the need for meaningful social connection provided by offline relationships. Individuals who feel like they *need* to go online for social support may be more likely to experience the short-term benefits of online social connection; however, in the long run, exchanging face-to-face for computer-mediated interactions often increases feelings of depression and loneliness (Kraut et al., 1998). Individuals who live a life online are particularly vulnerable to these potential costs of online interactions; when attempts to find social support online backfire—when the social "paradise" of the Internet turns out to be no more than a mirage—individuals who depend on the Internet for this support experience even less social support, report a lower quality of life, and exhibit more symptoms of depression than before turning to online sources of social connection (Korkeila, Kaarlas, Jääskeläinen, Vahlberg, & Taiminen, 2010; Weidman et al., 2012). For individuals who have nowhere else to go, the "solution" to these failures of social connection (turning to the Internet) simply exacerbates the problem (feelings of loneliness), potentially creating a self-defeating and self-reinforcing cycle of dependence on impoverished online relationships (Kim, LaRose, & Peng, 2009).

This cycle may explain why a need for social connection and dependence on media for social relationships is associated with addiction to online social networks (Baek, Bae, & Jang, 2013). Research suggests that, just like gambling or alcohol, Internet use can become a destructive addiction (Young, 1996). Internet addiction, also known as problematic Internet use (Morrison & Gore, 2010), can result in significant impairment in daily functioning (Hsu, Wen, & Wu, 2009; Lo, Wang, & Fang, 2005; Mitchell, Becker-Blease, & Finkelhor, 2005; Young, 2009). As with many other addictions, disconnecting from the Internet only enhances desire. Daily users who abstain from Facebook for just 48 hours report feeling an absence of social connection, and these feelings of missing out predict increases in subsequent Facebook use (Sheldon, Abad, & Hinsch, 2011)—much like the cravings of an addict in withdrawal may lead to subsequent overcompensation and overdose. This may explain, for example, why students who use Facebook spend less time studying than those who do not and, as a consequence, tend to have significantly lower GPAs (Kirschner & Karpinski, 2010). Despite the negative consequences for social, academic, and general well-being, individuals suffering from social problems persist in their preference for online over face-to-face interactions (Caplan, 2002, 2005). Taken together, the data paint a troubling picture for individuals who look online for solutions to their social problems (Kim et al., 2009).

Long-Term Consequences

Despite the gloom and doom suggested for those who use the Internet as a replacement for face-to-face social interactions, the full body of research conducted thus far paints a nuanced picture of the relationship between online connections, offline relationships, social well-being, and adaptive functioning. Across the board, it seems clear that we are motivated to pursue online social interactions; we post, tweet, and otherwise disclose information about ourselves, and we also attend to the information provided by others—although not always in the ways that typify face-to-face interactions. However, these online social interactions seem to create different outcomes for those who use online interactions to *augment* well-functioning offline relationships versus those who use online interactions to *replace* unsatisfying (or missing) offline relationships. Online social interactions that serve as extensions of offline relationships can help individuals increase social capital—for example, by maintaining connections with geographically or relationally distant friends and family. These interactions can be enjoyed for what they are without being criticized for what they are not. However, when online interactions are used as a replacement for offline relationships, the effects seem overwhelmingly negative (Kraut et al., 2002, 1998). People who expect online interactions to fulfill the need to connect often end up sorely disappointed when these expectations exceed reality. The impoverished nature of online interactions not only fails to fulfill the need to connect, but often exacerbates the feelings of social exclusion that motivate many people to seek digital connection in the first place. Online social interactions seem to make the rich richer, and the poor poorer.

A longitudinal study of social media mirrors these conclusions: individuals who used the Internet to connect with friends and family experienced positive effects of social media use on well-being, while individuals who used the Internet to meet new people experienced decreases in well-being (Bessière, Kiesler, Kraut, & Boneva, 2008). These negative consequences of misguided social media use may affect even casual users. For example, recent studies showed that Facebook use leads to increased feelings of loneliness and decreased life satisfaction (Kross et al., 2015; Verduyn, Lee, Park, Shablack, Orvell, et al., 2015). These studies are not simply indicative of a link between one specific social media site and one specific outcome; as indicated by a meta-analysis of 40 studies (Huang, 2010), the preponderance of evidence to date suggests that social media use undermines well-being.

Though social media use has both positive and negative implications for well-being, some of these data paint a bleak picture of its long-term consequences. Research in this area is still in its infancy, but the potential long-term consequences of social media for human welfare highlight a pressing need for further inquiry into this area; people are unlikely to suddenly turn away from social media as a form of interpersonal connection. Further research may at least allow us to ensure that the positive outcomes associated with this new way of communicating, connecting, and belonging outweigh the negatives.

The Future

We are social creatures, driven by a desire for social connection. Elements of our social minds, from the dopaminergic reward system to our unique ability to mentalize about others, serve to motivate and maximize our social connectedness. Our modern world encourages us to use these systems not only in face-to-face interactions, but also in interactions mediated by television, Facebook, Twitter, and other digital media. These opportunities to connect through a screen feed our social desires, but they may not truly satiate our hunger for connection.

This concept—that "old" adaptive systems acting in "new" technological environments can result in previously unseen and possibly maladaptive outcomes—suggests media may be a prime example of a "supernormal" stimulus. Supernormal stimuli are exaggerated versions of the stimuli that shaped our neural structures and cognitive tendencies over the course of evolution. They are products of the modern world that hijack adaptive systems and set them on a path toward unexpected ends (Barrett, 2010; Ward, 2013). In the case of new media, our social-seeking minds allow television programs and computer screens to serve up readily available social stimulation without the dangers of rejection or the costs of effort. Instead of an easy solution, they have the potential to become an easy escape with a high price.

The disconnection between adaptive systems and adaptive outcomes created by the application of "old" systems in "new" environments raises a deeper philosophical question about what it truly means for a behavior or an outcome to be "adaptive." The adaptive functions of social connection—and processes supporting these functions—are largely tied to issues of mate choice, food acquisition, and resistance to predation that are significantly less applicable in New York City than in the African savannahs of the Pleistocene (Tooby & Cosmides, 1990). True, failure to achieve social connection may result in feelings of loneliness or depression (Kraut et al., 1998; Weidman et al., 2012); but these feelings may be yet more cues leading us to achieve outcomes that no longer hold any essential adaptive qualities. The overall trend toward negative outcomes of social media use suggests that the majority of social media users may be using these potentially positive sources of social connection maladaptively—they are not augmenting offline relationships, but replacing them. As the social landscape continues to change—as older individuals continue to adopt social media as a form of interpersonal communication and as new generations are born into a world in which these sites, apps, and services are the norm—there is a distinct possibility that more people will not only be using social media, but that they will be doing so in ways that undermine social connection, quality of life, and general well-being.

At the same time, as new media continue to evolve to produce more abundant and more realistic stimuli to fulfill our own desires, these stimuli may become more capable of satiating our social urges. If this is the case—if mediated social "connection" develops such that the internal, psychological effects of engaging with these forms of connection are *identical* to those offered by face-to-face connection, even if the external effects remain vastly different—is this connection still impoverished? Or is a social life filtered through television screens, computer applications, or immersive virtual environments just as valid as one lived through birthday parties and barbecues?

Whatever the answer, the question is one that must be considered. As social networks continue to grow in popularity (Brenner, 2013; Tancer, 2008), leaving less time for and perhaps less interest in face-to-face communication (Wallsten, 2013), they will become an ever-increasing aspect of our daily lives. And as we glue ourselves to screens, huddle around monitors, and cradle mobile devices, we do not just affect our own social worlds—we model these behaviors for children (Turkle, 2013), a new generation growing up in a world where "new media" are not new at all, and where mediated communication is not an alternative but the norm.

We suggest that our most appropriate response may simply be awareness. Our desire to connect via social media stems from adaptive urges, but may lead us to maladaptive outcomes—or at least outcomes inconsistent with maximizing actual social capital. Our social minds are not likely to change course and revolt against mediated connection overnight; nor are social media likely to disappear in the blink of an eye. Our task, then, is not to fight the future, but to recognize what is happening—to know why we are drawn to our television screens and smartphones, and to manage our use of these devices such that we do not lose sight of the people around us, do not exchange our family at the dinner table for a rerun of *All in the Family*, do not replace face-to-face communication with another hour on Facebook, and do not allow social media to replace social connection.

REFERENCES

Aharon, I., Etcoff, N., Ariely, D., Chabris, C. F., O'Connor, E., & Breiter, H. C. (2001). Beautiful faces have variable reward value: fMRI and behavioral evidence. *Neuron, 32*(3), 537–551.

Ahn, D., & Shin, D.-H. (2013). Is the social use of media for seeking connectedness or for avoiding social isolation?: Mechanisms underlying media use and subjective well-being. *Computers in Human Behavior, 29*(6), 2453–2462.

Aron, A., Fisher, H., Mashek, D. J., Strong, G., Li, H., & Brown, L. L. (2005). Reward, motivation, and emotion systems associated with early-stage intense romantic love. *Journal of Neurophysiology, 94*(1), 327–337.

Baek, Y. M., Bae, Y., & Jang, H. (2013). Social and parasocial relationships on social network sites and their differential relationships with users' psychological well-being. *Cyberpsychology, Behavior, and Social Networking, 16*(7), 512–517.

Bargh, J. A., & McKenna, K. Y. A. (2004). The Internet and social life. *Annual Review of Psychology, 55*(1), 573–590.

Barrett, D. (2010). *Supernormal stimuli: How primal urges overran their evolutionary purpose.* New York: Norton.

Baumeister, R. F., & Leary, M. R. (1995). The need to belong: Desire for interpersonal attachments as a fundamental human motivation. *Psychological Bulletin, 117*(3), 497–529.

Berridge, K. C. (1996). Food reward: Brain substrates of wanting and liking. *Neuroscience and Biobehavioral Reviews, 20*(1), 1–25.

Bessière, K., Kiesler, S., Kraut, R., & Boneva, B. S. (2008). Effects of Internet use and social resources on changes in depression. *Information, Community and Society, 11*(1), 47–70.

Bohnet, I., & Frey, B. S. (1999). Social distance and other-regarding behavior in dictator games: Comment. *American Economic Review,* 335–339.

Bowles, S., & Gintis, H. (2002). Prosocial emotions. *The Economy as a Evolving Complex System, 3,* 339–364.

Brenner, J. (2013). *Instagram, Vine, and the evolution of social media.* Washington, DC: Pew Research Center.

Buckner, R. L., & Carroll, D. C. (2007). Self-projection and the brain. *Trends in Cognitive Sciences, 11*(2), 49–57.

Buckner, R. L., & Krienen, F. M. (2013). The evolution of distributed association networks in the human brain. *Trends in Cognitive Sciences, 17*(12), 648–665.

Caplan, S. E. (2002). Problematic Internet use and psychosocial well-being: Development of a theory-based cognitive behavioral measurement instrument. *Computers in Human Behavior, 18*(5), 553–575.

Caplan, S. E. (2005). A social skill account of problematic Internet use. *Journal of Communication, 55*(4), 721–736.

Cozby, P. C. (1972). Self-disclosure, reciprocity and liking. *Sociometry,* 151–160.

Cozby, P. C. (1973). Self-disclosure: A literature review. *Psychological Bulletin, 79*(2), 73–73.

Derrick, J. L., Gabriel, S., & Hugenberg, K. (2009). Social surrogacy: How favored television programs provide the experience of belonging. *Journal of Experimental Social Psychology, 45*(2), 352–362.

Dunbar, R. I. M., Marriott, A., & Duncan, N. D. C. (1997). Human conversational behavior. *Human Nature, 8*(3), 231–246.

Dunbar, R. I. M., & Shultz, S. (2007). Evolution in the social brain. *Science, 317*(5843), 1344–1347.

Ellison, N. B., Steinfield, C., & Lampe, C. (2007). The benefits of Facebook friends: Social capital and college students, use of online social network sites. *Journal of Computer-Mediated Communication, 12*(4), 1143–1168.

Emler, N. (1990). A social psychology of reputation. *European Review of Social Psychology, 1*(1), 171–193.

Emler, N. (1994). Gossip, reputation, and social adaptation. In R. F. Goodman & A. Ben-Ze'ev (Eds.), *Good gossip* (pp. 117–133). Lawrence: University Press of Kansas.

Epley, N., Akalis, S., Waytz, A., & Cacioppo, J. T. (2008). Creating social connection through inferential reproduction: Loneliness and perceived agency in gadgets, gods, and greyhounds. *Psychological Science, 19*(2), 114–120.

Epley, N., Waytz, A., & Cacioppo, J. T. (2007). On seeing human: A three-factor theory of anthropomorphism. *Psychological Review, 114*(4), 864–885.

Finn, S., & Gorr, M. B. (1988). Social isolation and social support as correlates of television viewing motivations. *Communication Research, 15*(2), 135–158.

Forest, A. L., & Wood, J. V. (2012). When social networking is not working: Individuals with low self-esteem recognize but do not reap the benefits of self-disclosure on Facebook. *Psychological Science, 23*(3), 295–302.

Gardner, W. L., Pickett, C. L., & Knowles, M. (2005). Social snacking and shielding. In K. D. Williams, J. P. Forgas, & W. Von Hippel (Eds.), *The social outcast: Ostracism, social exclusion, rejection, and bullying* (pp. 227–241). New York: Psychology Press.

Gingrich, B., Liu, Y., Cascio, C., Wang, Z., & Insel, T. R. (2000). Dopamine D_2 receptors in the nucleus accumbens are important for social attachment in female prairie voles (Microtus ochrogaster). *Behavioral Neuroscience, 114*(1), 173–183.

Greenwood, D. N. (2008). Television as escape from self: Psychological predictors of media involvement. *Personality and Individual Differences, 44*(2), 414–424.

Greenwood, D. N., & Long, C. R. (2010). Attachment, belongingness needs, and relationship status predict imagined intimacy with media figures. *Communication Research, 38*(2), 278–297.

Hartmann, T., & Goldhoorn, C. (2011). Horton and Wohl revisited: Exploring viewers' experience of parasocial interaction. *Journal of Communication, 61*(6), 1104–1121.

Helliwell, J. F., & Putnam, R. D. (2004). The social context of well-being. *Philosophical Transactions—Royal Society of London, Series B: Biological Sciences*, 1435–1446.

Holt-Lunstad, J., Smith, T. B., & Layton, J. B. (2010). Social relationships and mortality risk: a meta-analytic review. *PLoS Medicine, 7*(7). Horton, D., & Wohl, R. R. (1956). Mass communication and para-social interaction: Observations on intimacy at a distance. *Psychiatry, 19*(3), 215–229.

Hsu, S. H., Wen, M.-H., & Wu, M.-C. (2009). Exploring user experiences as predictors of MMORPG addiction. *Computers and Education, 53*(3), 990–999.

Huang, C. (2010). Internet use and psychological well-being: A meta-analysis. *Cyberpsychology, Behavior, and Social Networking, 13*(3), 241–249.

Hughes, D. J., Rowe, M., Batey, M., & Lee, A. (2012). A tale of two sites: Twitter vs. Facebook and the personality predictors of social media usage. *Computers in Human Behavior, 28*(2), 561–569.

Jonason, P. K., Webster, G. D., & Lindsey, A. E. (2008). Solutions to the problem of diminished social interaction. *Evolutionary Psychology, 6*(4), 637–651.

Kareiva, P., Watts, S., McDonald, R., & Boucher, T. (2007). Domesticated nature:

Shaping landscapes and ecosystems for human welfare. *Science, 316*(5833), 1866–1869.

Kim, J., LaRose, R., & Peng, W. (2009). Loneliness as the cause and the effect of problematic Internet use: The relationship between Internet use and psychological well-being. *CyberPsychology and Behavior, 12*(4), 451–455.

Kirschner, P. A., & Karpinski, A. C. (2010). Facebook and academic performance. *Computers in Human Behavior, 26*(6), 1237–1245.

Knowles, M. L. (2007). *The nature of parasocial relationships.* Unpublished doctoral dissertation, Northwestern University, Evanston, IL.

Korkeila, J., Kaarlas, S., Jääskeläinen, M., Vahlberg, T., & Taiminen, T. (2010). Attached to the web: Harmful use of the Internet and its correlates. *European Psychiatry, 25*(4), 236–241.

Kraut, R., Kiesler, S., Boneva, B., Cummings, J., Helgeson, V., & Crawford, A. (2002). Internet paradox revisited. *Journal of Social Issues, 58*(1), 49–74.

Kraut, R., Patterson, M., Lundmark, V., Kiesler, S., Mukophadhyay, T., & Scherlis, W. (1998). Internet paradox: A social technology that reduces social involvement and psychological well-being? *American Psychologist, 53*(9), 1017–1031.

Kross, E., Verduyn, P., Demiralp, E., Park, J., Lee, D. S., Lin, N., et al. (2013). Facebook use predicts declines in subjective well-being in young adults. *PLoS One, 8*(8).

Landis, M. H., & Burtt, H. E. (1924). A study of conversations. *Journal of Comparative Psychology, 4*(1), 81–89.

Lee, E.-J., & Jang, J.-w. (2013). Not so imaginary interpersonal contact with public figures on social network sites: How affiliative tendency moderates its effects. *Communication Research, 40*(1), 27–51.

Leiner, B. M., Cerf, V. G., Clark, D. D., Kahn, R. E., Kleinrock, L., Lynch, D. C., et al. (2009). A brief history of the Internet. *ACM SIGCOMM Computer Communication Review, 39*(5), 22–31.

Lo, S.-K., Wang, C.-C., & Fang, W. (2005). Physical interpersonal relationships and social anxiety among online game players. *CyberPsychology and Behavior, 8*(1), 15–20.

Malle, B. F. (2005). Folk theory of mind: Conceptual foundations of human social cognition. In R. R. Hassin, J. D. Uleman, & J. A. Bargh (Eds.), *The new unconscious* (pp. 225–255). New York: Oxford University Press.

Malle, B. F., & Hodges, S. (2005). Other minds. New York: Guilford Press.

Mars, R. B., Neubert, F.-X., Noonan, M. P., Sallet, J., Toni, I., & Rushworth, M. F. S. (2012). On the relationship between the "default mode network" and the "social brain." *Frontiers in Human Neuroscience, 6.*

Matthews, M. (1994). *The horseman: Obsessions of a zoophile*: Amherst, NY: Prometheus Books.

Meshi, D., Morawetz, C., & Heekeren, H. R. (2013). Nucleus accumbens response to gains in reputation for the self relative to gains for others predicts social media use. *Frontiers in Human Neuroscience, 7.*

Mitchell, K. J., Becker-Blease, K. A., & Finkelhor, D. (2005). Inventory of problematic internet experiences encountered in clinical practice. *Professional Psychology: Research and Practice, 36*(5), 498–509.

Mobbs, D., Greicius, M. D., Abdel-Azim, E., Menon, V., & Reiss, A. L. (2003). Humor modulates the mesolimbic reward centers. *Neuron, 40*(5), 1041–1048.

Mobbs, D., Yu, R., Meyer, M., Passamonti, L., Seymour, B., Calder, A. J., et al. (2009). A key role for similarity in vicarious reward. *Science, 324*(5929), 900.

Morrison, C. M., & Gore, H. (2010). The relationship between excessive Internet use and depression: A questionnaire-based study of 1,319 young people and adults. *Psychopathology, 43*(2), 121–126.

Naaman, M., Boase, J., & Lai, C. H. (2010, February). *Is it really about me?: Message content in social awareness streams.* Paper presented at the Proceedings of the 2010 ACM Conference on Computer Supported Cooperative Work, New York, NY.

Nielsen. (2014). An era of growth. Retrieved from *www.nielsen.com/content/dam/corporate/us/en/reports-downloads/2014 Reports/nielsen-cross-platform-report-march-2014.pdf.*

Nowak, M. A., & Sigmund, K. (2005). Evolution of indirect reciprocity. *Nature, 437*(7063), 1291–1298.

Oettingen, G., & Mayer, D. (2002). The motivating function of thinking about the future: expectations versus fantasies. *Journal of Personality and Social Psychology, 83*(5), 1198–1212.

Orr, E. S., Sisic, M., Ross, C., Simmering, M. G., Arseneault, J. M., & Orr, R. R. (2009). The influence of shyness on the use of Facebook in an undergraduate sample. *CyberPsychology and Behavior, 12*(3), 337–340.

Pani, L. (2000). Is there an evolutionary mismatch between the normal physiology of the human dopaminergic system and current environmental conditions in industrialized countries? *Molecular Psychiatry, 5*(5), 467–475.

Papacharissi, Z., & Rubin, A. M. (2000). Predictors of Internet use. *Journal of Broadcasting and Electronic Media, 44*(2), 175–196.

Park, N., Kee, K. F., & Valenzuela, S. N. (2009). Being immersed in social networking environment: Facebook groups, uses and gratifications, and social outcomes. *CyberPsychology and Behavior, 12*(6), 729–733.

Pempek, T. A., Yermolayeva, Y. A., & Calvert, S. L. (2009). College students' social networking experiences on Facebook. *Journal of Applied Developmental Psychology, 30*(3), 227–238.

Rainie, L., Fox, S., & Duggan, M. (2014). *The web at 25 in the U.S.* Washington, DC: Pew Research Center.

Rand, D. G., Greene, J. D., & Nowak, M. A. (2012). Spontaneous giving and calculated greed. *Nature, 489*(7416), 427–430.

Rand, D. G., Peysakhovich, A., Kraft-Todd, G. T., Newman, G. E., Wurzbacher, O., Nowak, M. A., et al. (2014). Social heuristics shape intuitive cooperation. *Nature Communications, 5.*

Reeves, B., & Greenberg, B. S. (1977). Children's perception of television characters. *Human Communication Research, 3*(2), 113–127.

Reeves, B., & Lometti, G. E. (1979). The dimensional structure of children's perceptions of television characters: A replication. *Human Communication Research, 5*(3), 247–256.

Reeves, B., & Nass, C. (1996). *The media equation: How people treat computers, television, and new media like real people and places.* New York: SLI Publications and Cambridge University Press.

Rilling, J. K., Gutman, D. A., Zeh, T. R., Pagnoni, G., Berns, G. S., & Kilts, C. D. (2002). A neural basis for social cooperation. *Neuron, 35*(2), 395–405.

Rose, R. L., & Wood, S. L. (2005). Paradox and the consumption of authenticity through reality television. *Journal of Consumer Research, 32*(2), 284–296.

Rubin, A. M., Perse, E. M., & Powell, R. A. (1985). Loneliness, parasocial interaction, and local television news viewing. *Human Communication Research, 12*(2), 155–180.

Russell, D., Cutrona, C. E., Rose, J., & Yurko, K. (1984). Social and emotional loneliness: An examination of Weiss's typology of loneliness. *Journal of Personality and Social Psychology, 46*(6), 1313–1321.

Ryan, T., & Xenos, S. (2011). Who uses Facebook? An investigation into the relationship between the Big Five, shyness, narcissism, loneliness, and Facebook usage. *Computers in Human Behavior, 27*(5), 1658–1664.

Scannell, P. (1996). Radio, television, and modern life: A phenomenological approach. New York: Blackwell.

Schilbach, L., Eickhoff, S. B., Rotarska-Jagiela, A., Fink, G. R., & Vogeley, K. (2008b). Minds at rest? Social cognition as the default mode of cognizing and its putative relationship to the default system of the brain. *Consciousness and Cognition, 17*(2), 457–467.

Shaw, L. H., & Gant, L. M. (2002). In defense of the Internet: The relationship between Internet communication and depression, loneliness, self-esteem, and perceived social support. *CyberPsychology and Behavior, 5*(2), 157–171.

Sheldon, K. M., Abad, N., & Hinsch, C. (2011). A two-process view of Facebook use and relatedness need-satisfaction: Disconnection drives use, and connection rewards it. *Psychology of Popular Media Culture, 1,* 2–15.

Sheldon, P. (2008). The relationship between unwillingness-to-communicate and students' Facebook use. *Journal of Media Psychology: Theories, Methods, and Applications, 20*(2), 67–75.

Sherif, M., Harvey, O. J., White, B. J., Hood, W. R., & Sherif, C. W. (1961). *Intergroup conflict and cooperation: The Robbers Cave experiment* (Vol. 10). Norman, OK: University Book Exchange.

Steijn, W. M. P., & Schouten, A. P. (2013). Information sharing and relationships on social networking sites. *Cyberpsychology, Behavior, and Social Networking, 16*(8), 582–587.

Steinfield, C., Ellison, N. B., & Lampe, C. (2008). Social capital, self-esteem, and use of online social network sites: A longitudinal analysis. *Journal of Applied Developmental Psychology, 29*(6), 434–445.

Tamir, D. I., & Mitchell, J. P. (2012). Disclosing information about the self is intrinsically rewarding. *Proceedings of the National Academy of Sciences, 109*(21), 8038–8043.

Tamir, D. I., & Mitchell, J. P. (2014). [Receiving social information]. Unpublished raw data.

Tamir, D. I., Zaki, J., & Mitchell, J. P. (2014). *Informing others is associated with behavioral and neural signatures of value.* Unpublished working paper.

Tancer, B. (2008). *Click: What millions of people are doing online and why it matters.* New York: Hyperion.

Tomasello, M. (1999). *The cultural origins of human cognition.* Cambridge, MA: Harvard University Press.

Tooby, J., & Cosmides, L. (1990). The past explains the present: Emotional adaptations and the structure of ancestral environments. *Ethology and Sociobiology, 11*(4), 375–424.

Tricomi, E., Rangel, A., Camerer, C. F., & O'Doherty, J. P. (2010). Neural evidence for inequality-averse social preferences. *Nature, 463*(7284), 1089–1091.

Tsao, J. (1996). Compensatory media use: An exploration of two paradigms. *Communication Studies, 47*(1–2), 89–109.

Turkle, S. (2013). What should we be worried about? *Edge* website, retrieved from *http://edge.org/response-detail/23795.*

Valkenburg, P. M., & Peter, J. (2007). Preadolescents' and adolescents' online communication and their closeness to friends. *Developmental Psychology, 43*(2), 267–277.

Valkenburg, P. M., Peter, J., & Schouten, A. P. (2006). Friend networking sites and their relationship to adolescents' well-being and social self-esteem. *CyberPsychology and Behavior, 9*(5), 584–590.

Verduyn, P., Lee, D., Park, J., Shablack, H., Orvell, A., Bayer, J., et al. (2015). Passive Facebook usage undermines affective well-being: Experimental and longitudinal evidence. *Journal of Experimental Psychology: General.*

Vernberg, E. M., Abwender, D. A., Ewell, K. K., & Beery, S. H. (1992). Social anxiety and peer relationships in early adolescence: A prospective analysis. *Journal of Clinical Child Psychology, 21*(2), 189–196.

Wallsten, S. (2013). *What are we not doing when we're online* (NBER Working Paper No. 19549). Cambridge, MA: National Bureau of Economic Research.

Ward, A. F. (2013). Supernormal: How the Internet is changing our memories and our minds. *Psychological Inquiry, 24*(4), 341–348.

Ward, A. F., Leimgruber, K., Norton, M. I., Olson, K., Gray, K., & Santos, L. (2014). *Paying forward prosocial behavior: People are selfish, but only in secret.* Unpublished working paper.

Waytz, A., Morewedge, C. K., Epley, N., Monteleone, G., Gao, J.-H., & Cacioppo, J. T. (2010). Making sense by making sentient: The neural bases of seeking understanding through anthropomorphism. *Journal of Personality and Social Psychology, 99*(3), 410–435.

Waytz, A., Zaki, J., & Mitchell, J. P. (2012). Response of dorsomedial prefrontal cortex predicts altruistic behavior. *Journal of Neuroscience, 32*(22), 7646–7650.

Weaver, J. B. (2003). Individual differences in television viewing motives. *Personality and Individual Differences, 35*(6), 1427–1437.

Weidman, A. C., Fernandez, K. C., Levinson, C. A., Augustine, A. A., Larsen, R. J., & Rodebaugh, T. L. (2012). Compensatory Internet use among individuals higher in social anxiety and its implications for well-being. *Personality and Individual Differences, 53*(3), 191–195.

Wellman, B., Haase, A. Q., Witte, J., & Hampton, K. (2001). Does the Internet increase, decrease, or supplement social capital? Social networks, participation, and community commitment. *American Behavioral Scientist, 45*(3), 436–455.

Wilder, D. A., & Thompson, J. E. (1980). Intergroup contact with independent manipulations on in-group and out-group interaction. *Journal of Personality and Social Psychology, 38*(4), 589–603.

Yamaguchi, S., Greenwald, A. G., Banaji, M. R., Murakami, F., Chen, D., Shiomura, K., et al. (2007). Apparent universality of positive implicit self-esteem. *Psychological Science, 18*(6), 498–500.

Young, K. S. (1996). Psychology of computer use: XL. Addictive use of the Internet: a case that breaks the stereotype. *Psychological Reports, 79*(3), 899–902.

Young, K. S. (2009). Internet addiction: Diagnosis and treatment considerations. *Journal of Contemporary Psychotherapy, 39*(4), 241–246.

Zaki, J., & Mitchell, J. P. (2013). Intuitive prosociality. *Current Directions in Psychological Science, 22*(6), 466–470.

Index

Note. Italics in page numbers indicate figures or tables.